PROGRESS IN BRAIN RESEARCH

VOLUME 80

AFFERENT CONTROL OF
POSTURE AND LOCOMOTION

PROGRESS IN BRAIN RESEARCH

VOLUME 80

AFFERENT CONTROL OF POSTURE AND LOCOMOTION

EDITED BY

J.H.J. ALLUM

*Division of Experimental Audiology and Neurootology, Department of Otorhinolaryngology,
University Hospital, Basel, Switzerland*

and

M. HULLIGER

Department of Clinical Neurosciences, University of Calgary, Alberta, Canada

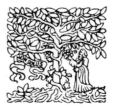

ELSEVIER
AMSTERDAM – NEW YORK – OXFORD
1989

© 1989, Elsevier Science Publishers B.V. (Biomedical Division)

ISBN 0-444-81225-3 (volume)
ISBN 0-444-80104-9 (series)

This book is printed on acid-free paper

Published by:
Elsevier Science Publishers B.V. (Biomedical Division)
P.O. Box 211
1000 AE Amsterdam
The Netherlands

Sole distributors for the USA and Canada:
Elsevier Science Publishing Company, Inc.
655 Avenue of the Americas
New York, NY 10010
USA

Library of Congress Cataloging-in-Publication Data

Afferent control of posture and locomotion.

(Progress in brain research ; v. 80)
Includes bibliographical references.
1. Locomotion. 2. Posture. 3. Afferent pathways.
I. Allum, J. H. J. II. Hulliger, M. III. Series.
QP376.P7 vol. 80   612′.82S   89-25903
[QP301]   [599′.01′88]
ISBN 0-444-81225-3 (alk. paper)

Printed in The Netherlands

List of Contributors

Allum
PD Dr Biomed. Eng. John H.J., Labor für experimentelle Neurootologie, HNO Universitätsklinik, Kantonsspital Basel, CH-4031 Basel, Switzerland
Tel.   +41 61 / 25 25 25 (Ext. 18522)
Fax   +41 61 / 25 74 05
pp. 399 – 409

Amjad
Dr Abdul M., Departments of Statistics and Physiology, University of Glasgow, Glasgow G12 8QQ, Scotland UK
Tel.   +44 41 / 339 8855 (Ext. 4759)
Fax   +44 41 / 330 4100
E-Mail GPAA07@VME.GLA.AC.UK
pp. 243 – 255

Bacher
Dr Michael, Neurologische Universitätsklinik, Eberhard-Karls-Universität, Kliniken Schnarrenberg, Hoppe-Seylerstrasse 3, D-7400 Tübingen, Federal Republic of Germany
Tel.   +49 7071 / 29 21 42
pp. 481 – 488

Banovetz
Dr James, Department of Physiology, The Medical School, Northwestern University, 303 East Chicago Avenue, Chicago, IL 60611, USA
Tel.   +1 312 / 908 7990
Fax   +1 312 / 908 5101
pp. 363 – 371

Behrens
Dr Frank, Physiologisches Institut, Freie Universität Berlin, Arnimallee 22, D-1000 Berlin 33, Federal Republic of Germany
Tel.   +49 30 / 838 25 55
E-Mail GRUESSER@ZEDAT.FU-BERLIN.DSP.DE2
pp. 183 – 196

Berger
Dr Wiltrud, Neurologische Universitätsklinik, Abteilung für Neurophysiologie, Hansastrasse 9a, D-7800 Freiburg i.Br., Federal Republic of Germany
Tel.   +49 761 / 270 72 10
Fax   +49 761 / 203 43 69
pp. 419 – 423

Berthoz
Dr Alain, Laboratoire de Physiologie Neurosensorielle, C.N.R.S., 15 Rue de l'Ecole de Médecine, F-75270 Paris Cédex 06, France
Tel.   +33 1 / 4329 61 54
Fax   +33 1 / 4354 16 53
pp. 377 – 383

Bessou
Prof Paul, Laboratoire de Physiologie, U.A. C.N.R.S. 649, Faculté de Médecine, 133 Route de Narbonne, F-31062 Toulouse, France
Tel.   +33 61 / 53 23 13 (Ext. 333)
Fax   +33 61 / 55 64 70 (Tel.): UNIPSAB 521880 F
pp. 37 – 45

Black
Dr F. Owen, Neurological Science Institute, 1120 NW 20th Avenue, Portland, OR 97209, USA
Tel.   +1 503 / 229 8163
pp. 411 – 418

Borel
Dr Liliane, Laboratoire de Psychophysiologie, U.A. C.N.R.S. 372, Université Aix-Marseille I, Centre de Saint Jérôme, Avenue Escadrille Normandie Niemen, F-13397 Marseille Cédex 13, France
Tel.   +33 91 / 28 84 60
Fax   +33 91 / 02 05 50
pp. 385 – 393

Breeze
Dr Peter, Department of Statistics, University of Glasgow, Glasgow G12 8QQ, Scotland, UK
Tel.   +44 41 / 330 4047
Fax   +44 41 / 77 7070
E-Mail GATA15@EDINBURGH.AC.UK
pp. 243 – 255

Brodin
Dr Lennart, Nobel Institute for Neurophysiology, Karolinska Institute, Solnavägen 1, Box 604 00, S-104 01 Stockholm, Sweden
Tel.   +46 8 / 728 69 11
Fax   +46 8 / 31 11 01
E-Mail PVTRH@SEQZ21.BITNET
pp. 321 – 327

Cabelguen   Dr Jean-Marie, Université P. et M. Curie, Institut des Neurosciences, Département de Neurophysiologie Comparée, Bâtiment B, 6ème étage, 9 Quai Saint Bernard, F-75005 Paris, France
Tel.   +33 14 / 4336 25 25 (Ext. 3254)   pp. 37 – 45

Caputi   Dr Angel A., Department of Clinical Neurosciences, University of Calgary, Health Sciences Centre, 3330 Hospital Drive N.W., Calgary, Alberta, Canada T2N 4N1
Tel.   +1 403 / 220 4595
Fax   +1 403 / 283 4740   pp. 75 – 85

Chen   Dr Dao-Fen, Department of Physiology and Biophysics, University of Washington, School of Medicine, I-421 Health Sciences Building, SJ-50, Seattle, 98195, USA
Tel.   +1 206 / 543 0440
Fax   +1 206 / 545 0305   pp. 431 – 436

Cheney   Dr Paul D., Dept. of Physiology, University of Kansas, Kansas City, KS 66103, USA
Tel.   +1 913 / 588 7403
E-Mail   PRU06@UKANMED.BITNET   pp. 437 – 449

Christenson   Johan, Nobel Institute for Neurophysiology, Karolinska Institute, Solnavägen 1, Box 604 00, S-104 01 Stockholm, Sweden
Tel.   +46 8 / 728 69 11
Fax   +46 8 / 31 11 01
E-Mail   PVTRH@SEQZ21.BITNET   pp. 321 – 327

Collewijn   Dr Han, Department of Physiology I, Faculty of Medicine, Erasmus University Rotterdam, P.O. Box 1738, NL-3000 DR Rotterdam, The Netherlands
Tel.   +31 10 / 408 75 60   pp. 197 – 209; 373 – 375

Conway   Dr Bernard A., Institute of Physiology, University of Glasgow, Glasgow G12 8QQ, Scotland, UK
Tel.   +44 41 / 339 8855 (Ext. 4759)
Fax   +44 41 / 330 4100
E-Mail   GPAA32@VME.GLA.AC.UK   pp. 243 – 255

Crommelinck   Dr Marc, Laboratoire de Neurophysiologie, Faculté de Médecine, Université de Louvain, UCL 5449, 54 Avenue Hippocrate, B- 1200 Bruxelles, Belgium
Tel.   +32 2 / 764 55 74
Fax   +32 2 / 764 53 22   pp. 351 – 362

Davey   Dr Nicholas G., Department of Physiology, Charing Cross and Westminster Medical School, Fulham Palace Road, London W6 8RF, England, UK
Tel.   +44 1 / 846 7284
Fax   +44 1 / 846 7338   pp. 19 – 25

Day   Dr Brian L., MRC Human Movement and Balance Unit, University Dept. of Clinical Neurology, Institute of Neurology, Queen Square, London, WC1N 3BG, England, UK
Tel.   +41 1 / 829 8759
Fax   +41 1 / 278 9836   pp. 467 – 472

Decostre   Dr Marie F., Laboratoire de Neurophysiologie, Faculté de Médecine, Université de Louvain, UCL 5449, 54 Avenue Hippocrate, B- 1200 Bruxelles, Belgium
Tel.   +32 2 / 764 54 47
Fax   +32 2 / 764 53 22   pp. 351 – 362

Dichgans   Prof Johannes, Neurologische Universitätsklinik, Eberhard-Karls-Universität, Kliniken Schnarrenberg, Hoppe-Seylerstrasse 3, D-7400 Tübingen 1, Federal Republic of Germany
Tel.   +49 7071 / 29 20 49   pp. 481 – 488

Dickson   Dr Michael, Institute of Physiology, University of Glasgow, Glasgow G12 8QQ, Scotland, UK
Tel.   +44 41 / 339 8855 (Ext. 4577)
Fax   +44 41 / 330 4100
E-Mail   GPAA21@VME.GLA.AC.UK   pp. 9 – 17

Diener   Prof Hans-Christoph, Neurologische Universitätsklinik, Eberhard-Karls-Universität, Kliniken Schnarrenberg, Hoppe-Seylerstrasse 3, D-7400 Tübingen 1, Federal Republic of Germany
Tel.   +49 7071 / 29 65 04   pp. 465 – 466; 481 – 488

Dietz   Prof Volker, Neurologische Klinik, Abteilung für Neurophysiologie, Hansastrasse 9a, D-7800 Freiburg i.Br., Federal Republic of Germany
Tel.   +49 761 / 270 72 10
Fax   +49 761 / 203 43 69   pp. 419 – 423

Illert   Prof Michael, Physiologisches Institut der Universität Kiel, Olshausenstrasse 40, D-2300 Kiel 1, Federal Republic of Germany
Tel.   +49 431 / 880 20 32
Fax   +49 431 / 880 20 72   pp. 273−281

Jankowska   Dr. Elzbieta, Department of Physiology, University of Göteborg, Medicinaregatan 11, Box 33031, S-400 33 Göteborg, Sweden
Tel.   +46 31 / 85 35 08   pp. 299−303

Joffroy   Dr Michel, Laboratoire de Physiologie, U.A.-C.N.R.S. 649, Faculté de Médecine, 133 route de Narbonne, F-31062 Toulouse, France
Tel.   +33 61 / 53 23 13 (Ext. 330)
Fax   +33 61 / 55 64 70 (Tel.): UNIPSAB 521880 F   pp. 37−45

Keshner   Dr Emily, Department of Physiology, The Medical School, Northwestern University, 303 East Chicago Avenue, Chicago, IL 60611, USA
Tel.   +1 312 / 908 2228
Fax   +1 312 / 908 5101   pp. 363−371

Kiehn   Dr Ole, Institute of Neurophysiology, The Panum Institute, University of Copenhagen, Blegdamsvej 3C, DK-2200 Copenhagen N, Denmark
Tel.   +45 31 / 35 79 00
Fax   +45 31 / 35 95 77   pp. 257−267

Lacour   Prof Michel, Laboratoire de Psychophysiologie, U.A. C.N.R.S. 372, Université Aix-Marseille I, Centre de Saint Jérôme, Avenue Escadrille Normandie Niemen, F-13397 Marseille Cédex 13, France
Tel.   +33 91 / 28 84 60
Fax   +33 91 / 02 05 50   pp. 385−393

Langenbach   Petra, Neurologische Universitätsklinik, Eberhard-Karls-Universität, Kliniken Schnarrenberg, Hoppe-Seylerstrasse 3, D-7400 Tübingen, Federal Republic of Germany   pp. 481−488

Lansner   Dr Anders, Department of Numerical Analysis and Computing Science, Royal Institute of Technology, S-100 44 Stockholm, Sweden
Tel.   +46 8 / 790 62 10
Fax   +46 8 / 790 09 30
E-Mail   ALA@BION.KTH.SE   pp. 321−327

Lefort   Dr Loïc, Lab. de Physiologie Neurosensorielle, C.N.R.S., 15 Rue de l'Ecole de Médecine, F-75270 Paris Cédex 06, France
Tel.   +33 1 / 4329 61 54
Fax   +33 1 / 4354 16 53   pp. 377−383

Leonard   Dr Christopher S., Department of Physiology and Biophysics, New York University Medical Center, 550 First Avenue, New York, NY 10016, USA
Tel.   +1 212 / 340 5410
Fax   +1 212 / 689 9060
E-Mail   LEONARD@NYUMED.BITNET   pp. 213−223

Maier   Marc A., Brain Research Institute, University of Zürich, August-Forel-Strasse 1, CH-8029 Zürich, Switzerland
Tel.   +41 1 / 385 63 54
Fax   +41 1 / 385 65 04
E-Mail   K298001@CZHRZU1A.BITNET   pp. 451−463

Maier   Dr Verena, Buchholzstrasse 127, CH-8053 Zürich, Switzerland
Tel.   +41 1 / 53 91 27   pp. 431−436

Marsden   Prof C. David, MRC Human Movement and Balance Unit, University Dept. of Clinical Neurology, Institute of Neurology, Queen Square, London, WC1N 3BG, England, UK
Tel.   +41 1 / 837 3611
Fax   +41 1 / 278 9836   pp. 467−472

Matthews   Prof Peter B.C., University Laboratory of Physiology, Parks Road, Oxford OX1 3PT, England, UK
Tel.   +44 865 / 272 500
Fax   +44 865 / 272 469   pp. 3−7; 103−112

Sugiuchi Dr Yuriko, Department of Physiology, School of Medicine, Tokyo Medical and Dental University, 1-5-45 Yushima 1-chome, Bunkyo-ku, Tokyo, 113 Japan
Tel. +81 3 / 818 71 72 pp. 137 – 147

Tan Joep, Department of Anatomy, Erasmus University, P.O. Box 1738, NL-3000 DR Rotterdam, The Netherlands
Tel. +31 10 / 408 73 01 or 408 73 08
Fax +31 10 / 436 28 41 pp. 213 – 223

Taylor Prof Anthony, United Medical and Dental Schools of Guy's and St. Thomas's Hospitals, Sherrington School of Physiology, St. Thomas's Campus, Lambeth Palace Road, London SE1 7EH, England, UK
Tel. +44 1 / 928 9292 (Ext. 3718)
Fax +44 1 / 928 0729 pp. 27 – 35; 239 – 242

Thompson Dr Philip D., MRC Human Movement and Balance Unit, University Dept. of Clinical Neurology, Institute of Neurology, Queen Square, London WC1N 3BG, England, UK
Tel. +41 1 / 829 8759
Fax +41 1 / 278 9836 pp. 467 – 472

Trend Dr Patrick, University Dept. of Clinical Neurology, Institute of Neurology, Queen Square, London, WC1N 3BG, England, UK pp. 61 – 74; 87 – 101

Van der Steen Dr Johannes, Department of Physiology I, Faculty of Medicine, Erasmus University Rotterdam, P.O. Box 1738, NL-3000 DR Rotterdam, The Netherlands
Tel. +31 10 / 408 75 58
Fax +31 10 / 436 28 41
E-Mail NETMAIL@HROEUR51.BITNET pp. 213 – 223

Vedel Dr Jean Pierre, Laboratoire de Neurosciences Fonctionnelles – U3, Equipe de Neurophysiologie de la sensorimotricité chez l'homme, C.N.R.S., 31 Chemin Joseph Aiguier, B.P. 71, F-13402 Marseille Cédex 9, France
Tel. +33 91 / 22 40 37 pp. 113 – 123

Vincent Steve, Department of Physiology, University of Alberta, Edmonton, Alberta, Canada T6G 2H7
Tel. +1 403 / 492 3783
Fax +1 403 / 492 8915
E-Mail USERSJVI@UALTAMTS.BITNET pp. 61 – 74

Waespe Dr Walter, Neurologische Klinik, Universitätsspital Zürich, Frauenklinikstrasse 26, CH-8091 Zürich, Switzerland
Tel. +41 1 / 255 55 10 pp. 225 – 236

Wallén Dr Peter, Nobel Institute for Neurophysiology, Karolinska Institute, Box 60400, S-104 01 Stockholm, Sweden
Tel. +46 8 / 728 69 13
Fax +46 8 / 31 11 01
E-Mail PVTRH@SEQZ21.BITNET pp. 321 – 327

Wannier Dr Thierry M.J., Department of Physiology, School of Medicine, Tokyo Medical and Dental University, 1-5-45 Yushima 1-chome, Bunkyo-ku, Tokyo, 113 Japan
Tel. +81 3 / 818 71 72 pp. 451 – 463

Ward James, Institute of Physiology, University of Glasgow, Glasgow G12 8QQ, Scotland, UK
Tel. +44 41 / 339 8855 (Ext. 4577)
Fax +44 41 / 330 4100
E-Mail GPAA21@VME.GLA.AC.UK pp. 9 – 17

Wiesendanger Prof Mario, Institut de Physiologie, Pérolles, CH-1700 Fribourg, Switzerland
Tel. +41 37 / 82 63 31
Fax +41 37 / 82 65 19 pp. 431 – 436

Wietelmann Dr Detlef, Physiologisches Institut der Universität Kiel, Olshausenstrasse 40, D-2300 Kiel 1, Federal Republic of Germany
Tel. +49 431 / 880 20 32
Fax +49 431 / 880 20 72 pp. 273 – 281

Wilson Prof Victor J., The Rockefeller University, 1230 York Avenue, New York, NY 10021-6399, USA
Tel. +1 212 / 570 8599
Fax +1 212 / 570 7974 pp. 149 – 157

Windhorst   Prof Uwe, Physiologisches Institut, Zentrum Physiologie und Pathophysiologie, Georg-August-Universität Göttingen, Humboldtallee 23, D-3400 Göttingen, Federal Republic of Germany
                 Tel.   +49 551 / 39 96 76
                 Fax   +49 551 / 39 96 12   pp. 283 – 294; 315 – 319
Wolfensberger   Dr Markus, ORL Klinik, Universitätsspital Zürich, Rämistrasse 100, CH-8091 Zürich, Switzerland   pp. 225 – 236

Afferent Control of POSTURE

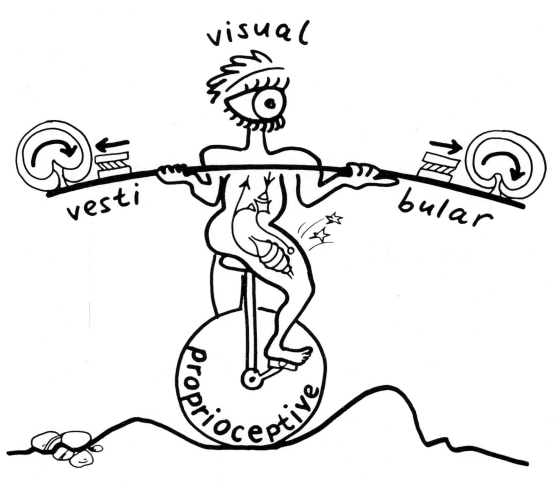

and

LOCOMOTION

Preface

As the cartoon on the facing page succinctly illustrates, man's stability when standing, in locomotion, or when *controlling* the motion of a vehicle is intimately dependent on spinal and supraspinal nervous systems' *integration* of sensory signals from proprioceptive, visual and vestibular receptor systems. These integrated signals then provide the basis for *motor commands.*

How then are these functions of control, integration and generation of motor commands performed by the brain? To answer this question we may view the motor systems of the brain as hierarchically organized structures, where neurone populations and simple reflex pathways form elementary building blocks. These lower order circuits are parts of neuronal loops which are connected both with intermediate motor centres in the brainstem and diencephalon, and with the higher order motor systems of the cortex and cerebellum. In turn, these higher structures send their output into descending pathways, and thus back to lower order circuits.

Simply by bringing the terms "control", "integration" and "generation of motor commands" into the forefront of a book on motor systems we are emphasizing a need to broaden our understanding of motor systems.

We use the term *control,* but what precisely does this encompass? The central nervous system seems to use a number of different control operations. On the one hand, it appears to use feedback signals much as they are used in analogue feedback circuitry. On the other hand, there are logical switching operations, triggered by critical events, which set or reset the responsiveness of neuronal circuits (as envisaged in the notion of "motor set"). Nature, however, probably employs a range of intermediate modes of control.

When discussing *integration,* what functions are we describing? Obviously, integration means more than linear summation of inputs to generate an output. It mostly refers to manifestation of emerging properties, which result from an interaction of several inputs and which cannot immediately be predicted from individual inputs. But until we can predict these emerging properties, from network structure and neuronal characteristics, we cannot claim to have understood the particular integrative process under investigation.

We refer to a *motor command,* but is it a single entity? Normally commands are synthesized in the distributed activity of neurone populations in motor centres and descending pathways. But what do these commands specify, what are the motor codes? For example, are movements coded in terms of trajectories, joint angles, desired length changes, or muscle activation patterns? If all these possible codes are employed in a single motor act, how and where are they transformed as the command descends through the motor hierarchy?

However one chooses to answer the questions raised above, the essential elements of these questions are so fundamental to our urge to understand brain function, that one can be assured of differing viewpoints in the quest for answers.

Some neurophysiologists assert that it is more important to understand the mechanisms of sensory transduction and of the afferent encoding of the time course of muscle length, retinal image slip or head acceleration, before embarking on a more general study of how motor control is organized to transform these signals into muscle action. Others predict that major advances in our understanding of how the central nervous system plans and regulates movement will only occur once the details of spinal and brainstem neuronal circuitry are more thoroughly understood. Still others believe that the key to unravel the complexity of human posture and locomotion will be apparent when the detailed function of higher order, cortical and subcortical, structures are known with mathematical precision. Yet another approach is to study human or animal postural and locomotive behaviour, looking for influences that act to select one of several potential motor patterns or strategies under a given set of circumstances. In this the selection procedure may prove to be highly dependent on particular sensory signals and the behavioural context, or it may mimic patterns demonstrated by known spinal or more central neuronal circuitry and thus lead to an immediate insight into the design of human motor control.

Each of these viewpoints has its strengths – and weaknesses! The strengths can be enhanced if the protagonists of such different approaches can interact with each other, on the basis of their common interest in motor control mechanisms, and if they formulate and receive constructive criticism, thereby preparing the ground for productive new extensions of current research. For this very purpose a group of scientists, who by their imagination, intuition, astute observation and theoretical acumen could be considered to be at the forefront of research on the afferent control of posture and locomotion, gathered in Rheinfelden, Switzerland, during September 1988 to present their research and have it openly criticized and discussed. This book represents the scientific outcome of this meeting. Its subject matter, which encompasses the material presented by each selected speaker, reflects closely the different approaches outlined above: current research on sensory transduction, spinal integration, and higher order neuronal and behavioural control.

The necessity of having a better understanding of the receptor mechanisms and spinal actions, and of the central fusimotor control of proprioceptive feedback from muscle spindles, when considering the control problems of posture and locomotion, is repeatedly advocated in Section I – *Control and Actions of Proprioceptive Feedback*. This section illustrates particularly clearly the intimate interdependence of complex central, and specific peripheral, motor control mechanisms. Section II – *Control and Actions of Vestibular and Visual Inputs* – is intended to highlight aspects of motor control, which have become increasingly clear in recent years, namely that postural and locomotive muscle activity is also highly dependent on vestibular and visual sensory signals. Thus, before a central command can be generated proprioceptive, vestibular and visual sensory signals must be integrated together. There are a number of possible ways to study this integration process. Some of these are presented in Section III – *Spinal Integration*. One such approach concentrates on investigating the exact details of coupling between various reflex pathways, whose actions merge in the spinal cord. Another line of research is concerned with the analysis and understanding of relatively simple neuronal networks. In this the close interplay of experimental approaches and the use of formal models emerges as a promising tool for the understanding of more complex systems. Yet another approach is to search for clues to the hierarchy and types of interaction in muscle responses to various sensory stimuli. This constitutes the main thread of Section IV – *Interaction of Visual, Vestibular and Proprioceptive Inputs*. The different ways in which a postural or locomotive motor output may be expressed depend on the context perceived by cerebral cortical structures. In contrast to spinal and brainstem neuronal circuits, which perhaps respond in a more machine-like fashion, Section V – *Higher Order Control of Posture and Locomotion* – demonstrates the particular flexibility and context dependence that cortical structures add to motor behaviour.

This book is focused on the primary objective of motor behaviour, as illustrated in our cartoon, on the purposeful orientation of the body parts in space and on the stabilization of the body and of perception. The movements of the monocyclist must be finely tuned so that leg, trunk, head and eye movements are fully coordinated, to avoid instability. To help the reader align his focus with that of the book, groups of 2 – 5 papers on related topics within each section are preceded by an overview and critique. This format led to a very lively and stimulating discussion when the papers were first presented orally at the international meeting in Rheinfelden. Naturally, at this meeting each critique followed rather than preceded the presentations. Using this technique of overview and critique of each group of papers we hope that also the non-specialist reader can easily grasp the issues involved and the directions for further research in motor control.

One of the leading lights in the field of motor control, Prof. Ian Alexander Boyd, unfortunately died in the fall of 1987, just as the meeting and structure for this book were being prepared. His contribution on the physiology of the muscle spindle would have been first in this volume. For this reason, this book is dedicated to his memory.

J.H.J. Allum, *Basel*
M. Hulliger, *Calgary*

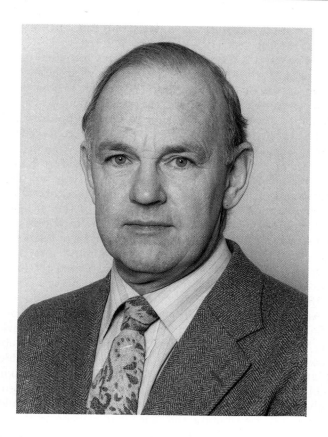

Ian Alexander Boyd

Born, 23rd May 1927. Died, 14th September 1987.

This symposium with its concern for proprioception and the muscle spindle follows in a distinguished line of earlier meetings of which a notable one was four years ago in Glasgow, when Ian Boyd was one of the principal hosts. It is a very great sadness that he is not, as usual, here with us today. He died almost this time last year while on holiday in Wales. He went for a gentle walk by himself but failed to return and was found sitting dead by the path, having suffered an unexpected and massive coronary thrombosis. The sense of shock remains vivid; those in the department first heard of it on the local radio. He was only just 60, with his scientific work still in full flood.

Career. Ian was a Scot and very conscious of it. He was born in Glasgow and then spent most of the rest of his life there from medical student to Professor of Physiology, much of the latter as chairman of a large and busy department. He qualified in Medicine and did a year as a Junior Hospital Doctor before turning to research. He seems to have been very conscious of the need for a background of hard science, for while experimenting on joint receptors for his Ph.D., he was also studying privately for an external degree from London in Physics and Maths. He sat his finals for this and presented his doctoral thesis in the same year (1954) when he was just 28.

By the age of 39 he was a full Professor in a system which does not promote lightly. This was no sinecure and when Margaret Thatcher launched the first of her attacks on British Universities he took early retirement. This was in 1983 when he was still only 56, and of course it was not a retirement from research but just from administration. He kept his lab and had been told he could remain there until he was 70, and he continued successfully in the struggle for grants. So we all expected the world to go on just the same for ever, as it was in our youth.

In his early years there was time for nothing but work, and for his one other interest of helping youth by running Scottish Schoolboys Clubs, where not surprisingly he rose to be Vice-Chairman of the Central Council. He didn't marry until 1971 when he was 44 and already chairman of Physiology. His wife was of similar age and they hoped to adopt children but in our bizarre society they were felt to be unsuitably old, so instead they took on two foster children to whom they gave a most tremendous amount.

It may be noted that he might have gone in quite another direction, since both his father and his brother practised Homeopathic Medicine and for the 10 years before becoming Professor Ian combined his normal University job with being director of the Boyd Medical Research Institute, which seems to have been oriented towards Homeopathy. Among Ian's published papers is a moving address to the British Homeopathic Society, telling them that they would never be believed by orthodox practitioners, as he clearly wished them to be, unless they could establish a scientific rationale for their therapy or at least carry out statistically acceptable trials.

Science. But Ian himself turned in full measure to exact and painstaking science, with the muscle spindle at the centre. His first paper on the spindle was published in 1958 and the last with his name on it has probably yet to appear. It would take too long to review and assess his contribution and place it in relation to that of others, but I would like to emphasize that Ian's great strength was to combine the physiological and histological study of the muscle spindle. This was shown at the very beginning by two separate notes he published on his own in 1958. The first, was entitled "The innervation of the neuromuscular spindle" and clearly described two kinds of intrafusal muscle fibre; the second was called "An isolated muscle spindle preparation" and was the prelude of so much to come. The histological work came to its major fruition in 1962 with a long, beautifully illustrated paper which firmly put bag and chain fibres on the map as separate entities. The isolated spindle work took rather longer to mature, and perhaps shows its major success in the paper with Gladden, McWilliam and Ward in 1976 which played a crucial part in the characterization of the nuclear bag fibres into two types, with one belonging to the dynamic system and the other to the static system; others, of course, contributed crucially to this unfolding story. It is perhaps most appropriate to give you Ian's own comment on this, written in 1981:

"Looking back over 25 years the author finds it hard to believe that it took so long, and needed so many different techniques to establish with certainty that there are three different types of intrafusal fibre and to elucidate the nature of their innervation. Nor is that the end of the story, by any means."

Character. Ian was a very private man, who was not easy to get to know. On a public stage he gave the most masterly and lucid presentation, but if you wanted to argue about the details he tended to retreat into himself. His approach seems to have been moulded by his early years, so that he concentrated on the relation between structure and function within the spindle, without wishing to go downwards to the underlying biophysics or upwards to the role of the spindle in relation to motor and sensory performance. But what he did, and what he left behind in new knowledge is enough for any man and we admire him unreservedly for it.

But now is not the time to attempt to analyse him further, especially as in his mid-thirties he wrote a most revealing article on *Medical Research as a Career* which gives us some insight as to what drove him on; it may also strike a chord in many of you as it applies so strongly to our particular branch of science and hardly at all to the Biochemical Empires that are now growing all around us. Let me quote a few excerpts:

"Tackling a research problem is like a dog worrying at a bone, gnawing at it, approaching it from different angles, shaking it, turning it over, retiring to have another look at it from a distance, and then returning to the fray. It requires great patience and persistence; the capacity to keep on at it no matter how frustrating or unrewarding it may seem. Occasionally we all have to admit defeat, but it is rare for any well-planned investigation to be completely unrewarding if tackled with sufficient persistence."

And, in like vein:

"To persistence we may add endurance . . . complicated experiments are frequently limited by the powers of endurance of the experimenter. The most crucial results are usually obtained near the end of the experiment and to have steady hands and a clear head after twelve hours continuous use of both requires exceptional staying power."

In a lighter mood:

"An attractive aspect of a research career is its variety . . . you have to be your own surgeon, engineer, electrician, author, artist, photographer and plumber. While all great discoveries are not made like that of Archimedes actually in a bath, many are undoubtedly made while wading in a sea of Ringer's fluid."

And, right to the heart:

"A difficult experiment successfully completed brings a deep sense of satisfaction and well-being. To that we may add the great thrill of making a new observation, of obtaining the experimental proof of a cherished theory or original idea."

Finally, let us hear Ian himself, speaking at the beginning of his teaching film "The Muscle Spindle" which I still regularly use and which rightly won many prizes. If he were with us now, he would doubtless be showing us a new film with new results which had become such a regular feature of our meetings. (The address closed with a video-showing of the opening sequences of the film.)

P.B.C. Matthews (Oxford, England)

BIBLIOGRAPHY

His first scientific work:
Boyd, I.A. (1953) Nerve impulses from proprioceptors in the knee joint of the cat. J. Physiol. (London), 119: 8 – 9P.

His first work on the muscle spindle:
Boyd, I.A. (1958) The innervation of mammalian neuromuscular spindles. J. Physiol. (London), 140: 14 – 15P.

His major histological paper:
Boyd, I.A. (1962) The structure and innervation of the nuclear bag muscle fibre system and the nuclear chain muscle fibre system in mammalian muscle spindles. Phil. Trans. Roy. Soc. B, 245: 81 – 136.

A crucial paper on the isolated spindle:
Boyd, I.A., Gladden, M.H., McWilliam, P.N. and Ward, J. (1977) Control of dynamic and static nuclear bag fibres and nuclear chain fibres by gamma and beta axons in isolated cat muscle spindles. J. Physiol. (London), 265: 133 – 162.

His attitude to Homeopathy:
Boyd, I.A. (1971) Homeopathy through the eyes of a Physiologist. Brit. Homeopathic Journal, vol. 60, No. 1.

His attitude to research, published in Surgo, which is apparently the Journal of the Glasgow medical students:
Boyd, I.A. (1963) Medical Research as a career. Surgo, 30: 14 – 17.

His historical survey of the unfolding story of the analysis of the 'wiring diagram' of the spindle:
Boyd, I.A. (1981) The muscle spindle controversy. Sci. Prog., Oxford, 67: 205 – 221.

Acknowledgements

The academic, scientific and personal support of the then Rectors of the Universities of Basel and Zürich, Prof. C.R. Pfaltz and Prof. K. Akert, was crucial in the organization and successful completion of this book. Invaluable secretarial and organization assistance was provided by Mrs Wanda Brunetti (Basel).

The generous and most valuable financial support of the following organizations is gratefully acknowledged:
Bank Julius Baer, Zürich
Basler Kantonalbank, Basel
Department of Education, Canton Aargau
Department of Education, Canton Zürich
Digitana AG, Horgen
Elbatex AG, Wettingen
Heinz Senn AG, Oftringen
Hoffmann-La-Roche AG, Basel
Muehlethaler Computer Systems AG, Attiswil
Nicolet Biomedical Instruments GmbH, Offenbach, FRG
Patria Life Insurance Company, Basel
Ringier Publishers, Zofingen and Zürich
Sandoz Wander AG, Basel
Siemens-Albis Medical Electronics AG, Zürich
SKAN AG, Basel
Swiss Academy of Sciences, Bern
Swiss Life Insurance and Pension Company, Zürich
Swiss National Science Foundation, Bern
Swiss Physiological Society, Bern
Toennies Medical Electronics KG, Freiburg i.Br., FRG

Our cartoon was drawn by Eva Hochreutener-Schneider based on a sketch which originally appeared as Fig. 1 of an article entitled 'Der neurologische Patient und der Schwindel' by Prof. M. Mumenthaler, Bern. The article was published in a book 'Der Schwindel aus interdisziplinärer Sicht', editor Prof. K. Karbowski, Springer, Berlin 1981. Peter Schneider drew the original sketch.

Contents

Section V – Higher Order Control of Posture and Locomotion

SECTION I

Control and Actions of Proprioceptive Feedback

J.H.J. Allum and M. Hulliger (Eds.)
Progress in Brain Research, Vol. 80
© 1989 Elsevier Science Publishers B.V. (Biomedical Division)

Overview and critique of Chapters 1 – 5

P.B.C. Matthews

Oxford, England

First, congratulations to all five authors on the high level of personal expertise they have shown by bringing off experiments of such complexity. If you go into a laboratory working on one of the trendy subjects like gene cloning the actual experimental manipulations tend to be quite simple, and are being carried out by a technician or a doctoral student. With us the principal investigator is involved to the hilt, and it is most impressive. But beyond this there is little common ground between the various sets of experiments I have to comment on. It would be possible to weigh in with a detailed criticism of each paper, but I feel no urge to be aggressive when I know how difficult everything is. Instead, I will mainly try to put the work in context.

Dickson et al. The first paper, given by Margaret Gladden, is a continuation of the work attempting to understand the spindle per se, as an isolated piece of machinery. It gets away from the continuing dialogue of which intrafusal fibre is responsible for what and turns to the classical question of how much of spindle behaviour can be explained in mechanical terms, leaving the rest to be explained by transducer mechanisms. The precise question attacked is whether the bag_1 fibre is excited by stretch to give some kind of active response, as well as behaving as a passive arrangement of springs and dashpots. Poppele and Quick (1981) produced evidence that it did respond actively, but the present work has as yet failed to find evidence for this under their particular conditions; however, it is certainly premature to exclude its occurrence, especially as I understand that so far only a single

spindle has been studied in detail.

So once again in the spindle field we have confusion, which may perhaps be traceable to differences in technique. You might feel that Poppele's positive observation of a shortening of intrafusal sarcomere spacing during continued stretch closes the matter, and proves that there is indeed an active process; and I wish I could feel that this was so, since the idea is highly attractive. However, while entirely accepting his observations, given the mechanical complexities of the situation his interpretation need not be taken as final.

I would also like to make one point on nomenclature. The term "stretch activation" has been chiefly used by those working on muscle to describe a direct response of the myofibrils to a mechanical stimulus. What we see in the spindle may well be due to this, making the term entirely appropriate for us. But Boyd's suggestion was that there might be an effect mediated via a depolarization of the membrane, as in smooth muscle; if so, a different name would be needed and the term "stretch activation" would have to be discarded. Meanwhile, since we are groping in the dark, we must be particularly careful not to add to the confusion by using other peoples' words inappropriately.

Davey and Ellaway. Turning next to the paper delivered by Peter Ellaway, I would note first how satisfying it is to see the reflex actions of the cutaneous system being fractionated by the use of physiological stimulation. It is really surprisingly late for us as reflexologists to be made aware that the central effects of the different types of cutaneous afferent differ, since on the sensory side most physiologists have long held this as an article of faith. Electrical stimulation of nerve trunks has lumped all the cutaneous afferents together for far too long, and is perhaps about as useful for the analysis of their coordinated reflex action as it has been for their contribution to conscious sensation.

But we have to be quite clear on just what is the difference that we have been told about. It would seem to be a combination of strength of action and directness of action, that the type I slowly adapting receptors are unique by acting on γ motoneurones by a synaptic pathway that is both short and powerful; this is the prerequisite for seeing an effect with spike triggered averaging. It has not been shown that under physiological conditions these receptors have the greatest effect on the γ motoneurones, since a stronger effect mediated via a longer synaptic pathway need not have shown itself with spike triggered averaging. In addition, as the authors well recognize, their findings are for one particular preparation; the relative potency of various pathways could well be altered by supraspinal control, so that under different conditions different reflex actions might come to the fore. We have to remember also that they are working right against the noise level, for this is how they explain away their finding no effect from over half the SA1 receptors studied; but, perhaps there are also further functional sub-divisions to be detected. For example, are static and dynamic gammas affected differentially? It will also be interesting to hear what happens when they investigate afferents from a wider area of skin. Will these prove to have the same excitatory action, when the effect would seem relatively non-specific, or will their action have a high degree of local sign and even reverse to inhibition, as described long ago with grosser methods? There is certainly plenty more waiting to be done.

Taylor and Donga. Turning now to the paper given by Anthony Taylor we find the question of central specificity being tackled on the efferent side, by recording simultaneously from spindles in two widely separated muscles in order to compare their pattern of fusimotor activation. It is fascinating to see how they sometimes behaved similarly and sometimes dissimilarly. My only comment here is that it would be helpful to have the data arrayed so as to compare the two muscles more directly. This should help them to establish how far the areas they were stimulating have a widespread non-specific "alerting" action on static and/or dynamic fusimotor systems and how far they are fractionated into components with local sign, different for each muscle. We have to remember that those studying spindle discharge in behaving animals can see a wide variety of responses, suggesting large differences of fusimotor drive, for spindles of a given muscle during a given motor task. The occurrence of such variation in the stimulation experiments would greatly complicate the comparison of the behaviour of spindles in different muscles, though on their showing such variability was not great.

There is the further point of interest, namely whether the situation is suitable for distinguishing between bag_2 and chain action on the spindle, and so enable one to recognize two distinct sorts of "static" centres, if they exist. My personal view is that it is premature to try and cast everything in this mould. The starting point justifying the attempt is the idea that the bag_2 and chain intrafusal fibres are under separate control. As we have just been reminded, Ian Boyd certainly believed that this was so, and asserted it with increasing force with the passage of time. However, Barker's group has had continuing reservations as to how far the peripheral machinery is available, as recently reiterated by Banks (1989). There certainly are differences in the degree to which individual static axons activate bag_2 and chain fibres, but for me at any rate it remains sub judice as to whether this goes to the level of there being separate systems with separate CNS control. Ironically, a quarter of a century ago it was Ian Boyd who was the "lumper" refusing to subdivide intrafusal muscle fibres into more than two types, while David Barker was the "splitter", arguing that this should be done. When stimulating the CNS electrically, as in the present experiments, the findings might happen to fall out so cleanly that they demanded to be explained in terms of two static systems; but the present sort of data would seem open to interpretation in other ways, and so does not help in trying to decide whether or not two such systems exist. This seems more likely to be resolved by work at the periphery. However, if there is a clear peripheral segregation, then we can expect it to be deployed to advantage by the CNS and for this central segregation also to be eventually demonstrable.

Bessou et al. On the next paper, given by Paul Bessou, I must say how nice it is to be shown the gamma firing directly, rather than having to deduce it from the pattern of afferent firing. At the same time one must sympathize with their inability to observe static and dynamic activity independently, and to have to attempt to deduce it like everybody else from the way the afferents are behaving. The differences between their muscles are interesting and fit with the cry of others, on the basis of single fibre recording, that each case needs to be taken on its own and that there is no one way that muscles and the fusimotor system are used. There is also the question whether the different arrangements used for studying the two muscles are responsible for some of the differences between them. The following papers on single fibre work make it unnecessary for me to labour the point that the present technique provides a valuable addition to our armamentarium, without in any way supplanting unitary recording.

Dutia and Price. This paper was delivered in a different session from the other four, but for the long-term record seemed more appropriately commented upon here. For those not immediately working upon the muscle spindle there may well be a sense of irritated bewilderment, as the complications mount and the subdivisions increase; but that is how the real world seems to be, and we cannot run away from it. For those more closely concerned, there is a sense of relief that physiological tools are being fashioned that enable the functions of

anatomically different elements to be studied; the historical cycle in which histological observation continually outruns the possibilities for functional analysis is a source of continued frustration. It is thus heartening to see how the systematic use of succinylcholine has enabled such a good case to be made out for the separation of the responses of primary afferents arising from spindle capsules with and without bag_1 intrafusal muscle fibres; one of the audience noted, however, that these capsules might also differ in whether or not they contained a "long chain" fibre. In the statistical sense, the classification must be at its most reliable for the neck muscles where both kinds of capsule are common. In muscles where the absence of a bag_1 fibre from a capsule is rare, there must be more chance that the odd response which deviates from the mean, even though in the expected direction, has arisen for some other reason.

The first fruit of the technique is to remind us of the importance of transducer mechanisms, over and above mechanical factors, in determining afferent behaviour. In line with much other work, the characteristic large Ia "dynamic response" of the passive spindle, reflecting the sudden change in afferent discharge on completion of stretching, cannot be attributed to the peculiar mechanical properties of the bag_1 intrafusal fibre, since similar behaviour is shown by all primary endings. This need not disturb us, since the early hope that all spindle behaviour could be attributed to the interaction of a variety of springs and dashpots has long been disappointed.

The main question is what to make of the very considerable differences between the behaviour shown by Ia afferents from the two kinds of capsule in the presence of fusimotor activity. The authors opt for what may be called the "individual" approach and suggest that there might be central mechanisms which can recognize the individuality of the two kinds of afferent, read them individually, and then operate on their different signals in various ways to abstract certain mechanically meaningful items of information. This is the classical approach, exemplified by many previous discussions on the relative functions of the primary and secondary spindle afferents. It is highly attractive, except for the increasing demands that it makes on the central reading apparatus each time a new peripheral sub-division is uncovered. In its present application, as given in Fig. 5, my only comment would be that if I wanted to design a spindle to give a rather "pure" dynamic response, uncontaminated by static effects (Fig. 5C), then I would leave out the bag_2 fibre (and probably chain fibres) and read off the desired value directly from the afferent, rather than leaving out the bag_1 fibre and having to settle down to compute the answer. To reply that there may be good reasons against using the simpler method, is to say no more than we do not know what is going on and so haven't got anywhere yet. Nonetheless, I am entirely in favour of playing such games and making such speculations.

The alternative to the "individual" approach may be called the "statistical" approach and, as just discussed, there is still the possibility that this is the way the different static gammas function to control the quite distinct bag_2 and chain intrafusal fibres. Peripheral differences certainly exist, but are not necessarily associated with discrete and independent central wiring rather than some kind of gradient of action. In the present context, this would avoid the need to postulate that Ia axons from the same muscle have to be connected up quite differently depending upon which of the two capsules of a tandem spindle they happen to come from. With "statistical" operation, the discrete information might perhaps just be thrown away and the various Ia discharges summed equally to produce an ensemble average which had the "desired" statistical properties (whatever these might be), even though derived from two separate sources neither of which of itself manifested the average behaviour. Alternatively, and this is the more appealing, there might be some gradient of central action (such as a distribution of terminals, or strength of synaptic action), possibly linked to the conduction velocity of the afferents concerned. Moreover, for some purposes the group II af-

ferents from the secondary endings might contribute to the same field of action. The present Fig. 4 provides a beautifully detailed example of what has long been appreciated, namely that plotting almost any measured variable of afferent responsiveness against conduction velocity yields a set of points which seem to be asking to be fitted by a single continuous curve rather than by a set of discrete functions, each applicable to a particular anatomical entity.

Resolution of such matters will not be easy or rapid, since the questions are different in kind from those that we have been tackling so far. The problem now is to understand how the analysing centres read the messages, and what they see in them, rather than just describing the signals set up by a variety of stimuli without particular regard as to how they are handled inside the CNS. Moreover, the motor control of the spindle and its sensory signalling probably need to be taken together in order to make sense of things, thus greatly increasing the complexity of the task. An elementary point is that those who are studying central connectivity, whether with the microscope or the micro-electrode, should remain alert to the possibility of differentiation within what have hitherto been thought of as unitary systems, such as the Ia fibres. For the β system, of course, thought has already been given to the matter with the view emerging that a mixed skeleto-fusimotor neurone receives much the same synaptic inputs as a purely skeletomotor neurone supplying a comparable set of extrafusal muscle fibers. I confess that my personal hope is that the muscle spindle will prove to operate within a set of general rules, applicable to a range of histologically distinct elements, and that we are not condemned to discover ever more functionally discrete subsystems and so forced to accept that the goal of wider understanding is receding faster than we are advancing.

Concluding remarks. Finally, I should like to stand back and ask what is the point of studies like the three on the CNS. Are they just piling on the data without increasing understanding, and are all such studies doomed at the outset to produce an infinite series of particular examples, incapable of generalization? However confusing things may look at the moment, I hope you will agree that the answer should still be No. Quite apart from the fact that we cannot hope to generalize until we have some data to start from, three specific kinds of thing are also being sought, often simultaneously but without mutual interference.

First, we are looking for truths about the spindle itself. The CNS can be expected to play upon the spindle more effectively than we are able to, and so central activation of the spindle may provide us with unique information about the periphery. This was classically so for the initial recognition of the static and dynamic systems, and as already discussed may provide a way of sub-dividing the static system.

Second, we are sorting out simple wiring diagrams, what connects with what by which interneurones and with what supraspinal control. At present we are thinking rather rigidly in terms of wiring diagrams labelled with the type of afferent fibre or fusimotor axon involved. In due course, the labels may change and progressively come to describe whole circuit blocks, each performing a particular function and comprising many separate anatomical elements. The wealth of interconnections has prevented us getting very far with this as yet.

Third, we are seeking meaning, and asking how these pathways are used in real life when an element of purpose is present; we are attempting to answer the question why, and not just how. But, of course, we can only usefully ask *why* is the spindle so complicated when we have a reasonable understanding of *how* it operates.

In all such experiments, we would seem in part to be travelling in hope, looking for inspiration as we go rather than just following a simple predetermined plan. But this is what makes our branch of science so fascinating, and why the Chiefs have to be so directly involved and can't just leave all the real work to the Indians, as in so many other areas of Biology.

References

Banks, R.W. (1988) Studies on the motor innervation of tenuissimus muscle spindles in the anaesthetized cat. *J. Physiol. (London)*, 406: 70P.

Poppele, R.E. and Quick, D.C. (1981) Stretch-induced contraction of intrafusal muscle in cat muscle spindle. *J. Neurosci.*, 1: 1069–1074.

J.H.J. Allum and M. Hulliger (Eds.)
Progress in Brain Research, Vol. 80
© 1989 Elsevier Science Publishers B.V. (Biomedical Division)

CHAPTER 1

Fusimotor mechanisms determining the afferent output of muscle spindles

M. Dickson, M.H. Gladden, D.M. Halliday and J. Ward

Institute of Physiology, Glasgow University, Glasgow G12 8QQ, U.K.

There is both direct and indirect evidence that stretch activation occurs in the dynamic bag$_1$ fibres of the mammalian muscle spindle and that it is responsible for maintaining the high sensitivity of primary sensory endings in stretches great enough to break the resting actomyosin bonds responsible for the short-range stiffness of muscle fibres. However the direct observations of dynamic bag$_1$ fibre behaviour during stretching were made on damaged fibres and during very slow stretches. Preliminary results of experiments employing faster stretches of intact muscle spindles are reported here. An image processing system is being developed to automate and facilitate analysis of sarcomere movements during stretch, release and activation of intrafusal fibres. Unequivocal evidence confirming the development of stretch activation has not yet been found. Boyd (1986a) believed that static bag$_2$ and chain fibres are controlled by separate populations of static γ motoneurones, while accepting that there is some degree of common innervation. His evidence and the functional implications are discussed.

Key words: Muscle spindle; Image analysis; Intrafusal muscle fibre; Sarcomere; Fusimotor neurone

Introduction

The responses of the primary and secondary sensory endings of muscle spindles depend not only upon muscle length and fusimotor stimulation, but also on the previous mechanical history of the muscle. Understanding the outcome, the sensory discharge, for a particular set of experimental parameters requires a knowledge both of the mechanical behaviour of the three types of intrafusal muscle fibre, and of how motor axons are "wired" in the spindle so that individual intrafusal fibres can be specifically activated.

The dynamic system

It is widely accepted that the increased sensitivity of the primary sensory ending to stretching seen during stimulation of dynamic γ axons occurs because these axons specifically innervate dynamic bag$_1$ (Db$_1$) intrafusal muscle fibres (Bessou and Pagès, 1975; Boyd et al., 1977). Contraction of the Db$_1$ fibre, maintained throughout a stretch, increases the rate of opening of the primary sensory spirals around this fibre relative to the opening rate in the passive fibre (Boyd et al., 1981). The opening and closing of these spirals in both active and passive states is governed by the unusual mechanical behaviour of the Db$_1$ fibre.

Boyd (1976) proposed that the Db$_1$ fibre becomes depolarized during passive stretching (stretch activation) and thought that the "creep" phenomenon which is characteristic of this type of fibre represented the decay of activation. Creep is a mechanical back-slippage of the Db$_1$ fibre sarcomeres towards the primary sensory ending seen immediately following stretch if the fibre is stretched and then held extended. The stretch activation hypothesis was used by Emonet-Dénand et al. (1985a,b) to explain the modulation of the responses of primary sensory endings of cats caused by conditioning stretches or by bursts of dynamic fusimotor stimulation. However, an alternative explanation (Morgan et al., 1984) is that these after-effects arise because the sensory endings respond to changes in muscle fibre stiffness brought about by the spontaneous formation of stable actomyosin cross-bridges (Hill, 1968). It is argued that these bridges are broken during stretching or contraction but spontaneously reform when the muscle length is held steady. The fibre stiffness and so the sensory response would thus depend upon the current number of cross-bridges and the muscle length at which the cross-bridges were established. Stretch after-effects are not confined to feline muscle spindles since human spindle afferent responses can also be modified similarly following stretch (Edin and Vallbo, 1988).

Direct evidence of stretch activation was reported by Poppele and Quick (1981) and Poppele (1985). During slow stretches, around $0.02 - 0.03$ resting lengths s^{-1}, the Db_1 fibre sarcomeres began to shorten as the stretching exceeded $2.5 - 3.0\%$, with a concomitant increase in the rate of tension development of the whole spindle. However the ends of the fibres in these experiments must have been damaged by puller chucks gripping them at the end of the capsular sleeve region.

Quantitative information on the movements of intrafusal muscle fibres has been limited partly because of the immense labour of analysing sequences of cine film taken of sarcomere movements, and because rapid movements occurring, for example during stretching, cause blurring of the images, and since defocusing occurs due to vertical movements of the muscle spindle relative to the microscope objective. We have partially solved these problems by using high-speed cine photography with strobe lighting and computerized image analysis of the cine film sequences. Our initial objective was to measure sarcomere lengths in intact Db_1 fibres during faster stretches than those employed by Poppele and Quick (1981). If stretch activation is responsible for the sensitivity

of the primary sensory endings to stretches of amplitudes greater than 0.2% once the resting actomyosin bonds have been broken, the mechanism would need to be engaged rapidly to be effective in fast stretches (Gladden, 1986).

The static system

Although static γ axons are regarded as a functionally single group they actually innervate two types of intrafusal muscle fibre, static bag_2 (Sb_2) and nuclear chain fibres. Both these fibre types have distinctive mechanical properties. When separately recruited their contraction has widely differing effects on both primary and secondary sensory discharges. Boyd believed that despite some overlap in innervation of the two fibre types each type could be activated largely independently and proposed that there are two types of static γ motoneurone, predominantly innervating either Sb_2 or chain fibres (Boyd, 1986a,b). Present evidence supporting Boyd's proposal is reviewed here in the Discussion.

Methods

Details about the equipment used and experimental arrangement were previously reported by Boyd et al. (1988a). Cine film of intrafusal fibre sarcomere movements during ramp and hold stretches of 0.1 resting lengths s^{-1} was taken at 32 frames s^{-1}. Both cine and video sequences (25 frames s^{-1}) were analysed using a Kontron IBAS Image Processing System. After digitizing the frames, each image in a sequence (Fig. 1A) was enhanced using a technique similar to that of high-pass filtering. This increased definition and enhanced the contrast between the A- and I-bands of the sarcomeres. The enhanced image (Fig. 1B) was further processed by threshold discrimination to give a binary white on black image, the A-bands remaining black. A narrow window was selected on the first image of each sequence encompassing up to 40 sarcomeres. The same sarcomeres were selected in subsequent images of the same sequence by compensating for any lateral or vertical movements of the whole spindle within the image plane. Thus the windows in Fig. 1 (black dashed lines in digitized images, Fig. 1A and C, white lines in enhanced images, Fig. 1B and D) all lie across the same sarcomeres although between images Fig. 1A,B and Fig. 1C,D the spindle has moved laterally relative to the microscope objective. The width and centre of each A-band in the window on the binary image was measured for every frame of a sequence. A sequential display of the windows (Fig. 2) gave a graphical representation of sarcomere width and displacement relative to the rest of the spindle during the sequence.

Although the sequential display indicated sarcomere displacements well during slow smooth movements the direction of displacement during irregular movements had to be established by determining the position of A-bands with distinctive features within successive windows. These features tended to change gradually during stretching, probably due to axial rotation of the fibre, necessitating appraisal of sarcomere patterns for each pair of consecutive images. Unfortunately the sarcomere banding in the Db_1 fibres frequently does not remain in register across the whole width of the fibre. This may lead to an error in sarcomere length measurements because twisting of the fibre during stretching may cause a section of the fibre where realignment of sarcomeres was taking place to cross the window. This restricts the number of sarcomeres which can be used to estimate average sarcomere length within a window. Thus the number of sarcomeres used to estimate the average sarcomere lengths shown in Fig. 3 was always less than 20, and this may have been why the total variability in average sarcomere length measurements was greater than that achieved by Poppele and Quick (1981), $\pm\ 0.05 - 0.075\ \mu$m compared with $\pm\ 0.025\ \mu$m. They measured $20 - 40$ sarcomere widths.

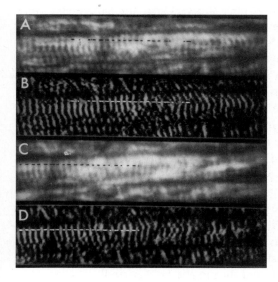

Fig. 1. A and C are digitized images of the dynamic bag_1 fibre in two cine frames, 20 frames apart in a sequence recording intrafusal muscle fibre movements at 32 frames s^{-1} during a pull of 0.1 resting lengths s^{-1}. B and D are the enhanced images of A and C respectively. Horizontal lines on each image indicate locations of windows. For further detail, see Methods.

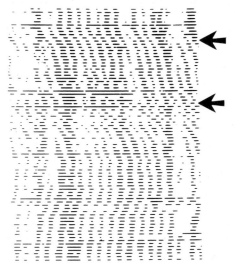

Fig. 2. From top to bottom, sequential display of windows encompassing selected adjacent sarcomeres of the dynamic bag_1 fibre, to illustrate the time course of sarcomere length change and displacement. On each line, the short horizontal bars show the length of the A-bands of individual sarcomeres falling within the analysis window at a given sampling time. The displacement of these sarcomeres relative to the spindle capsule is plotted in Fig. 3B. Arrows indicate windows displayed in Fig. 1.

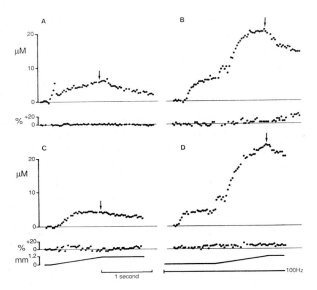

Fig. 3. Top traces: displacement in μm of dynamic bag₁ fibre sarcomeres in the polar direction. A, B: 0.3 mm from equator; C, D: 1.0 mm from equator. Timing of ramp and hold stretch of 10% shown by lowest traces in C and D applies also to A and B. Horizontal line below D: duration of fusimotor stimulation in B and D. Arrows indicate the end of stretch. Second traces: change in average sarcomere length (%).

Results

In our experiments not all Db_1 fibres exhibit creep in the passive state even when these spindles appear to be in good physiological condition. Sometimes creep occurs at one side of the equator only. Detailed results on one Db_1 pole are given below because pronounced creep was present in this pole in the passive state which was enhanced by γ dynamic activation. Thus, if creep represents the decay of stretch activation sarcomere shortening during stretch should have taken place in this fibre. Cine film of two positions along the fibre, 0.3 and 1.0 mm from the equator has been analysed.

Effects of stretch

It was known that the parts of the Db_1 fibre in the fluid space and adjacent part of the sleeve region move rapidly away from the primary sensory ending during stretch, and that this behaviour was not shared by the Sb_2 or chain fibres (Boyd et al., 1988a). Unexpectedly, in the passive fibre the time course of this displacement was strikingly different, 0.3 mm and 1.0 mm from the equator (Fig. 3A,C). The rapid displacement towards the pole at the very beginning of stretch in Fig. 3A (upper trace) was not seen further away from the equator (Fig. 3C, upper trace) and its termination may be due to the breaking of resting actomyosin bonds (Hill, 1968). However, the Db_1 sarcomeres 0.3 mm from the equator did not seem to be involved since there was surprisingly little change in sarcomere length (Fig. 3A, second trace). It was in this juxtaequatorial region that Poppele (1985) observed a shortening of sarcomeres of around 20% during passive stretch.

The data of Fig. 3B (lower trace), which were derived from recordings during dynamic γ stimulation, could be interpreted as demonstrating stretch activation since the sarcomeres do appear to be first lengthening and then shortening during stretch. However, the fact that the displacement (upper trace) reached a maximum well before the end of stretch suggests that the sarcomeres were giving way asynchronously.

Although high speed cine film of the equator during passive stretch was not taken, analysis of a video sequence revealed that the central primary spirals opened only about 7% during the first third of the stretch and then closed to return to the pre-stretch configuration during the rest of the hold phase of the ramp-and-hold stretch. In contrast to the adjacent part of the fibre only 0.3 mm away, there was practically no lateral displacement of the Db_1 sensory spirals. Fusimotor stimulation opened the same central spirals about 3% at the shorter length, and although the maximum extension during initial dynamic stretch was still around 7%, the extension persisted during the subsequent dynamic stretch and during the hold period.

Creep

Creep is usually seen close to the equator in the passive fibre but both its amplitude and the lateral extent of the creep can be increased by fusimotor activation or during a contracture induced by succinylcholine (Dickson et al., 1988). In the present example in the passive state creep was seen immediately after stretch 0.3 mm from the equator but was minimal at 1.0 mm (Fig. 3A,C, upper traces) while during fusimotor activation creep amplitude was increased at 0.3 mm and present at 1.0 mm but with a lesser amplitude (Fig. 3B,D, upper traces). The creep began after the end of the stretch in all cases. However in the Db_1 fibre of another spindle in which only slight creep was detected visually after the end of stretch 0.5 mm from the equator image analysis of the Db_1 behaviour during stretch showed that the creep began part way through the stretch, so that very little movement remained after the end of stretch. Similarly in a third Db_1 fibre in which no creep was visible after stretch, the creep had begun early during the stretch.

Effects of fusimotor activation

Displacement due to fusimotor activation occurred with a delay which was about 100 ms longer closer to the equator (Fig. 3B,D, upper traces). The fusimotor contraction site at this spindle pole was not seen, but was known to be more than 1.1 mm from the equator, and was most likely less than 2.0 mm from the equator. At the onset of the fusimotor tetanus at $100 \, s^{-1}$ the first junctional potential would begin about 2.0 ms after the muscle nerve was stimulated and the excitation contraction threshold would be exceeded probably during the rise time of the second junctional potential, so contraction should begin at the motor end plate with a delay of less than 20 ms (Gladden, unpublished observations). Conduction along the fibre is about 1 ms/mm but the peak potential falls with distance. The length constant in the polar direction is around $0.5-1.0$ mm and may be similar in the equatorial direction. Thus summation to threshold will be mainly responsible for the long delay before the onset of displacement which increases with distance from the motor end plate. This is in line with the observation of Bessou and Pagès (1975) that the onset of a displacement of a

Db_1 fibre was about 75 ms later when the stimulation frequency was $45 \, s^{-1}$ than with a frequency of $110 \, s^{-1}$.

Fusimotor stimulation increased the amplitude of displacement during stretch appreciably both at 0.3 mm and at 1.0 mm from the equator (Fig. 3B, D, first traces). However, both these displacements began with an irregularity suggesting that some structure was giving way in a jerky fashion. This may have been due to some mechanical interaction with the other spindle pole which also contracted because the fusimotor axon under investigation supplied both spindle poles.

Shortening of sarcomeres during fusimotor stimulation in the Db_1 fibre is marked only locally in the motor end plate region so that the lack of sarcomere shortening during the displacement caused by fusimotor contraction in Fig. 3B (lower trace) and D (middle trace) is not surprising. Stretching failed to change sarcomere spacing markedly, but there is a suggestion of lengthening during the creep in the juxtaequatorial region (Fig. 3B, lower trace).

It is important to appreciate that the responses in the two regions monitored (0.3 mm (Fig. 3A,B) and 1.0 mm (Fig. 3C,D) from the equator) were recorded consecutively, rather than simultaneously. However the sequences were chosen specifically because the previous mechanical history of the spindle was the same. Each was preceded by a ramp-and-hold stretch of 10%, terminating 6 s earlier. All the sequences were recorded within about 30 min and the behaviour of the Db_1 fibre was unchanged in any manner which could be detected visually.

Discussion

Stretch activation

Sarcomere shortening during stretching comparable to that observed by Poppele and Quick (1981) and Poppele (1985) in partly damaged fibres has not so far been seen in the intact Db_1 fibre. The sarcomere shortening towards the end of slow passive stretches they observed could have been due to a gradual giving way of stretched sarcomeres elsewhere in the fibre allowing the measured region to shorten. The simultaneous rise in spindle tension may have been caused by tightening of some passive element rather than an active process. However, this argument seems not entirely convincing for the particular example illustrated by Poppele (1985, Fig. 3). 20% shortening of Db_1 sarcomeres occurred in the juxtaequatorial region during stretching. These sarcomeres did not extend before the shortening began. The shortening proceeded smoothly as the stretch continued, and sarcomere lengthening began as soon as the spindle length was held constant. This behaviour indeed seems more consistent with an active contractile process. The phenomenon may be more easily detected in certain spindles and with improvements in sarcomere length measurements. Possibly initial length setting is an important factor. Poppele and Quick (1981) set the initial length of their spindles by the total spindle tension, but in the present experiments the initial length was adjusted up to the point where the nuclear chain fibres were just straightened.

It is well known that the primary sensory response to identical stretches is reproducible provided that length changes prior to the stretch follow the same pattern. So, with the present procedures (see Results), the Db_1 behaviour probably was identical during repeated trials. If this is assumed to be the case then late in the stretching phase the inner region must have continued to move outwards while the outer region had already stopped. This could be because the sarcomeres between these two regions had shortened, and could be interpreted as evidence for stretch activation. Alternatively, it may be argued that the outer region ceased to move outwards simply because sarcomeres in that region began to give way asynchronously. Asynchronous slippage is suggested by the displacement gradually levelling off in the outer region about half way through stretch (Fig. 3C, upper trace).

A simpler explanation is that the Db_1 fibre pole behaves initially like a calibrated elastic band which is held steady at one end (the equator) and pulled at the other (the pole). The band stretches most at the moving end. In the Db_1 fibre the sarcomeres nearer to the pole will reach their elastic limit before those closest to the equator. In the present example at 1.0 mm from the equator this occurred approximately half-way through the ramp stretch. Those very close to the equator may not in fact reach this limit, as in the case of the sarcomeres 0.3 mm from the equator. The difficulty with this argument is that the Db_1 fibre resting bonds would need to withstand a stretch much greater than 0.2% before breaking. The Db_1 fibre does not stretch equally along the length of the pole because the extracapsular region seems to be much stiffer than the portions in the sleeve region and fluid space. This leads to a maximum outward movement during stretch close to the polar end of the sleeve region (Boyd et al., 1988a).

Creep, if not due to stretch activation decay, probably occurs when the compliance of all or part of the striated section of the Db_1 fibre becomes greater than that of elements in the equatorial region, so that the parts of the fibre adjacent to the equator are drawn inwards towards it. The process may extend some sarcomeres as can be seen in Fig. 3C. The greater the extension of the equator the greater the stored potential energy, so the creep will be greater after a stretch during fusimotor stimulation or a succinylcholine-induced contracture. Local variations in structure no doubt play a part in determining the outcome in any specific set of experimental conditions. This interpretation is in line with the well known non-uniformity of histochemical reaction and ultrastructure along the length of the Db_1 fibre (Barker et al., 1976; Banks et al., 1977; Adal, 1985).

The opening of the primary spiral at the onset of stretch would be caused by the transmission of the pull along the Db_1 fibre which was initially stiff due to Hill's (1968) short range elasticity. But although the adjacent region, 0.3 mm away, moved away from the equator throughout the stretch, presumably when the stiffness fell, as the actomyosin cross-bridges broke early in the stretch, the pull was no longer transmitted to the spirals and these closed. The Ia response would thus be confined to a short burst as stretch was applied. As this seems unlikely to be the case other sensory terminals would respond to the continued stretch, i.e. terminals on the other intrafusal fibres or other terminals on the Db_1 fibre. Probably the central equatorial region of the Db_1 fibre where the measurements were made is itself very stiff but the flanking region, where the sensory terminals are not spiral in form (Banks et al., 1982) may be less stiff and more easily deformed. Several separate terminal branches of the Ia axon each supply short sections of the Db_1 equatorial region (Banks, 1986), an arrangement which seems designed to enable the receptor to detect displacement of any section independently of the others. Unfortunately the movement of the lateral part of the Db_1 equator was not accessible for recording at the pole for which most information is available, because it was obscured by Ia terminal branches. Therefore this interpretation remains speculative.

The static system

Gladden and McWilliam (1977) noted that in isolated muscle spindles with intact ventral roots contractions were observed in Sb_2 fibres during light anaesthesia in all spindles studied, indicating spontaneous activity in the static γ motoneurones controlling these fibres. Nuclear chain fibre activity occurred in about two-thirds of such preparations. This suggested that a group of static γ motoneurones might preferentially innervate Sb_2 fibres. These γ motoneurones could be involved in arousal (Gladden, 1981). There was no supporting histological evidence at that time that any static γ axon would innervate only Sb_2 fibres in several spindles.

Boyd (1986a) developed a new test for static γ action using a ramp frequency stimulation from 1 to 150 s^{-1} of single static γ axons while recording from the primaries and/or secondaries from as many spindles supplied by the axon as possible. Driving of the primary afferent occurred only if

chain fibres were involved. Responses due to Sb_2 with chain contraction departed from the typical patterns produced by each fibre type alone. The "diagnoses" were checked in some spindles by isolating them and observing the types of fibres activated during static γ stimulation, and also by following the motor axons to their destinations on intrafusal muscle fibres through serial sections combining light and electron microscopy (Boyd et al., 1988b). Remarkably Boyd found 11 static γs which innervated Sb_2 fibres in all the spindles supplied and 24 which supplied nuclear chain fibres. The position was weakened, however, by some degree of overlap. Particularly those γs innervating predominantly chain fibres tended to innervate, in some spindles, Sb_2 fibres as well.

Banks (1988) has recently reopened the debate by concluding that there is a continuous spectrum in which large diameter static γ axons tend to innervate Sb_2 fibres whilst smaller diameter axons innervate chain fibres. It should be noted however that he was not using Boyd's (1986a) classification test and that for his histological follow-up he used silver staining. Although his suggestion does raise the possibility that the CNS could control static effects by the size principle it is difficult to understand why the CNS would not need a much more precise control considering the diversity of static effects on both primary and secondary sensory afferent responses (Boyd, 1986b).

In one instance Boyd (1986a) found that a static γ axon innervated Sb_2 fibres in no less than six spindles, with no chain involvement. We know now that fusimotor innervation in newborn kitten tenuissimus muscles is highly non-selective (Gladden et al., 1989). At birth some fusimotor axons innervate both Db_1 and Sb_2 fibres, and others supply all three fibre types. As this innervation pattern occurs in adult cats extremely rarely, if ever, spindle development must entail some pruning or relocating of fusimotor endings. Thus the high degree of selectivity manifest in Boyd's example of an Sb_2-specific static γ axon is unlikely to arise randomly. Moreover Wand and Schwarz (1985) found that picrotoxin injection into the substantia nigra removed a component of static drive to primary sensory endings without changing the response of the secondary sensory endings, indicating an inhibition of those static γ motoneurones which specifically innervate Sb_2 fibres.

Static γ motoneurones which mainly innervate chain fibres are potentially very powerful because they can drive primary sensory endings while increasing the length sensitivity of the secondaries. Confusingly, stimulation of such a static γ axon may not increase the length sensitivity of secondaries in all the spindles innervated (Jami and Petit, 1978). However Jami et al. (1980) found that increasing the secondaries' length sensitivity might require the combined action of all chain fibres of at least one spindle pole. Since often only a few chain fibres are innervated per pole by one axon, they suggested that the full effect could be achieved by the simultaneous activity of several such γ motoneurones. Thus for a single muscle the total number of primaries exhibiting driving and of secondaries exhibiting increased length sensitivity could be controlled by adjusting the number of static γ motoneurones predominantly innervating chain fibres.

Acknowledgements

This work was supported by the Wellcome Trust. The authors deeply regret that Professor I.A. Boyd's untimely death deprived him of the pleasure of working on these first results of image analysis of the intrafusal fibre movements which he filmed.

References

Adal, M.N. (1985) Variation of the T-system in different types of intrafusal muscle fibre of cat spindles. In I.A. Boyd and M.H. Gladden (Eds.), *The Muscle Spindle,* Macmillan, London, pp. 35 – 38.

Banks, R.W. (1986) Observations on the primary sensory ending of tenuissimus muscle spindles in the cat. *Cell Tissue Res.,* 246: 309 – 319.

Banks, R.W. (1988) Studies on the motor innervation of cat tenuissimus muscle spindles in the anaesthetised cat. *J. Physiol. (London),* 406: 70P.

Banks, R.W., Harker, D.W. and Stacey, M.J. (1977) A study of mammalian intrafusal muscle fibers using a combined histochemical and ultrastructural technique. *J. Anat.,* 123: 783 – 796.

Banks, R.W., Barker, D. and Stacey, M.J. (1982) Form and distribution of sensory terminals in cat hindlimb muscle spindles. *Phil. Trans. Roy. Soc. B,* 299: 329 – 364.

Barker, D., Banks, R.W., Harker, D.W., Milburn, A. and Stacey, M.J. (1976) Studies of the histochemistry, ultrastructure, motor innervation and regeneration of mammalian intrafusal muscle fibres. *Prog. Brain Res.,* 44: 67 – 88.

Bessou, P. and Pagès, B. (1975) Cinematographic analysis of contractile events produced in intrafusal muscle fibres by stimulation of static and dynamic fusimotor axons. *J. Physiol. (London),* 252: 397 – 427.

Boyd, I.A. (1976) The response of fast and slow nuclear bag fibres and nuclear chain fibres in isolated cat muscle spindles to fusimotor stimulation, and the effect of intrafusal contraction on the sensory endings. *Quart. J. Exp. Physiol.,* 61: 203 – 254.

Boyd, I.A. (1986a) Two types of static γ-axon in cat muscle spindles. *Quart. J. Exp. Physiol.,* 71: 307 – 327.

Boyd, I.A. (1986b) Intrafusal muscle fibres in the cat and their motor control. In W.J.P. Barnes and M.H. Gladden (Eds.), *Feedback and Motor Control in Invertebrates and Vertebrates,* Croom Helm, London, pp. 123 – 144.

Boyd, I.A., Gladden, M.H., McWilliam, P.N. and Ward, J. (1977) Control of dynamic and static nuclear bag fibres and nuclear chain fibres by gamma and beta axons in isolated cat muscle spindles. *J. Physiol. (London),* 265: 133 – 162.

Boyd, I.A., Gladden, M.H. and Ward, J. (1981) The contribution of mechanical events in the Db_1 intrafusal fibre in cat muscle spindles to the form of the Ia discharge. *J. Physiol. (London),* 317: 80 – 81P.

Boyd, I.A., Gladden, M.H., Halliday, D. and Dickson, M. (1988a) Stroboscopic cinematographic and videorecording of dynamic bag_1 fibres during rapid stretching of isolated cat muscle spindles. In P. Hnik, T, Soukup, R. Vejsada and J. Zelena (Eds.), *Mechanoreceptors: Development, Structure and Function,* Plenum, New York, pp. 215 – 220.

Boyd, I.A., Sutherland, F.I. and Arbuthnott, E.R. (1988b) Fusimotor endings responsible for chain fibre "driving" of primary sensory endings in cat muscle spindles. In P. Hnik, T. Soukup, R. Vejsada and J. Zelena (Eds.), *Mechanoreceptors: Development, Structure and Function,* Plenum, New York, pp. 221 – 222.

Dickson, M., Gladden, M.H., Halliday, D.W. and Ward, J. (1988) Creep and reverse creep in the dynamic bag_1 fibre of muscle spindles isolated from the tenuissimus muscle of the cat. *J. Physiol. (London),* 406: 73P.

Edin, B.B. and Vallbo, Å.B. (1988) Stretch sensitization of human muscle spindles. *J. Physiol. (London),* 400:

101 – 111.

Emonet-Dénand, F., Hunt, C.C. and Laporte, Y. (1985a) Fusimotor after-effects on responses of primary endings to test dynamic stimuli in cat muscle spindles. *J. Physiol. (London),* 360: 187 – 200.

Emonet-Dénand, F., Hunt, C.C. and Laporte, Y. (1985b) Effects of stretch on dynamic fusimotor after-effects in cat muscle spindles. *J. Physiol. (London),* 360: 201 – 213.

Gladden, M.H. (1981) The activity of intrafusal muscle fibres during central stimulation in the cat. In A. Taylor and A. Prochazka (Eds.), *Muscle Receptors and Movement,* Macmillan, London, pp. 109 – 122.

Gladden, M.H. (1986) Mechanical factors affecting the sensitivity of mammalian muscle spindles. *Trends Neurosci.,* 9: 295 – 297.

Gladden, M.H. and McWilliam, P.N. (1977) The activity of intrafusal fibres during cortical stimulation in the cat. *J. Physiol. (London),* 273: 28 – 29P.

Gladden, M.H., Spike, R.C. and Sutherland, F.I. (1989) Immaturity of fusimotor innervation at birth in the cat. *J. Physiol. (London),* 412: 12P.

Hill, D.K. (1968) Tension due to interaction between the sliding filaments in resting striated muscle. The effect of stimulation. *J. Physiol. (London),* 199: 637 – 684.

Jami, L. and Petit, J. (1978) Fusimotor actions on sensitivity of spindle secondary endings to slow muscle stretch in cat peroneus tertius. *J. Neurophysiol.,* 41: 860 – 869.

Jami, L., Lan-Couton, D. and Petit, J. (1980) A study with the glycogen-depletion method of intrafusal distribution of gamma axons that increase sensitivity of spindle secondary endings. *J. Neurophysiol.,* 43: 16 – 26.

Morgan, D.L., Prochazka, A. and Proske, U. (1984) The after-effects of stretch and fusimotor stimulation on the responses of primary endings of cat muscle spindles. *J. Physiol. (London),* 356: 465 – 477.

Poppele, R.E. (1985) Relation between intrafusal fibre mechanics and the sensitivity of spindle sensory endings. In I.A. Boyd and M.H. Gladden (Eds.), *The Muscle Spindle,* Macmillan, London, pp. 167 – 171.

Poppele, R.E. and Quick, D.C. (1981) Stretch-induced contraction of intrafusal muscle in cat muscle spindle. *J. Neurosci.,* 1: 1069 – 1074.

Wand, P. and Schwarz, M. (1985) Two types of cat static fusimotor neurones under separate central control? *Neurosci. Lett.,* 58: 145 – 149.

J.H.J. Allum and M. Hulliger (Eds.)
Progress in Brain Research, Vol. 80
© 1989 Elsevier Science Publishers B.V. (Biomedical Division)

CHAPTER 2

Segmental influence of slowly-adapting cutaneous mechanoreceptors on γ motoneurones revealed by cross-correlation of unit discharges in the cat

N.J. Davey and P.H. Ellaway

Department of Physiology, University College London, London WC1E 6BT, England

Cross-correlations between the discharges of individual cutaneous afferents and γ motoneurones have been constructed in the spinal, decerebrated cat. The discharges of single receptors in the sural nerve field from the heel were recorded in dorsal root ganglia. Background discharges of γ motoneurones and the responses to heel stimulation were recorded from cut filaments of the muscle nerve to gastrocnemius medialis of the same leg. Slowly-adapting afferents were stimulated by steady application of a probe to the receptive field whereas rapidly-adapting afferents required continuous movement to sustain discharge of a receptor. Cross-correlation between the discharges of 17 out of 39 slowly-adapting, type-1 (SA1) mechanoreceptors and γ motoneurones revealed sharp increases in probability of γ motoneurone discharge that were delayed with respect to the afferent discharge. The peaks were of short duration with widths at half maximum in the range 2 – 7 ms and rise times of 1 to 4 ms. Deducting peripheral conduction times gave central delays of 3 – 6.5 ms for γ motoneurone facilitation. These delays were comparable to those of γ motoneurone excitation seen in response to electrical stimulation of the sural nerve at 1.5 to 4 times threshold. No short duration peaks were seen in correlograms between hair follicle ($n = 29$) or slowly-adapting type-2 (SA2) ($n = 11$) afferents and γ motoneurones. It is concluded that a single impulse from a SA1 afferent from the hairy skin of the heel is able to facilitate the discharge of γ motoneurones to the ipsilateral gastrocnemius muscle. The characteristics of the correlogram peaks between single afferent and efferent neurones suggest that the coupling involves at least one interneurone at a segmental level. The role of this pathway is discussed in relation to the type of stimuli that excite SA1 receptors.

Key words: Mechanoreceptor; γ Motoneurone; Cross-correlation analysis

Introduction

The proprioceptive feedback from muscle spindles is modulated by numerous reflex actions that impinge upon γ motoneurones and these reflex actions themselves are subjected to supraspinal control. Electrical stimulation of cutaneous nerves can have powerful excitatory and inhibitory effects on γ motoneurones (Grillner, 1969; Appelberg et al., 1977; Catley and Pascoe, 1978; Johansson and Sojka, 1985) as does mechanical stimulation of the skin (Hunt, 1951; Eldred and Hagbarth, 1954). However, the nature of the cutaneous receptors responsible for reflex modulation of γ motoneurone discharge has not been disclosed. The present study has used the technique of cross-correlation analysis to investigate the segmental connections between single cutaneous afferents and γ motoneurones supplying muscles closely associated with that skin area. We have shown that the discharges of slowly-adapting type-1 mechanoreceptors (Brown and Iggo, 1967; Burgess et al., 1968) in the sural nerve field cause tightly coupled increases in probability of discharge of γ motoneurones to the underlying gastrocnemius muscle. Hair follicle afferents and other mechanoreceptors showed no such connectivity.

Methods

Cats of either sex were anaesthetized with halothane $(1 - 3\%)$ in oxygen and decerebrated by intercollicular section of the brainstem and removal of the hemispheres. Following decerebration the anaesthetic was discontinued and the animals paralysed with gallamine triethiodide (Flaxedil) and respired artificially. The spinal cord was cut across at T9 or T10. The dorsal root ganglia of segments lumbar seven (L7) and sacral one (S1), the dorsal and ventral roots L7 and S1 and certain peripheral nerves were exposed for recording purposes. The leg of the cat was clamped by metal pins which gripped bone at the pelvis and base of the femur. A retort clamp supported the foot close to the plantar cushion. The fur of the heel and part of the foot was trimmed close to the skin. Functionally single γ motoneurones showing a background discharge in the absence of intentional stimulation were isolated by dissecting filaments of a nerve fascicle to the gastrocnemius medialis muscle. Axonal conduction velocities were determined and ranged from 12 to 44 m/s. Other criteria for identifying γ motoneurones were based on discharge characteristics which have been described previously (Ellaway and Trott, 1978). The discharges of single cutaneous afferents innervating the sural nerve field were recorded with a tungsten wire electrode from dorsal root ganglia. Axonal conduction velocity was measured using conduction delays assessed from back averaging a sural nerve recording from trigger spikes recorded in the dorsal root ganglion. Forward averages to a dorsal root recording were used in order to verify continuity of conduction of the afferent from the dorsal root ganglion on to the spinal cord.

Cross-correlation analysis was performed using a 1 ms time resolution up to 128 ms from the time of an impulse in either of two trains of spikes. A continuous 10-s period of analysis was used to con-

struct a cross-correlogram. The correlation computation was extended by summing successive correlograms, based on 10-s periods of discharge, up to a total of 160 to 320 s. The location of a peak of increased probability of discharge in a cross-correlogram was judged by eye and by use of the cumulative sum derivative (cusum) of the correlogram (Davey et al., 1986). Assessment of the statistical significance and amplitude of a peak in a correlogram have been described elsewhere (Ellaway and Murthy, 1985; Davey et al., 1987).

Results

The background discharges of between 1 and 6 γ motoneurones to the gastrocnemius medialis muscle were recorded in each of 21 spinal (T9 – 10) cats. Innocuous mechanical stimulation of the ip-

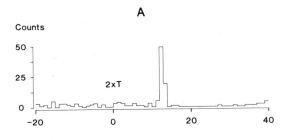

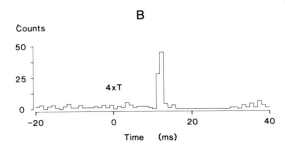

Fig. 1. Excitation of a γ motoneurone to the gastrocnemius medialis muscle in response to electrical stimulation of the sural nerve in the decerebrated, spinal cat. A, B: Peri-stimulus time histograms (PSTH) of the discharge of the γ motoneurone in response to electrical stimulation at 2 times threshold (A) and 4 times threshold (B). Stimuli delivered at time zero. Each PSTH is the result of 100 stimuli delivered at the rate of 1 per s. Conduction velocity of the γ efferent axons was 26 m/s.

silateral heel always facilitated γ motoneurone discharge.

Fig. 1 illustrates the response of a γ moto-neurone to electrical stimulation of the ipsilateral sural nerve at two stimulation strengths. The results are presented in the form of peri-stimulus time histograms (PSTHs) each of which comprises 100 stimuli. At twice the electrical threshold (2T) for the most excitable axons (Fig. 1A) stimulation excited the γ motoneurone at fairly fixed latency on 73% of trials. Raising the stimulus strength to 4T did not substantially alter the amount of the response (87%) but shortened the response latency (12 ms). Similar results were obtained for all γ motoneurones and we can confirm, in the spinal cat, that low threshold Aβ axons in the sural nerve elicit powerful excitation of the ipsilateral gastrocnemius γ motoneurones (Grillner, 1969; Catley and Pascoe, 1978; Johansson and Sojka, 1985). Subtracting the peripheral conduction times in the afferent and efferent limbs of the response in Fig. 1 gave a central delay of 3.0 – 3.5 ms. 3 – 4 ms was the modal value of the distribution of central delays of γ excitation in response to sural nerve stimulation (range 2 to 6.5 ms, $n = 36$).

In the same series of cats we cross-correlated the discharges of slowly adapting (SA) mechano-receptors ($n = 61$) in the sural nerve field with the discharges of individual gastrocnemius γ motoneurones. Seventeen afferents were found to have tightly-coupled correlations with one or more γ motoneurones. Fig. 2 illustrates cross-correlo-grams between the discharges of two different slowly-adapting mechanoreceptors and a γ motoneurone in the same cat. The γ motoneurone is the same as that used to provide data in Fig. 1. The correlograms were constructed from a number of recordings each of 10 s duration using steady pressure within the receptive field of the particular afferent applied by a hand held probe. Sampling of the data stream was not begun until after the ap-plication of the probe. This procedure avoided the synchronizing influence that the probe would have on a number of different afferents at the moment of contact with the skin. The receptors used in the

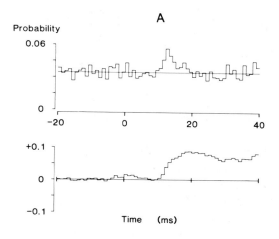

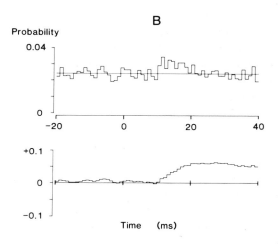

Fig. 2. Correlations between the discharges of single slowly-adapting type-1 mechanoreceptors and a γ motoneurone. A, B: correlograms (above) and cusums (below) of 1 ms bin width constructed from 160 s (A) and 320 s (B) periods of recording during the application of steady pressure to the afferent fields. Average rates of discharge were 10 i.p.s. for the SA1 afferents in A (axon velocity 60 m/s) and 10 i.p.s. for the SA1 afferent in B (62 m/s). The γ motoneurone had average discharge rates of 32 i.p.s. in A and 24 i.p.s. in B. Correlograms: the abscissae give time before and after the occurrence of afferent spikes. The ordinates give the probability of a γ motoneurone spike occur-ring in a 1 ms bin. Cusums: the ordinates of the cusums of the correlograms give the deviation from expected cumulative pro-bability of a γ motoneurone spike. This value rises from ap-proximately zero to 0.08 in A and 0.06 in B over periods of 8 and 10 ms with latencies of about 12 ms following an afferent spike. Same γ motoneurone as in Fig. 1.

experiment that provides data for Fig. 2 both proved to be slowly-adapting type-1 mechanoreceptors (SA1) according to criteria established by Brown and Iggo (1967) and Burgess et al. (1968). A peak is evident in both correlograms (Fig. 2) 12 ms after the time of occurrence of an afferent trigger spike (time zero). The peaks in the correlograms are statistically significant ($P < 0.001$). Below each correlogram is the equivalent cumulative sum. The deviation from the expected cumulative probability of an impulse in γ motoneurone discharge, given an impulse in the afferent (see Davey et al., 1987), is indicated by the total excursion of the cusum through the bins which constitute the peak. The values for the two correlograms are 0.08 and 0.06. Thus, on average, during the time span of the peak there were 0.08 γ efferent discharges above those expected by chance alone for each SA1 afferent discharge in Fig. 2A and 0.06 for the SA1 afferent in Fig. 2B.

If the correlograms are read from left to right then the peaks are delayed with respect to the time of the afferent discharge. Also, the peaks then show more sharply rising than falling phases. The peaks have latencies of 12 ms to the afferent trigger spike, rise times of approximately 2 ms and widths of 8 and 10 ms. If the peripheral conduction times are subtracted from the latencies of the peaks then the central delays of the raised probability of γ efferent discharge to the afferent spikes were approximately 3 to 3.5 ms. These are comparable to the central delay in the case of excitation of the γ motoneurone in response to electrical stimulation of the sural nerve (Fig. 1).

Twenty-five instances of increased probability of γ efferent discharge were observed involving 17 afferents. The distribution of central delays of this facilitation ranged from 2.7 to 6.5 ms with a modal value 3 to 3.5 ms. The rise times for correlogram peaks ranged from 1 to 4 ms ($n = 9$) with a mean of 1.9 ms. The widths of peaks of afferent/efferent coupling ranged from 2 to 11 ms with a mean of 6.5 ms.

All 17 afferents that gave tightly coupled excitation of γ motoneurone discharge were identified as slowly-adapting type-1 (SA1) mechanoreceptors (Brown and Iggo, 1967; Burgess et al., 1968). No evidence of a correlation was found in the case of 22 other SA1 afferents. The conduction velocities of the 17 axons ranged from 53 to 75 m/s. All gave a sustained discharge in response to a blunt probe pressed lightly against the skin. The adaptation of the discharge in response to constant pressure could show a prominent dynamic component or simply a steady, slow adaptation that continued for many seconds. None of the afferents showed a background discharge in the absence of intentional stimulation. Most SA1 receptors responded to light displacement of hairs and gave a brief, high frequency discharge (> 100 impulses/s (i.p.s.)) as a blunt probe was dragged across their receptive field. The size of the receptive fields varied from a point-like location to an area several millimetres across. Units that possessed large fields often had one or more discrete low threshold points within the field. During sustained pressure the discharges tended to be irregular with coefficients of variation of interspike intervals ranging from 0.22 to 0.61.

In contrast, 11 slowly-adapting mechanoreceptors were classified as type-2 (SA2) and distinguished from SA1 receptors principally on the basis of their more regular discharge trains. The coefficients of variation of interspike intervals for the 11 receptors ranged from 0.06 to 0.19. The receptors often exhibited a background discharge which was also regular. Correlations between the discharges of SA2 receptors and γ motoneurones revealed no peaks. Eleven SA receptors could not be categorized positively as SA1 or SA2 but none of these showed correlations with γ motoneurones.

No sharp correlations were found for a total of 29 hair follicle afferents in 34 pairings with γ motoneurones. In order to elicit a persistent discharge from hair follicle afferents hairs had to be continuously moved. Broad trends lasting tens of milliseconds were often seen in the resultant correlograms. The trend of increased probability of γ motoneurone discharge started before the time of impulse generation in the hair follicle afferent and was attributed to concomitant excitation of other afferents. The experiments with SA2 and hair afferents included 7 cats in which sharp correlations were seen between SA1 mechanoreceptors and γ motoneurones.

Discussion

This chapter presents direct evidence, based on cross-correlation of single unit discharges, that activation of SA1 mechanoreceptors facilitates the discharges of γ motoneurones.

17 of the 39 afferents that were categorized as SA1 units according to the criteria of Brown and Iggo (1967) and Burgess et al. (1968) gave closely-coupled facilitation of γ motoneurone discharge. These 17 were distributed among 10 out of 18 cats in which the afferent/efferent connections were examined. We suggest, therefore, that such correlations are a relatively frequent occurrence. Nevertheless, in most cats a larger number of negative interactions were encountered and the reason for this may be that the connectivity between some SA1 afferents and γ motoneurones is too weak to be revealed by the technique of cross-correlation. We tentatively conclude that this study has revealed relatively strong interactions between SA1 afferents and γ motoneurones but that weaker connections may have been missed.

Broad correlations spanning tens of milliseconds were sometimes observed between hair follicle afferents and γ efferents. These broad peaks did not show a preferred latency to afferent impulses. In fact, the observed increase in probability of efferent discharge could occur in advance of the precise time of individual afferent impulses. Neither was there any sign of a sharp increase in probability superimposed upon the broad correlation. Broad correlations most probably resulted from the excitatory action of other receptors, including SA1 afferents, that were stimulated (by the imposed rhythmic hair movements described above) at about the same time as the individual hair follicle afferent used to construct the correlogram.

None of the 11 SA2 receptors gave correlations

with γ motoneurones even though six were studied in experiments in which SA1 correlations were observed. However, we refrain from concluding that facilitatory actions on γ motoneurones from SA2 afferents or hair follicle afferents do not exist. Light pressure and hair movement on the heel of the spinal cat cause facilitation of γ efferent discharge that is evident as a gross change in frequency. These manoeuvres excite discharges in hair follicle and SA2 afferents as well as SA1 afferents. It is possible that the cross-correlation technique fails to reveal a connection from hair follicle and SA2 afferents to γ motoneurones due to the limitation in its resolving power.

Any averaging technique, such as cross-correlation, can produce a spurious relation between afferent and efferent neurone if the afferent is activated synchronously with others in the afferent population (Hamm et al., 1985). In our paradigm, we know from direct recordings that a number of different cutaneous receptors were excited when a stimulus was applied to the receptive field of the particular afferent under study. However, we have evidence from direct recording and cross-correlation of the discharges of pairs of afferents with overlapping or adjacent fields that afferent synchrony does not occur with the stimuli used to reveal SA1/γ efferent interactions (Davey and Ellaway, 1985).

The distribution of central delays for the raised probability of γ efferent discharge had a modal value of 3 to 3.5 ms and these figures were not substantially different from the central delays obtained for the response of γ motoneurones to electrical stimulation of the sural nerve. This makes it probable that at least one interneurone is involved in the coupling between afferent and efferent neurones. However, the tight nature of the coupling, as exemplified by the sharp onset and short duration of the correlogram peaks, show that there is a high probability of discharge of a γ motoneurone given a single spike in an individual SA1 afferent. Similar types of coupling have been observed between cutaneous afferents and propriospinal neurones (Tapper and Wiesenfeld,

24

1980; Brown et al., 1987).

Skin inputs have potent effects on γ moto-neurones in certain reduced or anaesthetized preparations but there is no coherent pattern of activation (Johansson and Sojka, 1985). However, no previous studies have been selective in the type of cutaneous receptor stimulated and the diversity of action on γ motoneurones may simply reflect the fact that electrical stimulation of nerves or gross mechanical stimulation of the skin excites afferents of several different modalities. In this study we have been able to identify a specific excitatory action of slowly-adapting, type-1, mechanorecep-tors (SA1) in the sural nerve field on gastrocnemius γ motoneurones. It remains to be discovered whether such tightly coupled connectivity exists between other populations of fusimotor neurones and SA1 afferents of specific skin areas as might be expected from the earlier findings (Eldred and Hagbarth, 1954) of association between certain skin areas and fusimotor populations.

The functional significance of the excitatory action of SA1 afferents on γ efferents has to take account of the diverse responses of the receptors. The discharge characteristics and receptive field organization of SA1 afferents make them well suited for detecting position and intensity of events on the skin surface (Johansson, 1978). However, hair movement or substantial stretch of the skin may provoke the discharge of SA1 receptors. These properties add up to a picture of SA1 receptors as highly sensitive afferents that are likely to be discharged during locomotion or maintenance of posture and not simply by direct contact with external objects (see Hulliger et al., 1979).

Finally, it should be pointed out that the SA1 coupling with γ motoneurones that we have reveal-ed in the spinal cat would normally be under the control of a powerful, supraspinal inhibitory pathway. We have evidence (Davey and Ellaway, unpublished observations) that the coupling with SA1 afferents causes short term synchrony of discharge of γ motoneurones via shared inputs. This synchrony is suppressed completely in the decerebrated cat if the dorsolateral funiculus of the spinal cord is intact (Davey and Ellaway, 1988).

Acknowledgements

We thank Maria Catley for her technical assistance, Alan Ainsworth for tungsten electrodes and Jim Pascoe for his computer programs for time series analysis. This work was supported by the National Institutes for Health grant NS19215 and the Wellcome Trust.

References

Appelberg, B., Johansson, H. and Kalistratov, G. (1977) The influence of Gp II muscle afferents and low threshold skin afferents on dynamic gamma motoneurones to the triceps surae of the cat. *Brain Res.*, 132: 153 – 158.

Brown, A.G. and Iggo, A.A. (1967) A quantitative study of cutaneous receptors and afferent fibres in the cat and rabbit. *J. Physiol. (London)*, 193: 707 – 733.

Brown, A.G., Koerber, H.R. and Noble, R. (1987) Excitatory actions of single impulses in single hair follicle afferent fibres on single spinocervical tract cells in the cat. *J. Physiol. (London)*, 382: 291 – 312.

Burgess, P.R., Petit, D. and Warren R. (1968) Receptor types in cat hairy skin supplied by myelinated fibres. *J. Neurophysiol.*, 31: 833 – 848.

Catley, D.M. and Pascoe, J.E. (1978) The reflex effects of sural nerve stimulation upon gastrocnemius fusimotor neurones of the rabbit. *J. Physiol. (London)*, 276: 32P.

Davey, N.J. and Ellaway, P.H. (1985) The nature of the reflex coupling between skin afferents and gamma motoneurones in the cat. *J. Physiol. (London)*, 366: 127P.

Davey, N.J. and Ellaway, P.H. (1988) Control from the brainstem of synchrony of discharge between gamma motoneurones in the cat. *Exp. Brain Res.*, 72: 249 – 263.

Davey, N.J., Ellaway, P.H. and Stein, R.B. (1986) Statistical limits for detecting change in the cumulative sum derivative of the peristimulus time histogram. *J. Neurosci. Methods*, 17: 153 – 166.

Davey, N.J., Ellaway, P.H. and Friedland, C.L. (1987) Quantitative assessment of the degree of synchrony between the discharges of neurones. *J. Physiol. (London)*, 390: 10P.

Eldred, E. and Hagbarth, K.-E. (1954) Facilitation and inhibition of gamma efferents by stimulation of certain skin areas. *J. Neurophysiol.*, 17: 59 – 64.

Ellaway, P.H. and Murthy, K.S.K. (1985) The source and distribution of short term synchrony between gamma motoneurones in the cat. *Quart. J. Exp. Physiol.*, 70: 233 – 247.

Ellaway, P.H. and Trott, J.R. (1978) Autogenetic reflex action on to gamma motoneurones by stretch of triceps surae in the decerebrated cat. *J. Physiol. (London)*, 276: 49 – 66.

Grillner, S. (1969) The influence of DOPA on the static and the dynamic fusimotor activity to the triceps surae of the spinal cat. *Acta Physiol. Scand.*, 77: 490 – 509.

Hamm, T.M., Reinking, R.M., Roscoe, D.D. and Stuart, D.G. (1985) Synchronous afferent discharge from a passive muscle of the cat: significance for interpreting spike triggered averages. *J. Physiol. (London),* 365: 77 – 102.

Hulliger, M., Nordh, E., Thelin, A.-E. and Vallbo, Å.B. (1979) The responses of afferent fibres from the glabrous skin of the hand during voluntary finger movements in man. *J. Physiol. (London),* 291: 233 – 249.

Hunt, C.C. (1951) The reflex activity of mammalian small nerve fibres. *J. Physiol. (London),* 115: 456 – 469.

Johansson, H. and Sojka, P. (1985) Actions on gamma motoneurones elicited by electrical stimulation of cutaneous afferent fibres in the hind limb of the cat. *J. Physiol. (London),* 366: 343 – 364.

Johansson, R.S. (1978) Tactile sensibility in the human hand: Receptive field characteristics of mechanoreceptive units in the glabrous skin area. *J. Physiol. (London),* 281: 101 – 123.

Tapper, D.N. and Wiesenfeld, Z. (1980) A dorsal spinal neural network in cat. I. responses to single impulses in single type I cutaneous input fibres. *J. Neurophysiol.,* 44: 1190 – 1213.

J.H.J. Allum and M. Hulliger (Eds.)
Progress in Brain Research, Vol. 80
© 1989 Elsevier Science Publishers B.V. (Biomedical Division)

CHAPTER 3

Central mechanisms of selective fusimotor control

A. Taylor and R. Donga

Sherrington School of Physiology, U.M.D.S., St. Thomas's Hospital, London SE1 7EH, U.K.

Experiments on anaesthetized cats have confirmed the existence of regions of the midbrain from which dynamic fusimotor effects can be produced by electrical stimulation. Simultaneous recording from hindlimb and jaw muscle spindles has shown that both of these widely different muscle groups are affected from identical or closely related regions. The anatomical structure common to many of the pathways, which are likely to be involved at the sites of effective stimulation is the fasciculus retroflexus and it is suggested that this indicates that the habenulo-interpeduncular system may be involved in generating "dynamic fusimotor set" at the onset of movements, as a possible function of its place as an output pathway for the limbic system. The results are discussed in relation to the other well known source of dynamic control of spindles, namely the MesADC.

Key words: Muscle spindle; Fusimotor control; Habenula nucleus; Fasciculus retroflexus; Mid-brain; Dynamic control; Fusimotor set; Jaw muscle; Hindlimb muscle; Brain stimulation

Introduction

Mammalian muscle spindles contain three intrafusal fibre types, the activation of which permits control over the static and dynamic properties (see Boyd, 1985). If the great potentiality for flexibility of movement control, which this suggests, is to be realized, it should be possible to find CNS centres or pathways exerting a degree of selective influence over each intrafusal fibre type which at least to some extent should be separate from pathways to α motoneurones. The elucidation of such central mechanisms has both theoretical and practical importance. Thus the ability to excite fusimotor neurones generally, separate from α motoneurones, has forced a revision of the concept of universal "α-γ linkage" (Granit, 1955) to the simple descriptive term of "α-γ co-activation" to refer to those occasions on which α and γ activities are observed to be positively correlated (Matthews, 1972, p. 523). From the earliest experiments of

Granit and Kaada (1952) evidence has continued to accrue that many widely separated areas in the CNS can exert some separate control over fusimotor neurones, often predominantly either static or dynamic (fully reviewed by Matthews, 1972), and this indicates that a wide range of different motor activities may normally each have its own pattern of fusimotor accompaniment. From the practical viewpoint the finding of areas from which static or dynamic effects can be produced separately by electrical stimulation (e.g. Appelberg, 1981) can be exploited to identify fusimotor neurones, as one or the other type. This has been used first to determine their pattern of reflex connections (well summarized by Johansson, 1981), and secondly to identify the fusimotor types showing particular patterns of discharges during movements (Donga et al., 1988).

The work to be described in this paper originated from the latter study, making use of stimulation of midbrain areas giving selective dynamic fusimotor effects, that is the region close to the red nucleus designated the MesADC (mesencephalic area for dynamic control) by Appelberg and Jeneskog (1972). The practical objectives of this study were realized, but the interesting additional observation was made that an area very effective for eliciting dynamic fusimotor output was just rostral to the red nucleus and extended dorsally from this point coincident with the fasciculus retroflexus (FR). This is a large bundle of fibres linking the habenular nuclear complex with the interpeduncular nucleus (IPN) and other midbrain structures. Since the habenular nuclei have extensive inputs from the limbic system which may be expected to be involved in arousal in preparation for a motor task, the possibility arises that the enhanced dynamic fusimotor drive characteristic of this state (dynamic "fusimotor set", Hulliger et al., 1985) might originate from this source. Here we describe the results of stimulating in and around the FR while assessing fusimotor effects by spindle afferent recording during controlled muscle stretch.

Methods and Results

Cats were prepared under halothane followed by chloralose (50 mg/kg) or under sodium pentobarbitone (35 mg/kg). In either case small i.v. supplements of pentobarbitone were given to maintain a level of anaesthesia with no spontaneous movements but with flexion withdrawal reflexes present.

Muscle spindle afferents were recorded from two widely separated muscle groups, namely the jaw-closing muscles and the triceps surae. The jaw spindle activity was recorded from the first order afferent cell bodies in the mesencephalic trigeminal nucleus (MeV) as described by Cody et al. (1972) using glass-coated tungsten electrodes with tip inclined caudally at 10° to the vertical. Ramp and hold muscle stretches were applied via a servo puller attached to a screw in the symphysis menti. Stretches were of 10° amplitude at 15 or 30°/s occurring every 6 s and lasting 2 s. This corresponds

to approximately 4 mm stretch of the midpart of the masseter muscle. Afferents were designated as primary or secondary according to their dynamic index (DI) after infusion of succinylcholine (200 mg/kg). The dynamic indices of 33 units were bimodally distributed indicating that those with dynamic index less than 50 impulses per s (i.p.s.) were probably secondary afferents ($n = 18$) and those with higher values probably primary afferents ($n = 15$). Spindle afferents from medial gastrocnemius (MG) were recorded from dorsal root filaments and characterized by muscle twitch and by conduction velocity. Usually two or three MG afferents were recorded of which one was generally a secondary. A second servo puller applied the same waveform of stretch to MG as to the jaw but with amplitude 5 mm at 15 or 7.5 mm/s. The starting length corresponded to the midposition of the ankle joint.

In order to obtain fusimotor responses from brainstem stimulation it is necessary to keep anaesthesia light, but under these contitions there is a marked fluctuation of spontaneous activity. This makes observation of single stretch responses with the usual instantaneous frequency display an unreliable way of systematically relating stimulation site with fusimotor effects. Consequently, the procedure has been adopted of recording on tape between 5 and 10 ramp stretch responses of spindle afferents before, during and after stimulation. Subsequently cycle histograms were plotted with 100 ms bin widths and calibrated in terms of equivalent firing frequency. Because of the smoothing which this introduces the peak frequencies using this method are lower than those conventionally seen with frequencygrams because the latter are dominated by the exceptionally short interspike intervals.

Stimulation was delivered unipolarly through a stainless steel electrode sheathed in glass with a core of metal exposed, which was $30-50$ μm in diameter at its base and $100-300$ μm long. Constant voltage negative pulses of 0.1 ms duration were used generally at 50 per s and 5 V. Electrode tracks were tilted 33° to the vertical, tip caudally in a parasagittal plane. Iron marks were made in each useful track and visualized by perfusion with formal saline and 1% potassium ferrocyanide. Track reconstructions were made from parasagittal sections projected on copies of the best fitting plate from Berman's (1968) atlas.

Medial tegmental regions producing dynamic effects

Extensive studies by Appelberg and his collaborators (see especially Appelberg and Jeneskog, 1972; Jeneskog, 1974) have identified two medial tegmental regions which when stimulated produce selective hindlimb fusimotor effects. The regions were designated dorsal and ventral. The dorsal region was co-extensive with the red nucleus and extended caudally from it in the region of the medial longitudinal fasciculus. It evoked rather pure dynamic effects carried via the contralateral funiculus of the cord and its stimulation simultaneously evoked climbing fibre responses in the paramedian lobule of the cerebellum. These features together have been taken since to define the so-called MesADC (mesencephalic area for dynamic control). The other, more ventral region, in the vicinity of the interpeduncular nucleus, was said to have more mixed effects but often predominantly static. The pathway for these effects was in the lateral and ventrolateral funiculus of the cord respectively.

We have been able to reproduce these findings, at least in part, for jaw muscle spindles (Donga et al., 1985). In that work, based on 44 experiments in which the medial tegmentum was explored widely (to be reported in full elsewhere) dynamic effects were found scattered around the red nucleus. Some regions certainly corresponded to the MesADC,

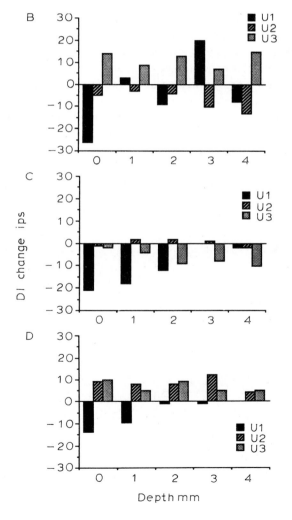

Fig. 1. Changes in dynamic index (DI) of spindle afferents during stimulation in the tracks indicated in A. In B, C and D ordinates are changes in DI relative to mean control values. U1: jaw muscle spindle primary afferent; U2: MG secondary; U3: MG primary. Plots B, C and D relate to tracks 10, 11 and 12 respectively. Stimulus 6 V, 50 per s. RN, red nucleus; PAG, periaqueductal grey; 3N, 3rd nerve.

dorsal and caudal to the red nucleus. An example from the present series with simultaneous recording from a jaw muscle primary and a gastrocnemius (MG) primary and secondary spindle afferent is shown in Fig. 1. The strongest dynamic enhancements are seen from track 10, dorso-caudal to the red nucleus, with the MG primary being affected from a wider area than the jaw primary afferent. The relatively small effects seen here with stimulation at 50 per s could probably be greatly increased with stimulation at 300 per s, as generally used by others. Lower frequencies were used here because of the need to control for stimulus artefact at the nearby MeV recording site. In addition to the sensitivity-enhancing effects, reductions in DI also occur in all tracks mainly corresponding to the rostral periaqueductal grey and subjacent reticular formation.

The series of jaw spindle experiments, however, showed a predominance of dynamic effects (pure dynamic effects in 23 out of 44 observations) elicited from rostral and ventral to the red nucleus as illustrated in Fig. 2. The most prominent effects correspond anatomically to stimulation at the location of the fasciculus retroflexus (FR). The increases in DI must be due to γ_d action rather than to reduction of spontaneous γ_s drive because the initial frequency (IF) clearly increases.

Stimulation directed specifically at the habenulo-interpeduncular system

In a series of 6 experiments stimulating tracks were directed to cross the FR at various points. In all cases strong dynamic effects were produced at points close to this fibre tract. Fig. 3 indicates that stimulation close to the termination of the FR in the interpeduncular nucleus (IPN) has a clear dynamic influence on an MG primary (cf. C with B) but not on a jaw unit (F and G). At the same depth, stimulation in a track 1.0 mm laterally

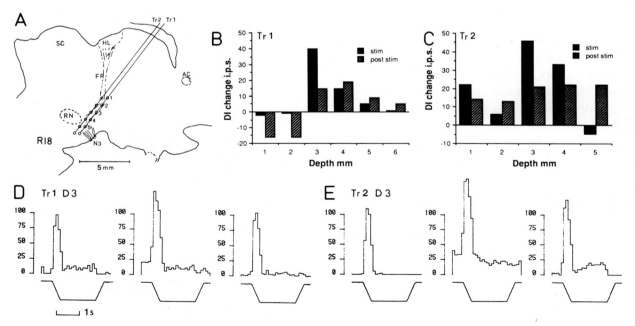

Fig. 2. Effects of stimulating rostral to the red nucleus (RN) on the DI of a jaw spindle primary afferent. A: drawing to show stimulating tracks 1 and 2 which correspond to plots B and C and to histograms D and E respectively, in which ordinate scale is mean frequency in i.p.s. D and E show successively control, stimulation period and post-stimulation periods. The displacement waveform is shown below with stretch downwards. SC, superior colliculus; HL, lateral habenular nucleus; AC, anterior commissure; FR, fasciculus retroflexus; RN, red nucleus. Histogram ordinates: frequency in i.p.s. Stimuli: 4 V, 0.2 ms, 50 per s.

selectively excited the jaw spindles (cf. E with D).

A track intersecting the FR near its midpoint is illustrated in Fig. 4. There is a strong dynamic effect on an MG primary at depth 40 with smaller effects 1 mm on either side. The jaw spindle afferent recorded (not shown) was a secondary and showed no significant effects.

In the case illustrated in Fig. 5 the stimulating electrode was aimed at the lateral habenular nucleus (HL) and passed immediately adjacent to its rostral margin. There are mixed effects with predominant fusimotor inhibition (shown by the reduction in IF) in the more dorsal parts (positions 41 – 43), and excitation in the deeper parts (44 – 47). This excitatory effect was probably due to dynamic action because the MG primary ending showed an increase in DI though the jaw spindle was unaffected. However the outstanding effect was a large increase in DI for the jaw unit when the stimulating point was immediately below the surface of the thalamus in the striae medullaris (depth 42). This effect has been confirmed on two other occasions and is particularly interesting because the striae medullaris represent the chief input pathways to the habenular nuclei from the limbic system.

Static fusimotor effects

Although the data presented here are consistent with the proposal that stimulation of the habenulo-interpeduncular system primarily excites dynamic fusimotor output there are many cases of variable and mixed effects, such as those just seen in Fig. 5. A possible explanation is that there are other adjacent structures which when stimulated have mainly γ_s effects. In fact stimulation along tracks through the dorsomedial tegmentum between those shown in Figs. 4 and 5 often gives strong, relatively pure static effects as shown in Fig. 6.

Here the track passed 1 mm rostral to that of Fig. 5 with depth 31.5 of Fig. 6 representing the point of crossing with the FR. The important dif-

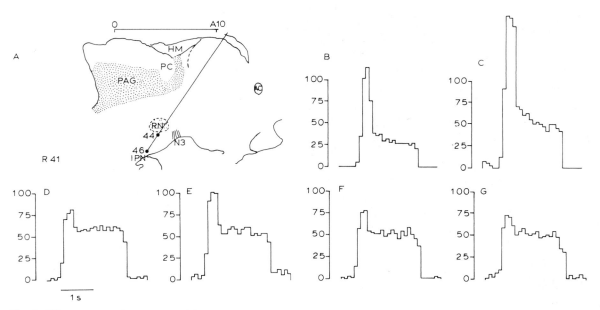

Fig. 3. Effects on stretch responses of jaw muscle and hindlimb spindle primary afferents of stimulation in the region of the interpeduncular nucleus (IPN). B and C control and stimulation responses of MG primary to stimulation at point marked 46. F and G are similar responses for jaw muscle spindle primary. D and E responses of the latter tested again with stimulation 1 mm further laterally. Histogram ordinates: frequency i.p.s. Stimuli: 8 V, 0.1 ms, 50 per s. PAG, periaqueductal grey; PC, posterior commissure; HM, medial habenular nucleus; RN, red nucleus.

ference however is that here the track passed 0.65 mm medial to the FR within the periaqueductal grey (PAG). The large rise in IF of primaries coupled with reduction of DI indicate contraction of bag$_2$ fibres. Static γ fibres to nuclear chains were probably not involved because spindle secondaries were little affected (e.g. U3 in Fig. 6). During stimulation in this region there were large rises of blood pressure and extension of forelimbs. Stimulation symmetrically on the other side (ipsilateral to the spindles) gave identical effects.

Discussion

Assessment of fusimotor effects

The criteria for recognizing static (γ_s) and dynamic (γ_d) fusimotor action are well set out by Matthews (1972) and more recently by Hulliger (1979). Primary afferents show the precence of γ_d activity by marked increase in dynamic sensitivity to stretch and increased dynamic index (DI) with relatively little increase in initial frequency (IF). Silencing during shortening is not generally

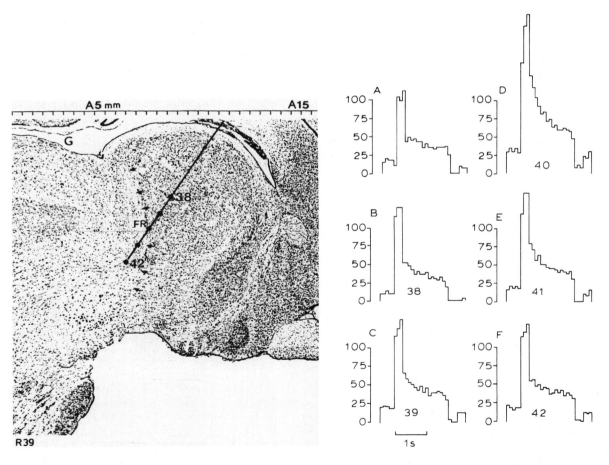

Fig. 4. Responses of MG spindle primary to stimulating along a track intersecting the fasciculus retroflexus (FR) near its mid-point. A: control. B to F: responses during stimulation (7 V, 0.1 ms, 50 per s) at the points indicated by the numbers 38 to 42 (mm along track from an arbitrary reference point). Histogram ordinates frequency in i.p.s.

prevented (but see Morgan et al., 1985) and γ_d effects on secondary endings are uncommon. Primary afferents show the presence of γ_s activity

by reduction in dynamic sensitivity and DI, by marked increase in IF and by permitting firing to continue during the stretch release. The firing of secondary endings is increased.

Several problems arise in applying these criteria in essentially intact animals under light anaesthesia. First the effects described above relate predominantly to work in which spindles have no background fusimotor activity because of de-efferentation or deep anaesthesia. Secondly, the effects are due to activation of single γ_s or γ_d axons. Complications arise when both types are active together. Finally, in natural conditions, all the fusimotor fibres of one type may be expected to be active rather than a single one.

Another problem of a quite different kind is the need to take account of separate static innervation of nuclear bag$_2$ and nuclear chain fibres (Boyd and Ward, 1975; Boyd, 1985). Activation of chain fibres has a powerful driving action on primary afferents which thereby loose their sensitivity to stretch. They also have a far more powerful excitatory effect on secondary endings than do the

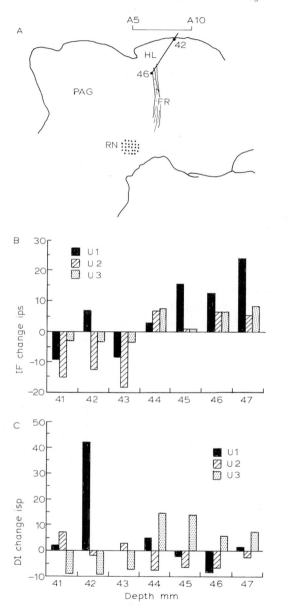

Fig. 5. Changes in initial frequency (IF) and dynamic index (DI) of a jaw spindle primary (U1), an MG secondary (U2) and an MG primary (U3) during stimulation along the track indicated in A. Plots B and C show changes in IF and DI respectively. Stimuli: 5 V, 50 per s. Numbers 41–47, mm along track (in A) from an arbitrary reference point.

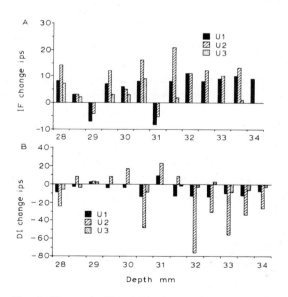

Fig. 6. Changes in IF and DI of two primary MG spindle afferents U1 and U2, and one MG secondary U3. The stimulating electrode track was 1 mm rostral to that of Fig. 5, but passed 0.65 mm medial to the FR. Stimuli: 5 V, 0.1 ms, 50 per s.

bag$_2$ fibres (Boyd, 1981). The classical γ_s fusimotor system now seems to comprise two distinct subpopulations. Boyd (1985) summarizes: "Static bag γ motor neurones bias the group Ia discharge in all the spindles they supply, and sometimes the discharge from secondary endings at any innervated pole; ... Static chain γ motor neurones bias the group Ia discharge of all the spindles they supply, and the discharge from secondary endings at any innervated pole". It now seems wise therefore to diagnose the intrafusal changes responsible for particular afferent effects in terms of bag$_1$, bag$_2$ or chain fibre contraction.

In the present work a number of measures of the ramp responses were available, but for simplicity's sake we report only IF and DI. Using these for primaries it seems possible in most cases to be quite confident in recognizing changes in bag$_1$ and bag$_2$ action. Monitoring EMG in a number of cases showed no significant extrafusal activation which could have accounted for the observed effects by β innervation.

In these terms it is evident that the present results provide good circumstantial evidence for activation of bag$_1$ fibres of spindles in widely different muscle groups by stimulation of the habenulo-interpeduncular system. Evidence of this kind can never be conclusive because other adjacent structures might be responsible or at least involved, if multiple sources of dynamic drive exist. However, the circumstantial case for the involvement of the habenular pathway is made more attractive because the habenulo-interpeduncular pathway appears to be one important efferent route from the limbic system (Lake, 1973) which may influence motor centres in the lower brainstem and spinal cord as well as the ascending reticular activating system. Activation of this pathway in preparation for movement could then seem a reasonable way by which the "dynamic fusimotor set" observed in active cats (Hulliger et al., 1985) may arise. Recording from the habenular system under such conditions would be necessary however to give any substance to this hypothesis.

Another matter of interest is the relationship of the habenular system and the MesADC. We have not recorded from the cerebellar paramedian lobules to look for climbing fibre responses which are regarded as an essential accompaniment of MesADC activation, nor do we yet know the pathways by which the dynamic drive from the habenular system reaches the lower brainstem and spinal cord. However it is known (Brodal, 1985) that the FR projects not only to the IPN but also to the substantia nigra and mesencephalic reticular formation. Clearly it would be possible to excite FR fibres via any of their collaterals to these regions. This could therefore provide an explanation for the widely diverse regions in the midbrain from which some MesADC-like effects were obtainable.

Finally the present work provides further evidence that central structures can provide independent control of the separate intrafusal system (see also Gladden, 1981). Here we have seen the habenular system like the MesADC apparently specifically exciting bag$_1$ fibres, and the periaqueductal grey exciting bag$_2$ fibres. No region exciting chain fibres has been observed in the present work.

Acknowledgements

We are grateful for support from the Research Endowments Committee of St. Thomas's Hospital. Mr. M.A. Bosley and Mr. A.P.S. Smale provided expert assistance.

References

Appelberg, B. (1981) Selective central control of dynamic gamma motoneurones utilized for the functional classification of gamma cells. In A. Taylor and A. Prochazka (Eds.), *Muscle Receptors and Movement,* Macmillan, London, pp. 97 – 108.

Appelberg, B. and Jeneskog, T. (1972) Mesencephalic fusimotor control. *Exp. Brain Res.,* 15: 97 – 112.

Berman, A.L. (1968) *The Brain Stem of the Cat.* University of Wisconsin Press, Madison, 175 pp.

Boyd, I.A. (1981) The action of three types of intrafusal fibres in isolated cat muscle spindles on the dynamic and length sensitivities of primary and secondary sensory endings. In A. Taylor and A. Prochazka (Eds.), *Muscle Receptors and*

Movement, Macmillan, London, pp. 17–32.

Boyd, I.A. (1985) Internal working of muscle spindles. Review. In I.A. Boyd and M.H. Gladden (Eds.), *The Muscle Spindle,* Macmillan, London, pp. 129–150.

Boyd, I.A. and Ward, J. (1975) Motor control of nuclear bag and nuclear chain intrafusal fibres in isolated living muscle spindles of the cat. *J. Physiol. (London),* 244: 83–112.

Brodal, A. (1985) *Neurological Anatomy, 4th Edn.* Oxford University Press, Oxford, 1053 pp.

Cody, F.W.J., Lee, R.W.H. and Taylor, A. (1972) A functional analysis of components of the mesencephalic nucleus of the fifth nerve in the cat. *J. Physiol. (London),* 226: 249–261.

Donga, R., Gottlieb, S., Juch, P.J.W. and Taylor, A. (1985) The influences of red nucleus stimulation on fusimotor activity of jaw muscles of the cat. *J. Physiol. (London),* 372: 25P.

Donga, R., Gottlieb, S., Juch, P.J.W. and Taylor, A. (1988) The use of mid-brain stimulation to identify jaw muscle fusimotoneurones in reflex movements in anaesthetised cats. *J. Physiol. (London),* 398: 39P.

Gladden, M.H. (1981) The activity of intrafusal fibres during central stimulation in the cat. In A. Taylor and A. Prochazka (Eds.), *Muscle Receptors and Movement,* Macmillan, London, pp. 109–122.

Granit, R. (1955) *Receptors and Sensory Perception,* Yale University Press, New Haven, 369 pp.

Granit, R. and Kaada, B. (1952) Influence of stimulation of central nervous structures on muscle spindles in cat. *Acta Physiol. Scand.,* 27: 130–160.

Hulliger, M. (1979) The responses of primary spindle afferents to fusimotor stimulation at constant and abrubtly changing rates. *J. Physiol. (London),* 294: 461–482.

Hulliger, M., Zangger, P., Prochazka, A. and Appenteng, K. (1985) Simulations reveal large variations in fusimotor action in normal cats: "fusimotor set". In I.A. Boyd and M.H. Gladden (Eds.), *The Muscle Spindle,* Macmillan, London, pp. 311–315.

Jeneskog, T. (1974) A descending pathway to dynamic fusimotor neurones and its possible relation to a climbing fibre system. *Umeå* University Medical Dissertations, No. 14.

Johansson, H. (1981) Reflex control of γ-motoneurones. *Umeå* University Medical Dissertations, New Series, No. 70.

Lake, N. (1973) Studies of the habenulo-interpeduncular pathway in cats. *Exp. Neurol.,* 41: 113–132.

Matthews, P.B.C. (1972) *Mammalian Muscle Receptors and their Central Actions.* Arnold, London, 630 pp.

Morgan, D.L., Prochazka, A. and Proske, U. (1985) Action of single dynamic fusimotor neurones on cat soleus Ia afferents during muscle shortening. *Exp. Brain Res.,* 58: 56–61.

J.H.J. Allum and M. Hulliger (Eds.)
Progress in Brain Research, Vol. 80
© 1989 Elsevier Science Publishers B.V. (Biomedical Division)

CHAPTER 4

Discharge patterns of γ motoneurone populations of extensor and flexor hindlimb muscles during walking in the thalamic cat

P. Bessou, Ph. Dupui, J.M. Cabelguen, M. Joffroy, R. Montoya and B. Pagès

UA CNRS 649, Laboratoire de Physiologie, Faculté de Médecine de Toulouse, 133, Route de Narbonne, 31062 Toulouse Cédex, France

Two monopolar recordings of the whole activity in a fine nerve branch innervating the gastrocnemius lateralis (GL) or the sartorius medialis (SM) muscle were obtained during spontaneous walking in thalamic cats. Using a special electronic device, the potentials of several groups of efferent (α and γ) and afferent (I and II) fibres constituting the whole nerve activity were separated. In the present paper we compare the data obtained for an ankle extensor (GL) and a hip-knee flexor (SM) during the step cycle. In both muscles the γ motoneurone population is activated in parallel with the α motoneurone population. Usually, between the cyclic locomotor discharges, the GL γ neurones are tonically active whereas the SM γ neurones are silent. During muscle contraction, the group I and II afferent discharges are both length and γ dependent, but the prevailing factor is the muscle shortening for the GL afferents and the cyclic γ drive for the SM afferents. Both dynamic and static fusimotor efferents appear to be activated during muscle contraction, but on indirect evidence it is suggested that dynamic action prevails in GL spindles whereas static action dominates in SM spindles.

Key words: Fusimotor neurone; Muscle spindle; Muscle afferent; Locomotion; Thalamic cat

Introduction

A great deal is now known about the discharge pattern of cat α motoneurones during locomotion (see Grillner, 1981). By contrast, the equivalent information about γ motoneurones is scanty (Severin, 1970; Perret, 1976; Sjöström and Zangger, 1976; Murphy et al., 1984). The shortage of data on γ neurones results from the technical difficulty of recording directly from these small neurones in moving animals.

The technique of direct recording from single γ efferents suffers from several limitations. It does not permit accurate deductions about the activity level and recruitment order in a pool of γ neurones during locomotion because of the difficulty to acquire a large sample of γ units supplying a given muscle under homogeneous experimental conditions. Direct recording from a limited number of γ motoneurones does not allow to deduce the consequences of a multi-unit fusimotor outflow to a muscle spindle population. Recordings of single γ efferents are usually made from isolated filaments in cut muscle nerves, i.e. after the sensorimotor loops that control the contraction of the muscle under study have been opened. The denervation reduces afferent inputs to the CNS and then may lead to abnormal discharge of γ motoneurones.

The behaviour of γ motoneurones during locomotion thus requires a re-investigation with more comprehensive techniques. With this in mind, we have developed a technique which permits to record and sort the potentials of different groups of efferent (α and γ) and afferent (group I and group II) fibres from the ensemble activity of an intact fine branch of a muscular nerve (Bessou et al., 1981). We have previously used this technique to study the discharge patterns of small populations of neurones supplying an extensor (Bessou et al., 1986) or a flexor (Bessou et al., 1988) hindlimb muscle during spontaneous walking of the thalamic cat. The records of the discharges of the four fibre groups of the nerve studied, simultaneously monitored with electromyographical (EMG) and mechanical (joint angle displacements) events in the hindlimb, allowed the analysis during the step cycle of the discharge pattern of the γ motoneurone population supplying the muscle, its relationship with α motoneurone activity, and inferences on the γ action on the discharge of group I and II muscle afferents. In the present paper we will review and compare our previous data obtained for extensor and flexor hindlimb muscles during spontaneous walking of the thalamic cat in an attempt to better understand the role of fusimotor neurones during locomotor movements.

Methods

Surgical procedures

The experiments were performed on 32 adult cats (2.5 – 4.5 kg), anaesthetized with halothane (fluothane, I.C.I. Ltd.) in a 50% oxygen-air mixture. After tracheotomy, the cat was suspended in a prone position, the head fastened in a non-traumatic head-holder and the spinal column fixed in a frame by clamping the spinous process of the 7th lumbar vertebrae.

In 15 cats, the left hindlimb was partially denervated by cutting femoral and hamstring muscle nerves as well as sural and lateral femoral cutaneous nerves. A fine natural branch of the nerve of the gastrocnemius lateralis (GL) or medialis (GM) muscle (anatomically ankle extensor and knee flexor) of this hindlimb was dissected in continuity over a distance of 8 – 10 mm (Bessou et al., 1981). The foot of the studied limb did not contact the experimental table surface, and the

walking movements of the left hindlimb, because of its denervation, were reduced to the extension (plantar flexion) and flexion (dorsal flexion) of the ankle joint (for details see Bessou et al., 1986).

In 17 cats, the finest of the nerve branches innervating the sartorius medialis (SM) muscle of the left hindlimb was dissected in continuity over a distance of 8 – 10 mm. The SM was selected because it flexes hip and knee and exhibits a typical flexor EMG burst during the step cycle (Forssberg et al., 1980; Perret and Cabelguen, 1980; Hoffer et al., 1987). In these experiments no denervation was performed.

After the initial surgery, the entire cerebral cortex was removed and then the anaesthesia was discontinued. The resulting thalamic preparation could show spontaneous locomotor activity with well coordinated movements of the four limbs (Orlovskii, 1969; Perret and Buser, 1972). As the head and the pelvic girdle of the cat were fixed and the limbs were not on a treadmill belt, the height of the animal was adjusted so that during the stance phase of the step cycle the pads of the 3 limbs in GL or GM experiments and the four limbs in SM experiments were free to slip backward on the flat surface of the experimental table smeared with paraffin oil.

Recordings

Two monopolar recordings of the whole activity of the fine nerve branch selected for study were obtained with two electrodes separated by 4 mm. The action potentials of different groups of efferent (α and γ) and afferent (I and II) fibres were separated, according to their propagation directions and conduction velocities by electronic processing (Joffroy, 1975). The firing frequency of each fibre population was measured by a frequency-meter (time constant 0.1 s). Details of the recording and sorting of action potentials as well as the limits of performance of the sorting process have been presented in a previous study (Bessou et al., 1981).

In the experiments on the GL or GM, the EMG activity of this muscle and the electroneurographic

(ENG) activity of the whole sartorius nerve were recorded and the variations of the ankle angle were monitored. During slow and moderate gaits, like those considered in the present study, the SM and GL each exhibit a single (flexor and extensor, respectively) burst of EMG activity per step cycle, especially when the amplitude of the locomotor movements of the studied hindlimb is limited (Perret, 1976; Perret and Cabelguen, 1980).

In the experiments on the SM, the EMG activity of this muscle and that of gluteus maximus muscle (anatomically a hip extensor) were recorded and the variations of the hip angle were monitored. The gluteus maximus muscle exhibits a single (extensor) burst of EMG activity per step cycle (Rasmussen et al., 1978; Perret and Cabelguen, 1980).

Results

Fig. 1 shows the records obtained during two step cycles of the left hindlimb in two experiments, one on the GL muscle (left column) and the other on the SM muscle (right column). The mean walking cadence was in GL 72.4 and in SM 68.2 step cycles/min. The duration of the flexor burst was approximately 40% of that of the step cycle. These features were those of a slow walk (Goslow et al., 1973; Halbertsma, 1983). The amplitude of the angle displacements of hip and ankle joints were quite similar to those measured during overground locomotion at the same speed in the intact cat (Goslow et al., 1973). However, since in GL experiments the foot did not contact the ground, the E_2 phase (Philippson, 1905) was absent and the ankle was dorsiflexed only once per step cycle.

Extensor and flexor efferent discharges

During the step cycle the cyclic discharges of GL and SM γ motoneurones were in phase with, and had a similar time course to the locomotor discharges of the corresponding α motoneurones (Fig. 1). So, there was a clear cyclic coactivation of α and γ motoneurones of extensor and flexor muscles during walking. In either case, the γ

motoneurones were activated during shortening contraction of the muscle they supplied.

Since knee movements were absent in the gastrocnemius experiments (cf. Methods), the GL lengthened (downward deflexion in Fig. 1, left column) during the first third of ankle (dorsi-) flexion in spite of a concomitant activation of its γ motoneurones. The GL lengthening contraction

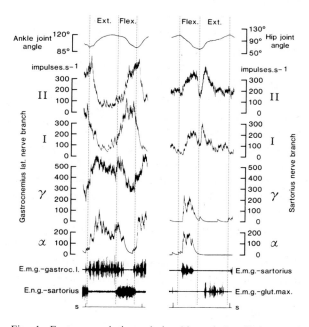

Fig. 1. Features and time-relationships of the discharge of populations of α and γ efferent axons and of group I and II afferent fibres in an intact thin branch of the gastrocnemius lateralis nerve (left column) and of the sartorius medialis nerve (right column) during spontaneous step cycles in two walking thalamic cats. Identical arrangement in both columns. First trace: joint angle, left, ankle plantar-flexion (upward deflexion, Ext) and dorsi-flexion (downward deflexion, Flex); right, hip flexion (downward deflexion, Flex) and extension (upward deflexion, Ext). Second and third traces: firing frequency of II and I afferent fibre populations, respectively. Fourth and fifth traces: firing frequency of γ and α efferent axon populations, respectively. Sixth and seventh traces: left, electromyogram of the gastrocnemius lateralis muscle (e.m.g., gastroc.l.) and electroneurogram of the sartorius nerve (e.n.g., sartorius); right, electromyogram of the sartorius medialis (e.m.g., sartorius) and electromyogram of the gluteus maximus (e.m.g., glut. max). Eighth trace, time marker, 1 s calibration. The dotted lines indicate the onsets of the extension and the flexion phases of both joints.

was accompanied by a second peak of γ activity. That suggests that the α-γ co-activation occurs, whatever the conditions (shortening or lengthening) of the muscular contraction in the step cycle. A similar proposal has been made by Prochazka et al., (1977) from records of the discharge pattern of single spindle afferents of triceps surae and the whole-length of the parent muscle in the freely moving cat. However, it is difficult to draw safe inferences about the discharge pattern of fusimotor neurones from such recordings alone (but see Prochazka et al., 1985).

Between the rhythmic bursts of activation the GL and GM γ populations often (12 out of 15 experiments) exhibited a sustained activity while the SM γ populations were often (12 out of 17 experiments) silent as the α populations of both muscles always were. This discharge pattern of the gastrocnemius γ populations might result from recruitment of individual γ motoneurones showing tonic and phasic patterns of activity during locomotion (Murphy et al., 1984; see also Prochazka et al., 1985, for tonic firing patterns). The residual activity of gastrocnemius γ at the end of the ankle dorsiflexion might explain, partly, why the cyclic increase of the firing rate of γ motoneurones often preceded those of α motoneurones.

Extensor and flexor afferent discharges
Active muscle shortening. During muscle contraction, the discharge patterns of group I and II afferents were different in extensor and flexor muscles.

The firing rate of GL afferents (I and II) decreased steeply during the active shortening of the parent muscle (Fig. 1, left column, Ext.), in spite of the concomitant discharge of the γ motoneurones. However, this γ discharge was powerful enough to slow down the drop and usually to prevent silencing of the discharge of GL spindle afferents. Indeed, following a curarization of α and γ neuromuscular junctions, a similar passive shortening of the muscle elicited a steeper drop and it caused prolonged silence in the firing of I and II

muscle afferents.

On the contrary, the firing rate of SM afferents (I and II) increased, often markedly, during the periods of active shortening of the parent muscle (Fig. 1, right column, Flex.). So, the concomitant γ discharge overcompensated the unloading of spindle afferents.

These results showed that during muscle contraction the prevailing factor was the muscle length change for the GL and GM spindles and the fusimotor drive for the SM spindles.

Passive muscle lengthening. During lengthening of the GL or SM, due to the contraction of the antagonistic muscles, the discharge of their I and II afferents increased but with different time course.

The discharge of GL afferents (I and II) (Fig. 1, left column, Flex.) consisted of: (i) a small initial increase during the early part of the ankle dorsiflexion while the GL length change was small and the γ activity still high; (ii) a large increase resulting from the fast lengthening of the muscle in spite of the simultaneous decrease of the γ activity; (iii) a small and slow increase or a plateau of discharge due to both a small and slow muscle lengthening and a low level of the γ activity at the end of ankle dorsiflexion. In 3 out of 15 experiments, the GL γ motoneurones were silent during the flexor contraction. Then the discharge of GL afferents was determined by the features of the muscle lengthening alone.

The discharge of the SM afferents (I and II) during lengthening of the muscle (Fig. 1, right column, Ext.) featured: (i) a low firing rate at the onset of hip extension because the muscle was still short and the γ motoneurones were silent at this time; (ii) a rapid increase and a peak of impulse rate during the first part of hip extension exclusively elicited by the fast lengthening of the muscle since γ were silent throughout hip extension; (iii) a release of the discharge occurring when the SM relaxed and was only slowly lengthened by contractions of antagonistic muscles (Severin et al., 1967). Thus, the firing rate of SM afferents was low when the muscle was at its greatest length during the step cycle. That evidenced the low "static" responsiveness of the spindle endings when the γ activity was depressed.

Discussion

Comments concerning the preparation

In the present paper we have not compared the afferent and efferent activities in a nerve branch of the gastrocnemius muscle with the corresponding activities in a nerve branch of a relevant antagonistic muscle (i.e. an ankle flexor). Indeed, preliminary experiments performed on the tibialis anterior muscle revealed two main drawbacks: (i) to reach the nerve branches it was necessary to remove the peroneus longus and extensor digitorum longus muscles, which degraded walking movements of the ankle; (ii) the nerve branches were too thick (diameter > 0.2 mm) to obtain a signal-to-noise ratio which would have kept counting errors of the sorting device below 5 – 10% (Joffroy, 1975). We have chosen the SM, a hip and knee flexor, because its EMG activity during walking has approximately the same timing as that of ankle flexors, especially during slow or moderate gaits like those considered in our study (Forssberg et al., 1980; Perret and Cabelguen, 1980; Perret, 1983). Moreover, one of the nerve branches which supply the SM was thin enough (diameter < 0.2 mm) to minimize the counting errors of the sorting device.

Acute recordings were performed in the thalamic cat because with chronically implanted electrodes in intact cats it was difficult to avoid mechanical injury of thin nerve branches and to obtain stable recordings during locomotor movements. Moreover, the thalamic preparation exhibits spontaneous locomotor movements which were broadly similar to those of the intact cat (Perret, 1983), although the length variations, especially in GM, were slightly abnormal (see above, Methods).

In the group I afferent population discharge it was not possible to separate Ia from Ib potentials because the conduction velocities of the two types of fibres largely overlap. But, the group I afferent discharge probably was dominated by potentials from spindle primary endings on the following grounds: the firing rate of the group I afferents varied in parallel with that of the group II afferents, the latter being a reliable index of the spindle activity since group II afferent discharge almost exclusively comes from spindle secondary endings; the tendon organ activity was probably low in our experiments because the SM during the swing phase and the GL and GM during the ankle plantar flexion were contracting against minimal load. However, it cannot entirely be ruled out that the – very low level – group I discharge during GM shortening (Fig. 1, left, Ext.) was partly due to activity from Ib afferents, given their exquisite sensitivity to active muscle force (Houk and Henneman, 1967).

Discharge of different afferent populations

The discharge patterns of small populations of afferent fibres derived from the same muscle gives a more accurate picture of muscle afferent signals returned to the CNS during walking than unitary recordings obtained by chronically implanted micro-electrodes (Prochazka et al., 1976, 1977; Loeb and Duysens, 1979; Loeb et al., 1985) or averaged rate profiles of a few muscle afferents (Dürmüller et al., 1987; Prochazka et al., 1989, this volume). Indeed, the firing patterns of single spindle afferents show a great degree of variability because afferents come from spindles located in different regions of the muscle, or from a given muscle group composed of muscles having not exactly the same function and EMG pattern during walking, or from different animals. In addition, this variability might reflect important peripheral events for the CNS and its suppression by the method of averaging of the rate profiles of single units recorded in different circumstances is questionable.

The discharge patterns of group I and II afferent populations in the walking thalamic cat are, nevertheless, very similar to those of single spindle afferents during unrestrained walking in the intact cat. Thus, the firing rates of single spindle afferents are clearly modulated in close relation to the length changes of the parent muscle (see references above) although some discrepancies between afferent firing rate and parent muscle length appear for ankle flexors (tibialis anterior and peroneus longus) and hip flexors (sartorius medialis and sartorius lateralis) (Loeb and Duysens, 1979; Loeb et al., 1985). These discrepancies have been attributed to fusimotor activation, but it should be pointed out that when the afferent firing rate and the parent muscle length increase or decrease in parallel one cannot conjecture anything about the activity in the fusimotor system without direct recording of the γ activity, or without quantitative tests of simulation methods to deduce fusimotor action from afferent recordings (Hulliger and Prochazka, 1983; Hulliger et al., 1987 and 1989, this volume).

The afferent discharges from the GL and GM, because of their close relation with the muscle length changes, can provide the CNS with convenient information on the execution of the step cycle. The discharge of the afferents from the SM increasing as a result of the cyclic γ activity during the active muscle shortening can play a suitable role in a mechanism of servo-assistance (Matthews, 1970) of the swing movement of the limb. Moreover, it appears that the sensory message conveyed individually by group I and II afferents from the SM cannot contain any straightforward information on muscle position alone, and that more involved central mechanisms ("computations") are required to extract the appropriate signal.

Co-activation of α and γ motoneurones

We provide direct evidence that during walking of the thalamic cat the γ motoneurones are activated in parallel with the α motoneurones. The observation of α-γ coactivation in several types of rhythmic and voluntary movements (see Hulliger, 1984) and the existence of skeleto-fusimotor (β) neurones that send out the same command signal to spindles and motor units (see Laporte et al., 1981) suggest that the CNS may link the fusimotor

and the skeletomotor commands to adapt muscle spindle responsiveness to muscular activity. The presence in mammals of α motoneurones, in addition to β motoneurones innervating specifically extrafusal muscle fibres unbalances skeletomotor versus fusimotor control. The balance can only be retrieved by the development of a γ fusimotor system activated in parallel with the α system. The advantage of a central control of the α and γ pathways is to provide more flexibility than the linkage of the two effectors through a single efferent (β) pathway. Previous results indeed suggest that the locomotor command acts on α and γ motoneurones through two separate pathways (Murphy et al., 1984; Bessou et al., 1986).

Dynamic and static γ activation

The separate sorting of the potentials of the dynamic and static γ axons is impossible with our electronic device because their ranges of conduction velocities completely overlap (see Matthews, 1972). However, the firing patterns of group I and II afferents during shortening contractions of the parent muscle provide some information about the type of γ neurones that contribute to the whole γ discharge.

For the GL and GM muscles, the inability of the rhythmic γ discharge to overcome the unloading effects of muscle shortening on group I afferent discharge suggests that dynamic γ are activated (Lennerstrand and Thoden, 1968). Moreover, the brief bursts of discharge of group I afferents accompanying segmented EMG activity point to a great dynamic sensitivity of the spindle primary endings during muscle contraction (Bessou et al., 1986). The decrease to a low level of the firing rate of the group I and II afferents during muscle shortening suggests that static γ efferents do not contribute much in the whole γ discharge. However, by curarizing selectively α motor endplates, we have provided indirect evidence for the presence of static γ firing, contributing to the whole γ discharge (Bessou et al., 1986). Hence the dynamic and static components of the γ system appear to be activated in parallel with the α system, but dynamic usually outclass static effects. This could provide a sensitization of Ia afferents to small disturbances that may occur during the stance phase.

Similar conclusions can be drawn from 5 out of the 17 experiments on the SM muscle. In the remaining 12 experiments, the cyclic γ discharge was able to overcome the unloading effects of active muscle shortening on the group I and II afferents. This indicated that strong static fusimotor activation occurred at this time. However, rhythmically modulated dynamic γ firing may also have contributed, since dynamic γ are also capable of overcoming the effects of shortening during slow alternating movements (Rioult-Pedotti et al., 1988).

To sum up, our results suggest a differential fusimotor control of functionally different muscles during walking. On indirect grounds, quite similar conclusions have been drawn in the walking thalamic cat (Perret and Buser, 1972; Perret and Berthoz, 1973; Cabelguen, 1981) and during treadmill locomotion in the unrestrained intact cat (Loeb and Duysens, 1979; Loeb et al., 1985). Yet our conclusions concerning ankle extensors are, at least partly, at variance with those drawn by Taylor et al. (1985) from spindle afferent discharges in the walking premammillary cat.

Motoneurone recruitment

The α motoneurones are recruited orderly according to the size principle (Henneman et al., 1965 a,b). The principle presumably also applies to β motoneurones which are α motoneurones according to the conduction velocity of their axons. Jami et al. (1982) showed that the conduction velocities of the dynamic β motoneurones, innervating extrafusal motor units of the slow type (Barker et al., 1977), are slower than those of static β motoneurones, innervating extrafusal motor units of the fast type (Jami et al., 1979). Consequently, the dynamic β neurones will be recruited before the static β neurones. In contrast, the recruitment of γ motoneurones according to size is functionally meaningless because of the extensive

overlap of the range of conduction velocities of the dynamic and static γ axons (Matthews, 1972).

The recruitment of motoneurones is presumably better correlated with the functional properties of their muscle effectors rather than their size per se, in relation with the presynaptic organization of the synaptic input to motoneurones and with neuromuscular trophic influences, as was suggested by Burke (1981) for the α motoneurones. For instance, the velocity of contraction of muscular fibres distinguishes between slow and fast extrafusal fibres (Gordon and Phillips, 1953) as well as between slow and fast intrafusal fibres (Boyd, 1976). In each contracting system, the extrafusal and intrafusal components contract together as a result of the activation of β motoneurones and, probably, as a result of any central co-activation of α and γ motoneurones. The dynamic β motoneurones act on slow extrafusal fibres and slow intrafusal bag$_1$ fibres (Barker et al., 1977, 1980) and the static β motoneurones on fast extrafusal and fast intrafusal chain fibres (Jami et al., 1978, 1979, 1982). Bessou and Pagès (1975) and Boyd et al. (1977) have shown that the dynamic γ axons innervate slow intrafusal fibres (bag$_1$) while the static γ axons innervate fast intrafusal fibres (bag$_2$ and/or chain). Therefore, since in routine behavioural activities, such as walking, several mechanisms ascertain that slow motor units are preferentially activated and recruited before the fast motor units (see review of Buchthal and Schmalbruch, 1980), the recruitment of slow α motoneurones innervating slow motor units will be coupled with the activation of dynamic β and γ motoneurones, whereas the recruitment of fast α motoneurones innervating fast motor units will be coupled with the activation of static β and γ motoneurones. On this view, it is worth noting that the active shortening of ankle extensors during the stance phase is much slower than that of ankle flexors during the swing phase (Goslow et al., 1973) and that the relative strength of dynamic and static fusimotor influences on their spindles indeed is different.

Acknowledgements

This investigation was supported by a research grant from the Fondation pour la Recherche Médicale.

References

Barker, D., Emonet-Dénand, F., Harker, D.W., Jami, L. and Laporte, Y. (1977) Types of intra- and extra-fusal muscle fibre innervated by dynamic skeleto-fusimotor axons in cat peroneus brevis and tenuissimum muscle, as determined by the glycogen depletion method. *J. Physiol. (London), 266:* 713 – 726.

Barker, D., Emonet-Dénand, F., Laporte, Y. and Stacey, M.J. (1980) Identification of the intrafusal endings of skeleto-fusimotor axons in the cat. *Brain Res., 185:* 227 – 237.

Bessou, P. and Pagès, B. (1975) Cinematographic analysis of contractile events produced in intrafusal muscle fibres by stimulation of static and dynamic fusimotor axons. *J. Physiol. (London), 252:* 397 – 427.

Bessou, P., Joffroy, M. and Pagès, B. (1981) Efferents and afferents in an intact muscle nerve: Background activity and effects of sural nerve stimulation in the cat. *J. Physiol. (London), 320:* 81 – 102.

Bessou, P., Cabelguen, J.M., Montoya, R. and Pagès, B. (1986) Efferent and afferent activity in a gastrocnemius nerve branch during locomotion in the thalamic cat. *Exp. Brain Res., 64:* 553 – 568.

Bessou, P., Dupui, Ph., Joffroy, M., Montoya, R. and Pagès, B. (1988) Modulation au cours de la marche de l'activité efférente et afférente d'un muscle fléchisseur chez le chat thalamique. *Arch. Int. Physiol. Biochim., 96 (3):* A102.

Boyd, I.A. (1976) The response of fast and slow nuclear bag fibres and nuclear chain fibres in isolated cat muscle spindles to fusimotor stimulation, and the effect of intrafusal contraction on the sensory endings. *Q. J. Exp. Physiol., 61:* 203 – 254.

Boyd, I.A., Gladden, M.H., McWilliam, P.N. and Ward, J. (1977) Control of dynamic and static nuclear bag fibres and nuclear chain fibres by gamma and beta axons in isolated cat muscle spindles. *J. Physiol. (London), 265:* 133 – 162.

Buchthal, F. and Schmalbruch, H. (1980) Motor-units of mammalian muscle. *Physiol. Rev., 60:* 90 – 142.

Burke, R.E. (1981) Motor units: anatomy, physiology and functional organization. In J.M. Brookhart, V.B. Mountcastle and V.B. Brooks (Eds.), *Handbook of Physiology, Sect. 1, The Nervous System, Vol. II Motor Control, Part 1,* American Physiological Society, Bethesda, pp. 345 – 422.

Cabelguen, J.M. (1981) Static and dynamic fusimotor controls in various hindlimb muscles during locomotor activity in the decorticate cat. *Brain Res., 213:* 83 – 97.

Dürmüller, N., Hulliger, M., Prochazka, A. and Trend, P. St. J. (1987) Ensemble proprioceptive activity in feline gait. *J. Physiol. (London), 392:* 63P.

Forssberg, H., Grillner, S. and Halbertsma, J. (1980) The locomotion of the low spinal cat. 1 - Coordination within a hindlimb. *Acta Physiol. Scand., 108:* 269 – 281.

Gordon, G. and Phillips, C.G. (1953) Slow and rapid components in a flexor muscle. *Q. J. Exp. Physiol., 38:* 35 – 45.

Goslow, Jr. G.E., Reinking, R.M. and Stuart, D.G. (1973) The cat step cycle: Hindlimb joint angles and muscle lengths during unrestrained locomotion. *J. Morphol., 141:* 1 – 41.

Grillner, S. (1981) Control of locomotion in bipeds, tetrapods and fish. In J.M. Brookhart, V.B. Mountcastle and V.B. Brooks (Eds.), *Handbook of Physiology, Sect 1, The Nervous System, Vol II, Motor Control, Part 2,* American Physiological Society, Bethesda, pp. 1179 – 1236.

Halbertsma, J. (1983) The stride cycle of the cat: The modelling of locomotion by computerized analysis of automatic recordings. *Acta Physiol. Scand.,* suppl. 521: 1 – 75.

Henneman, E., Somjen, G. and Carpenter, D.O. (1965b) Functional significance of cell size in spinal motoneurones. *J. Neurophysiol., 28:* 560 – 580.

Henneman, E., Somjen, G. and Carpentier, D.O. (1965a) Excitability and inhibitability of motoneurones of different sizes. *J. Neurophysiol., 28:* 599 – 620.

Hoffer, J.A., Loeb, G.E., Sugano, N., Marks, W.B., O'Donovan, M.J. and Pratt, C.A. (1987) Cat hindlimb motoneurones during locomotion. III, Functional segregation in sartorius. *J. Neurophysiol., 57:* 554 – 562.

Houk, J. and Henneman, E. (1967) Responses of Golgi tendon organs to active contractions of the soleus muscle of the cat. *J. Neurophysiol., 30:* 466 – 481.

Hulliger, M. (1984) The mammalian muscle spindle and its central control. *Rev. Physiol. Biochem. Pharmacol., 101:* 1 – 110.

Hulliger, M. and Prochazka, A. (1983) A new simulation method to deduce fusimotor activity from afferent discharge recorded in freely moving cats. *J. Neurosci. Methods, 8:* 197 – 204.

Hulliger, M., Horber, F., Medved, A. and Prochazka, A. (1987) An experimental simulation method for iterative and interactive reconstruction of unknown (fusimotor) inputs contributing to known (spindle afferent) responses. *J. Neurosci. Methods, 21:* 225 – 238.

Hulliger, M., Dürmüller, N. Prochazka, A. and Trend, P. (1989) Flexible fusimotor control of muscle spindle feedback during a variety of natural movements. In J.H.J. Allum and M. Hulliger (Eds.), *Afferent Control of Posture and Locomotion, Prog. Brain Research Vol. 80,* Elsevier, Amsterdam, pp. 87 – 101.

Jami, L., Lan-Couton, D., Malmgren, K. and Petit, J. (1978) "Fast" and "Slow" skeleto-fusimotor innervation in cat tenuissimum spindles: a study with the glycogen-depletion method. *Acta Physiol. Scand., 103:* 284 – 298.

Jami, L., Lan-Couton, D., Malmgren, K. and Petit, J. (1979) Histophysiological observations on fast skeleto-fusimotor axons. *Brain Res.*, 164: 53 – 59.

Jami, L., Murphy, K.S.K. and Petit, J. (1982) A quantitative study of skeleto-fusimotor innervation in the cat peroneus tertius muscle. *J. Physiol. (London)*, 325: 125 – 144.

Joffroy, M. (1975) Méthode de discrimination des potentiels unitaires constituant l'activité complexe d'un filet nerveux non sectionné. *J. Physiol. (Paris)*, 70: 239 – 252.

Laporte, Y., Emonet-Dénand, F. and Jami, L. (1981) The skeleto-fusimotor or β-innervation of mammalian muscle spindles. *Trends Neurosci.*, 4: 97 – 99.

Lennerstrand, G. and Thoden, U. (1968) Position and velocity sensitivity of muscle spindles in the cat. II. Dynamic fusimotor single-fibre activation of primary endings. *Acta Physiol. Scand.*, 74: 16 – 29.

Loeb, G.E. and Duysens, J. (1979) Activity patterns in individual hindlimb primary and secondary muscle spindle afferents during normal movements in unrestrained cats. *J. Neurophysiol.*, 42: 420 – 440.

Loeb, G.E., Hoffer, J.A. and Pratt, C.A. (1985) Activity of spindle afferents from cat anterior thigh muscles. I. Identification and patterns during normal locomotion. *J. Neurophysiol.*, 54: 549 – 564.

Matthews, P.B.C. (1970) The origin and functional significance of the stretch reflex. In P. Andersen and J.K.S. Jansen (Eds.), *Excitatory Synaptic Mechanisms,* Universitets Forlaget, Oslo, pp. 301 – 315.

Matthews, P.B.C. (1972) *Mammalian Muscle Receptors and their Central Actions.* Arnold, London, 630 pp.

Murphy, P.R., Stein, R.B. and Taylor, J. (1984) Phasic and tonic modulation of impulse rate in gamma motoneurones during locomotion in premammillary cats. *J. Neurophysiol.*, 52: 228 – 243.

Orlovskii, G.N. (1969) Spontaneous and induced locomotion of the thalamic cat. *Biophysics,* 14: 1154 – 1162.

Perret, C. (1976) Neural control of locomotion in the decorticate cat. In R.M. Herman, S. Grillner, P. Stein and D.G. Stuart (Eds.), *Neural Control of Locomotion,* Plenum, New York, pp. 587 – 615.

Perret, C. (1983) Centrally generated pattern of motoneurone activity during locomotion in the cat. In A. Roberts and B. Roberts (Eds.), *Neural Origin of Rhythmic Movements,* Cambridge University Press, Cambridge, pp. 405 – 422.

Perret, C and Berthoz, A. (1973) Evidence of static and dynamic fusimotor actions on the spindle response to sinusoïdal stretch during locomotor activity in the cat. *Exp. Brain Res.*, 18: 178 – 188.

Perret, C. and Buser, P. (1972) Static and dynamic fusimotor activity during locomotor movements in the cat. *Brain Res.,* 40: 165 – 169.

Perret, C. and Cabelguen, J.M. (1980) Main characteristics of the hindlimb locomotor cycle in the decorticate cat with special reference to bifunctional muscles. *Brain Res.,* 187: 333 – 352.

Philippson, M. (1905) L'autonomie et la centralisation dans le système nerveux des animaux, *Trav. Lab. Physiol. Inst. Solvay Bruxelles,* 7: 1 – 208.

Prochazka, A., Westermann, R.A. and Ziccone, S.P. (1976) Discharges of single hindlimb afferents in the freely moving cat. *J. Neurophysiol.*, 39: 1090 – 1104.

Prochazka, A., Westermann, R.A. and Ziccone, S.P. (1977) Ia afferent activity during a variety of voluntary movements in the cat. *J. Physiol. (London),* 268: 423 – 448.

Prochazka, A., Hulliger, M., Zangger, P. and Appenteng, K. (1985) "Fusimotor set": new evidence of α-independent control of γ-motoneurones during movement in the awake cat. *Brain Res.,* 339: 136 – 140.

Prochazka, A., Trend, P., Hulliger, M. and Vincent, S. (1989) Ensemble proprioceptive activity in the cat step cycle: towards a representative look-up chart. In J.H.J. Allum and M. Hulliger (Eds.), *Afferent Control of Posture and Locomotion, Prog. Brain Research, Vol. 80,* Elsevier, Amsterdam, pp 61 – 74.

Rasmussen, S., Chan, A.K. and Goslow, Jr. G.E. (1978) The cat step cycle: electromyographic patterns for hindlimb muscles during posture and unrestrained locomotion. *J. Morphol,* 155: 253 – 270.

Rioult-Pedotti, M.S., Kohen, R. and Hulliger, M. (1988) On the ability of static and dynamic γ-motoneurones to maintain spindle Ia firing during muscle shortening. *Eur. J. Neurosci. Suppl.,* 1: 269.

Severin, F.V. (1970) The role of the gamma motor system in the activation of the extensor alpha motor neurones during controlled locomotion. *Biophysics,* 15: 1138 – 1145.

Severin, F.V., Orlovskii, G.N. and Shik, M.K. (1967) Work of the muscle receptors during controlled locomotion. *Biophysics,*12: 575 – 586.

Sjöström, A. and Zangger, P. (1976) Muscle spindle control during locomotor movements generated by the deafferented spinal cord. *Acta Physiol. Scand.*, 97: 281 – 291.

Taylor, J., Stein, R.B. and Murphy, P.R. (1985) Impulse rates and sensitivity to stretch of soleus muscle spindle afferent fibers during locomotion in premammillary cats. *J. Neurophysiol.*, 53: 341 – 360.

J.H.J. Allum and M. Hulliger (Eds.)
Progress in Brain Research, Vol. 80
© 1989 Elsevier Science Publishers B.V. (Biomedical Division)

CHAPTER 5

Physiological properties of tandem muscle spindles in neck and hind-limb muscles

R.F. Price and M.B. Dutia

Department of Physiology, University Medical School, Teviot Place, Edinburgh EH8 9AG, U.K.

Although tandem muscle spindle complexes are found in small but significant numbers in most muscles, experimental investigation of their properties has been problematic because of the difficulty of distinguishing their afferents from those of "normal" single spindles. Of particular interest are the afferents from b_2c capsules of tandem spindles, which unlike normal spindles contain only a static b_2 nuclear bag fibre and some nuclear chain fibres. The absence of a dynamic b_1 nuclear bag fibre from b_2c spindles has engendered much speculation as to their response properties and their possible role in motor control. We have recently developed a method for the identification of afferents from b_2c spindles in electrophysiological experiments, using infusion or topical application of succinylcholine (SCh). SCh causes the contraction of the dynamic b_1 and static b_2 nuclear bag intrafusal fibres, and paralyses the nuclear chain fibres. Afferents from b_2c spindles are characterized by a strong "biasing" of their discharge rate to about 100 impulses per second (i.p.s.) when activated by SCh (reflecting the contraction of the static b_2 fibre), while primary afferents from normal b_1b_2c spindles show a large increase in dynamic sensitivity as well as "biasing" (reflecting the contraction of both dynamic b_1 and static b_2 bag fibres). Histological examination of tenuissimus spindles activated by SCh has confirmed this relationship between the pattern of activation by SCh and the number of intrafusal nuclear bag fibres in the spindle. In this paper we review the value of SCh as a means of testing spindle afferents for functional inputs from sensory terminals on the nuclear bag fibres, and discuss the properties of b_2c afferents from tandem spindles in the context of their possible function.

Key words: Muscle spindle; Muscle spindle afferent; Succinylcholine; Tandem spindle; Muscle afferent

Introduction

The classic view of the mammalian muscle spindle is that of a single encapsulated sensory structure containing a bundle of specialized intrafusal muscle fibres, a central sensory zone and a characteristic pattern of motor and sensory innervation (Boyd, 1981a; Matthews, 1981a,b; Hulliger, 1984). However, it has long been appreciated that muscle spindles can occur in two main forms of complexes. The first, which was recognized by Sherrington and called the "compound muscle-spindle", occurs when several single spindles lie in close apposition in the muscle but still remain separate entities. The second occurs when two or more capsules are formed in series along an intrafusal fibre bundle, with some of the intrafusal fibres of one capsule extending into the others. This latter morphology was named the "tandem spindle" by Cooper and Daniel (1956) but had been seen before by others in mammals and amphibia (for a brief review of the early literature see Barker and Ip, 1961).

Tandem spindle complexes occur in relatively small but significant numbers in most muscles, and are found in particularly high density in the dorsal extensor muscles of the neck in the cat (Richmond et al., 1985). Most commonly, tandem spindles have two capsules linked in series ("double tandem", Barker and Ip, 1961), but chains of up to five have been described. In a double tandem spindle, one capsule is generally about twice as long as the other and contains several nuclear bag and nuclear chain intrafusal fibres, whereas the smaller capsule contains only a single nuclear bag fibre and a few chain fibres. The large capsule receives sensory innervation from both primary (group I) and secondary (group II) axons, whereas the smaller one generally only receives a primary axon, which may have an unusual terminal morphology (Barker and Ip, 1961; Richmond et al., 1986). Like single spindles, the large capsules of tandem spindles were shown by histochemistry to contain one bag_1 fibre, one bag_2 fibre and $3-10$ chain fibres (Bakker and Richmond 1981; Banks et al., 1982; Kucera, 1982; Walro and Kucera, 1985; Richmond et al., 1986), leading to the use of the term "b_1b_2c spindle" to describe this type of capsule. On the other hand, the smaller capsule consistently lacks the dynamic bag_1 fibre, and such capsules are therefore called "b_2c spindles". The capsules of a double tandem spindle are linked by the long bag_2 fibre which extends through both capsules.

Various possible roles have been proposed for spindle complexes, particularly tandem spindles. However investigation of the properties of tandem spindles has been difficult first because their incidence in hind-limb muscles is usually around 10% of the total (Richmond et al., 1985) and secondly because there has not been a means of differentiating between afferents from single and tandem spindles during electrophysiological experiments. In relation to the first of these problems, the detailed morphological examination of the muscles of the cat neck by Richmond, Abrahams and their co-workers has shown them to contain a high density of spindles and a relatively high proportion of tandem spindle units (e.g. up to 50% in the biventer and complexus muscles (Richmond and Abrahams, 1975b; Bakker and Richmond, 1981)). The neck muscles are therefore a useful preparation in which to examine the proper-

ties of tandem spindles (Richmond and Abrahams, 1979; see also Chan et al., 1987). We have recently developed a method for the identification of tandem spindle afferents in electrophysiological experiments, using infusion or topical application of succinylcholine (SCh) (Price and Dutia, 1987). In this paper we review the usefulness of SCh as a means of activating muscle spindles, and the recent data on the properties of identified tandem muscle spindle afferents in the context of their proposed functions.

Excitation of hind-limb muscle spindles by succinylcholine

Acetylcholine (ACh), and its analogue SCh, when applied to the isolated tenuissimus spindle cause the dynamic bag_1 and the static bag_2 nuclear bag fibres to go into contracture, while the nuclear chain fibres, like extrafusal muscle fibres, are paralysed (Gladden, 1976; Boyd, 1985). The dynamic bag_1 fibre appeared to have a lower threshold than the static bag_2 fibre. Subsequently SCh has been used in the isolated spindle preparation as an alternative to γ fusimotor stimulation for producing bag intrafusal fibre contraction selectively (e.g. Boyd, 1985; Dickson et al., 1988).

Primary and secondary endings

Dutia (1980) following upon the experiments of Rack and Westbury (1966), examined the response of soleus spindle afferents to ramp stretches during intra-arterial infusions of SCh. While Rack and Westbury had shown that intravenous administration of SCh increased the dynamic sensitivity of soleus primary endings very markedly (presumably because of the contracture of the dynamic bag_1 fibre), with intra-arterial SCh infusion this dynamic activation (Fig. 1A, middle panel) was followed by a further stage of excitation when an increase in position sensitivity was superimposed on the high dynamic response (Fig. 1A, bottom), presumably as a result of the subsequent additional contracture of the static bag_2 fibre. Thus when fully activated by SCh the response of the soleus primary spindle afferent was similar to that obtained with combined strong dynamic and static fusimotor stimulation (Emonet-Dénand et al., 1977). However it subsequently became apparent from Boyd's work on isolated tenuissimus spindles that γ efferents innervating the static bag$_2$ fibre cause a marked increase in the primary afferent discharge rate ("biasing"), rather than an increase in position sensitivity (Boyd, 1981b, 1986; see also below).

The afferent discharge of secondary afferents from soleus spindles was gradually facilitated during intra-arterial SCh infusion, without marked changes in the dynamic or position sensitivities (e.g. Fig. 1B, Dutia, 1980). This is consistent with the predominant termination of group II afferents

on the nuclear chain fibres. Golgi tendon organ afferents, and possibly joint afferents, are also facilitated by SCh infusion in a similar manner (Dutia and Ferrell, 1980). These non-specific effects are likely to be the consequence of the significant release of potassium ions from the depolarized extrafusal muscle fibres (Paintal, 1964; Kidd and Vaillant, 1974; but see Gregory and Proske, 1987). The different effects of SCh on the responsiveness to stretching of primary and secondary endings have been exploited in a number of studies in which other, classical, means of classifying spindle afferents could not be employed (e.g. Inoue et al., 1981).

"Intermediate" endings

In addition to the characteristic effects of SCh on primary and secondary afferents as illustrated in Fig. 1, Dutia (1980) found a significant number of soleus afferents which showed "intermediate" patterns of excitation in the presence of SCh. The discharge of intermediate endings was at first gradually facilitated as for secondary endings (Fig. 1B), but then showed a clear increase in dynamic or position sensitivity. The magnitude of this increase was always substantially less than that for typical primary endings. Such intermediate afferents had axonal conduction velocities in the 60 – 80 m/s range, intermediate between those of typical soleus primary and secondary afferents. Dutia (1980) suggested that the likely morphology underlying the behaviour of intermediate afferents was that of a juxtaequatorial secondary ending with significant collateral terminations on the dynamic (b$_1$) or static (b$_2$) nuclear bag fibres. Subsequently, however, it was proposed by Banks, Barker and Stacey (1982) that such intermediate behaviour might be shown by afferents from b$_2$c capsules of tandem muscle spindles. In the light of our recent experiments on the effects of SCh on spindle afferents from neck and hind-limb muscles (below), it is now clear that afferents from b$_2$c spindles have a different and very characteristic response to SCh that permits their identification and further study.

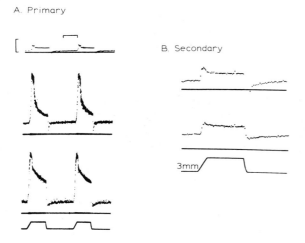

A. Primary

B. Secondary

3mm

Fig. 1. Examples of the effects of SCh on the responses to ramp stretches of a primary (Ia) afferent (A) and a secondary (group II) afferent (B) from soleus. In A the top panel shows the control responses of the Ia afferent to repeated ramp stretches (3 mm amplitude) before the start of intra-arterial SCh infusion (100 μg/kg/min). After the start of infusion the dynamic response increased very markedly (A, middle). With continued infusion the position response (the discharge rate at the extended muscle length, before the release of the ramp stretch) also increased, without change in the dynamic response (A, bottom). The secondary afferent (B) did not show similar changes in sensitivity, and its overall discharge rate gradually increased during SCh infusion (upper, control response; lower, maximally activated response). Calibration bars: A, 100 i.p.s., 1 s; B, 50 i.p.s., 0.5 s.

Excitation of neck muscle spindles by succinylcholine

Primary and secondary afferents

In experiments on the neck extensor muscle biventer cervicis, out of 72 muscle spindle afferents isolated in the muscle nerves about 1/3 were relatively weakly excited by SCh in the same way as typical hind-limb secondary (group II) afferents (Price and Dutia, 1987). A further 1/3 were activated by SCh as illustrated in Fig. 2A, developing an increased dynamic sensitivity (indicating an input from an contracted bag_1 fibre) and a marked biasing of·their discharge to 80 – 100 impulses per second (i.p.s.), similar to that produced by static γ axons innervating bag_2 fibres in tenuissimus spindles (Boyd, 1981b, 1986). These changes are interpreted as the consequence of the combined contracture of the bag_1 and bag_2 fibres on primary afferents from b_1b_2c spindle capsules in the neck muscle. Thus, in the neck spindles, contracture of the bag_2 fibre biased the primary afferent discharge instead of increasing the position sensitivity as in the soleus spindles. This difference may reflect variations in the nature of signals from the Ia sensory terminals on the two bag fibres or in their interaction in generating the Ia afferent discharge, and remains to be investigated. In later experiments on medial gastrocnemius and tenuissimus Ia afferents, we have observed both types of effects of b_2 fibre contraction, biasing being more common than an increase in position sensitivity.

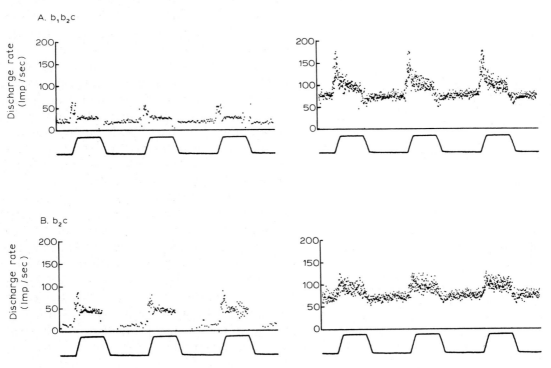

Fig. 2. A: activation of a neck primary (b_1b_2c) afferent by SCh. Left panel, control responses to 3 mm ramp stretches. Right panel, maximum activation. Note increase in dynamic response, superimposed on a strong "biasing" of the discharge rate to about 85 i.p.s. B: activation of a tandem b_2c afferent from tenuissimus. Left panel, control responses. Right, maximum activation. Note biasing, without an increased dynamic response. Histological examination confirmed that this afferent came from a single-bag spindle (see Fig. 3). In each section of the figure the stretch was held constant for 1 s before being released to the original muscle length for 1.5 s.

b₂c Primary afferents

The remaining 1/3 of neck muscle spindle afferents were strongly biased to around 100 i.p.s., but without an increase in dynamic sensitivity, as illustrated by the afferent in Fig. 2B. These spindle afferents therefore showed a different response to SCh from any seen in the soleus experiments, and revealed a strong input from an activated static bag₂ fibre (causing the biasing), without any input from an activated dynamic bag₁ fibre (absence of an increased dynamic response). This pattern of SCh activation corresponds exactly to the known morphology of the b₂c units of tandem spindles which lack a dynamic bag₁ fibre (Richmond and Abrahams, 1975b; Bakker and Richmond, 1981; Richmond et al., 1986), and was interpreted as

characteristic of primary afferents from b₂c spindle units (Price and Dutia, 1987). Our subsequent experiments, designed to correlate the pattern of SCh activation with the morphology of the activated spindle, have confirmed this interpretation.

Morphological confirmation of the identification of tandem spindles using succinylcholine

In recent experiments we have isolated afferents from muscle spindles in the tenuissimus muscle, which on average contains 15 muscle spindles (Boyd, 1956) of which 6% (i.e. 0 or 1 in any one muscle) are b₂c capsules of tandem spindles (Kucera, 1982). The spindle afferents were isolated in lumbosacral dorsal root filaments in the conven-

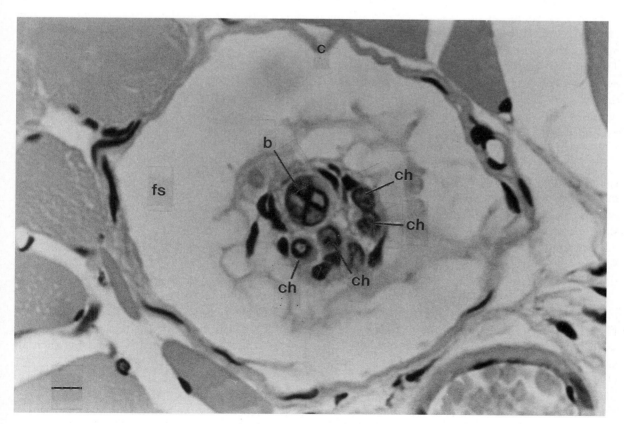

Fig. 3. Photomicrograph of a transverse section through the spindle of origin of the tenuissimus b₂c afferent whose response to SCh is shown in Fig. 2B. Note the single large-diameter intrafusal fibre containing four nuclear profiles in section (b), and the smaller nuclear chain fibres containing single nuclei in section (ch). fs, fluid space; c, capsule. Calibration bar, 10 μm.

tional manner. Units with relatively short conduction delays (< 2 ms) were sampled preferentially in order to exclude secondary (group II) afferents which were not of interest.

The intramuscular location of each of the spindles from which an afferent was available, was determined as accurately as possible by local probing and by stimulating the intramuscular nerve branches at various points along the muscle with a pair of surface electrodes (Bessou and Laporte, 1962). The spindle was then activated by topically applying SCh (100 μg/ml) from a syringe to the surface of the overlying muscle. In the fourth of seven experiments, one spindle afferent was found that was activated by SCh in the same way as the presumed b_2c afferents in the neck muscle, and is shown in Fig. 2B. The location of this spindle was marked with epimysial sutures. At the end of the experiment the block of tissue incorporating the markers was excised, fixed (buffered formal saline, 48 h) and processed for paraffin wax embedding. Serial 6 μm transverse sections were cut through the blocks and every twentieth section was mounted, stained (haematoxylin and eosin), and examined.

Fig. 3 shows a photomicrograph of a transverse section through the equatorial region of the only spindle which was found in the area of muscle marked during the experiment. The spindle capsule is seen to contain a large-diameter intrafusal fibre showing four nuclear profiles in section (a nuclear bag), accompanied by several smaller intrafusal fibres each containing only a single nuclear section. This spindle therefore contained only one nuclear bag fibre and four nuclear chain fibres; although we did not perform enzyme histochemistry to confirm that the bag fibre was a static bag_2 fibre, it is known that virtually all single-bag spindles are in fact b_2c units. (Kucera (1982) found a single b_1c spindle capsule in a sample of 341 tenuissimus spindle capsules; see also Banks et al., 1982; Richmond et al., 1986; Kucera and Walro, 1987). Thus, our "diagnosis" of this spindle as a b_2c capsule, based on the pattern of activation of its afferent by SCh, was confirmed

morphologically. Similarly, the "diagnosis" of seven further b_1b_2c afferents by means of their excitation by SCh, was also confirmed by histological demonstration of their origin in spindles containing a pair of bag fibres and a number of chain fibres.

Properties of identified b_2c spindle afferents

Passive properties

De-efferented b_2c afferents from the biventer muscle, identified by their pattern of SCh activation, had characteristics rather similar to those of b_1b_2c afferents from that muscle (Price and Dutia, 1987). Thus, their sensitivity to 1 Hz sinusoidal stretching ranged from about $5-75$ i.p.s./mm, higher than that of secondary endings but overlapping with that of the b_1b_2c afferents. Their discharge could be "driven" 1:1 by small-amplitude vibration at frequencies of $60-200$ Hz, a range similar to that of b_1b_2c afferents but significantly higher than that of secondary afferents. The coefficients of variation of their resting discharge rates ranged from 0.02 to 0.07, overlapping those of secondary and b_1b_2c afferents ($0.18-0.035$ and $0.025-0.105$ respectively). These measurements show that in the *passive* spindle (i.e. without γ fusimotor activity or SCh activation) b_1b_2c and b_2c afferents could not be distinguished on the basis of their response to muscle stretching, despite the lack of the b_1 fibre in the b_2c capsules (cf. Richmond and Abrahams, 1979). Banks, Ellaway and Scott (1980), in a survey of a large number of primary axons from peroneal spindles, also found no systematic differences in their responses to stretch that might have been attributed to b_2c afferents, although they did not have a means of identifying such afferents.

Conduction velocity

In further experiments on spindle afferents from the medial gastrocnemius muscle, in which some 24% of spindles may be of the tandem type (Swett and Eldred, 1960), we attempted to determine whether b_2c afferents could be distinguished from b_1b_2c and secondary afferents on the basis of their axonal conduction velocity. Fig. 4 shows the results from 82 medial gastrocnemius afferents tested with intra-arterial infusions of SCh, where each symbol indicates the "diagnosis" of the afferent on the basis of its excitation by SCh. The distribution of conduction velocities demonstrates clearly the recognized distinction between the vast majority of b_1b_2c ($\times$, $80-120$ m/s) and secondary ($\diamondsuit$, $30-60$ m/s) endings. However, the conduction velocities of b_2c afferents ($\blacktriangledown$) overlap with those of the slower b_1b_2c afferents ($70-95$ m/s), and could therefore not be separated from them on this basis. Fig. 4 also shows the range of conduction velocities of "intermediate" afferents ($\blacksquare$), whose pattern of excitation by SCh indicates their origin as secondary endings with collateral terminations on one or both nuclear bag fibres (Dutia, 1980). The results shown in Fig. 4 demonstrate the difficulty in using the classical test of afferent conduction velocity as a means of differentiating primary and secondary spindle af-

ferents (even in hind-limb muscles), and emphasize the value of SCh as a tool for revealing functional inputs from the b_1 and b_2 nuclear bag fibres in the discharge of spindle afferents. In particular, the pattern of activation by SCh appears to be a valuable test for identifying afferents from b_2c units of tandem spindles, for further study in electrophysiological experiments.

Discussion

The earliest suggestion as to the role of tandem spindles was that, because of their greater length, tandem spindles could provide a more generalized signal of extrafusal muscle status than that provided by single spindles (Swett and Eldred, 1960; Barker and Ip, 1961). It was not clear, however, what extra information might be provided by a tandem spindle in which some intrafusal fibres were shared over and above that provided by a compound muscle spindle with several spindles aligned in close proximity end-to-end, and this suggestion has not reappeared in recent literature.

The absence of a bag$_1$ fibre from the b_2c spindle units has been presumed to give the b_2c primary afferent a reduced dynamic sensitivity (e.g. Boyd and Gladden, 1985; Richmond et al., 1985). In line with this, it has been proposed that primary-like afferents from neck and masseter muscles with dynamic sensitivities intermediate between those of primary and secondary endings are b_2c afferents (Richmond and Abrahams, 1979; Inoue et al., 1981). However, the work summarized above, and that of Banks, Ellaway and Scott (1980) suggests that in the de-efferented, passive spindle, there is no clear borderline between the dynamic sensitivities on b_2c and b_1b_2c primary afferents (see Fig. 4 above; Price and Dutia, 1987). It is only in the activated spindle that a significant contribution from the dynamic b_1 fibre is revealed, which can then be used as the basis for differentiating between the two types of afferent.

The similarity in response characteristics of identified b_2c and b_1b_2c afferents, indicates that the b_1 fibre is not the major determinant of

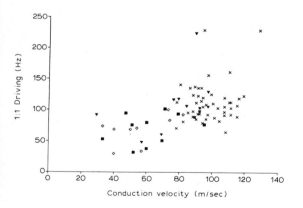

Fig. 4. Plot of the maximum frequency to which afferents from medial gastrocnemius could be "driven" 1:1 by small-amplitude vibration, against their axonal conduction velocity. Each afferent was categorized by means of its pattern of activation by SCh as either primary (b_1b_2c, $\times$), secondary ($\diamondsuit$), "intermediate" ($\blacksquare$), or tandem (b_2c, $\blacktriangledown$). Note the good correspondence between the characterization of primary and secondary afferents by SCh and their conduction velocities, and the overlap between the conduction velocities of b_2c afferents with the slower primary afferents.

dynamic responsiveness in the passive spindle. It would seem that the dynamic response of the Ia afferent in the passive spindle does not depend on a local stretch-induced contraction ("stretch-activation") of the b_1 fibre (Poppele and Quick, 1981).

Banks et al. (1982) suggested that b_2c primary afferents might provide a signal with enhanced static sensitivity, and that this might help in the control of tonically active anti-gravity muscles such as the neck extensors. An analogous suggestion has been made for other muscles whose spindles appear relatively rich in elements of the dynamic system as a specialization appropriate to fine control (e.g. lumbrical muscles, Walro and Kucera, 1985). However, as indicated by Richmond et al. (1986), the observed distribution of tandem spindles in different muscles does not fit well with this idea. Thus, in the cat neck, the biventer muscle has the major anti-gravity function, but splenius, which is a head rotator, is just as rich in tandem spindles (Richmond and Abrahams, 1975b). Similarly soleus, a major hindlimb anti-gravity muscle, is not particularly rich in tandem spindles. Within a muscle, tandem spindles tend to be more common near myotendinous junctions (Bakker and Richmond, 1981; Kucera and Walro, 1987), and it may be that their higher in-

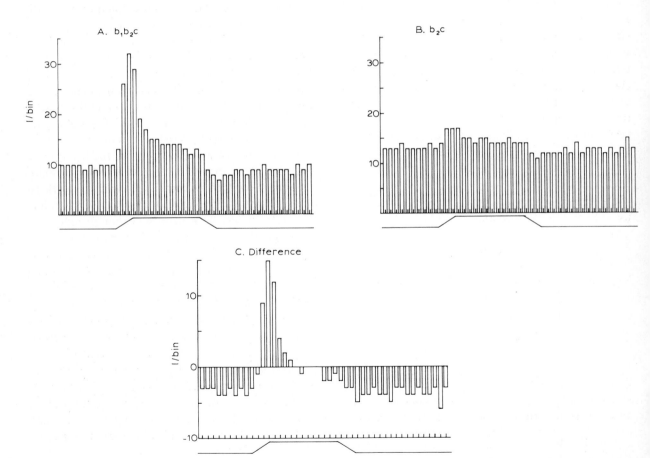

Fig. 5. Comparison of the response to stretching of a primary afferent from medial gastrocnemius (A), with that of a tandem b_2c afferent (B). The histograms show the number of spikes counted in 100 ms-wide bins, during one ramp stretch applied when the afferents were maximally activated by SCh. C shows the result of subtracting the b_2c response (B) from the b_1b_2c response (A).

cidence in certain muscles is related more to a greater area of myotendinous contact. The dorsal neck extensor muscles of the cat are divided into serial compartments by several transverse tendinous inscriptions (Richmond and Abrahams, 1975a) and so have a relatively large myotendinous contact area; analogous considerations may also apply to pennate muscles (e.g. medial gastrocnemius) with large aponeuroses of origin or insertion.

The major difference between the b_1b_2c and b_2c primary afferents would therefore appear to be in the nature of their fusimotor control, and their responsiveness to natural stimulation in the presence of fusimotor activity. b_1b_2c spindle units receive several static and dynamic, γ and β axons, whereas the b_2c spindle units receive only a few static fusimotor axons which innervate the bag$_2$ and chain fibres (Bakker and Richmond, 1981; Banks et al., 1982; Richmond et al., 1986; Kucera and Walro, 1987). As a consequence, the properties of b_1b_2c and b_2c primary afferents would be very differently affected by fusimotor and skeletofusimotor activity during movements. Dynamic fusimotor activity will not have any influence on the responsiveness of b_2c afferents, whose sensitivity would be exclusively controlled by the activity of static fusimotor neurones. By contrast, the responsiveness of primary afferents from b_1b_2c spindles will be determined by the activity of both dynamic and static fusimotor neurones, and by interactions between their effects at the level of the intrafusal fibres and the afferent nerve terminals. Richmond et al. (1986) have proposed that the CNS might employ the afferent signal from b_2c spindles as a "benchmark" against which the b_1b_2c afferent activity could be compared. As illustrated in Fig. 5 using data from medial gastrocnemius spindles maximally activated by SCh, subtraction of the b_2c afferent response to a ramp stretch (Fig. 5B) from the b_1b_2c response to the same stretch (Fig. 5A) could allow the nervous system to extract a signal with high dynamic sensitivity (Fig. 5C), even under conditions of strong static biasing due to the maximal contracture of the static b_2 nuclear bag fibre. Such a computation would be valuable in selectively maintaining dynamic sensitivity, controlled by the efferent activity in the dynamic fusimotor system, independently of variations in the level of co-activation of static fusimotor neurones controlling the same spindles. For such a subtraction to take place it would seem necessary to process the afferent signals from b_1b_2c and b_2c spindles differently, perhaps routing the b_2c signal through an inhibitory interneurone before it converges with the b_1b_2c signal onto higher-order cells in the spinal cord. Given the ability to test for, and identify, afferents from b_2c spindles by means of their response to SCh, further experimental investigation of such proposals can be envisaged.

Acknowledgements

This work was supported by a grant from the UK Medical Research Council. We thank Edinburgh University and Stonyhurst College for additional financial support.

References

Bakker, G.J. and Richmond, F.J.R. (1981) Two types of muscle spindles in cat neck muscles: A histochemical study of intrafusal fibre composition. *J. Neurophysiol.,* 45: 973–986.

Banks, R.W., Ellaway, P.H. and Scott, J.J. (1980) Responses of de-efferented muscle spindles of peroneus brevis and tertius muscles in the cat. *J. Physiol. (London),* 310: 53P.

Banks, R.W., Barker, D. and Stacey, M.J. (1982) Form and distribution of sensory terminals in cat hindlimb muscle spindles. *Phil. Trans. R. Soc. Lond. B,* 299: 329–364.

Barker, D. and Ip, M.C. (1961) A study of single and tandem types of muscle-spindle in the cat. *Proc. Roy. Soc. Lond. B,* 154: 377–397.

Bessou, P. and Laporte, Y. (1962) Responses from primary and secondary endings of the same neuromuscular spindle of the tenuissimus muscle of the cat. In D. Barker (Ed.), *Symposium on Muscle Receptors,* Hong Kong University Press, Hong Kong, pp. 105–119.

Boyd, I.A. (1956) The tenuissimus muscle of the cat. *J. Physiol. (London),* 133: 35–36P.

Boyd, I.A. (1981a) The isolated mammalian muscle spindle. *Trends Neurosci.,* 3(11): 258–265.

Boyd, I.A. (1981b) The action of the three types of intrafusal fibre in isolated cat muscle spindles on the dynamic and

56

length sensitivities of primary and secondary sensory endings. In A. Taylor and A. Prochazka (Eds.), *Muscle Receptors and Movement,* Macmillan, London, pp. 17–32.

Boyd, I.A. (1985) Intrafusal muscle fibres in the cat and their motor control. In W.J.P. Barnes and M.H. Gladden (Eds.), *Feedback and Motor Control in Invertebrates and Vertebrates,* Croom Helm, London, pp. 123–144.

Boyd, I.A. (1986) Two types of static gamma axon in cat muscle spindles. *Q. J. Exp. Physiol.,* 71 (2): 307–327.

Boyd, I.A. and Gladden, M.H. (1985) Morphology of mammalian muscle spindles. Review. In I.A. Boyd and M.H. Gladden (Eds.), *The Muscle Spindle,* Macmillan, London, pp. 3–22.

Chan, Y.S., Kasper, J. and Wilson, V.J. (1987) Dynamics and directional sensitivity of neck muscle spindle responses to head rotation. *J. Neurophysiol.,* 57: 1716–1729.

Cooper, S. and Daniel, P.M. (1956) Human muscle spindles. *J. Physiol., (London),* 265: 133–162.

Dickson, M., Gladden, M.H., Halliday, D.M. and Ward, J. (1988) Creep and reverse creep in the dynamic bag$_1$ fibre of muscle spindles isolated from the tenuissimus muscle of the cat. *J. Physiol. (London),* 406: 73P.

Dutia, M.B. (1980) Activation of cat muscle spindle primary, secondary and intermediate sensory endings by suxamethonium. *J. Physiol. (London),* 304: 315–330.

Dutia, M.B. and Ferrell, W.R. (1980) The effect of suxamethonium on the response to stretch of Golgi tendon organs in the cat. *J. Physiol. (London),* 306: 511–518.

Emonet-Dénand, F., Laporte, Y., Matthews, P.B.C. and Petit, J. (1977) On the subdivision of static and dynamic fusimotor actions on the primary ending of the cat muscle-spindle. *J. Physiol. (London),* 268: 827–861.

Gladden, M.H. (1976) Structural features relative to the function of intrafusal muscle fibres in the cat. In S. Homma (Ed.), *Understanding the Stretch Reflex, Prog. Brain Res., Vol. 44,* Elsevier, Amsterdam, pp. 51–59.

Gregory, J.E. and Proske, U. (1987) Responses of muscle receptors in the kitten to succinylcholine. *Exp. Brain Res.,* 66: 167–175.

Hulliger, M. (1984) The mammalian muscle spindle and its central control. *Rev. Physiol. Biochem. Pharmacol.,* 101: 1–110.

Inoue, H., Morimoto, T. and Kawamura, Y. (1981) Response characteristics and classification of muscle spindles of the masseter muscle in the cat. *Exp. Neurol.,* 74: 548–560.

Kidd, G.L. and Vaillant, C.H. (1974) The interaction of K$^+$ and stretching as stimuli for primary muscle spindle endings in the rat. *J. Anat.,* 119: 196.

Kucera, J. (1982) One-bag-fiber muscle spindles in tenuissimus muscles of the cat. *Histochemistry,* 76: 315–328.

Kucera, J. and Walro, J.M. (1987) Heterogeneity of spindle units in the cat tenuissimus muscle. *Am. J. Anat.,* 178: 269–278.

Matthews, P.B.C. (1981a) Evolving views on the internal operation and functional role of the muscle spindle. *J. Physiol. (London),* 320: 1–30.

Matthews, P.B.C. (1981b) Muscle spindles: Their messages and their fusimotor supply. In J.M. Brookhart, V.B. Mountcastle and V.B. Brooks (Eds.), *Handbook of Physiology – The Nervous System, Vol. II, Motor Control, Part 1,* American Physiological Society, Bethesda, pp. 189–228.

Paintal, A.S. (1964) Effects of drugs on vertebrate mechanoreceptors. *Pharm. Rev.,* 16(4): 341.

Poppele, R.E. and Quick, D.C. (1981) Stretch-induced contraction of intrafusal muscle in cat muscle spindle. *J. Neurosci.,* 1: 1069–1074.

Price, R.F. and Dutia, M.B. (1987) Properties of cat neck muscle spindles and their excitation by succinylcholine. *Exp. Brain Res.,* 68: 619–630.

Rack, P.M.H. and Westbury, D.R. (1966) The effects of suxamethonium and acetylcholine on the behaviour of cat muscle spindles during dynamic stretching, and during fusimotor stimulation. *J. Physiol. (London),* 186: 698–713.

Richmond, F.J.R. and Abrahams, V.C. (1975a) Morphology and enzyme histochemistry of dorsal muscles of cat neck. *J. Neurophysiol.,* 38: 1312–1321.

Richmond, F.J.R. and Abrahams, V.C. (1975b) Morphology and distribution of muscle spindles in dorsal muscles of the cat neck. *J. Neurophysiol.,* 38: 1322–1339.

Richmond, F.J.R. and Abrahams, V.C. (1979) Physiological properties of muscle spindles in dorsal neck muscles of the cat. *J. Neurophysiol.,* 42: 604–617.

Richmond, F.J.R., Stacey, M.J., Bakker, G.J. and Bakker, D.A. (1985) Gaps in spindle physiology: Why the tandem spindle? In I.A. Boyd and M.H. Gladden (Eds.), *The Muscle Spindle,* Macmillan, London, pp. 75–81.

Richmond, F.J.R., Bakker, G.J., Bakker, D.A. and Stacey, M.J. (1986) The innervation of tandem muscle spindles in the cat neck. *J. Comp. Neurol.,* 245: 483–497.

Swett, J.E. and Eldred, E. (1960) Comparisons in structure of stretch receptors in medial gastrocnemius and soleus muscles of the cat. *Anat. Rec.,* 137: 461–473.

Walro, J.M. and Kucera, J. (1985) Rat muscle spindles deficient in elements of the static system. *Neurosci. Lett.,* 59: 303–307.

J.H.J. Allum and M. Hulliger (Eds.)
Progress in Brain Research, Vol. 80
© 1989 Elsevier Science Publishers B.V. (Biomedical Division)

Overview and critique of Chapters 6 – 10

P.H. Ellaway

London, England

The five papers in this group set out to examine the nature of proprioceptive feedback and the role that it might play in the intact animal or human being. This critique will select specific parts of those papers for discussion and, in each case, pose certain questions that arise either from the techniques used or the results gained in the experiments described by the particular authors.

The last decade has seen a plethora of recordings made of the discharge of individual proprioceptors during natural movements, both in animals and man. Individual reports have presented intriguing glimpses of the patterns of afferent activity but the interpretation of what such input is signalling has suffered from the fragmentary nature of the data. The paper by *Prochazka and his colleagues* is their latest and laudable attempt to present an ensemble profile of muscle afferent discharge during a specific motor act — medium paced walking in the cat. In this task, they have tackled the considerable problem of non-uniformity in the step cycle duration of the cat by selecting a number of trigger points from which to average the afferent discharges of Ia, II and Ib afferents. They take the reasonable view that the turning points in the length changes of muscles provide trigger points that are least likely to obscure or "smear" the transient but consistent changes in afferent discharge that occur at these times. The authors acknowledge that the data presented is incomplete but will be updated by further work. In continuing with this task it is important that they do not become too dogmatic in their statements concerning the ensemble afferent profile during a motor

act. My concern is that, although other laboratories will be aware of the nature of the generalizations being made, those who review the field and write the textbooks will be tempted to lift statements without qualification. For example, the assertion in the summary that "Net ensemble Ia rates ... exceed 25 kilo-impulses/second..." is information that is likely to be misused unless due consideration is given to the time profile of the ensemble. One other criticism is that the authors state that a "fairly clear picture of ensemble motor output" of muscle is available in the EMG. This is not so. This generalization ignores the division of motor units into fast and slow types, and the fact that different muscles have different proportions of these motor unit types. Gross EMG recordings may give undue emphasis to large, fast motor units when recruited and the envelope of activity will not give a clear picture of the activity of either type. Even α motoneurones of the same modality do not fire identically, a situation that is acknowledged by the authors for afferent discharge. It may be that activity of both efferent and afferent neurones will depend on their location within a muscle, and that the relationship between individual afferents and motor units (Windhorst and Schwestka, 1982) is as important as the ensemble afferent input to the CNS.

The papers presented by *Hoffer et al.* and by *Hulliger et al.* will be discussed together since the main point raised by Hoffer's findings appears to cast doubt upon the viability of the methods used by Hulliger and his colleagues. The principal aims of both authors were to measure and interpret muscle spindle discharge during natural movement. Spindle discharge is determined partly by fusimotor drive and partly by length changes resulting from active and passive movements of the parent muscle. Recordings of the discharge of fusimotor neurones in intact animals (and man) have not been achieved to date despite the experience and success that both laboratories have had with recording discharges from larger myelinated fibres. The lack of success with fusimotor neurones appears to be related directly to the small size of γ motoneurone axons. An alternative approach to assessing fusimotor activity by direct recording is the simulation used by Hulliger, Prochazka and their colleagues. The essence of their technique is to correct any mismatch between the spindle discharge seen in acute and chronic recordings. In the acute experiment recordings are made from an anaesthetized cat. The length of the spindle bearing muscle is constrained to follow that previously seen in a chronic recording from an intact cat. The difference in spindle discharge is attributed to absence of fusimotor drive in the acute preparation. Fusimotor neurone axons are then stimulated according to a pattern which is altered during an iterative procedure until the match is optimal. The final pattern is assumed to be the best approximation to the actual discharge that occurred during the original chronic recording.

Hoffer set out to ascertain whether the length changes imposed upon a skeletal muscle in the cat during lengthening and shortening are, in reality, communicated to the muscle spindle end organs in that muscle. He raises the doubt that length changes of the whole muscle, as measured from tendinous origin to insertion, will result in comparable spindle length changes during both passive movements and active contraction of the parent muscle. If his doubts are founded, then the simulation studies of Hulliger and Prochazka, where passive movements in their acute preparation are compared with active movements in chronic cats, may be invalid. Hoffer uses an invasive technique to position a pair of piezoelectric crystals near the origin and insertion of muscle fibres within a cat

skeletal muscle. He explains in his article how these crystals may be used to measure the length of a bundle of fibres at one particular location. His results reveal an intriguing situation (see his Fig. 2) that a restricted bundle of fibres may not follow the length changes experienced by the muscle as a whole, particularly during active lengthening and passive shortening. The reasons proposed for this discrepancy are that muscle becomes stiffer than tendon during active contraction resulting in the tendon being stretched disproportionally more than the active muscle fibres or that alterations in muscle fibre pinnation angle lead to discrepancies between whole muscle and muscle fibre length. The claim is made that muscle spindles lying in parallel with such a restricted bundle of extrafusal muscle fibres will similarly not follow the length change of the whole muscle.

These studies therefore raise certain questions. Are the simulation experiments of Hulliger et al. inventing fusimotor drive that does not exist? This might be the case during passive shortening if the spindles are not, in fact, shortening. Alternatively, is fusimotor drive being underestimated during yield of the active muscle if the spindles are not lengthening? These questions are asked on the assumption that Hoffer's results do indeed show that spindles regularly experience less mechanical displacement than the whole muscle. Before this generalization can be accepted we should wait for confirmation of the findings. The results presented in Hoffer's contribution to this meeting appear to come largely from one cat and one pair of implanted transducers. It would also be important to know whether other bundles of muscle fibres in a skeletal muscle show the same restricted length changes. Indeed, it is possible that some extrafusal fibres may be stretched disproportionally more than would be expected from the length changes of the whole muscle. If the actions of the gastrocnemius muscle are based upon compartmentalization of the muscle then such differences in the amount of internal stretch will be relevant to control of the individual compartments. Alternatively, the aggregate input from muscle spindles will be important in the reflex control of motoneurone discharge. In either case it is necessary to know how the internal length changes are distributed. If it is possible to implant more than one pair of crystals in a muscle without causing damage, do the different regions behave similarly? It should also be asked whether the assumption made by Hoffer, that measurement of the distance between the implanted crystals represents spindle length, is correct. The method provides an indirect measure of distance between two points that approximate to the origin and insertion of extrafusal muscle fibres. This appears to have an average value of about 20 mm. However, direct measurements of spindles in gastrocnemius medialis give lengths ranging from 4 to 6 mm (Swett and Eldred, 1960a,b).

In conclusion, it is of considerable interest that localized regions of skeletal muscle do not follow the overall length changes. However, corroborative evidence and a more direct measure of spindle length are now needed before these results can be regarded as invalidating the simulations created by Hulliger and his colleagues.

The contribution to this section by *Matthews* concerned the debate as to the origin and central mechanisms of the human "long latency stretch reflexes". He presents evidence that implicates a long loop pathway for some components of the long latency responses in some muscles. The difficulty with assessing work in this field is that the arguments for and against different mechanisms are based on so many different systems. Some muscles appear to lack the shortest-latency, stretch reflex response expected from the monosynaptic connection of primary spindle afferents with motoneurones. Other muscles do not have clearly defined M2 and M3 responses. Nevertheless, by judicious choice of muscle and stimulation parameters Matthews has presented convincing arguments for the participation of several mechanisms. But does the emphasis lie in a particular one? Matthews himself is now changing the emphasis on the plausible mechanisms in the light of his new results. His conclusions stress the point

that slowly conducting group II axons from secondary endings cannot be the sole mechanism responsible for the long latency responses. Even that statement may need further dissection as we heard at this same meeting that secondary endings from muscle spindles do not all behave in the same way. In the cat, at least, there exist intermediate secondary endings (Price and Dutia, 1989, Chapter 5, this volume). The afferent axon conduction velocities span the upper group II and lower group I range which, if they exist in man, would confound the cooling experiments reported by Matthews. In man the afferent innervation of spindles is poorly understood but is likely to be very different from the cat. It does not, therefore, come as any surprise that human long latency stretch responses continue to be difficult to interpret.

The work presented by *Roll, Roll and Vedel* is in support of the argument that vibration of skeletal muscle in man induces kinaesthetic illusions and that the body attempts to correct for these illusions by producing associated motor responses. There is no doubting the claims made in their work and, indeed, the author of this critique has experienced some of the "illusions" himself. The difficulty that I have with the work is in accepting that the illusions and motor responses are due to altered kinaesthetic appreciation of the muscle stimulated by vibration. Before coming to this conclusion the authors have to convince us that the "illusions" are not, in fact, real movements of the image on the retina.

The following example will illustrate the problem. The authors maintain that vibration of the superior rectus muscles of the eyes results in postural sway forward. In fact, what they measure is force in a number of strain gauges under the feet. That certainly does occur in a direction which would result in sway forward if the body moved. However, they state that body movements were prevented by a mechanical device fixed at the neck so it is unclear whether movement did occur at joints such as the hip, knee and ankle, which presumably were free to move. However, that is not the main issue. The brain would have received increased proprioceptive input from muscle spindles during vibration of the superior rectus muscles. Such an input would normally be received if the muscles had been stretched, i.e. if the eyeball had been rotated downwards. In order to retain a fixed image on the retina one would expect the body to sway backwards. In fact, it sways forward. Alternatively, if vibration of the muscle had resulted in contraction and the eyeball was rotated upwards one would indeed expect the body to attempt to sway forward in order to preserve the image in the same place on the retina. Of course, with many degrees of freedom for movement in the body there may be other plausible responses to vibration and other expectations. Consideration of just the two described above suggests that the response (sway forward) may be a reaction to a real alteration of position of images on the retina rather than the illusion of eye movement. In order to strengthen the claim that vibration induces altered kinaesthetic appreciation of position of the eye rather than real movement, it would be useful to monitor eye movement, perhaps by recording the electro-oculogram. It would also be helpful to know exactly what movement could occur at various positions and joints in the body.

A second example of their work where real displacements of an image on the retina may have accounted for the "illusion" of movement was the experiment involving vibration of the soleus tendon. The subject stood in the dark with body movement restricted at the shoulders. Vibration of the soleus muscle produced an apparent downward movement of a visual target. There are several reasons why this should have occurred. (1) The author's interpretation is that an illusion of movement occurs due to a vibration-induced proprioceptive pattern that is interpreted as forward whole body movement. This is a perfectly reasonable explanation. If the subject has the impression that he has leant forward his expectation is that the light target would now appear higher in his visual field. Since it does not, and if the body has not moved, then the subject would experience the sensation that the target has moved

downwards. However, consider now what might happen if some movement of the eyes occurs. (2) If the eye rotates upward to compensate for the illusion of forward tilt of the body then a real shift of the image of the target on the retina occurs and the target will appear to move downwards. But this is not an illusion. The position of the image on the retina has altered. Finally, since movement of the body is restrained only at the shoulders contraction of soleus may have produced displacement at certain joints. (3) It is quite possible that vibration will have induced a vibration reflex in soleus causing backward tilt of the body. The gaze of the eyes would therefore be shifted upwards and the position of the image of the target on the retina would change. The target would appear to move downwards, as experienced by the subject, but this would again be due to a real shift in position of the image of the retina.

In conclusion, the authors are asked whether the reactions of the subjects are due to illusions of movement that result from the altered proprioceptive input or whether they could be a result of actual movements of part of the body or the eyes. Whatever the answer their experiments have revealed that the proprioceptive input important for orientating the body with respect to the visually perceived world does not come solely from muscles acting at skeletal joints but also from the extraocular muscles themselves.

References

Price, R.F. and Dutia, M.B. (1989) Physiological properties of tandem muscle spindles in neck and hind-limb muscles. In J.H.J. Allum and M. Hullinger (Eds.), *Afferent Control of Posture and Locomotion, Prog. Brain Res., Vol. 80,* Elsevier, Amsterdam, pp. 47–56.

Swett, J.E. and Eldred, E. (1960a) Distribution and numbers of stretch receptors in medial gastrocnemius and soleus muscles of the cat. *Anat. Rec.,* 137: 453–460.

Swett, J.E. and Eldred, E. (1960b) Comparisons in structure of stretch receptors in medial gastrocnemius and soleus muscles of the cat. *Anat. Rec.,* 137: 461–473.

Windhorst, U. and Schwestka, R. (1982) Interactions between motor units in modulating discharge patterns of primary muscle spindle endings. *Exp. Brain Res.,* 45: 417–427.

J.H.J. Allum and M. Hulliger (Eds.)
Progress in Brain Research, Vol. 80
© 1989 Elsevier Science Publishers B.V. (Biomedical Division)

CHAPTER 6

Ensemble proprioceptive activity in the cat step cycle: towards a representative look-up chart

A. Prochazka[1], P. Trend[2], M. Hulliger[3] and S. Vincent[1]

[1]Department of Physiology, University of Alberta, Edmonton, Canada; [2]Department of Physiology, St. Thomas's Hospital, London, U.K.; and [3]Brain Research Institute, University of Zürich, Switzerland

Analysis of the control of movement in tasks such as stepping is severely restricted by the lack of quantitative data on the ensemble activity of afferents in the numerous muscles involved. We have started to build up a quantitative "look-up-chart" of the ensemble afferent and efferent profiles in the cat step cycle. To this end, we have developed software which allows us to digitize afferent firing, muscle length and electromyogram (EMG) activity, and to align segments for averaging by choosing one or more reference points in the step cycle. The ensemble firing of triceps surae Ia afferents showed lower than expected mean and peak rates, whereas triceps group II and Ib afferents were more active than predicted. There were small but significant transients in Ia firing at foot-off and touch-down which could not be explained in terms of origin-to-insertion length alone. They were most likely caused by propagated mechanical transients or tendon compliance effects giving rise to small differences between the origin-to-insertion length and the intramuscular length "seen" by spindles. Net ensemble Ia rates, based on previous estimates of spindle populations, probably exceed 25 kilo-impulses/second (ki.p.s.) in some muscles. Inputs as large as this are likely to contribute significantly to reflex control.

Key words: Proprioception; Reflex; Motor Control; Muscle afferent

Introduction

During voluntary movement, the central nervous system receives simultaneous input from tens of thousands of proprioceptors in each limb (Chin et al., 1962; Boyd and Smith, 1984). Single α motoneurones receive monosynaptic input typically from $60 - 100$ synergistic Ia afferents (Eccles et al., 1957; Mendell and Henneman, 1971; Nelson and Mendell, 1978; Fleshman et al., 1981) and polysynaptic input from many other receptors (Matthews, 1972).

Before any reliable systems analysis of specific motor tasks is possible, it is important to have quantitative information on ensemble inputs and outputs rather than on the activity of individual afferents or motor units. Technically, it is reasonably straightforward to record ensemble motor output, either as EMG activity, or as limb force or movement. Over the years comprehensive information on the EMG profiles of the main leg muscles during locomotion has been collected in humans, and more recently in cats, dogs and other species. Fig. 1 brings the cat and human data together in the form of look-up charts. The human chart is reproduced from Carlsöö (1972) and we constructed the cat chart to the same format using data from the publications listed in the figure legend.

Some interesting points emerge from Fig. 1. Despite the fact that human gait is bipedal and plantigrade, whereas feline gait is quadrupedal and digitigrade, there are striking similarities in both the joint angle profiles and the temporal relation-

62

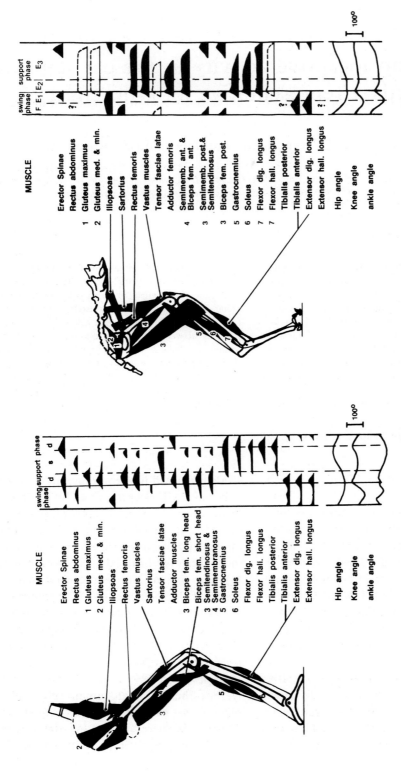

Fig. 1. Electromyographic (EMG) activity profiles of muscles in human leg (left) and cat hindlimb (right) in the step cycle. Support phase in humans divided into double support (d: both feet on ground) and single ipsilateral support (s). Cat step cycle according to Philippson (1905), swing phase: flexion(F), first extension (E₁); support phase: yield (E₂), final extension (E₃). The human EMG profiles are after Carlsöö (1973) and Winter (1987); length profiles are schematics based on our own goniometric recordings. The cat EMG data were drawn from: Engberg (1964), Engberg and Lundberg (1969), Prochazka et al. (1976), Rasmussen et al. (1978), Carlson et al. (1979), Forssberg (1979), Halbertsma (1983) and Abraham et al. (1985). Dashed lines indicate incomplete or conflicting data. Muscle length profiles are schematics based on our own recordings.

ships between muscle activities. The main disparity is in the calf muscles, which in humans provide forward propulsion and passive knee flexion at the end of the stance phase of the step cycle, whereas in cats they counteract the ankle dorsiflexion which would occur as a result of weight-bearing at the onset of stance. It is evident that foot-off and foot-contact are associated with major transitions in EMG and joint angle profiles, these being particularly abrupt in the cat. The control of these transitions is likely to depend upon afferent feedback, a point which will be taken up again later.

In contrast to the fairly complete picture of ensemble motor output, the data on ensemble afferent input is very scanty. There is no afferent equivalent to the EMG. The nearest thing, the multi-unit neurogram recorded from peripheral nerve, is made up of discharges of α and γ motoneurones as well as spindle, tendon organ and other afferents in varying and unknown proportions.

Recordings from single muscle afferents during voluntary movement should in principle provide scaled down versions of the ensemble firing. But afferents of the same modality and in the same muscle do not fire identically even during stereotyped tasks such as locomotion (e.g. Loeb et al., 1985a). This is partly because the stretch sensitivity of afferents is dependent on their location within a muscle (Stuart et al., 1972; Meyer-Lohmann et al., 1974), and also because different muscle spindles receive different strengths of fusimotor action. The technical difficulties of obtaining afferent recordings during voluntary movement and the lack of analytical tools to deal with the variability in such data have so far hindered the collation of quantitative ensemble firing profiles.

We recently began assembling a quantitative "look-up-chart" of Ia, II and Ib firing during the step cycle in various key hindlimb muscles in the conscious cat (Dürmüller et al., 1987), and in this paper we will present the material as it currently stands. As will be seen our most complete data are for triceps surae and hamstring afferents. Initial entries have also been made for plantaris, peroneus

longus, extensor digitorum longus, gluteus medius and semimembranosus anterior afferents. In general, the ensemble Ia profiles are closely related to, and phase-advanced on origin-to-insertion muscle length. Most muscle afferents, irrespective of location, showed abrupt firing transitions at foot touch-down, and to a lesser extent at lift-off. The ensemble triceps Ia profile showed a slightly augmented response to E_2 stretch, suggesting some phasic fusimotion. Group II profiles followed muscle length very closely, with mean firing rates and modulation depths comparable to those of Ia afferents.

Methods

The afferent recording techniques have been described in detail elsewhere (Prochazka and Hulliger, 1983), and are only summarized here.

Implantation

In one surgical procedure, performed with pentobarbital anaesthesia (40 mg/kg i.p., then i.v. maintenance doses), and with antiseptic precautions, a prefabricated loom of four 17 μm diameter enamelled Nickel-chrome micro-wires was implanted so that the de-insulated, bevelled tips of the wires were positioned in the L7 dorsal root ganglion, the connecting cable leading subcutaneously to an acrylic headpiece. Pairs of EMG wires were tied into the lateral gastrocnemius and posterior biceps femoris muscles and also led subcutaneously to the headpiece. Nylon monofilaments were embedded into the bony points of origin and insertion of these muscles, emerging percutaneously along the line of the muscle, to provide attachments for external saline-in-rubber length gauges. A silicone rubber cannula was inserted into the right external jugular vein and led to a port embedded in the headpiece, allowing antibiotics or short-acting anaesthetic to be administered in the days following recovery. Cats recovered from the procedures over a 12 to 24 h period. After 1 – 3 days, when the effects of the anaesthetic had fully worn off, they bore the small implants with no sign of discomfort or motor deficit.

Chronic recordings

Single-fibre neuronal recordings depended upon the electrode tips slowly migrating into favourable positions near cell bodies or axons in the dorsal root ganglion. Following recovery the electrodes were checked daily by attaching a small 3-channel telemeter to the headpiece and monitoring activity with a nearby FM receiver. When a single unit was present, a saline length gauge was attached to the appropriate monofilaments, the fine connecting wires (Cooner AS632) were led to the telemeter, and taped to the skin of the leg and back. The telemeter's EMG input was mated up with the appropriate socket in the headpiece. The cat was then allowed to move freely about the floor of a room ca. 4 m × 3 m.

Identification

Much importance was attached to accurate localization and identification of the afferent ending. When enough voluntary movement data had been obtained from a given afferent, the cat was anaesthetized (i.v. thiopental until muscle tone was abolished). The receptor was located by palpation and joint manipulation. Afferent responses to length changes of various waveforms applied manually were then recorded. When enough such data had been collected, suxamethonium (200 μg/kg) was administered i.v., and in the subsequent 3 – 4 min, the muscle stretching was repeated. Spindle primary and secondary afferents and tendon organ afferents are differently affected by suxamethonium, so this procedure is useful in differentiating between them (Prochazka and Hulliger, 1983). Typically these tests took 15 – 45 min.

Analysis

Telemetered data were de-coded and recorded onto cassette tapes with a TEAC R61 instrumentation recorder. All trials were video-taped (Sony C7 Video-recorder). Subsequent analysis consisted of initial viewing on a storage oscilloscope (Tektronix 5111). Selected segments including 10 – 50 step cycles per afferent were then stored digitally with a Cambridge Electronic Design 1401 interface operating via BBC, IMB PC or Olivetti M28 host micro-computers. Software was developed which allowed us to scroll through these data and select desired reference points in each cycle (usually maxima or minima in the length trace) for subsequent averaging. Averages were of muscle length, EMG and accumulated instantaneous frequency (frequencygram) with the event occurrence histogram superimposed. Each afferent contributed equal numbers of cycles to a given average.

Results

The quantitative data in this paper were obtained in 17 chronically implanted cats (T series: 6, 16, 23, 29 and HPT series: 5 – 11, 13, 14, 17, 19, 20, 21). Afferents were: triceps surae (9 Ia, 2 II, 4 Ib), plantaris (2 Ia, 2 II, 1 Ib), hamstrings (6 Ia, 2 Ib), and single Ia and Ib afferents from flexor and extensor digitorum longus and gluteus medius.

Alignment of averages

In freely walking cats, step cycle durations varied considerably. Furthermore, in combining data from different cats, we were faced with systematic differences in walking speed and muscle length profiles. Even when we restricted the choice of cycles to those with periods between 650 and 750 ms (corresponding to walking speeds of 0.5 to 0.65 m/s) and swing durations within the range 250 – 300 ms, alignment of averages at a single reference point inevitably resulted in "smear" at other points in the cycle, this effect increasing with increasing pre- or post-reference interval. Fig. 2 shows four averages of gastrocnemius EMG, length and the firing of a single gastrocnemius Ia ending. Each average comprises the same four step cycles, but with different reference points. There are subtle, but potentially important differences between the averages. For example, the increase in Ia firing just after swing onset is more abrupt in

Fig. 2C than in Fig. 2A, and whereas in Fig. 2B, C and D the Ia rate declines to zero just before foot contact, in Fig. 2A this minimum is smeared out.

We rejected normalization of cycle duration as a solution to the problem, as this would result in a loss of temporal information, and yet "smear" would still occur because of the inconstancy of the ratio of swing to stance durations. As a compromise, we decided to choose two or three reference points in the step cycle which were likely to be important from a reflex or control point of view, and we constructed composite averages

about these points (see below and Fig. 4). Firing transients associated with these key points were thereby represented with minimal distortion in the histograms even though they occurred at widely separated parts of the cycle.

Triceps surae afferents

There were considerable differences in the firing profiles of different Ia afferents in the same muscle or group of muscles. This has been noted before (Prochazka et al., 1976; Loeb et al., 1985a) and is presumably due to differences in fusimotor action,

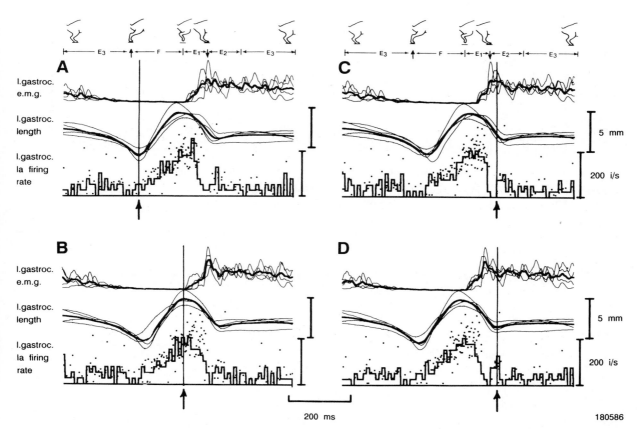

Fig. 2. Influence on step cycle averages of reference points of alignment. Four averages, each of the same four step cycles. In each case, top trace: rectified filtered gastrocnemius EMG (single sweeps thin lines, average profiles thick lines); middle trace: gastrocnemius origin-to-insertion length; bottom trace: superimposed instantaneous frequency (frequencygram) of single gastrocnemius Ia afferent, and the associated event histogram, bin width 10 ms. The calibration of the event histograms in terms of mean rates was checked with averages of known time courses of instantaneous rate. Alignment to length minimum in swing phase (A); length maximum in swing phase (B); first action potential in Ia burst signalling foot touch-down (C); length minimum in stance phase (D).

66

and to a lesser extent to individual receptor sensitivity and location within the muscle. In Fig. 3 we have arranged averages from nine triceps surae Ia afferents (Fig. 3A – I) in order of modulation depth. Fig. 3D and F were probably soleus endings as they were unresponsive to knee rotation. The remainder were identified as gastrocnemius endings. For clarity, the contributing individual traces (as shown in Fig. 2) were omitted. However, a given afferent tended to fire very similarly in step cycles of similar duration. The averages show that individual triceps Ia afferents were modulated through 100 to 200 impulses per second (i.p.s.),

with firing generally peaking at maximally 250 i.p.s. in the swing phase of the step cycle.

Within the swing phase, peaks occurred at substantially different times in different endings. This has an important bearing on the location and magnitude of the peak in the ensemble triceps Ia firing rate histogram, shown in Fig. 4. Here we decided upon three reference points for alignment, indicated by the small vertical arrows in Fig. 4B, C and D. The points were at the minimum of gastrocnemius length in early swing (E_3/F: Fig. 4B), the length maximum at the F/E_1 transition (Fig. 4C), and the length minimum in early stance

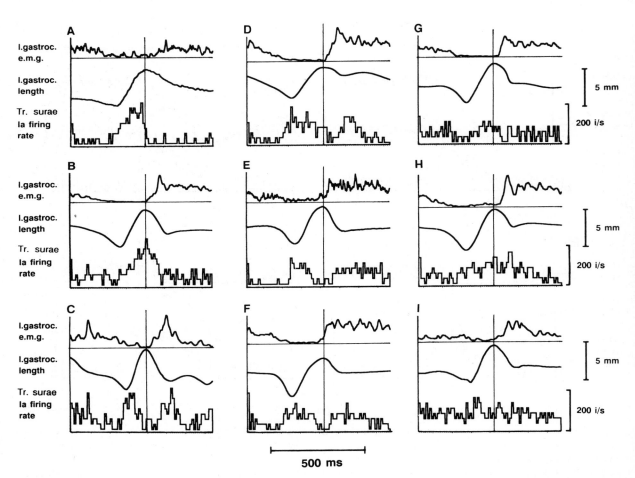

Fig. 3. Nine triceps surae Ia endings, each averaged over four step cycles. Traces as in Fig. 2, except that single sweeps were omitted for clarity. Averages A – I displayed in order of Ia modulation depth over the step cycle. Note the range of responses, and the variation in the position of peak firing during the swing phase. Event histograms: 8 ms bin widths.

(E₁/E₂: Fig. 4D). Our aim was to optimize the resolution of the composite averages and impulse histogram at foot-off, mid-swing and touchdown, on the assumption that afferent input at these moments in the step cycle is likely to be especially important for movement control. We also tried using the EMG peak in early E_2 and the first Ia action potential in the burst at foot touchdown in E_1 as references (not illustrated), but abandoned this when we found that these features were indistinct or absent in some step cycles.

Some interesting and rather unexpected results emerge from Fig. 4. First, the Ia firing transitions at foot-off and touchdown are 30–40 ms advanced upon the length minima which we and others had taken to be coincident with these events. These advances had puzzled us for some time, as they were not reproduced by Ia afferents subjected to identical length variations in acute simulation experiments (e.g. Prochazka and Hulliger, 1983). We then observed similar advances in the responses of cutaneous afferents of the paw, and so in separate experiments we recorded the moments of touchdown and foot-off with the use of aluminium foil taped to the footpad and signalling contact as the cat walked on metal

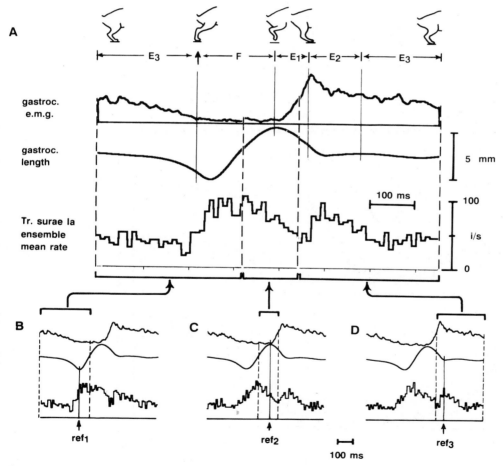

Fig. 4. Grand average of 9 triceps surae Ia afferents each contributing 4 step cycles. Same source data as in Fig. 3, but the grand average (A) is constructed from 3 segments of separate averages B, C and D of the same 36 single cycles, aligned at the vertical arrows, the relevant segments being demarcated by vertical dashed lines. Note the low modulation depth, and the phase advance of Ia firing on muscle length.

sheeting. We found that the gastrocnemius length minima were indeed always delayed by 30 – 40 ms with respect to touchdown and foot-off (Dür-müller et al., 1987; Elek, Llewellyn, Prochazka and Trend, in preparation).

The mean firing per triceps Ia afferent was 54 i.p.s. over the full step cycle, and the depth of modulation was between 90 and 100 i.p.s., depending upon how the reference points were chosen (90 i.p.s. in Fig. 4). Peak rates (ca. 100 i.p.s.) occurred halfway through F and at foot contact. Assuming a total population of 150 triceps Ia af-

ferents, net triceps Ia modulation depth was 100 × 150 = 15 kilo-impulses per second (ki.p.s.), step cycle mean was 8.1 ki.p.s. and peak was 15 ki.p.s.

We have only rarely recorded from triceps surae group II spindle afferents. Fig. 5 shows data from two such afferents, each contributing ten step cycles. The time course of mean firing rate followed origin-to-insertion length closely. We were surprised that the modulation depth and peak rate (both 135 i.p.s.) exceeded those of the Ia afferent profile, though admittedly more group II data are needed before this comparison can be considered

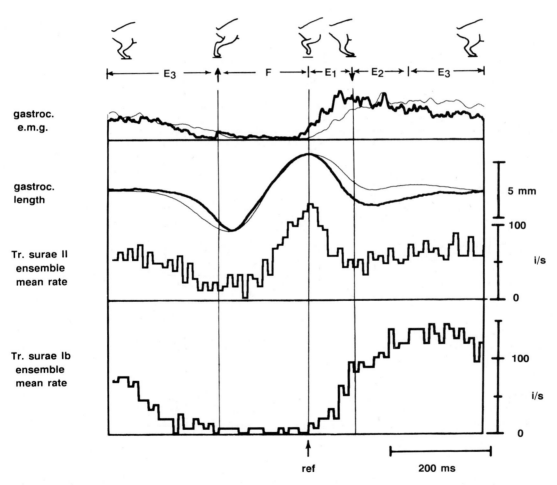

Fig. 5. Triceps surae, averages of 2 group II endings (10 cycles each) and 4 group Ib endings (4 cycles each). EMG and length: thick traces from group II data, thin traces from Ib data. Note close correspondence between group II profile and origin-to-insertion muscle length. Also note higher than expected mean Ib rate during stance.

reliable. The tendon organ profile in the bottom panel, based upon four afferents, also showed an unexpectedly high peak rate and modulation depth (both 145 i.p.s.). Each contributing Ib afferent fired with a characteristic time course over the step cycle, but there were significant differences between afferents. Furthermore, our sample may

have favoured lower-threshold tendon organs and so again more units must be included before values such as those given above can be considered representative. Data from several further triceps Ib afferents are available from previous tapes, and will be added to the histograms in the near future.

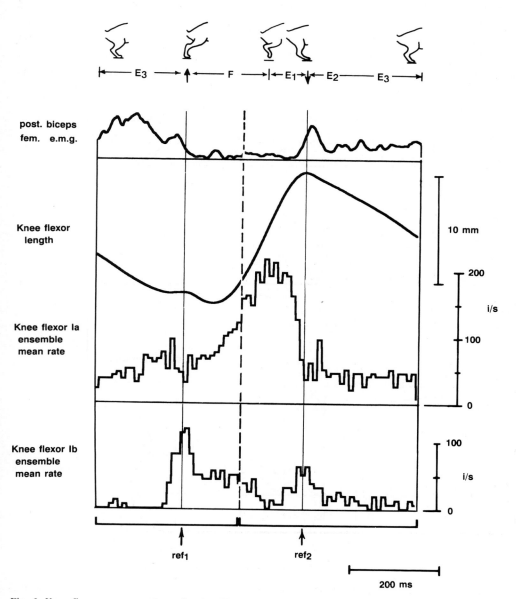

Fig. 6. Knee flexors: averages from five Ia afferents (4 cycles each) and 2 Ib afferents (8 cycles each). Note high peak rate of Ia profile during swing. Biceps femoris EMG was averaged from records corresponding to 3 of the afferent units only.

Hamstring afferents

The knee flexor components of the hamstring muscles (posterior biceps femoris, posterior semimembranosus and semitendinosus) undergo much larger length changes during the step cycle than do the triceps surae muscles. Fig. 6 shows the ensemble mean rate profiles of 5 Ia afferents and 2 Ib afferents. The Ia peak rate was 215 i.p.s. and modulation depth was 190 i.p.s. The Ib peak rate and modulation depth were both 140 i.p.s. It is worth noting the small length reversal and the associated surges in both Ia and Ib firing prior to the main F-phase lengthening. These were seen in most individual cycles and indeed had been illustrated without comment in previous descriptions of chronic hamstring afferent recordings (e.g. Prochazka et al., 1976; Loeb and Duysens, 1979). From the foot contact measurements described above, we confirmed that foot-off generally occurred at the peak of the small length reversal, as indicated schematically in Fig. 6.

Fig. 7 brings together some of our quantitative ensemble profiles and qualitative profiles of other hindlimb muscles (derived from Loeb and

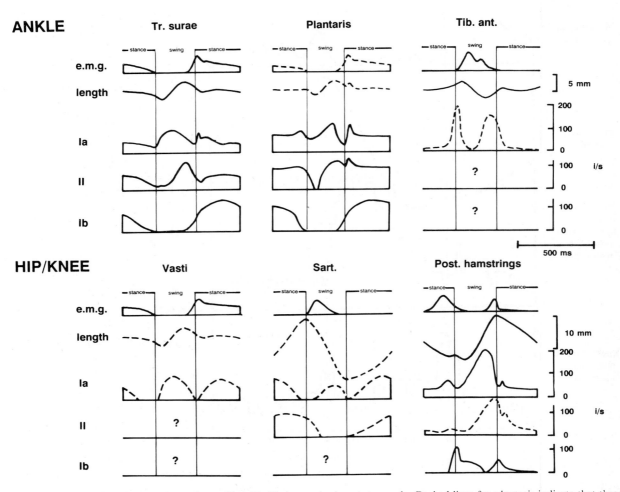

Fig. 7. Schematic of current look-up chart of key hindlimb muscles in cat step cycle. Dashed lines for plantaris indicate that these are qualitatively estimated time courses. Remaining dashed profiles are our own representations of the single-unit studies of Loeb and co-workers (see text).

Duysens, 1979; Loeb and Hoffer, 1985; Loeb et al., 1985a,b). Though fledgling ensemble histograms and anecdotal data exist for afferents in other muscles, e.g. extensor digitorum longus, peroneus longus, flexor digitorum longus, tibialis posterior, semimembranosus anterior, rectus femoris and the glutei, the schematics of Fig. 7 represent the bulk of the better established afferent profiles currently available in the normal cat.

Discussion

Alignment of ensemble averages

In the course of assembling the averages it became apparent that the choice of reference points for alignment had a significant effect on transients in the final profiles. The greater the temporal separation of a specific transient from a reference point, the more it was "smeared" in the ensemble average. To our knowledge this issue has not been addressed in gait analysis before, and yet it is a problem inherent in all signal averaging when single trigger points are used to align cycles. The normalization of cycle duration (e.g. Winter, 1987) tends to reduce, though not abolish the dispersion of phase-dependent transients provided that the relative durations of phases such as stance and swing remain constant. The latter is known not to hold in the cat step cycle (Halbertsma, 1983). Furthermore, temporal information is lost with normalization.

Ideally, one would want to trigger at every definable point in the step cycle, multiply each resultant average with an appropriate weighting function, and summate all of the weighted averages to form the final profile. As a compromise, we arbitrarily selected length turning points close to important transitions in the cycles, formed averages from cycles aligned to each of these, and combined them in segments to produce the final averages. Furthermore, we restricted ourselves to cycles of a 650–750 ms period. It was clear that with faster gait, the afferent profiles changed, generally having higher mean and peak rates and modulation depths. The present material

is therefore only representative of medium paced walking. Separate look-up charts would be required for an analysis of fast walking, trotting and galloping.

Afferent firing profiles: net ensemble rates

The triceps surae histrograms revealed some inaccuracies in earlier attempts at constructing ensemble afferent firing profiles (Prochazka, 1985, 1986). The 30–40 ms leads of foot-off and touchdown on triceps length minima, and the associated earlier firing of the Ia afferents had not been correctly anticipated. More importantly, mean peak rates and modulation depths were lower than predicted in the Ia afferents and higher than predicted in both group II and Ib afferents (though more data is required to confirm this).

The triceps surae are innervated by some 150 Ia afferents distributed as follows: medial gastrocnemius: 60; lateral gastrocnemius: 35; soleus: 55 (Chin et al., 1962). Thus on our evidence, medial gastrocnemius, the most richly endowed, would generate a peak Ia input to the spinal cord of about 6 ki.p.s. in early swing and again just prior to foot contact. The latter peak occurs during gastrocnemius activity and is therefore likely to contribute to homonymous and synergistic reflex control (Nichols, 1987). However, the F-phase peak could well contribute to reflex inhibition of the pretibial muscles (see decline in tibialis anterior Ia profile at swing onset in Fig. 7). The high and sustained Ib rates during stance are potentially very important for reflex control. The tentative finding that group II afferents may have higher ensemble rates than Ia afferents is also significant, but needs confirmation.

The close similarity between monitored length and group II firing in Fig. 5 indicates that spindles do not "see" as distorted a version of origin-to-insertion muscle length as suggested by Griffiths and Hoffer, 1987, and Hoffer et al., 1989, in this volume (see also Prochazka et al., 1988). In separate simulation experiments we found that tonic static action was necessary to recreate the high "bias" level of group II firing, and that this alone, without additional modulation, gave a good fit. There was no evidence of the pronounced α-linked increase in group II firing due to static fusimotion hypothesized by Lundberg et al. (1987), and this underlines the importance of establishing a firmly based afferent look-up chart for future hypotheses of central and peripheral interaction.

The group Ia lead on muscle length at foot-off and touchdown is more difficult to explain. Soleus Ia afferents showed some phase advance on length in reproduced step cycle length variations but even with concomitant tonic static fusimotor stimulation to prevent unloading, the increase in Ia firing at E_3/F and E_1/E_2 came $20-30$ ms later than in the chronic data. There are four possible explanations. First, tendon unloading (shortening) at E_3/F might slightly phase advance the internal muscle length "seen" by spindles (Prochazka et al., 1988; Hoffer et al., 1989, this volume). However at foot contact the tendons rather than the spindles would be stretched, and this is inconsistent with the observed E_1/E_2 phase advance. Second, sudden bursts of fusimotor action might accelerate spindle firing at these times. Various features, including the abruptness of Ia firing onset in E_1/E_2 militate against this explanation. Third, the jarring of the lower limb at foot-off and touchdown might propagate a pressure wave to which Ia afferents are responsive. Fourth, the sudden active contraction or loading of other muscles (e.g. hamstrings at foot-off and flexor digitorum and hallucis longus at touchdown) might distort nearby triceps compartments and briefly excite their spindle Ia endings.

In retrospect, the gastrocnemius records of Goslow et al. (1973) showed distinct lags of the E_3/F length minima on foot-off (20 ms or more: sampling interval was 20 ms), though no lags were evident at foot contact. The brief length reversal which we noticed in knee flexors (see Results) is also discernible in the records of Goslow et al. (1973). The delay in triceps lengthening is probably due to the initial yield (dorsiflexion) at the paw (Prochazka et al., 1977). We have consistently noticed that averaged gastrocnemius EMG shows an abrupt turning point $15-25$ ms after presumed foot contact (e.g. Fig. 4). A fuller description of afferent activity on foot-fall and its reflex consequences is in preparation (Elek, Llewellyn, Prochazka and Trend).

Hamstring afferents

The knee flexors are stretched more rapidly than the triceps surae during swing, and this is reflected in the high peak Ia rate and modulation depth. Semitendinosus is well endowed with spindles (ca. 120 Ia afferents: Barker, 1962; Chin et al., 1962), and so from Fig. 6, the peak ensemble Ia input from this muscle would be about 26 ki.p.s. Kirkwood and Sears (1982) and Kirkwood et al. (1984) estimated that 14 ki.p.s. of Ia input would bring motoneurones to threshold from rest, and 20 ki.p.s. would produce maintained discharge. On our data therefore, homonymous and synergistic Ia input must contribute significantly to the hamstrings EMG burst at the end of swing (the timing of which is atypically late in Fig. 6). Much debate has centred upon whether this burst is centrally or peripherally generated, and whether it is abolished by deafferentation or not (Grillner and Zangger, 1979). The second Ib burst in Fig. 6 evidently results from the knee flexor activation in late swing, and comes too late to compete reflexly with the Ia input. The large Ia peak, and the subsequent abrupt decline just prior to touchdown could be involved in the control of the transition from swing to stance (Rossignol et al., 1975). In this context, it is interesting that the decline in the hamstrings Ia profile was coincident with, and followed a similar time course to, the abrupt increase in gastrocnemius EMG anticipating foot contact (cf. Figs. 4 and 6).

The afferent look-up chart: future updating

It is clear from Fig. 7 that much remains to be done before a comprehensive quantitative picture of the ensemble afferent activity from the cat hindlimb can emerge. Hypotheses of the central control of the step cycle (e.g. Lundberg et al.,

1987) are still all too dependent upon results and theories derived in decerebrate or other reduced preparations. This is because the chronic data has tended to be anecdotal and lacking in unity. We feel that the analytical approach to quantifying ensemble afferent firing is the best way forward. Interestingly, a similar approach to characterizing neuronal ensembles is adopted by Fetz et al. (1989) in this volume. Specific histograms presented in this paper already offer a robust description of key afferent profiles. The data is stored digitally in a manner which readily allows for the addition of new material as it becomes available. The data can be shared with other laboratories involved in chronic afferent recordings in the future so that a central library of afferent profiles can be built up. In the meantime we have been using averaged Ia and II profiles in recent simulation experiments to deduce net fusimotor action during stepping.

Acknowledgements

This work was supported by the British MRC and the Alberta Heritage Foundation for Medical Research. We thank Dr K. Appenteng for his help in obtaining some of the early chronic data.

References

Abraham, L.D., Marks, W.B. and Loeb, G.E. (1985) The distal hindlimb musculature of the cat. Cutaneous reflexes during locomotion. *Exp. Brain Res.,* 58: 594 – 603.

Barker, D. (1962) The structure and distribution of muscle receptors. In D. Barker (Ed.), *Symposium on Muscle Receptors,* Hong Kong Univ. Press, Hong Kong, pp. 227 – 240.

Boyd, I.A. and Smith, R.S. (1984) The muscle spindle. In P.J. Dyck, P.K. Thomas, E.H. Lombert and R. Bunge (Eds.), *Peripheral Neuropathy, 2nd edn.,* Saunders, London, pp. 171 – 202.

Carlson, H., Halbertsma, J. and Zomlefer, M. (1979) Control of the trunk during walking in the cat. *Acta Physiol. Scand.,* 105: 251 – 253.

Carlsöö, S. (1973) *How Man Moves.* Heinemann, London, 117 pp.

Chin, N.K., Cope, M. and Pang, M. (1962) Number and distribution of spindle capsules in seven hindlimb muscles of the cat. In D. Barker (Ed.), *Symposium on Muscle Recep-*

tors, Hong Kong University Press, Hong Kong, pp. 241 – 248.

Dürmüller, N., Hulliger, M., Prochazka, A. and Trend, P.St.J. (1987) Ensemble proprioceptive activity in feline gait. *J. Physiol. (London),* 392: 63P.

Eccles, J.C., Eccles, R.M. and Lundberg, A. (1957) The convergence of monosynaptic excitatory afferents on to many species of alpha motoneurones. *J. Physiol. (London),* 137: 22 – 50.

Engberg, I. (1964) Reflexes to foot muscles in the cat. *Acta Physiol. Scand., 62 Suppl.* 235: 1 – 64.

Engberg, I. and Lundberg, A. (1969) An electromyographic analysis of muscular activity in the hindlimb of the cat during unrestrained locomotion. *Acta Physiol. Scand.,* 75: 614 – 630.

Fetz, E.E., Cheney, P.D., Mewes, K. and Palmer, S. (1989) Control of forelimb muscle activity by populations of corticomotoneuronal and rubromotoneuronal cells. In J.H.J. Allum and M. Hulliger (Eds.), *Afferent Control of Posture and Locomotion, Prog. Brain Res., Vol. 80,* Elsevier, Amsterdam, pp. 437 – 449.

Fleshman, J.W., Munson, J.B. and Sypert, G.W. (1981) Homonymous projection of individual group Ia-fibres to physiologically characterized medial gastrocnemius motoneurons in the cat. *J. Neurophysiol.,* 46: 1339 – 1348.

Forssberg, H. (1979) On integrative motor functions in the cat's spinal cord. *Acta Physiol. Scand., Suppl.* 474: 56 pp.

Goslow, G.E., Reinking, R.M. and Stuart, D.G. (1973) The cat step cycle: hind limb joint angles and muscle lengths during unrestrained locomotion. *J. Morphol.,* 141: 1 – 41.

Griffiths, R.I. and Hoffer, J.A. (1987) Muscle fibres shorten when the whole muscle is being stretched in the "yield" phase of the freely walking cat. *Soc. Neurosci. Abstr.,* 13: 124.

Grillner, S. and Zangger, P. (1979) On the central generation of locomotion in the low spinal cat. *Exp. Brain Res.,* 34: 241 – 261.

Halbertsma, J. (1983) The stride cycle of the cat: the modelling of locomotion by computerized analysis of automatic recordings. *Acta Physiol. Scand., Suppl.* 521: 75 pp.

Hoffer, J.A., Caputi, A.A., Pose, I.E. and Griffiths, R.I. (1989) Roles of muscle activity and load on the relationship between muscle spindle length and whole muscle length in the freely walking cat. In J.H.J. Allum and M. Hulliger (Eds.), *Afferent Control of Posture and Locomotion, Prog. Brain Res., Vol. 80,* Elsevier, Amsterdam, pp. 75 – 85.

Kirkwood, P.A. and Sears, T.A. (1982) Excitatory postsynaptic potentials from single muscle spindle afferents in external intercostal motoneurones of the cat. *J. Physiol. (London),* 322: 287 – 314.

Kirkwood, P.A., Sears, T.A. and Westgard, R.H. (1984) Restoration of function in external intercostal motoneurones of the cat following partial central deafferentation. *J. Physiol. (London),* 350: 225 – 251.

Loeb, G.E. and Duysens, J. (1979) Activity patterns in individual hindlimb primary and secondary muscle spindle afferents during normal movements in unrestrained cats. *J. Neurophysiol.,* 42: 420 – 440.

Loeb, G.E. and Hoffer, J.A. (1985) Activity of spindle afferents from cat anterior thigh muscles. II. Effects of fusimotor blockade. *J. Neurophysiol.,* 54: 565 – 577.

Loeb, G.E., Hoffer, J.A. and Pratt, C.A. (1985a) Activity of spindle afferents from cat anterior thigh muscles. I. Identification and patterns during normal locomotion. *J. Neurophysiol.,* 54: 549 – 564.

Loeb, G.E., Hoffer, J.A. and Marks, W.B. (1985b) Activity of spindle afferents from cat anterior thigh muscles. III. Effects of external stimuli. *J. Neurophysiol.,* 54: 578 – 591.

Lundberg, A., Malmgren, K. and Schomburg, E.D. (1987) Reflex pathways from group II muscle afferents. 3. Secondary spindle afferents and the FRA: a new hypothesis. *Exp. Brain Res.,* 65: 294 – 306.

Matthews, P.B.C. (1972) *Mammalian Muscle Receptors and their Central Actions.* Arnold, London, pp. 591 – 597.

Mendell, L.M. and Henneman, E. (1971) Terminals of single Ia fibres: location, density, and distribution within a pool of 300 homonymous motoneurons. *J. Neurophysiol.,* 34: 171 – 187.

Meyer-Lohmann, J., Riebold, W. and Robrecht, D. (1974) Mechanical influence of extrafusal muscle on the static behaviour of de-efferented primary muscle spindle endings in cat. *Pflügers Arch.,* 352: 267 – 278.

Nelson, S.G. and Mendell, L.M. (1978) Projection of single knee flexor Ia fibres to homonymous and heteronymous motoneurons. *J. Neurophysiol.,* 41: 778 – 787.

Nichols, T.R. (1987) A technique for measuring the mechanical actions of heterogenic (intermuscular) reflexes in the decerebrate cat. *J. Neurosci. Methods,* 21: 265 – 273.

Philippson, M. (1905) L'autonomie et la centralisation dans le système nerveux des animaux. *Trav. Lab. Inst. Solvay. Bruxelles,* 7: 1 – 208.

Prochazka, A. (1985) Afferent input during normal movements. In W.J.P. Barnes and M. Gladden (Eds.), *Feedback and Motor Control in Vertebrates and Invertebrates,* Croon Helm, London, pp. 169 – 172.

Prochazka, A. (1986) Proprioception during voluntary movement. *Can. J. Physiol., Pharmacol.,* 64: 499 – 504.

Prochazka, A. and Hulliger, M. (1983) Muscle afferent function and its significance for motor control mechanisms during voluntary movements in cat, monkey and man. In J.E. Desmedt (Ed.), *Motor Control Mechanisms in Health and Disease,* Raven, New York, pp. 93 – 132.

Prochazka, A., Westerman, R.A. and Ziccone, S. (1976) Discharges of single hindlimb afferents in the freely moving cat. *J. Neurophysiol.,* 39: 1090 – 1104.

Prochazka, A., Schofield, P., Westerman, R.A. and Ziccone, S. (1977) Reflexes in cat ankle muscle after landing from falls. *J. Physiol. (London),* 272: 705 – 719.

Prochazka, A., Elek, J., Hulliger, M., Vincent, S. and Waldon, V. (1988) Tendon stretch in cat gait estimated from muscle spindle firing in active and passive movements. *Soc. Neurosci. Abstr.,* 14: 262.

Rasmussen, S., Chan, A.K. and Goslow, G.E. (1978) The cat step cycle: electromyographic patterns for hindlimb muscles during posture and unrestrained locomotion. *J. Morphol.,* 155: 253 – 270.

Rossignol, S., Grillner, S. and Forssberg, H. (1975) Factors of importance for the initiation of flexion during walking. *Soc. Neurosci. Abstr.,*: 181.

Stuart, D.G., Mosher, C.G., Gerlach, R.L. and Reinking, R.M. (1972) Mechanical arrangement and transducing properties of Golgi tendon organs. *Exp. Brain Res.,* 14: 274 – 292.

Winter, D.A. (1987) *The Biomechanics and Motor Control of Human Gait.* University of Waterloo Press, Ontario, 72 pp.

J.H.J. Allum and M. Hulliger (Eds.)
Progress in Brain Research, Vol. 80
© 1989 Elsevier Science Publishers B.V. (Biomedical Division)

CHAPTER 7

Roles of muscle activity and load on the relationship between muscle spindle length and whole muscle length in the freely walking cat

J.A. Hoffer, A.A. Caputi, I.E. Pose and R.I. Griffiths

Departments of Clinical Neurosciences and Medical Physiology, University of Calgary, Faculty of Medicine, Calgary, Alberta T2N 4N1, Canada

The objective of this research was to compare the length of muscle spindles to the length of the whole muscle, during normal movements. Pairs of piezoelectric crystals were implanted near the origin and insertion of muscle fibres in the medial gastrocnemius (MG) muscle of cats. The distance between crystals was measured with pulsed ultrasound, the origin-to-insertion length of the MG muscle was measured with a transducer made of saline-filled silicone tubing, MG force was measured with a tendon force transducer and EMG activity was selectively recorded in the vicinity of implanted crystals. These signals were simultaneously recorded during posture or locomotion on a motorized treadmill. Three periods were identified in the step cycle, during which the relation between muscle length and spindle length changed dramatically. In *period I* (roughly corresponding to the late F and E_1 phases of swing), the MG muscle and spindles followed similar length changes: both were stretched and then shortened by about 6 mm. In *period II* (corresponding to the stance phase, $E_2 - E_3$) the MG muscle yielded under the weight of the body and was stretched by $1 - 3$ mm, whereas the MG spindles typically continued shortening. In *period III*, the MG muscle shortened rapidly by $6 - 8$ mm after the foot left the ground and then stretched again by about the same amount, whereas the spindles could remain nearly isometric. We attribute these large discrepancies in muscle and spindle length to the architecture of the MG muscle and the compliance of long tendinous elements in series with the spindles. We conclude that the length changes imposed on muscle spindles during voluntary movements are not simply related to the parent muscle length changes and cannot be estimated without taking into account the muscle architecture, the location of the spindle within the muscle, the level of muscle activation and the external load.

Key words: Muscle spindle; Muscle fiber; Muscle length; Cat locomotion; Fusimotor neuron

Introduction

Mammalian muscle spindles are stretch receptor organs whose afferent output is thought to reflect complex interactions between two kinds of time-dependent input: muscle length and fusimotor drive. In freely moving animals, the activity of identified fusimotoneurones has been impossible to record, due to their small size. Instead, fusimotor activity has been inferred by assuming it responsible for any features in spindle afferent ac-

tivity that depart from the "passive" responses of de-efferented spindles to similar changes in muscle length (e.g., Prochazka et al., 1976, 1979, 1985; Loeb and Duysens, 1979; Loeb and Hoffer, 1981; 1985; Hulliger, 1984; Hulliger et al., 1987).

In analysing spindle afferent discharge patterns in normal movements, it has generally been assumed that the changes in muscle length are equally imposed onto the muscle spindles and that the spindle movements can be replicated in the passive muscle. Implicit in this assumption is the concept that tendons are series elements that are either so stiff that their length remains essentially constant, or that their length varies as a constant fraction of the total muscle length during normal movements. However, whereas this assumption may be largely valid for *passive* muscles, it is likely to be invalid for *active* muscles. The stiffness of activated extrafusal muscle fibres increases markedly (e.g., Hoffer and Andreassen, 1981; Proske and Morgan, 1984), to the extent that it may meet or exceed the stiffness of the "entire tendinous component" (Rack and Westbury, 1984; see also Viidik, 1972; Morgan, 1977; Morgan et al., 1978; Griffiths, 1984). In pinnate muscles the angles of pinnation may change when the fibres are activated and a large, variable fraction of muscle stretch may be taken up by the aponeurotic sheets where the muscle fibres insert (viz., Otten, 1988). As a result, a distorted version of the muscle movement is likely to be registered by the muscle spindles. The complexity of the interplay between muscle and tendon stiffness is further compounded by the fact that muscle stiffness will vary in proportion to the number of fibres activated at any time, as well as their discharge rates (Proske and Morgan, 1984; Rack and Westbury, 1984).

The role of tendinous components is likely to be even more important in biarticular muscles, where muscle fibres and spindles typically span a small fraction of the length of a limb muscle. In wallabies hopping at high speed, Griffiths (1984) concluded from the mechanical properties of the medial gastrocnemius (MG) muscle and tendon that the MG fibres shortened in the early stages of muscle stretch. In cats, the rest-length of MG muscle fibres is of the order of $15 - 25$ mm (Walmsley and Proske, 1981), whereas the origin-to-insertion length of a large cat's MG muscle varies from some 115 to 125 mm (Goslow et al., 1973).

Although complex arrangements like, for example, "tandem" spindles have also been described (e.g., Banks et al., 1982), the typical MG spindles are arranged in parallel with extrafusal muscle fibres in the central region of the muscle (Swett and Eldred, 1960). Thus, a typical MG spindle is 15 – 25 mm long and is in series with some 100 mm of tendinous elements and in parallel with extrafusal fibres that have low stiffness when inactive and high stiffness when active.

In this study we tested the hypothesis that the length input to muscle spindles is not strictly related to the length of the parent muscle during voluntary movements. We used the ultrasound transit-time technique to measure muscle fibre and spindle length in central regions of the MG muscle. This technique has been widely used in cardiovascular research (viz., Rushmer et al., 1956) and in the study of diaphragm movements (reviewed by Newman et al., 1984). A method for using ultrasound to study muscle fibre length in the contracting MG muscle of anaesthetized cats was recently developed by Griffiths (1987). This approach gave preliminary data from one chronically implanted cat (Griffiths and Hoffer, 1987), prior to the present study.

Our results confirm the hypothesis that muscle spindles are not subjected to the same length changes as the parent muscle during normal locomotion, and suggest that the length of a muscle spindle is a complexly varying fraction of total muscle length that depends on the muscle architecture, the location of the spindle within the muscle, the extent of muscle activation and the external load.

Methods

Experimental design

Three large male cats (3.6 – 4.4 kg) were trained to walk or trot on a motorized treadmill enclosed within a Plexiglas box, set at level, uphill ($+ 10\%$ grade) or downhill ($- 10\%$ grade) positions, at a range of speeds from about 0.2 to over 2.0 m/s. After 4 – 6 weeks of daily training, each cat was deeply anaesthetized with halothane in oxygen/nitrous oxide mixture. The left hindlimb was prepared for surgical implantation of electrodes and transducers (described below). The leads from the implanted devices coursed subcutaneously and emerged in small bundles around a 40-pin connector (see Hoffer et al., 1987) attached to the cat's back with four size-2 subfascial Mersilene sutures. After surgery, the cats were administered a sedative (Atravet) and an analgesic (morphine sulfate, 0.1 mg/kg, subcutaneously every 8 h) for at least 24 h. Two or three days after surgery, the cats could be exercised on the treadmill for several minutes at slow speeds. Recordings were carried out starting on the sixth postsurgical day. The cats showed little or no sign of impairment and by the second week after implant they could walk for 30 min or more with periodic rest periods, and run at up to 2.2 m/s.

Measurement of MG muscle spindle length

The essence of our estimation of spindle length lies on the careful implantation of pairs of piezoelectric crystals near the origin and insertion of identified groups of muscle fibres (as in Griffiths, 1987) in central regions of the MG muscle (Fig. 1). Implicit in the measurement of transit

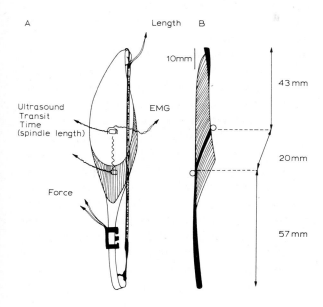

Fig. 1. A: schematic diagram of the left MG muscle, dorsal view, with implanted devices. B: diagram of the MG muscle, longitudinal cross-section, shows typical dimensions and orientation of its muscle and tendon fibres (adapted from Walmsley and Proske, 1981). The crystals recorded the length of muscle spindles in the highlighted region.

time of pulsed ultrasound bursts that are emitted by one crystal and received by the other, are two important assumptions: (1) that the velocity of ultrasound does not change much with the state of activation of the muscle (Hatta et al., 1988) and (2) that muscle fibres and spindles run straight between their origin and insertion. Fibres near the surface of a muscle can curve markedly during active shortening, but fibres in the central region of the MG muscle, where most spindles are located (Swett and Eldred, 1960), are likely to remain nearly straight (e.g., Otten, 1988, Fig. 15).

We used cylindrical crystals, 1.5 mm in diameter and 1.5 mm in length, having a natural frequency of 5 MHz (CY5-2; Triton Technology), fitted with Teflon-coated, multistrand, stainless steel leads (Cooner AS 631). Cylindrical crystals performed far better than disc crystals used in earlier experiments (Griffiths, 1987; Griffiths and Hoffer, 1987), mainly because disc crystals must be critically aligned when implanted and must remain well aligned through movement to obtain a useable signal, whereas the strength of the signal detected with cylindrical crystals is largely independent of rotational changes. In addition, the ultrasound-absorbing air gap that tended to be formed between disc crystals and muscle surface (viz., Griffiths, 1987, Fig. 1) was reduced or eliminated using cylindrical crystals. Since silicone rubber also absorbs ultrasound, we further improved the strength of the transmitted signal by adhering with epoxy a small piece of Dacron cloth to the top surface of each crystal, rather than using a silicone rubber block (viz., Griffiths, 1987).

Implantation of piezoelectric crystals

After both the deep and medial surfaces of the MG muscle belly were surgically exposed, the intended placement of one crystal of each pair was selected along the midline of the deep surface of the muscle and marked with a grain of Methylene blue (as in Griffiths, 1987). The orientation of tendinous fibres was used as a reference for orientation and placement of the crystals. The corresponding placement of the superficial crystal in each pair was determined by electrical microstimulation at the marked point (modified from Griffiths, 1987), using a concentric needle electrode (o.d. = 0.5 mm) and stimulating at 2 Hz using $40-70$ μA $\times$ 0.2 ms pulses. Upon each stimulus, a tiny dimple was observed on the medial surface, indicating the origin of the extrafusal fibres that were being stimulated near their distal end. A second grain of Methylene blue was placed at the dimple. A piezoelectric crystal was then positioned directly over each marked spot, such that the cylinder axis was perpendicular to the plane determined by the long axis of the MG muscle and the axis of the fibres to be measured (Fig. 1), and its Dacron cloth piece was sutured to the fascia using size 5-0 sutures. Either 12 or 13 piezoelectric crystals were implanted in each of three cats, strategically placed to measure the length of fibres and spindles in three regions of the MG muscle, as well as the length changes of segments of aponeurotic sheets in series with the muscle fibres and spindles of interest.

The amplitude of the recorded signals often improved markedly during the second week post-implant, suggesting that the crystals were being encapsulated by proliferating connective tissue and any remaining air was being absorbed. In post-mortem verification, each crystal left a precise imprint in the connective tissue on the muscle surface. This confirmed the position of the crystals and suggested that they were not displaced during movement.

Estimation of accuracy of muscle spindle length measurement with piezoelectric crystals

The measurement of distance between pairs of crystals was made with a Sonomicrometer 120 (Triton Technology) as described by Griffiths (1987). Our estimation of absolute muscle fibre and spindle length may have included a systematic error of the order of 1 mm, due to uncertainty in the placement of the crystals and the thickness of the aponeurotic sheets. A further source of occasional measurement uncertainty was a false trigger on other than the first wavefront in the received

burst. This tended to happen when signal strength declined for relatively long lengths, or when signal strength increased markedly for short lengths. A false trigger that skipped by one wavelength would cause an error in length measurement of 0.33 mm. A few examples of false triggers can be seen in the data in Figs. 2A and 3A, typically around the shortest and longest spindle length values recorded during walking. These false triggers were rare enough that they did not seriously distort the shape of the recorded signal. Assuming $1-2\%$ variations in the conduction velocity of ultrasound in active muscle (Hatta et al., 1988), the total uncertainty in the measurement of spindle length changes was generally less than $\pm$ 0.5 mm.

Measurement of whole muscle length

The origin-to-insertion length of the MG muscle was recorded with a length transducer made of saline-filled silicone tubing (Loeb and Hoffer, 1981, 1985). Heavy sutures tied to the ends of the transducer were passed through holes drilled in a sesamoid bone within the tendon of origin of MG, and the calcaneum. The transducer was connected to an AC bridge amplifier (Bak Electronics) driven at a constant frequency (25, 30 or 35 kHz). The DC output signal was low-pass filtered (5 ms time constant). In limited recordings, the length of the MG muscle was simultaneously measured with a pair of piezoelectric crystals attached to the sesamoid bone and to the proximal end of the force transducer (described below), although this measurement excluded the distal 30 mm of MG tendon. The length transducer records were calibrated for specific steps of interest, using joint angle measurements made from videotaped records (30 frames/s) and measurements of bone lengths. The cosine law was used to calculate MG length (viz., Goslow et al., 1973).

Measurement of muscle force and EMG

Force was recorded from the MG tendon by an implanted spring steel "E" transducer (Walmsley et al., 1978; Loeb and Hoffer, 1981, 1985). Force records were low-pass filtered at 100 Hz. The electromyogram was selectively recorded by bipolar electrodes consisting of a pair of Teflon-coated, multistrand, stainless steel wires (Cooner AS 631) with exposed ends. The two electrodes were sewn into the muscle at the sides of each of the superficial crystals, about 5 mm apart, such that one electrode was about 2 mm deep and the other was superficial. EMG records were amplified 1000-fold and filtered in the 50 – 5000 Hz range prior to tape-recording. To remove noise generated by the crystals, EMG records were further low-pass filtered at 250 Hz (18 dB/octave).

All signals were recorded on FM tape (10 kHz bandpass), along with a master time code (Datum) that was used for synchronization of videotaped images during data analysis. Data shown in Figs. 2 and 3 were played back into an electrostatic recorder with 25 kHz peak capture (Gould S1000).

Results

Relation between muscle length and muscle spindle length during locomotion

A consistent finding that emerged from our records was that the relationship between MG

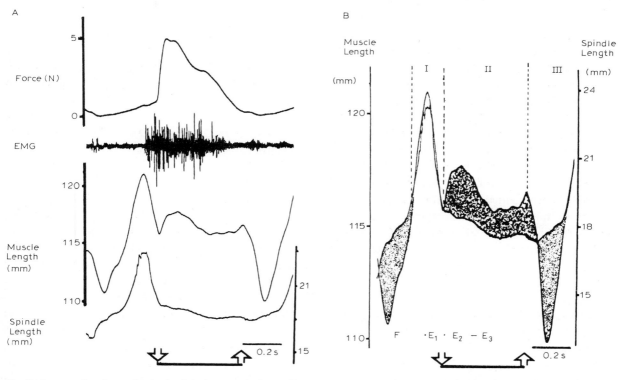

Fig. 2. A: example of records obtained during a typical step. From top, traces are: force recorded from the MG tendon by an implanted spring steel transducer; electromyogram recorded by bipolar electrodes sewn near the crystals; origin-to-insertion length of the MG muscle, recorded with a saline-filled silicone tubing transducer spanning from the sesamoid bone in the tendon of origin, to the calcaneum; length of muscle spindles in the central portion of MG, recorded by piezoelectrode crystals. *Horizontal bar* indicates weight-bearing period for the implanted hindlimb. *Arrows* indicate paw touchdown and liftoff. B: traces corresponding to the length of the MG muscle and the length of muscle spindles are superimposed to reveal three periods (I, II, III) of dissimilar relationship. The phases of the Philippson step cycle (F, flexion; E_1, E_2, E_3, extension) are also shown. Note that muscle and spindle length are very similar in period I, but the spindles are not stretched with the muscle in period II, and the spindles are not shortened with the muscle in period III.

muscle length and MG spindle length changed systematically and dramatically during locomotion. We identified three distinct periods in the step cycle, that overlapped roughly, though not exactly, with the four classic phases of the step cycle (F = flexion; E_1, E_2, E_3 = extension phases) described by Philippson (1905) from joint angle transitions. During period I, while the limb was unloaded during late swing, the muscle length and spindle length excursions had similar direction and shape, and comparable amplitude. During period II, while the limb was loaded during stance, the muscle was stretched while the spindles were not. During period III, in early swing, the muscle was first shortened considerably and then lengthened by about the same amount, while the spindles showed only modest changes in length.

Fig. 2A shows the MG force, EMG, muscle length and spindle length signals recorded from a cat taking one representative step at about 0.5 m/s on a level treadmill. Fig 2B shows again the muscle length and spindle length traces from the same step, now superimposed to highlight the principal similarities and differences. The weight-bearing phase (stance) for the instrumented hindlimb is shown by a horizontal bar. Arrows mark transitions between loaded and unloaded phases. It is apparent that the muscle and spindle length traces obey very different relations during the three periods, indicated in Fig. 2B as I, II and III.

Period I

This period comprises half of the swing phase, since it starts in the middle of the F phase and includes the E_1 phase. Initially the MG muscle is passively stretched by the action of antagonists. No EMG is present. The MG spindles are also stretched, and follow a very similar timecourse to the MG muscle length. At the F to E_1 transition, almost coincident with the onset of EMG, the MG fibres proceed to rapidly shorten against minimal load. The MG muscle also shortens, following an almost identical time course and extent as the spindles. The rapid muscle shortening phase comes to an abrupt end at the moment of foot contact, as

the limb is loaded (downward arrow in Fig. 2A, 2B), and here also ends period I.

Period II

This period consists of the E_2 and E_3 phases, the periods of load-bearing of the instrumented limb. As the weight is transferred, the MG muscle "yields" and stretches by a variable amount. In contrast, the muscle fibres typically do not yield during the E_2 phase. Rather, the fibres usually continue shortening during E_2 (viz., Griffiths, 1984), albeit at a considerably slower rate than during E_1. Thus, the MG spindles are typically not stretched during the E_2 phase, even though the MG muscle is. During the E_3 phase, the MG length record can show multiple inflexions. Active shortening usually follows the peak of yield. Toward the end of E_3 the muscle can be passively lengthened as its EMG activation declines and the knee extends maximally. In contrast, spindles in the central region of the MG muscle tend to remain fairly isometric, or experience only an attenuated version of the changes seen in the whole muscle length.

Period III

This period consists of the early F phase. Initially, the MG muscle is rapidly and passively shortened following the release of foot contact at the end of the stance phase (upward arrow in Fig. 2). The spindles do not follow the abrupt shortening of the MG muscle, probably because the pushoff is mediated by muscles other than MG (e.g. posterior tibial muscle; viz. Abraham and Loeb, 1985). As the ankle extends further but the knee starts to flex, the previously stretched MG tendon appears to take up the shortening, sparing the MG fibres and spindles from participating. Eventually, the MG length reaches a minimum and the MG muscle starts to be passively stretched by the action of ankle flexors. The fibres and spindles follow the stretch at an initially much reduced rate but, eventually (presumably once the tendon is sufficiently stretched), the rate of stretch of the spindles catches up with the whole muscle and a new Period I begins.

Comparison of length and velocity of MG muscle and spindles during the step cycle

From a 4.4 kg cat walking on a level belt at 0.5 m/s, the following observations were made from the data in Fig. 2.

Periods III and I, F phase

The origin-to-insertion length of the MG muscle changed by 10 to 12 mm, from about 110 to 120 mm (10% of MG rest-length). The length of the muscle spindles in the central portion of MG increased by about 7.5 mm, from 15.5 to 23 mm (35% of rest-length). During the final 100 ms of the F phase, the velocity of stretch of the MG muscle was 550 mm/s, or about 5 rest-lengths per second (RL/s; viz., Prochazka and Hulliger, 1983). At the beginning of stretch, still in period III, the spindles were slow to follow the stretching muscle, probably because the distal tendon started out slack. Mid-way through the F phase the spindles caught up with the muscle and their peak velocity of stretch was also about 550 mm/s, or about 25 RL/s, during period I.

Period I, E_1 phase

The amount of shortening during E_1 depends on the timing between the onset of EMG and the contact with the ground, and is in fact kept fairly constant, both for level walking and for up- or downhill walking (see further examples in Fig. 3). In the example of Fig. 2, the MG muscle shortened by 5 mm and the spindles by almost the same amount. The velocity of shortening of both the MG muscle and spindles during E_1 was about 800 mm/s, corresponding to about -8 RL/s for the muscle and -40 RL/s for the muscle spindles.

Period II, E_2 phase

In the example for Fig. 2, the MG muscle yielded by 2.0 mm during the first 100 ms after foot contact, whereas the MG spindles, pulled by fully activated extrafusal fibres, were shortened by an additional 0.25 mm during the same time. The rate of stretch of the MG muscle during E_2 was 20 mm/s

(0.2 RL/s), while the spindles shortened at a rate of 2.5 mm/s (-0.1 RL/s). The extent of muscle yield could be quite variable. In some steps the spindles could also experience some yield, although in such cases the extent of spindle yield was a small fraction of muscle yield (examples in Fig. 3). No systematic observations could be made on the extent and rate of length changes in the MG muscle during period II, E_3 phase, because of the high variability from step to step.

Period III, early F phase

A consistent observation was that the inactive MG muscle could shorten by as much as 8 mm following footlift and then stretch again by about the same amount, but the muscle fibres and spindles in the central region of MG experienced only a small amount of movement (< 1 mm).

Variations in the relation between muscle length and muscle spindle length during level, uphill and downhill locomotion

Fig. 3A shows raw records obtained from the same cat as in Fig. 2, during seven consecutive steps on a level treadmill belt set at 0.47 m/s. There was considerable variation in the MG tendon force amplitude and EMG (upper traces) as well as in the cycle durations of the steps shown, because the belt speed had been reduced from 0.77 m/s moments before, and the cat was adjusting to the new speed. Note that the excursions in MG muscle and spindle length during the unloaded phases (late F and E_1; period I) were strikingly similar from step to step. We will concentrate here on the differences between muscle and spindle length that occurred during the load-bearing phases (E_2 and E_3; period II).

The first six steps in Fig. 3A were all different from each other. In the first step, the MG muscle length "yielded" prominently upon touchdown and then decreased through mid-stance, whereas the MG fibres and spindles were held briefly isometric and then shortened all through E_2 and into E_3. In the second step, there was only a small yield and the muscle remained fairly isometric

82

through E_2 and E_3. The spindle length record shows an almost imperceptible yield, but then the spindles shortened steadily throughout the rest of the stance phase. The amount of muscle yield in the third step was again small, but note that the spindles followed a similar time course to the first step during E_1 and early E_2. The force in the third step was considerably larger. In the fourth step, the muscle showed little or no yield; muscle length and spindle length declined similarly. The fifth step showed larger yield and also larger force than the previous steps; still, the MG spindles continued to shorten during E_2 and E_3. The sixth step showed the largest yield of all and an intermediate

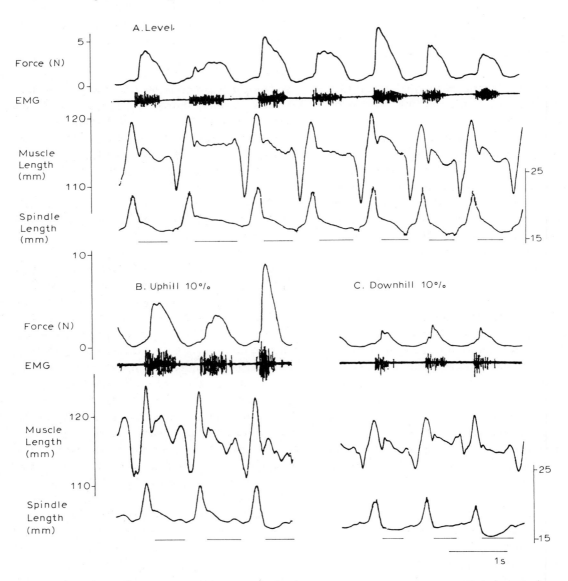

Fig. 3. A: examples of records obtained from a cat walking on a level treadmill at about 0.5 m/s, during seven consecutive steps. B: records obtained during uphill walking on a 10% grade at 0.4 m/s. C: same, for downhill walking on a 10% grade at 0.4 m/s. Traces as in Fig. 2.

force, but even here the spindles continued shortening. The last step shown in Fig. 3A, taken as the cat resumed a constant speed, looks fairly similar to the first step.

Fig. 3B shows records obtained from the same cat during uphill walking at 0.4 m/s. The same traces as in Fig. 3A are shown, and the calibrations are all the same. During uphill walking, the general shape of all the traces was roughly similar to level walking, but the amplitude of MG force, EMG and length changes were all larger. In contrast, the muscle spindle length records were almost identical to the level walking steps shown in Fig. 3A, except that the average length had shifted toward a somewhat longer value. The MG muscle yielded more prominently during uphill than level walking, but the muscle fibres and spindles did not yield any more than they did during level walking. Similarly, spindle length did not reflect the marked decline in MG muscle length at the end of stance. Thus, the characteristic dissociation between muscle and spindle length already observed during the E_2 and late E_3 phases of level walking (period II), was further exaggerated during uphill walking.

Fig. 3C shows records obtained from the same cat during downhill walking at 0.4 m/s. During downhill walking, the amplitude and duration of MG force and EMG were smaller than during level walking. The MG muscle yielded by varying amounts during E_2, and shortened less at the end of E_3. The muscle fibres and spindles did not yield, but they also did not shorten further at foot contact; rather, the spindles remained fairly isometric in two of the three steps shown and, in the third step, shortened markedly during E_2 and then lengthened during E_3, even while the muscle was shortening. Again, spindle length did not reflect muscle length during downhill walking, and the overall patterns were not quite the same as in level walking.

In summary, a comparison of level, uphill and downhill walking confirmed the finding that the relationship between the length of the MG muscle and its spindles changed systematically during three periods of the step cycle.

Discussion

Relation between spindle length and muscle length during active movements

The main conclusion from this study is that the length changes imposed on the MG muscle spindles do not directly reflect the length changes undergone by the parent muscle during most of the step cycle. Three periods in the step cycle were identified, during which the spindle length and muscle length were differently related. Only during one period, when the limb was unloaded, were the length changes in the muscle and its spindles well correlated. During the loaded period of the step cycle the muscle was stretched much more than its spindles, while at the early swing phase, the muscle shortened much more than its spindles.

The simplest interpretation of these observations is that the MG spindles are in series with long, compliant tendinous fibres that take care, during most of the step cycle, of a large fraction of the length changes seen from the origin to the insertion of the muscle. Early during period I, with the tendinous fibres relatively stiffer than the inactive muscle fibres, the spindles closely follow the length changes that are imposed on the muscle. As the MG muscle is activated in E_1 and starts to shorten in the absence of external load, the ends of the muscle are pulled in by the shortening fibres, and now it is the muscle that closely follows the length changes of the spindles. After foot contact, during early period II, the MG muscle is active and the limb is loaded, so the tendon is pulled from both ends. The action of external loads causes the muscle to yield during E_2, but the tendinous components undergo the stretching, not the muscle fibres and spindles. The muscle fibres continue to actively shorten, at further expense of the tendinous components, and so the spindles shorten, even though the muscle "yields". During E_3 the MG muscle and tendon shorten somewhat, and the tendon force declines. At the end of E_3, the MG muscle is often lengthened again by the action of the extending knee. During period III, the MG muscle is released as the foot gives up contact with the ground. This provides the opportunity for the still stretched tendinous elements to shorten. The now-inactive fibres, and spindles in parallel with them, do not participate in this shortening, and can in fact lengthen modestly as the muscle belly regains its shape.

Our data support prior suggestions by others, in particular by Rack and Westbury (1984), that spindles do not fully partake in the movements of their parent muscles, due to the compliance of tendinous series components. In addition, we have obtained preliminary recordings using piezoelectric crystals mounted along portions of the aponeurotic sheets of the MG muscle (Caputi, Hoffer and Pose, unpublished data) that further confirm this view. It should be noted that a recently published general muscle model by Otten (1988) includes several architectural features that are supported by our observations.

Need for re-interpretation of prior observations on spindle activity patterns during normal movements

Prior studies often assumed that fusimotor activity was responsible for any features in spindle afferent activity that departed from the "passive" responses of de-efferented spindles to similar changes in muscle length (e.g., Prochazka et al., 1976, 1979, 1985; Loeb and Duysens, 1979; Loeb and Hoffer, 1981, 1985; Hasan, 1983; Hulliger, 1984; Hulliger et al., 1987). As a consequence of this study, we now know that an estimation of muscle spindle length based on the length of the parent muscle is incorrect for most of the step cycle. For example, the amount of fusimotor action during the "yield phase" of extensor muscles is likely to have been greatly underestimated in simulation studies that assumed that spindle length changes in active muscles could be reproduced in passive muscles if whole muscle length was reproduced (e.g., Prochazka et al., 1985; Hulliger et al., 1987). Also, models of spindle response to stretch that were based on passive muscle properties (e.g., Hasan, 1983) must be modified if they are to be applicable to active muscles. Clearly,

future studies of natural spindle activity patterns will have to simultaneously include either the technique of pulsed ultrasound transit-time or some other, equivalent method of detection of actual spindle movement.

Acknowledgements

We thank T. Leonard and M. Stemler for expert assistance with training and caring after the cats. Funds were provided by grants from the Muscular Dystrophy Association of Canada, the Medical Research Council of Canada and the Spinal Cord Research Foundation (USA) to J.A.H. A.A.C. and R.I.G. were postdoctoral fellows of the Alberta Heritage Foundation for Medical Research.

References

Abraham, L.D. and Loeb, G.E. (1985) The distal hindlimb musculature of the cat: patterns of normal use. *Exp. Brain Res.*, 58: 580 – 593.

Banks, R.W., Barker, D. and Stacey, M.J. (1982) Form and distribution of sensory terminals in cat hindlimb muscle spindles. *Phil. Trans. R. Soc. Lond. B.*, 299: 329 – 364.

Goslow, G.E., Reinking, R.M. and Stuart, D.G. (1973) The cat step cycle: hind limb joint angles and muscle lengths during unrestrained locomotion. *J. Morphol.*, 141: 1 – 41.

Griffiths, R.I. (1984) *Mechanical Properties of an Ankle Extensor Muscle in a Freely Hopping Wallaby.* Ph.D. Thesis, Monash University, Melbourne, Australia.

Griffiths, R.I. (1987) Ultrasound transit time gives direct measurement of muscle fiber length in vivo. *J. Neurosci. Methods,* 21: 159 – 165.

Griffiths, R.I., Hoffer, J.A. (1987) Muscle fibres *shorten* when the whole muscle is being stretched in the "yield phase" of the freely walking cat. *Soc. Neurosci. Abstr.*, 13: 1214.

Hasan, Z. (1983) A model of spindle afferent response to muscle stretch. *J. Neurophysiol.*, 49: 989 – 1006.

Hatta, I., Sugi, H. and Tamura, Y. (1988) Stiffness changes in frog skeletal muscle during contraction recorded using ultrasonic waves. *J. Physiol. (London),* 403: 193 – 209.

Hoffer, J.A. and Andreassen, S. (1981) Regulation of soleus muscle stiffness in premammillary cats: intrinsic and reflex components. *J. Neurophysiol.*, 45: 267 – 285.

Hoffer, J.A., Loeb, G.E., Marks, W.B., O'Donovan, M.J., Pratt, C.A. and Sugano, N. (1987) Cat hindlimb motoneurons during locomotion. I. Destination, axonal conduction velocity and recruitment threshold. *J. Neurophysiol.*, 57: 510 – 529.

Hulliger, M. (1984) The mammalian muscle spindle and its central action. *Rev. Physiol. Biochem. Pharmacol.,* 101: 1 – 110.

Hulliger, M., Horber, F., Medved, A. and Prochazka, A. (1987) An experimental simulation method for iterative and interactive reconstruction of unknown (fusimotor) inputs contributing to known (spindle afferent) responses. *J. Neurosci. Methods,* 21: 225 – 238.

Loeb, G.E. and Duysens, J. (1979) Activity patterns in individual hindlimb primary and secondary muscle spindle afferents during normal movements in unrestrained cats. *J. Neurophysiol.,* 42: 420 – 440.

Loeb, G.E. and Hoffer, J.A. (1981) Muscle spindle function during normal and perturbed locomotion in cats. In A. Taylor and A. Prochazka (Eds.), *Muscle Receptors and Movement,* Macmillan, London, pp. 219 – 228.

Loeb, G.E. and Hoffer, J.A. (1985) Activity of spindle afferents from cat anterior thigh muscles. II. Effects of fusimotor blockade. *J. Neurophysiol.,* 54: 565 – 577.

Morgan, D.L. (1977) Separation of active and passive component of short-range stiffness of muscle. *Am. J. Physiol.,* 232: C45 – C49.

Morgan, D.L., Proske, U. and Warren, D. (1978) Measurements of muscle stiffness and the mechanisms of elastic storage of energy in hopping kangaroos. *J. Physiol. (London),* 282: 253 – 261.

Newman, S., Road, J., Beliemare, F., Clozel, J.P., Lavigne, C.M. and Grassino, A. (1984) Respiratory muscle length measured by sonomicrometry. *J. Appl. Physiol.,* 56: 753 – 764.

Otten, E. (1988) Concepts and models of functional architecture in skeletal muscle. *Exercise Sport Sci. Rev.,* 18: 89 – 137.

Philippson, M. (1905) L'autonomie et la centralisation dans le système nerveux des animaux. *Trav. Lab. Physiol. Inst. Solvay Bruxelles,* 7: 1 – 208.

Prochazka, A. and Hulliger, M. (1983) Muscle afferent function and its significance for motor control mechanisms during voluntary movements in cat, monkey and man. In J.E. Desmedt (Ed.), *Motor Control Mechanisms in Health and Disease,* Raven Press, New York, pp. 93 – 132.

Prochazka, A., Westerman, R.A. and Ziccone, S.P. (1976) Discharges of single hindlimb afferents in the freely moving cat. *J. Neurophysiol.,* 39: 1090 – 1104.

Prochazka, A., Stephens, J.A. and Wand, P. (1979) Muscle spindle discharge in normal and obstructed movements. *J. Physiol. (London),* 287: 57 – 66.

Prochazka, A., Hulliger, M., Zangger, P. and Appenteng, K. (1985) "Fusimotor set": new evidence for alpha-independent control of gamma-motoneurons during movement in the awake cat. *Brain Res.,* 339: 136 – 140.

Proske, U. and Morgan, D.L. (1984) Stiffness of cat soleus muscle and tendon during activation of part of muscle. *J. Neurophysiol.,* 52: 459 – 468.

Rack, P.M.H. and Westbury, D.R. (1984) Elastic properties of the cat soleus tendon and their functional importance. *J. Physiol. (London),* 347: 479 – 495.

Rushmer, R.F., Franklin, D. and Ellis, R. (1956) Left ventricular dimensions recorded by sonocardiometry. *Circ. Res.,* 4: 684 – 688.

Swett, J.E. and Eldred, E. (1960) Distribution and numbers of stretch receptors in medial gastrocnemius and soleus muscles of the cat. *Anat. Rec.,* 137: 453 – 460.

Viidik, A. (1972) Simultaneous mechanical and light microscopic studies of collagen fibres. *Z. Anat. Entwickl. Gesch.,* 136: 204 – 212.

Walmsley, B. and Proske, U. (1981) Comparison of stiffness of soleus and medial gastrocnemius muscles in cats. *J. Neurophysiol.,* 46: 250 – 259.

Walmsley, B., Hodgson, J.A. and Burke, R.E. (1978) Forces produced by soleus and medial gastrocnemius muscles during locomotion in freely moving cats. *J. Neurophysiol.,* 41: 1203 – 1216.

J.H.J. Allum and M. Hulliger (Eds.)
Progress in Brain Research, Vol. 80
© 1989 Elsevier Science Publishers B.V. (Biomedical Division)

CHAPTER 8

Flexible fusimotor control of muscle spindle feedback during a variety of natural movements

M. Hulliger[1], N. Dürmüller [1], A. Prochazka[2] and P. Trend[3]

[1]*Brain Research Institute, University of Zürich, August-Forel-Strasse 1, CH-8029 Zürich, Switzerland;* [2]*Department of Physiology, University of Alberta, Edmonton, Alberta, Canada T6G 2H7; and* [3]*Department of Physiology, St. Thomas's Hospital Medical School, Lambeth Palace Road, London SE1 7EH, U.K.*

A refined version of an experimental iterative simulation method is described, which was used to infer, from chronic spindle afferent recordings, type and time course of static and dynamic fusimotor activation during a variety of voluntary movements. When used to estimate overall fusimotor drive (without distinction between static and dynamic action) the method provides unique solutions. However, when generating independent γ_s and γ_d activation profiles, the solutions no longer are strictly unique. Yet the boundary conditions imposed by the type specific characteristics of γ-action nevertheless permit detection of powerful activation, especially of dynamic efferents. Extending the finding of selective dynamic fusimotor activation during unpredictably imposed and resisted stretches, evidence for powerful, often transient activation of dynamic efferents has now been obtained for three additional motor paradigms. First, initiation of walking was accompanied by mixed fusimotor action. Static drive was stepped up and then maintained, whereas dynamic drive declined after an initial abrupt peak. Second, corrective balancing on a narrow walk beam was characterized by largely maintained static background drive, whilst dynamic activation profiles often exhibited powerful surges or transients, when the animal crouched to regain balance. These preceded subsequent EMG bursts during the stretch phase of crouching by about 300 ms. Third, preparation for landing from rapid lowering featured prominent and possibly selective activation of dynamic fusimotor neurones, which peaked while the animal was in mid-air and declined upon landing, and which preceded the sharp onset of EMG after landing by several hundred milliseconds. In all cases the fusimotor activation profiles were unrelated to the parent muscle EMG and difficult to reconcile with the notion of $\alpha - \gamma$ linkage or coactivation. These findings then clearly support the concept of flexible central control, particularly of dynamic γ-motoneurones during certain motor tasks.

Key words: Muscle spindle; Fusimotor neuron; Efferent control; Motor adaptation; Motor control; Voluntary movement; Chronic recording; Experimental simulation; Iterative approximation

Introduction

Static and dynamic γ motoneurones are controlled from numerous sites in the central nervous system, including motor cortex, thalamus, cerebellum and various brainstem regions (reviewed in Matthews, 1972, and Hulliger, 1984). Whilst some of these structures appear to be non-selective, by acting on γ_d, γ_s, and α motoneurones indiscriminately, others exert more selective descending control. Mainly on the basis of experiments with electrical stimulation, some regions have been described from which γ motoneurones can be activated, uncontaminated by α activation. From other areas static γ motoneurones appear to be activated selectively (reviews above, and Schwarz et al., 1984). Until recently only a single area exerting exclusive control of dynamic γ motoneurones was known (MesADC, mesencephalic area for dynamic control; Appelberg, 1981). But with the discovery of the selective dynamic fusimotor effects elicited from the habenulo-interpeduncular system (Taylor and Donga, 1989, this volume) the CNS' known capacity of selective and flexible control of γ efferents and of muscle spindle feedback has now been further expanded.

In spite of the undeniable potential of flexible central control of fusimotor neurones, experimental evidence to demonstrate its use during movement has only slowly accumulated. The technical difficulties of direct recordings from γ motoneurones have certainly contributed to this (see Prochazka and Hulliger, 1983). Direct recordings from fully identified γ efferents have so far only been achieved in reduced preparations, but even in these identification of type (static vs dynamic) mostly was impossible or uncertain. Moreover, in freely moving animals and man fusimotor activity had to be inferred from recordings of spindle afferent discharge. Yet this is fraught with uncertainty, given the higly nonlinear properties of the muscle spindle and given the fact that none of the distinguishing characteristics of fusimotor action apply universally. For instance, at short muscle length static efferents activated at low rates can augment the sensitivity to stretches, and at long length dynamic efferents can reduce it (see Hulliger, 1984, 1987). Also, until recently it was taken for granted that spindle afferent firing during muscle shortening was a hallmark of static fusimotor action. Yet there is mounting evidence that in their ability to maintain spindle firing during shortening static and dynamic efferents differ only quantitatively (Morgan et al., 1985), since modulated γ_d action is quite capable of provoking appreciable Ia firing during shortening, for sinusoidal movements up to about 3 Hz (Rioult-Pedotti et al., 1988).

The patterns of γ activity, which have been recorded or inferred, cover a wide spectrum, ranging from strict $\alpha - \gamma$ linkage (Granit, 1955) or somewhat looser $\alpha - \gamma$ coactivation (e.g. Vallbo et al., 1979) to a high degree of $\alpha - \gamma$ independence (e.g. Vallbo and Hulliger, 1981; Schieber and Thach, 1985; reviewed in Hulliger, 1987). For rhythmic movements some degree of $\alpha - \gamma$ coupling has often been emphasized. Sjöström and Zangger (1976) described tight linkage in flexor and extensor muscles during fictive spinal locomotion. Perret and Berthoz (1973), Cabelguen (1981) and Bessou et al. (1989, this volume) inferred $\alpha - \gamma_s$ for flexor and $\alpha - \gamma_d$ coactivation for extensor muscles for locomotion in the thalamic cat. A similar, if more cautious, line was taken by Loeb et al. (1985) and Loeb and Hoffer (1985) in interpreting spindle firing patterns during treadmill locomotion in chronically implanted cats. But experimental simulations, based on chronic spindle afferent recordings from freely moving cats, failed to confirm the general applicability of these γ activation patterns (Prochazka et al., 1985; Hulliger et al., 1986a, b).

From the outset it has always been known that γ motoneurones could also be tonically activated during rhythmic movements (e.g. Eklund et al., 1964). More recently this has been further emphasized both in studies on reduced preparations and on freely moving animals. In decerebrate cats static γ efferents were found to be activated tonically, whilst dynamic efferents fired rhythmically (in phase with α motoneurones). This was true for hindlimb locomotor (Murphy et al., 1984; Taylor et al., 1985) and intercostal respiratory muscles (Greer and Stein, 1986). Moreover, for respiratory movements dynamic action was optional or task-dependent, in that it was only manifest when respiratory drive was increased. Yet the reverse pattern (tonic γ_d firing with $\alpha - \gamma_s$ coactivation) was described for jaw movements in anaesthetized cats (Appenteng et al., 1980; Gottlieb and Taylor, 1983). This contradiction will probably only be resolved in additional recordings during natural movements. Yet for the time being it remains a distinct possibility that even for relatively uniform rhythmic movements fusimotor strategies are task-dependent.

Prochazka, Hulliger and colleagues used an experimental simulation method (see Methods) to analyse the fusimotor activation profiles underlying chronically recorded spindle firing patterns during spontaneous movements in unrestrained cats. In line with the above, they concluded that fusimotor activity during rhythmic movements had a significant tonic component. Moreover, it was found to switch from largely static, during routine steps, to predominantly dynamic, during imposed and then resisted stretches. Finally, it could undergo slow gradual changes, during unfamiliar motor performance. The term "fusimotor set" was coined to describe these features and the concept of task-dependence of fusimotor control (Hulliger et al., 1985; Prochazka et al., 1985; reviewed in Prochazka, 1989). However, the experimental evidence to support this notion was qualified by the limited number of motor paradigms that were investigated, and by restricted numbers of predefined γ-activation profiles, whose actions were assessed experimentally.

An improved experimental simulation technique has now been used to assess chronically recorded spindle afferent firing patterns (target responses) from a wider range of movements. This method permits target reproducing stimulation patterns to be approximated iteratively, by recourse to the error between simulated and chronic target responses, and it no longer relies on tests of explicit or predefined γ-activation profiles. The preliminary findings, which are reported here, confirm the earlier observations and further emphasize that the fusimotor strategies, which are adopted during natural movements, indeed are flexible and strongly task-dependent.

Methods

Apart from the extended iterative simulation technique, most aspects of the experimental methods have previously been described in detail (Hulliger and Prochazka, 1983; Hulliger et al., 1987) and are therefore summarized only briefly. The simulation approach combines chronic recordings in freely moving cats with acute experiments in separate anaesthetized cats. In the chronic experiments responses of muscle spindle afferents are recorded, whilst the animals perform a variety of movements. In the acute experiments the fusimotor activation profiles underlying the

chronically recorded responses are reconstructed by matching test spindle responses with the target spindle responses of the chronic experiment, using an iterative procedure where, in successive response (or iteration) cycles, the former gradually approximates the latter, as the fusimotor stimulation profiles are optimized in successive attempts. Methodologically the only new feature of the present report are the dual channel iterations which are described in more detail below (see also Fig. 2).

Chronic recordings

In a single aseptic operation under pentobarbital anaesthesia cats were implanted with tungsten microwires, placed in the L7 dorsal root ganglion, and with EMG wires placed in the lateral gastrocnemius muscle. Connectors for external length gauges were inserted into the bony points of origin and insertion of the same muscle. After recovery from surgery neurogram, EMG and length signals were recorded at regular intervals, using telemetry. During such recording sessions, especially when single unit activity from a suspected muscle spindle afferent was detected, the cats were allowed to perform various spontaneous movements, including self-paced walking at various speeds and initiation and cessation of

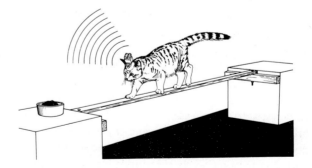

Fig. 1. Chronically implanted cat walking on a narrow beam for food reward. The telemeter, mounted onto an implanted headpiece, was used to monitor ankle extensor (lateral gastrocnemius) EMG and length and single unit activity recorded with micro-wires from the L7 dorsal root ganglion. See also text and Prochazka (1984), and Prochazka et al. (1989b).

locomotion. Alternatively they were enticed (with food rewards) to walk or balance on narrow beams of selectable width (mostly 4 cm), which were mounted on two pedestals 2 m apart and about 50 cm above the floor (see Fig. 1), or they were brought to make preparations for landing, when they were picked up from a bench by the experimenter to be rapidly returned without actually falling (referred to below as "rapid lowering"). At the end of a single unit recording session, the afferent was carefully identified during thiopental anaesthesia (presumed fusimotor silence). Various movements (staircase, sinusoidal or trapezoidal stretches) were applied by hand by the experimenter, both before and after intravenous infusion of succinylcholine, to differentiate between primary and secondary muscle spindle and Golgi tendon organ afferents. For further detail on the above procedures see Prochazka (1984) and Prochazka et al. (1989a, b). Subsequently spindle discharge, length, and EMG signals from representative segments of recording were digitized and stored on computer diskettes, to be transferred to another laboratory for use in acute simulation experiments.

Acute simulation experiments

The stimulation studies were performed on separate, pentobarbital anaesthetized cats. After laminectomy and dorsal and ventral rhizotomy (L6 – S2) 10 – 12 soleus spindle afferents were micro-dissected in dorsal root filaments and mounted for parallel recording. The afferents were screened to identify those which had similar passive stretch response characteristics to one of the chronically recorded units, by monitoring their responses to imposed movements. These were originally recorded in a chronic experiment during deep anaesthesia (see above, unit identification) and were then passively reproduced in the acute experiment, using a hybrid signal generator and an electromagnetic stretcher. Afferents, which matched well the chronic target response to the same movement, were selected for further study. Up to five, functionally single, fusimotor efferents (static

or dynamic, in varying proportions), which acted on the chosen afferent, were then prepared. Saturation tests were performed to determine (for individual efferents, and for groups of γ fibres of the same type) the maximum effective stimulation rates.

Single channel iterations

Chronically recorded active movements where then also replicated with identical time course and amplitude and at the same mean muscle length. These segments were from the same data set (same chronically recorded afferent) as the imposed movements used for the screening of passive response properties (above). For each segment static and/or dynamic γ-activation profiles were sought which permitted a reconstruction of the original (or "target") response to this movement, as recorded in the chronic animal. This was not done simply by trial and error. Instead, in successive stimulation cycles the response (termed "current" response) of the selected spindle afferent to concomitant replicated movement and pulse rate modulated (static and/or dynamic) fusimotor stimulation was compared with the chronic target response. An error signal was then computed which could be incorporated (by subtraction) into the last stimulation profile to generate the stimulation profile of the next stimulation cycle (see Fig. 2, generation of the second stimulation profile using the error, e_1, of the first cycle). Whilst the replicated movement and the target response were invariant for a given sequence of stimulation cycles, the fusimotor stimulation profile was modified, iteratively, and optimized, until the essential features of the target response were matched by the current response. Instead of, or in combination with, the incorporation of the error signal to modify the stimulation profile, the user always had the option of redrawing segments or the entire profile by hand, using a digitizing tablet (Fig. 2, cycle 4, "graphics"). It has previously been shown (Hulliger et al., 1987) that target reconstructing stimulation profiles, which were generated in separate iteration se-

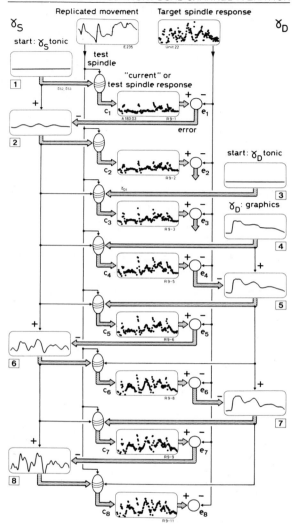

EXPERIMENTAL SIMULATION: DUAL CHANNEL ITERATION

quences and which started from different initial profiles, were identical. In other words, the procedure converged onto a single unique solution, provided that self-perpetuating (since ineffective) high frequency components (beyond the measured cut-off frequency of the $\gamma - $ Ia combinations studied) were removed by suitable low-pass filtering. In the same vein, it was found in the present experiments that care had to be taken to exclude similarly self-perpetuating (although low-frequency) components, which arose when stimulation profiles were allowed to project beyond the saturation limit, in order to secure unique solutions. In both cases this applied to the iterative generation of a single set of stimulation profiles, which was used for the activation of static or dynamic, or for the combined (but identical) activation of static and dynamic efferents, and which is referred to as "single channel" iteration.

ferents, these profiles were converted into rate modulated pulse trains, using voltage controlled oscillators. The data illustrated are from an acute simulation experiment, where two γ_s- and a single γ_d-axon, each mounted on a separate electrode, were stimulated independently. The test spindle of the acute simulation experiment (ellipsoid with sensory spirals) was subjected to concomitant variations of muscle length (replicated movement) and static and dynamic fusimotor drive (shown by arrows converging onto the spindle). The test responses ("current" response of each iteration cycle, $c_1 - c_8$) are illustrated in the centre column. Subtraction of the target from the current response provided an error signal ($e_1 - e_8$, summing points in the column below the target response) which, in most cycles, was used to generate a new stimulation profile for the next iteration cycle. For instance, the error of the first cycle (e_1) was used to generate the new γ_s-stimulation profile of the second cycle. With dual channel operation, two sets of stimulation profiles were generated independently (γ_s, left, γ_d, right). In each cycle the user had to decide which of the two channels the current error signal was to be directed to. This choice and the alternation of operation between channels is indicated by the broad stippled bands and arrows. In contrast, single solid lines and arrows indicate the flow of signals which did not change between cycles. Note that at the end of the 3rd cycle the error signal (e_3) was discarded, since the new γ_d stimulation profile for the 4th cycle was drawn by hand, using a digitizing tablet ("γ_d: graphics"). Finally, note the good match between the target response (top) and the last test response (c_8, bottom), compared with the striking mismatch of the first test spindle response (c_1). Cf. also text and Hulliger et al. (1987).

Fig. 2. Dual channel iteration sequence to reconstruct chronically recorded spindle firing in an acute simulation experiment. Each iteration cycle encompasses the generation of a test response to stretch and fusimotor stimulation, the computation of an error signal, and the generation of the fusimotor stimulation profile of the next cycle. The cycle numbers are indicated in the small square boxes at the left and right hand margins. The replicated movement (two steps and an episode of balancing during beam walking) and the chronic target response of a spindle Ia afferent (top panels) were invariant and used in each iteration cycle as stimulus and reference, respectively. The fusimotor stimulation profiles are shown in the left (γ_s) and right hand (γ_d) columns as analogue signals (driving functions). For stimulation of functionally single fusimotor ef-

Dual channel iterations

Fig. 2 gives an example of the iterative generation of two independent sets of stimulation profiles in two separate activation channels, as was most commonly used for independent stimulation of static and dynamic γ efferents. Individual iteration cycles are identical with those of the single channel procedure, in that a response to combined mechanical and fusimotor stimulation was compared with the target, providing an error signal which then could be incorporated into the fusimotor stimulation profile of the next cycle (cycles 2, 5–8 in Fig. 2). Alternatively this new profile could again be drawn by hand (4th cycle in Fig. 2). The new feature is that two efferent activation profiles could be iteratively modified in alternation and that at the end of each cycle the user had the choice of either continuing with the current or of switching to the other channel. Since in dual channel iterations two variables (X, Y; unknown fusimotor activation profiles) can be altered independently to generate a given target, it is not surprising that strictly unique solutions (in terms of X and Y) were not normally found. In spite of this, some functionally relevant general features of underlying fusimotor firing patterns (broad time course, range and limits) could nevertheless be defined (see Results).

Results

The present report is based on chronic recordings from 6 muscle spindle afferents (5 primaries, 1 secondary, from 5 animals) and on simulation experiments in 26 anaesthetized cats. In these 38 primary and 5 secondary spindle afferents (selected from more than 250 afferents, as screened in passive matching trials) were studied with selective

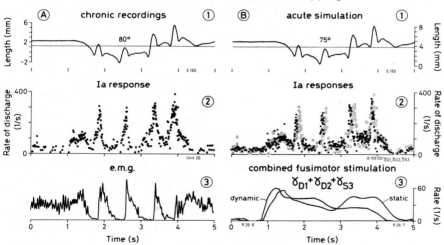

Fig. 3. Stepping episode beginning from quiet standing. A: chronic recordings. B: recordings from an acute simulation experiment. A1, length variations in parent muscle (lateral gastrocnemius), centred around a mean length of 1.3 mm (corresponding to an ankle joint angle of 80°). Calibration: 0 mm corresponding to 90° at the ankle. A2, muscle spindle Ia response. A3, parent muscle EMG. B1, same movement as in A1, replicated in the simulation experiment at 3.75 mm mean length (75° at the ankle; length calibration as in A1). Simulations were performed at this slightly longer mean length, since the passive responses of the two afferents (chronic and acute) to separate imposed movements were best matched (see Methods), when a length offset corresponding to 5° ankle angle offset was introduced. B2, chronic Ia response (large background raster dots) and simulated response (small black dots) during concomitant independent stimulation of two γ_d- and a single γ_s-axon. The simulated response was from the 7th and last cycle of a dual iteration sequence. B3, fusimotor stimulation profiles, as used to generate the response of B2. The dynamic profile was generated at the end of the 5th, and first used in the 6th cycle of the sequence, and then also used without further change in the 7th cycle. The static profile was first used in the 7th and last cycle of the sequence.

or combined stimulation of altogether 32 dynamic and 49 static fusimotor efferents.

Fusimotor wind-up with initiation of locomotion

Fig. $3A_2$ shows the response of a primary spindle afferent from triceps surae during an episode of spontaneous stepping, which started from rest and which was recorded in a chronically implanted cat. Just before the first step the parent muscle shortened (Fig. $2A_1$), as the animal rose from a slightly crouched position. Whilst this was not accompanied by a significant increase in EMG activity (Fig. $2A_3$), there was a clear step-like increase in the afferent's discharge rate, in spite of concomitant muscle shortening. Moreover, the afferent's responses to the four steps which followed were characterized by very high firing rates (peak rates 400/s or more) during muscle stretch (F phase). In contrast, during quiet standing (at the beginning and end of the recordings of Fig. 2A) Ia discharge rate was rather low (around 30/s), whilst mean EMG activity was highest. From these observations it can be inferred qualitatively, that with the onset of locomotion fusimotor drive was stepped up significantly and that, comparing rest with locomotion, the time course of α- and γ-activity was dissociated. However, any quantitative deductions concerning strength and type of fusimotor action would rest on uncertain grounds (see Introduction).

In simulation experiments it was first confirmed that mere passive reproduction of the chronic movement failed to elicit Ia responses that matched the chronic target response during stepping (not illustrated). In contrast, single channel iterations (with parallel activation of static and dynamic γ efferents) gave satisfactory matches of the target response (not illustrated). They indicated that overall fusimotor drive was suddenly increased (from an insignificant resting level) just before the commencement of locomotion, that it declined slightly during the stepping episode, and that it was reset to the low resting value at the end of the stepping sequence. Moreover, single channel iterations with activation of static efferents alone (up to three γ_s fibres stimulated simultaneously) failed to reproduce the first two discharge peaks of the chronic response during the F phase of the first two steps of Fig. 3 (not illustrated). Similarly, selective activation of dynamic fusimotor fibres, whilst reproducing peak discharge rates during the F phase of the steps, failed to maintain spindle firing during the periods of relatively rapid shortening just preceding the first step, and during the stance phase of the first and last step (not illustrated).

These observations confirmed the presence (inferred above) of a transient increase of overall fusimotor drive during the stepping episode of Fig. 3, and they indicate that both static and dynamic action must have contributed to the features of the chronically recorded response. This was further corroborated in dual channel iterations, when γ_s and γ_d efferents were stimulated independently, and when alternating iterations in two channels permitted generation of two different stimulation profiles. Fig. $3B_2$ illustrates the response of a primary afferent during combined activation of a static and two dynamic γ efferents with different patterns of rate modulated stimulation (Fig. $3B_3$). Apart from minor phase differences during the first three steps, the simulated response of Fig. $3B_2$ (black dots) gave a satisfactory approximation of the chronic target response (background raster profile). The successful stimulation profiles are illustrated in Fig. $3B_3$. Combined with other observations from simulations of the same segment, or other examples of initiation of locomotion, they indicate that at the beginning of a walking episode static fusimotor drive is stepped up from a low resting level and then maintained approximately constant, whilst dynamic drive tends to slowly decline after a pronounced initial transient peak.

The particular solution of the dual channel iteration of Fig. $3B_3$ was not unique, since in fine detail the successful stimulation profiles varied from one iteration sequence to the next. However, the main features, as emphasized above, were necessary components. For instance, the initial surge of γ_d drive was indispensable to reproduce the dynamic features of the chronic response during the first two steps (see above). The subsequent decline was also mandatory to avoid exaggerated dynamic responses during the subsequent steps. These took place at longer muscle length where the Ia afferent of Fig. 3B revealed the well known length dependence of sensitivity to stretch (see Hulliger, 1984).

The conclusion that at the beginning of a series of steps static fusimotor drive was stepped up and then maintained at an approximately constant level was further supported in iterative simulations of chronically recorded spindle group II responses. In the simulation experiments concerned the γ efferents, which acted on the selected (best matching) secondary afferent, were identified as static by virtue of their typical effect on separate Ia responses to large ramp and hold stretches (Emonet-Dénand et al., 1977).

Finally, it is evident that the successful stimulation profiles of Fig. $3B_3$ bore no resemblance to the time course of skeletomotor activity, as revealed by the EMG which accompanied the original movement (Fig. $3A_3$). Whilst the EMG showed the characteristic extensor bursts during the $E_1 - E_3$ phase of the step cycle (Philippson, 1905; see also Prochazka et al., 1989b) the static and dynamic fusimotor activation profiles both had dominant tonic components. Also, the superimposed modulation was unrelated to the locomotor rhythm. In a loose sense α and γ motoneurones were "coactivated", since both were active during the walking episode. However, as pointed out above, during the periods of rest at the beginning and end of the sequence α- and γ-activity was entirely dissociated (γ-silence), indicating a significant degree of $\alpha - \gamma$ independence.

Beam walking

When the animals walked on a narrow beam (Fig. 1) afferent discharge patterns often were in-conspicuous and firing rates were low (means well below 100/s, peaks below about 250/s). Spindle firing then was hardly distinguishable from that seen during walking on the floor. Previously, this was shown to be dominated by largely tonic static fusimotor action (Prochazka et al., 1985; Hulliger et al., 1986b). In the present experiments this was confirmed in the majority of cases in single and dual simulations of additional chronic stepping segments. The exception to this rule was a limited number of steps from one animal, where in iterative simulations the chronically recorded Ia response was best matched by steady γ_s combined with approximately EMG modulated γ_d drive, not unlike the pattern described by Murphy et al. (1984) for locomotion in the decerebrate cat.

However, when maintenance of equilibrium required the animal's attention (either due to spontaneous loss of balance or following intentional perturbation of the beam by the experimenter), the animals normally crouched in an attempt to regain equilibrium. Such periods of instability and balancing were frequently accompanied by abrupt surges or transients in spindle discharge rate.

Two examples of recordings during balancing on the beam are shown in Figs. 4 and 5. The chronic afferent recordings are illustrated in Fig. $4A_2$, B_2 and in Fig. 5_2 (background raster patterns). In either case the animal stopped walking and crouched, until balance was regained. Crouching was accompanied by triceps extension (about 4 mm in Fig. 4, and 2 mm in Fig. 5) which provoked dramatic spindle Ia responses, with peak firing rates around 500/s. In either case mere passive simulations (reproduction of the movement without concomitant γ-stimulation) clearly fell short of the chronic target response. This indicated that the balancing was accompanied by a major surge in fusimotor drive.

For both examples of balancing (Figs. 4 and 5) iterative simulations with either pure static action (up to three γ_s fibres stimulated together) or with pure dynamic action (one or two γ_d fibres activated) failed to reproduce important features of the chronic responses. Static action was consistently incapable of reproducing the dynamic transient of the chronic response, even when stimulation rates were allowed to peak at 200 to 300/s. Dynamic action failed to reproduce the high maintained firing rates during the crouch (note the slight shortening during the plateau, at long length) and particularly during the rapid shortening at the end of the crouching phase. These findings suggested that combined static and dynamic fusimotor drive was responsible for the transient

and the maintained increase of firing observed in the chronic recordings.

Fig. 4A is an example of a single channel iteration, where a static and a dynamic γ efferent always were activated with the same pattern of rate modulated stimulation. The successful profile is shown in Fig. $4A_3$ and strongly suggests that a major transient of fusimotor drive indeed accompanied the episode of balancing. However, whilst proving a useful indication of total underlying

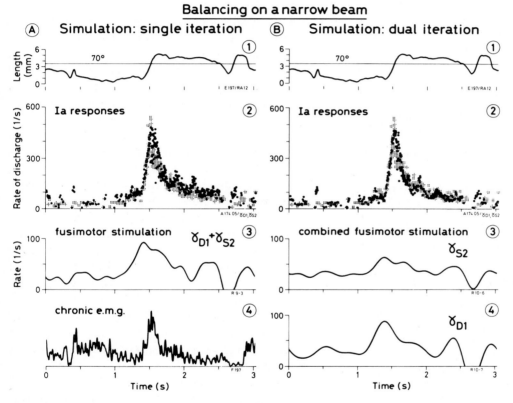

Fig. 4. Balancing on a narrow beam. A: single channel iteration with identical time course of stimulation of a single dynamic and a single static γ-axon. B: dual channel iteration with independent stimulation of the same efferents (see also Fig. 2). A1, B1, replicated movement, muscle stretch plotted upwards; calibration: 0 mm corresponding to an ankle joint angle of 90° in the acute simulation experiment; both in the chronic and the acute experiment the movement was centred around a mean length corresponding to a joint angle of 70° (fine reference line). A2, B2, chronic Ia response (large background raster dots), same in A and B, and simulated responses (small black dots) from two separate iteration sequences in the same experiment and with the same test spindle afferent. In A2, iterative simulation was terminated after three cycles. In B2, the target reproducing simulated response was reached after seven iterations. A3, B3, and B4, fusimotor stimulation profiles (same γ_d and γ_s fibres in A and B), in A3, 3rd iteration, in B3, 6th, and in B4, 7th iteration. A4, chronically recorded EMG of parent muscle (lateral gastrocnemius). In the chronic experiment the cat was about to lose balance at the beginning of the segment illustrated (top) and stopped walking. During the first 1.5 s, the animal stood quietly, at 1.5 s it crouched (rapid stretch), and after 2.5 s it resumed walking.

fusimotor drive, the finding permitted no conclusions regarding the distribution of action between static and dynamic efferents.

Fig. 4B illustrates the results of a dual channel iterative reconstruction of the same chronic

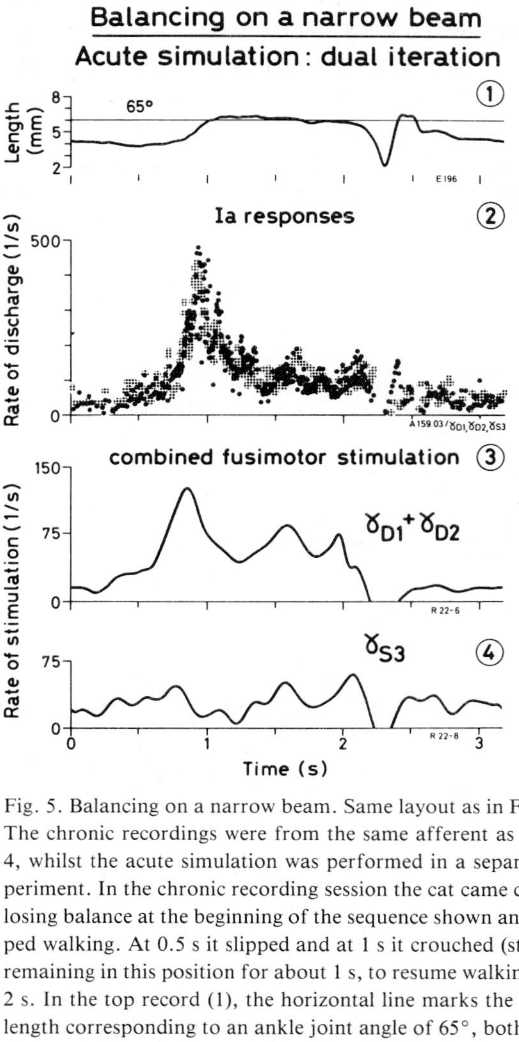

Fig. 5. Balancing on a narrow beam. Same layout as in Fig. 4B. The chronic recordings were from the same afferent as in Fig. 4, whilst the acute simulation was performed in a separate experiment. In the chronic recording session the cat came close to losing balance at the beginning of the sequence shown and stopped walking. At 0.5 s it slipped and at 1 s it crouched (stretch), remaining in this position for about 1 s, to resume walking after 2 s. In the top record (1), the horizontal line marks the muscle length corresponding to an ankle joint angle of 65°, both in the chronic and acute recordings. In the second panel, the best matching simulated response was reached in the 8th and last cycle of a dual channel iteration sequence, during concomitant variations of muscle length and static and dynamic fusimotor drive. The final dynamic stimulation profile (third panel, two γ_d-axons stimulated) was from the 6th iteration cycle, and the final static profile (bottom, a single γ_s-axon stimulated) from the 8th cycle.

response during balancing. The target reproducing stimulation profiles, which were generated independently, are shown in Fig. $4B_3$ and B_4. Both profiles exhibited a tonic background component and a superimposed transient of fusimotor drive, which in this and other examples of balancing on the beam was consistently larger for dynamic than for static efferents (cf. also Fig. 5). These transients preceded and overlapped the rapid stretch and the concomitant surge of Ia discharge during crouching by about 300 ms. Moreover, they preceded the surge of EMG by the same amount. A detailed comparison (Fig. $4A_2$ and B_2) of the degree of matching that was achieved, shows that independently generated (i.e. separate) static and dynamic activation patterns were more successful in reproducing the chronic response (note, e.g., the mismatch in Fig. $4A_2$ just before and during the decay of the peak of afferent firing).

Fig. 5 provides another example of a dual channel iterative reconstruction of a chronically recorded response during balancing. The successful γ_d- and γ_s-stimulation profiles (panels 3 and 4) illustrate the features emphasized above (Fig. 4) even more clearly. In spite of the smaller length excursion during the crouch (cf. Fig. 4) the afferent response was equally impressive. Its reconstruction was only possible with a powerful surge of dynamic fusimotor drive (note that two γ_d fibres were stimulated at up to 125/s). As in the example of Fig. 4, the increase in fusimotor drive preceded the stretch (at the beginning of crouching) and the concomitant surge in EMG (not illustrated) by about 300 ms.

Whilst the general features of the profiles illustrated in Figs. 4 and 5 were reproducible (within and between experiments) the details of the emerging patterns were not, since − within limits − power of fusimotor action could be redistributed between efferent channels. Hence, strictly, the solutions were not unique, but the functionally interesting features, i.e. the surge in overall drive, with a compulsory γ_d transient, were general. Moreover, the presence of largely tonic static fusimotor drive was further confirmed in simulations of chronic spindle secondary responses during beam walking. In these trials the fusimotor efferents were fully identified as static γ motoneurones by their unambiguous static effect on simultaneously recorded Ia responses to large stretches (Emonet-Dénand et al., 1977). In this case the simulations were single channel iterations and provided unique solutions (Hulliger et al., 1987).

Taken together, these observations then indicate that a major surge of fusimotor drive was initiated some 300 ms before the animal crouched in order to regain its balance. This surge was clearly more pronounced for dynamic than for static efferents. In either case the pattern and timing of activation differed significantly from the concomitant EMG. This further suggests that in these corrective reactions the control of α, γ_s, and γ_d motoneurones encompasses a significant measure of mutual independence.

Preparation for landing

When cats were lifted up from a bench by the experimenter and then rapidly returned, spindle Ia firing gradually increased whilst the animal was in mid-air (Fig. 6, chronic recording shown as background raster profile). This was accompanied by slow ankle extension and shortening of lateral gastrocnemius, the parent muscle of the afferent of Fig. 6. Upon landing, the muscle was stretched very rapidly under the sudden impact of the body weight, and the afferent showed a pronounced transient response, with discharge rate peaking around 500/s (Fig. 6).

Passive simulations of the length variations during lifting and rapid lowering were suboptimal, demonstrating that these manipulations were accompanied by activation of fusimotor neurones. Likewise, iterative simulations with pure static action failed to reproduce the characteristic transient peak of the chronic response (both not illustrated). However, good approximations were achieved in simulations with pure dynamic action. These yielded waxing and waning profiles (Fig. 6, bottom), where setting (i.e. an increase) of fusimotor drive in mid-air was followed by resetting (reduction) of

drive upon landing. Powerful dynamic action was required to achieve such matches, as is illustrated in the example of Fig. 6, where two γ_d fibres had to be activated at stimulation rates up to 75/s. When, in dual channel iterations, static action was allowed to contribute, comparable matches of the target response were obtained. The dynamic stimulation profiles then still peaked just before landing (as in Fig. 6, bottom), but the build-up of drive was somewhat delayed and then more abrupt.

Whilst on the evidence of simulation trials (as in Fig. 6) dynamic fusimotor drive peaked just before

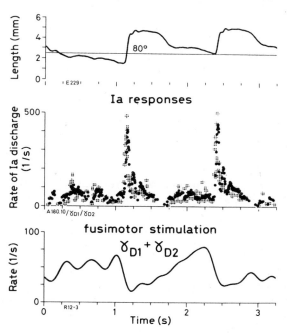

Fig. 6. Preparation for landing during rapid lowering. Same layout and calibrations as in Figs. 3B to 5. In the chronic recording session the animal was repeatedly lifted up by the experimenter and then rapidly returned to a laboratory bench. When it was in mid-air the parent muscle (lateral gastrocnemius) was only weakly activated, but since the body weight did not have to be supported it nevertheless shortened slightly (1st second and around 2 s). Upon impact from landing, the muscle was stretched very rapidly (top), and the EMG revealed a large synchronous peak (not illustrated).

impact on the supporting surface, the EMG of the parent muscle rose and fell strictly in phase with the afferents' dynamic peak during landing, whilst in mid-air it remained at a low steady level.

Taken together, these findings demonstrate a significant degree of $\alpha - \gamma$ dissociation and either selective (Fig. 6) or predominant (dual iterations) activation of dynamic efferents in preparation for landing. It appears therefore, that setting and resetting of fusimotor drive can take place within short periods of time (less than a second).

Discussion

The simulation method

Spindle afferent discharge during voluntary movement is determined by the length variations of the parent muscle and the type and time course of any concomitant fusimotor drive. In the present experiments an experimental iterative simulation method has been used to infer the patterns (amplitude, time course) of activation of static and dynamic fusimotor efferents from chronically recorded spindle afferent responses. The method is based on the reproduction of chronically recorded length variations in acute experiments, and on the correction of any mismatch between acute test responses and chronic target responses by adding appropriate amounts of tonic or phasic, static and/or dynamic fusimotor drive. In its present form the method has two main limitations. First, it fails to give strictly unique solutions, when static and dynamic drive are allowed to vary independently, and second, for the present data, it rests on the assumption that local spindle length variations are scaled versions of whole muscle length variations.

For functional considerations the lack of uniqueness of solutions is relative rather than absolute. It is true that for dual channel iterations (generating independent γ_s and γ_d profiles) the fusimotor power (as required for successful simulations) can, within limits, be redistributed between static and dynamic efferents. However, certain characteristic properties of these efferents

provide boundary conditions, which limit the range of possible solutions. In the present experiments extremely high Ia discharge rates (beyond $400 - 500/s$) during stretch could normally only be accounted for by activation of dynamic efferents, and discharge rates beyond about $100/s$ during fast shortening usually required static fusimotor action. Also, for reproducible behaviour static fusimotor drive can be estimated independently in simulations of chronically recorded spindle secondary responses, where single channel iterations provide unique solutions.

Estimates of local muscle spindle length variations, based on ultrasonic measurements of single muscle fibre − rather than whole muscle − length changes have provided evidence that the latter might be a poor approximation of the former (Hoffer et al., 1989, this volume). The discrepancies described have been attributed to effects of tendon compliance and of alterations in muscle fibre pinnation angle, both depending on the degree of activation of the muscle. If these effects are large and general, then the present experiments may have underestimated fusimotor drive during the active phases of the movements. Under these conditions spindles in the chronic recordings would then have been exposed to smaller internal length changes than were apparent externally. Moreover, in the simulations the chronically recorded active movements were replicated passively. However, some caution may be indicated, before whole muscle length recordings are entirely dismissed. Control experiments to assess the impact of distributed skeletomotor activation upon spindle Ia sensitivity to imposed movements have revealed rather small effects (Appenteng et al., 1983; Elek et al., 1989, and to be published). Moreover, if present they were only seen at short muscle lengths, whilst at longer lengths (as in Figs. $3 - 6$) they were hardly detectable.

Flexible fusimotor control

Earlier evidence from simulation studies indicated that spindle Ia responses to unpredictably imposed stretches were dominated by selective dynamic fusimotor activation (Hulliger et al., 1985; Prochazka et al., 1985), and that the sensitization of primary afferents in paw shake responses was due to similarly selective, waxing and waning dynamic fusimotor drive (Prochazka et al., 1989a). The purpose of the present experiments was to seek additional evidence for flexible fusimotor control in different types of movement, and to test the hypothesis that selective activation of dynamic γ efferents was related to the novelty or unfamiliarity of motor tasks.

It was confirmed that routine steady state stepping in a familiar environment was dominated by static fusimotor action. However, at the beginning of a stepping episode, fusimotor wind-up (as previously inferred by Loeb et al., 1985) involved dynamic as well as static fusimotor activation. Yet over a few step cycles dynamic drive gradually declined whilst static action was maintained, in agreement with the earlier results (above). Further, when cats came close to losing balance while walking on a narrow, occasionally perturbed beam, corrective reactions were accompanied by a significant transient increase of dynamic fusimotor drive, which strongly enhanced Ia sensitivity to stretch, e.g. when the animal crouched. Similar, and possibly selective, transient activation of dynamic efferents occurred in preparation of (and prior to) landing from rapid lowering. As in the case of beam walking, this strongly sensitized primary afferents to the rapid stretch (upon landing) of the ankle extensor muscles, in line with earlier descriptions of high afferent sensitivity after landing from free falls (Prochazka et al., 1977; Lewis et al., 1979). In all these cases the fusimotor activation profiles bore no resemblance to the time course of parent muscle EMG, as recorded chronically. This further corroborates that $\alpha - \gamma$ coactivation, even in its loosest sense, is not a general rule of fusimotor control (Hulliger et al., 1985; Prochazka et al., 1985).

These findings clearly provide further evidence for flexibility and selectivity of central control, particularly of dynamic fusimotor efferents. Yet it is equally evident that unfamiliarity or even novel-

ty of a motor task cannot be the only determinant of such selective activation. Landing from rapid lowering (a laboratory paradigm) and walking on a perturbed beam may be unfamiliar, but initiation of locomotion is not. However, the possibility remains that novelty is one of several factors promoting setting of dynamic fusimotor drive, to sensitize spindle feedback when this is required for accurate motor performance.

Acknowledgements

This work was supported by grants from the Swiss National Science Foundation, the Hartmann Müller Foundation for Medical Research, the Alberta Heritage Foundation for Medical Research, and the British Medical Research Council. We thank Werner Frey for competent technical assistance in the simulation experiments and Ruth Emch, Eva Hochreutener and Hans Künzli for their excellent art and photographic work.

References

Appelberg, B. (1981) Selective central control of dynamic gamma motoneurones utilized for the functional classification of gamma cells. In A. Taylor and A. Prochazka (Eds.), *Muscle Receptors and Movement,* Macmillan, London, pp. 97 – 108.

Appenteng, K., Morimoto, T. and Taylor, A. (1980) Fusimotor activity in masseter nerve of the cat during reflex jaw movements. *J. Physiol. (London),* 305: 415 – 431.

Appenteng, K., Hulliger, M., Prochazka, A. and Zangger, P. (1983) Distributed α- and γ-stimulation in anaesthetized cats during simulation of normal movements: matching of spindle afferent discharge patterns to deduce fusimotor action. *J. Physiol. (London),* 339: 10P.

Bessou, P., Dupui, P., Cabelguen, J.-M., Joffroy, M., Montoya, R. and Pagès, B. (1989) Discharge patterns of gamma motoneurone populations of extensor and flexor hindlimb muscles during walking in the thalamic cat. In J.H.J. Allum and M. Hulliger (Eds.), *Afferent Control of Posture and Locomotion, Prog. Brain Res., Vol. 80,* Elsevier, Amsterdam, pp. 37 – 45.

Cabelguen, J.-M. (1981) Static and dynamic fusimotor controls in various hindlimb muscles during locomotor activity in the decorticate cat. *Brain Res.,* 213: 83 – 97.

Eklund, G., von Euler, C. and Rutkowski, S. (1964) Spontaneous and reflex activity of intercostal gamma motoneurones. *J. Physiol. (London),* 171: 139 – 163.

Elek, J., Hulliger, M., Prochazka, A., Vincent, S. and Waldon V. (1989) Stretch of gastrocnemius tendons in cat step cycle inferred from muscle spindle responses to active and passive movements. *J. Physiol. (London), 414:* 18P.

Emonet-Dénand, F., Laporte, Y., Matthews, P.B.C. and Petit, J. (1977) On the subdivision of static and dynamic fusimotor actions on the primary ending of the cat muscle spindle. *J. Physiol. (London), 268:* 827 – 861.

Gottlieb, S. and Taylor, A. (1983) Interpretation of fusimotor activity in cat masseter nerve during reflex jaw movements. *J. Physiol. (London),* 345: 423 – 438.

Granit, R. (1955) *Receptors and Sensory Perception.* Yale University Press, New Haven, 369 pp.

Greer, J.J. and Stein, R.B. (1986) Tonic and phasic activity of gamma motoneurons during respiration in the cat. *Soc. Neurosci. Abstr.,* 12: 683.

Hoffer, J.A., Caputi, A.A., Pose, I.E. and Griffiths, R.I. (1989) Roles of muscle activity and load on the relationship between muscle spindle length and whole muscle length in the freely walking cat. In J.H.J. Allum and M. Hulliger (Eds.), *Afferent Control of Posture and Locomotion, Prog. Brain Res., Vol. 80,* Elsevier, Amsterdam, pp. 75 – 85.

Hulliger, M. (1984) The mammalian muscle spindle and its central control. *Rev. Physiol. Biochem. Pharmacol.,* 101: 1 – 110.

Hulliger, M. (1987) The role of muscle spindle receptors and fusimotor neurones in the control of movement. In R.J. Ellingson, N.M.F. Murray and A.M. Halliday (Eds.), *The London Symposia (EEG Suppl. 39),* Elsevier, Amsterdam, pp. 58 – 66.

Hulliger, M. and Prochazka, A. (1983) A new simulation method to deduce fusimotor activity from afferent discharge recorded in freely moving cats. *J. Neurosci. Methods, 8:* 197 – 204.

Hulliger, M., Zangger, P., Prochazka, A. and Appenteng, K. (1985) Fusimotor "set" vs. $\alpha - \gamma$ linkage in voluntary movement in cats. In A. Struppler and A. Weindl (Eds.), *Electromyography and Evoked Potentials, Adv. Applied Neurol. Sciences, Vol. 1,* Springer-Verlag, Heidelberg, pp. 56 – 63.

Hulliger, M., Prochazka, A. and Trend, P. (1986a) Applicability of the concept of "fusimotor set" during voluntary movement to biarticular hindlimb muscles. *Neurosci. Lett., Suppl.* 26: S164.

Hulliger, M., Prochazka A. and Zangger, P. (1986b) Fusimotor activity in freely moving cats. Tests of concepts derived from reduced preparations. In S. Grillner, P.S.G. Stein, D.G. Stuart, H. Forssberg and R.M. Herman (Eds.), *Neurobiology of Vertebrate Locomotion,* Macmillan, London, pp. 593 – 605.

Hulliger, M., Horber, F., Medved, A. and Prochazka, A. (1987) An experimental simulation method for iterative and interactive reconstruction of unknown (fusimotor) inputs contributing to known (spindle afferent) responses. *J. Neurosci. Methods, 21:* 225 – 238.

Lewis, M.McD., Prochazka, A., Sontag, K.-H. and Wand, P. (1979) Efferent and afferent responses during falling and landing in cats. In R. Granit and O. Pompeiano (Eds.), *Reflex Control of Posture and Movement, Prog. Brain Res., Vol. 50,* pp. 423 – 428.

Loeb, G.E. and Hoffer, J.A. (1985) Activity of spindle afferents from cat anterior thigh muscles. II. Effects of fusimotor blockade. *J. Neurophysiol.,* 54: 565 – 577.

Loeb, G.E., Hoffer, J.A. and Pratt, C.A. (1985) Activity of spindle afferents from cat anterior thigh muscles. I. Identification and patterns during normal locomotion. *J. Neurophysiol.,* 54: 549 – 564.

Matthews, P.B.C. (1972) *Mammalian Muscle Receptors and their Central Actions.* Arnold, London, 630 pp.

Morgan, D.L., Prochazka, A. and Proske, U. (1985) Action of single dynamic fusimotor neurones on cat soleus Ia afferents during muscle shortening. *Exp. Brain Res.,* 58: 56 – 61.

Murphy, P.R., Stein, R.B. and Taylor, J. (1984) Phasic and tonic modulation of impulse rates in γ-motoneurons during locomotion in premammillary cats. *J. Neurophysiol.,* 52: 228 – 243.

Perret, C. and Berthoz, A. (1973) Evidence of static and dynamic fusimotor actions on the spindle responses to sinusoidal stretch during locomotor activity in the cat. *Exp. Brain Res.,* 18: 178 – 188.

Philippson, M. (1905) L'autonomie et la centralisation dans le système nerveux des animaux. *Trav. Lab. Physiol. Inst. Solvay Bruxelles,* 7: 1 – 208.

Prochazka, A. (1984) Chronic techniques for studying neurophysiology of movement in cats. In R. Lemon (Ed.) *Methods of Neuronal Recording in Conscious Animals, IBRO Handbook Series, Methods in the Neurosciences, Vol. 4,* Wiley, Chichester, pp. 113 – 128.

Prochazka, A. (1989) Sensorimotor gain control: a basic strategy of motor systems? *Prog. Neurobiology,* in press.

Prochazka, A. and Hulliger, M. (1983) Muscle afferent function and its significance for motor control mechanisms during voluntary movements in cat, monkey, and man. In J.E. Desmedt (Ed.), *Motor Control Mechanisms in Health and Disease, Adv. Neurol.* 39, pp. 93 – 132.

Prochazka, A., Westerman, R.A. and Ziccone, S.P. (1977) Ia afferent activity during a variety of voluntary movements in the cat. *J. Physiol. (London),* 268: 423 – 448.

Prochazka, A., Hulliger, M., Zangger, P. and Appenteng, K. (1985) "Fusimotor set": new evidence of α-independent control of γ-motoneurones during movement in the awake cat. *Brain Res.,* 339: 136 – 140.

Prochazka, A., Hulliger, M., Trend, P., Llewellyn, M. and Dürmüller, N. (1989a) Muscle afferent contribution to control of paw shakes in normal cats. *J. Neurophysiol.,* 61: 550 – 562.

Prochazka, A., Trend, P., Hulliger, M. and Vincent, S. (1989b) Ensemble proprioceptive activity in the cat step cycle: towards a representative look-up chart. In J.H.J. Allum and

M. Hulliger (Eds.), *Afferent Control of Posture and Locomotion, Prog. Brain Res., Vol. 80,* Elsevier, Amsterdam, pp. 61–74.

Rioult-Pedotti, M.S., Kohen, R. and Hulliger, M. (1988) On the ability of static and dynamic γ-motoneurones to maintain spindle Ia firing during muscle shortening. *Eur. J. Neurosci. Suppl.,* 1: 269.

Schieber, M.H. and Thach, W.T. (1985) Trained slow tracking. II. Bidirectional discharge patterns of cerebellar nuclear, motor cortex, and spindle afferent neurons. *J. Neurophysiol.,* 54: 1228–1270.

Schwarz, M., Sontag, K.-H. and Wand, P. (1984) Nondopaminergic neurones of the reticular part of substantia nigra can gate static fusimotor action onto flexors in cat. *J. Physiol. (London),* 354: 333–344.

Sjöström, A. and Zangger, P. (1976) Muscle spindle control during locomotor movements generated by the deafferented spinal cord. *Acta Physiol. Scand.,* 97: 281–291.

Taylor, A. and Donga, R. (1989) Central mechanisms of selective fusimotor control. In J.H.J. Allum and M. Hulliger (Eds.), *Afferent Control of Posture and Locomotion, Prog. Brain Res., Vol. 80,* Elsevier, Amsterdam, pp. 27–35.

Taylor, J., Stein, R.B. and Murphy, P.R. (1985) Impulse rates and sensitivity to stretch of soleus muscle spindle afferent fibers during locomotion in premammillary cats. *J. Neurophysiol.,* 53: 341–360.

Vallbo, Å.B., Hagbarth, K.-E., Torebjörk, H.E. and Wallin, B.G. (1979) Somatosensory, proprioceptive, and sympathetic activity in human peripheral nerves. *Physiol. Rev.,* 59: 919–957.

Vallbo, Å.B. and Hulliger, M. (1981) Independence of skeletomotor and fusimotor activity in man? *Brain Res.,* 223: 176–180.

J.H.J. Allum and M. Hulliger (Eds.)
Progress in Brain Research, Vol. 80
© 1989 Elsevier Science Publishers B.V. (Biomedical Division)

CHAPTER 9

Analysis of human long-latency reflexes by cooling the peripheral conduction pathway; which afferents are involved?

P.B.C. Matthews

University Laboratory of Physiology, Parks Road, Oxford OX1 3PT, U.K.

This chapter first outlines current views on the afferents of origin of human "long-latency stretch reflexes", and especially whether they are fast or slow. Attention is concentrated on methodology; other approaches can be found elsewhere with appropriate bibliography (Marsden et al., 1983; Matthews, 1985, 1986a; Wiesendanger, 1986). Recent experiments involving cooling of the human arm are then described. They were performed on the abductor digiti minimi and first dorsal interosseus muscles. The arm was cooled from wrist to axilla by circulating cold water through a tube wrapped round it. Cooling slows conduction by a constant proportion, hence the conduction delay introduced by cooling a segment of nerve is greater for small slow axons than for large fast ones. On this basis it was concluded that group I muscle afferents (presumably Ia) can elicit a long-latency reflex with a long central delay, as also can fast cutaneous afferents. No evidence was found for a long-latency reflex with the delay introduced peripherally by conduction along slow axons (i.e. spindle group II afferents). However, the co-existence of such a mechanism has yet to be excluded.

Key words: Cold; Conduction velocity; Muscle spindle; Muscle stretch; Muscle reflex; Stretch reflex; Reflex; Temperature; Tendon jerk; Vibration

Introduction and survey of methodology

It is now some 30 years since Hammond (1960), using biceps, first recorded the complex EMG responses that are evoked in a human muscle when it is forcibly stretched while it is being contracted voluntarily. Following his lead, all have continued to agree that any initial short-latency component (M1) is attributable to the excitation of Ia afferents from the spindle primary endings which then excite the motoneurones via mono- or oligo-synaptic spinal pathways. However, confusion still reigns over the origin of the later (M2, M3) components of the response, and in spite of many bold words there has been little improvement on Hammond's original suggestions that either "it might be carried by slower afferents" or that the effects of fast afferents are delayed by their being mediated via "a longer route in the central nervous system".

For some years attention was diverted away from Hammond's original dichotomy by what now appears to have been a side issue, namely could the supposed delayed response be due simply to a continued Ia short-latency action with the reflex fortuitously segmented into a series of apparently separate responses by adventitious factors (such as muscle resonances breaking up a continuing Ia discharge into a series of bursts). This can now be readily accepted as playing an important part in determining the precise waveform of the EMG response. But it can be dismissed as the origin of everything that is otherwise attributable to genuine long-latency action, distinct from the monosynaptic reflex.

Unloading response

The strongest evidence for such a curt dismissal of an important factor is obtained by shifting attention away from the effects of stretching the contracting muscle to the effects of releasing it, and observing what happens on reducing the ongoing reflex drive rather than increasing it. The resultant unloading response, consisting of a reduction of the pre-existing EMG activity, can be considered as the mirror image of the stretch response and the same questions asked about the origin of its various components, in so far as they can again be recognized. For the long flexor of the thumb, the long-latency component of the unloading response occurs virtually on its own, uncontaminated by a short-latency component, thus testifying to its distinctiveness by eliminating the possibility of attributing it to successive bursts of Ia firing (Matthews, 1984a). Slow stretch may also evoke a relatively pure long-latency response, but it is then much harder to rule out the possibility that this might be due to the need for temporal summation of the central effects of a slowly incrementing afferent discharge. Rapid stretch evokes a clear short-latency response, whereas changing the velocity of release has little or no effect on the latency of the unloading response.

Flexor digitorum profundus has recently been shown to behave similarly to flexor pollicis longus and this has allowed a further possibility to be dismissed, namely that the long-latency unloading response might represent an active inhibition evoked from the excitation of proprioceptors in the stretched antagonist, rather than a disfacilitation due to a reduction of afferent firing from receptors in the agonist on its release (Matthews and Miles, 1988a,b). The distinction was made possible by the ability to position the hand so that the extensor tendons are mechanically disengaged from acting at the terminal interphalangeal joint while the deep flexor tendon remains engaged; this has long been known to anatomists and has already been exploited to study proprioception (Gandevia et al., 1983).

Paucity of experimental methods

The reason for the failure of a plethora of papers to establish where all the time disappears in a long-latency reflex is basically due to the paucity of techniques available to attack the problem at its heart. There are plenty of observations of the EMG responses evoked by a variety of differing waveforms of stretch applied to a variety of muscles. These certainly suggest the important principle that different muscles may be controlled differently, being influenced in different degree by short and long latency pathways; but that is only a beginning.

In both animals and man, stimulation at, and recording from, a variety of sites within the CNS have established both that the requisite circuitry exists, and that there is indeed plenty of time available for Ia activity elicited by muscle stretch to reach the motor cortex and then be reflected back to the muscle in question to produce a "long-latency" response of the observed latency. The study of patients with a variety of lesions typically shows that long-latency responses are eliminated by damage to the postulated long-loop pathway to the motor cortex and back; but this does not prove whether the effect is direct, by interrupting the reflex pathway itself, or indirect, by interfering with circuits which control the responsiveness of lower reflex centres (notably those in the spinal cord). Moreover, in some animal work late responses have persisted after ablating the higher centres, arguing that the loss of time can be produced other than by transmission to and from the cerebral cortex.

Local anaesthesia and multiple pathways

One current impediment to clear thinking is that too few words are being used for too many things; partly through a poverty of vocabulary, somewhat similar responses are liable to be equated instead of being distinguished as separate entities. There is no reason why distinct responses, with quite different underlying mechanisms, should not have much the same latency and be evoked by the same crude stimulus. In human studies, what tends to be thought of simply as "muscle stretch" in fact means joint displacement, with its consequential afferent input from joint receptors and surrounding skin; the relative balance between cutaneous and muscular reflexes could well vary both with the precise details of stimulation and with the central "set" of the subject. However, it has been amply proved that cutaneous/joint afferents cannot be held uniquely responsible for long-latency responses, since these may persist after the moving part has been rendered insentient by local anaesthesia while the more distant controlling muscle remains unaffected.

It bears emphasis, since there has been some confusion about the matter, that the early observations on the long thumb flexor which suggested that such local anaesthesia inevitably abolishes all long-latency action (Marsden et al., 1972) has not been upheld by subsequent work; the late thumb responses have now been repeatedly observed to survive both in the original two subjects after continued experimentation (Marsden et al., 1977) and in a variety of other subjects, naive or otherwise (Marsden et al., 1979; Matthews, 1984a; Loo and McCloskey, 1985). For all other muscles long-latency responses have regularly been found to persist after eliminating cutaneous and joint inputs by local anaesthesia (big toe, Marsden et al., 1977; foot, Iles, 1977, Chan et al., 1979; wrist, Bawa and McKenzie, 1981; finger, Matthews and Miles, 1988b).

The reported abolition (Darton et al., 1985) of a late response from the first dorsal interosseus muscle seems likely to be a testimony to the power of cutaneous reflexes from the human hand, and certainly cannot be taken to argue against the existence of long-latency muscular reflexes for other muscles. Electrical stimulation of digital nerves produces powerful long-latency responses which

much evidence suggests are mediated transcortically (Jenner and Stephens, 1982). It seems likely that cutaneous and muscular responses are often superimposed to produce a compound response. For the flexor digitorum profundus, local anaesthesia may remove a late component of the overall responses, while leaving the earlier components unaffected (Matthews and Miles, 1988b).

Slow afferents

Until recently, relatively little attention was paid to the possible role of slow afferents. Then a series of experiments comparing the effects of stretch and vibration were used to argue that slow afferents provide a large and perhaps exclusive contribution to the muscular component of the long-latency response (Matthews, 1984a). The essential observation was that vibration fails to elicit a long-latency response that is at all comparable with that elicited by stretch. In comparison with stretch, vibration only weakly excites the group II afferents from the spindle secondary endings thus suggesting that these relatively slow afferents might be responsible for the long-latency response. Alternative explanations can fairly readily be constructed to cover the different effects at the onset of a stretch or a period of vibration, so the group II hypothesis has not gained universal acceptance. However, such alternative explanations cannot be readily extended to cover the effects of cessation of stimulation: mirroring the contrast seen at the commencement of stimulation, release of stretch gives a long-latency unloading response while cessation of vibration gives a short-latency reduction of EMG activity. So both of Hammond's original suggestions remain very much alive.

Comparison of the latency of the long-latency responses evoked from different muscles might seem to offer a promising way of determining whether the delay of the long-latency reflex was introduced peripherally or centrally. On comparing muscles in the same limb, the excess delay of the long over the short latency response should be the same if the delay occurred centrally (through long-loop transmission), but greater for peripheral muscles if the delay occurred peripherally (by virtue of conduction in slow afferents). On the other hand, on comparing muscles in the upper and lower limbs, at the same distance from the spinal cord, the excess delay should be the same for a spinal reflex activated by slow afferents, but greater for the leg than the arm for a transcortical reflex dependent upon fast afferents. Unfortunately, such experiments have failed to produce an agreed answer. This is largely because of the difficulty of ensuring that equivalent reflexes are indeed being compared for the different muscles; such complications have already been discussed (Matthews, 1984b). It may be emphasized that the well known comparison of responses of muscles controlling the jaw, thumb and big toe (Marsden et al., 1976b) does nothing to resolve the problem, since the lengths of both the central and the peripheral conduction pathways alter in parallel.

Cooling

Darton et al. (1985) introduced cooling of the limb as a completely independent way of testing whether the afferent limb of the reflex depends upon fast or upon slow afferent fibres. The rationale is provided by the demonstration, by single fibre recording in the cat, that cooling reduces the conduction velocity of medullated axons by a constant proportion of the normal warm value, irrespective of their size and initial conduction velocity (Paintal, 1965; Franz and Iggo, 1968). Thus the the extra time taken to traverse a given section of cooled nerve, over and above the normal value, is greater for slow than for fast fibres, since their initial conduction time is the greater. Darton et al. (1985) used cooling to study the responses recorded from the first dorsal interosseus muscle on tapping the index finger. They stated that the early and late components of response were slowed by the same absolute amount by cooling, and concluded that they had thereby excluded any contribution from slow afferents to their particular long-latency response; they extended this conclusion to cover all other long-latency responses, including those studied by Matthews (1984a) for the thumb flexor.

It is the thesis of this chapter that cooling does indeed provide a powerful tool for attacking the question, but that Darton et al. (1985) failed to deploy it under sufficiently discriminating conditions for their statements to be accepted at face value, even though some of their conclusions are probably correct. Two major points need to be made about their experiments. First, judging by their illustrated example, it seems doubtful whether the latency of their long-latency response could be measured with sufficient accuracy to permit a definitive conclusion on the relative slowing of the two components of reflex response. The particular problem is that the late response follows hard on the heels of the early response, so that its precise beginning cannot be decided upon with sufficient certainty; this would not matter if the waveform of the responses remained constant during cooling (since the latency of any other two points could then be compared), but this was not so.

The second point arises from the probability, on their own showing on the basis of further experiments, that the particular long-latency response they studied was cutaneous rather than muscular in origin (vide supra). If this is accepted, then their cooling experiment becomes uninterpretable in terms of afferent fibre size. This is because of the anatomically complex innervation of the hand so that the skin overlying a muscle may be supplied by a different nerve from the muscle itself. In their particular case, the skin of the index finger is supplied by the median nerve whereas the first dorsal interosseus muscle is supplied by the ulnar nerve. Thus the efferent limb of their reflexes was invariably in the ulnar nerve, whereas the afferent limb might have been either in the ulnar nerve (for a muscular reflex) or in the median nerve (for a cutaneous reflex). This would not matter if cooling affected the two nerves equally; however, by virtue of lying more deeply, the median nerve might be expected to be cooled appreciably the less. Thus without further study it is quite inappropriate to use the short-latency muscular reflex as the standard by which to compare the slowing of the long-latency, possibly cutaneous, reflex.

The effects of cooling thus appeared ripe for re-examination, as described below. Some of the findings have already been described in brief (Matthews, 1986b, 1987), but full publication awaits the performance of further experiments. The present account provides more detail and discussion than before so as to highlight the basic argument, but no attempt has been made to provide full documentation or illustration.

Present methodology

The difficulties with the previous cooling experiments were largely circumvented as follows: –
(1) For one series of experiments the abductor digiti minimi (ADM) muscle was used; this has the advantage that both it and its overlying skin are supplied by the ulnar nerve.
(2) The ADM was found to lack an appreciable short latency response so that the beginning of its long-latency response could be determined, and its latency measured, with much greater certainty than when it immediately follows an earlier response.
(3) Ramp displacements were used as well as taps. These produced relatively little short latency response from the first dorsal interosseus (FDI) muscle, thus enabling the latency of its long-latency response also to be determined with reasonable certainty.
(4) The F wave was used as the standard to indicate the amount of slowing of large axons produced by the cooling; the F wave is the recurrent discharge elicited from a small number of motoneurones on exciting them antidromically on stimulating their axons peripherally. On the reasonably safe assumption that afferents behave similarly to efferents of comparable size, the slowing of the F wave induced by stimulating the ulnar nerve at the wrist gives the slowing to be expected of a muscular reflex dependent upon fast afferents. Recent control experiments confirm that the use of the F wave is not vitiated by any prolongation of the refractory period of the motor axons on cooling (Matthews, 1988; unlike the reflex, the returning orthodromic volley responsible for the F wave might have shown significant additional slowing by virtue of travelling in the relative refractory period).

The use of the F wave was essential for ADM, since its short-latency response was never good enough to provide a reference. It also proved preferable to the use of the short-latency response of FDI, by virtue of normally being easier to measure. It had the further merit that it could be applied equally to axons travelling in the median nerve by recording from the median-innervated muscles of the thenar eminence on stimulating the median nerve at the wrist.

Cooling

Fig. 1 illustrates the experimental arrangement. The arm was cooled by circulating water at 10°C through a thin-walled rubber tube which was wrapped around it from wrist to axilla. This was done for up to 1.5 h by which time the surface temperature of the arm under the tubing had fallen to around 12 – 15°C; the thermocouple used for the measurement was placed on the skin and protected from the direct effect of the cooling by cotton wool. The hand was kept warm by radiant heat and its surface temperature normally remained

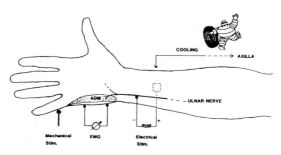

Fig. 1. The experimental arrangement used for studying abductor digiti minimi.

well above 30°C. Even with cooling of both arm and hand for 1.5 h the depths of the arm are known to remain very appreciably warmer than its surface (Barcroft and Edholm, 1943); the deep temperature can be expected to have been even better maintained in the present experiments by virtue of warm venous blood returning from the hand. It follows that the nerves must have been cooled to a very different extent at different points along their length.

The remaining methods were standard (cf. Matthews, 1984a). With the aid of a visual monitor of the force exerted, normal human subjects made a steady voluntary contraction of 10 – 20% maximum of the muscle studied; this was either the abductor digiti minimi or the first dorsal interosseus muscle, both of which are supplied by the ulnar nerve. The muscle was stretched by an electromechanical stretcher which pressed upon the finger (usually at the level of the proximal interphalangeal joint) on its side away from the other fingers. The subject was instructed to maintain a constant effort against the stretcher and to avoid responding voluntarily to the mechanical stimulus; the stimuli were normally repeated every 800 ms. The EMG was recorded with surface electrodes placed immediately over the muscle, and then rectified and averaged for 64 to 256 trials. Displacements of 2 – 5° were applied at around 100°/s for the ramp stretch and at about 10-times this speed for taps; the tap stimulus was completed within 10 ms.

Results and Discussion

Experiments on abductor digiti minimi

Both tap and ramp stretch elicited a well marked reflex response with a latency of about 60 ms and a well-defined beginning. These may both be taken to be long-latency responses since the short-latency response of the comparably located flexor pollicis brevis occurs at about 35 ms (Matthews, 1984b). At their peak the level of EMG was increased to about twice its initial value. Stimulation of the ulnar nerve at the wrist elicited an F wave with a latency of just over 30 ms. These responses are illustrated in Fig. 2; the tap also elicited a small inhibitory response, probably due to the excitation of cutaneous afferents (cf. Jenner and Stephens, 1982).

On commencing cooling the latency of all three responses increased steadily and more or less in parallel, so that after 1 – 1.5 h cooling they had increased by 15 – 25 ms from their initial value. The precise amount of the increase varied between experiments, particularly between those performed on different subjects (two thickset subjects showed appreciably less slowing than two slender ones). Thus at the height of cooling, the latency of the F wave had increased to about 50 ms and that of the reflexes to about 80 ms.

The observation that the latency of the reflexes increased by the same amount as that of the F wave provides a rather convincing demonstration that they must have been mediated by fast afferents; on anatomical considerations these can be safely presumed to run in the ulnar nerve. It follows that the central delay has to be long, since an oligosynaptic spinal response would have a latency only slightly above that of the F wave, whereas there would seem to be at least an additional 20 ms available for central processes. However, these observations on ADM do nothing to show whether the responsible afferents arise from skin, or from muscle (or from both).

Appropriate cutaneous reflexes certainly exist. Electrical stimulation of the digital nerves by ring electrodes placed round the little finger elicited a complex reflex response analogous to that already described for the FDI (Jenner and Stephens, 1982). The pronounced E_2 excitatory component had a latency of 60 ms and very similar to that of the reflex responses elicited by mechanical stimulation. This E_2 response behaved in just the same way as the two other reflexes on cooling, and slowed by the same amount as them and the F wave. This provides strong supporting evidence for the pre-existing view that these electrically induced reflexes depend upon fast afferents acting with a sufficiently long central delay for transcortical transmission to be a very strong possibility. However, cutaneous afferents seem unlikely to be solely responsible for the response evoked by displacing the little finger, since on a single occasion the mechanically elicited responses persisted virtually unchanged after anaesthetizing the finger by injecting local anaesthetic at its base. But this cannot be judged conclusive, since cutaneous and joint afferents associated with the metocarpo-phalangeal joint were probably still being excited by the imposed displacement.

Experiments on the first dorsal interosseus

Rapid displacement of the index finger evoked a clear short latency response with a latency of around 35 ms, and of an amplitude varying markedly between subjects. This was typically followed by a series of complex waves. With slower ramp displacement this short-latency response became much smaller, and usually no longer interfered with the recognition of the beginning of the long-latency response which normally retained a sharp beginning. As explained below, this delayed response is believed to be a compound event containing both cutaneous and muscular components, with the muscular component beginning slightly earlier and so usually determining the overall latency.

On cooling the arm the short-latency response elicited by a tap behaved as hoped and showed the same slowing as the F wave induced by ulnar stimulation, again around 20 ms as for ADM. This

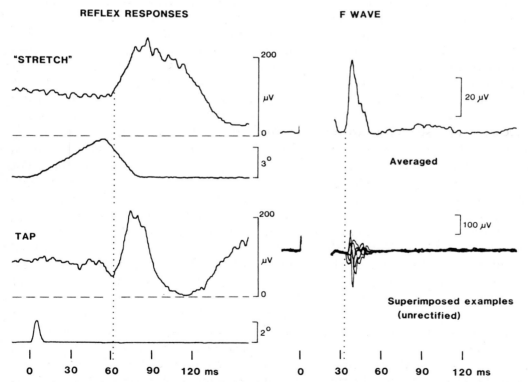

Fig. 2. Typical responses recorded from ADM in the absence of cooling. Left, reflex responses evoked by mechanical displacement of the little finger in the direction required to stretch ADM (the EMG was rectified then averaged, $n = 510$; the movement of the servo-controlled stimulator is shown below). Right, the F wave recorded from ADM on stimulating the ulnar nerve at the wrist. Top, averaged rectified responses ($n = 255$); bottom, sample of individual responses before rectification. The much larger M wave elicited by the stimulus has been removed and the tracing left blank (this was done electronically).

helps further validate the use of the F wave as a standard for assessing the slowing of large fast axons. Moreover, the finding makes it very unlikely that large afferent fibres could behave differently from large motor axons.

In two of the three subjects, the long-latency response behaved similarly and equally simply (the third has yet to be investigated in detail) and slowed by the same amount as the F wave induced by ulnar stimulation. However, the interpretation of this finding for FDI requires a knowledge of the amount of slowing of large axons in the median nerve, as well as that of those in the ulnar nerve. This was determined by recording the F wave evoked in thenar muscles on stimulating the median nerve at the wrist. It was regularly found to be far less than that of the ulnar motor fibres of comparable velocity; typically the median axons slowed only one-quarter to one-third as much as the ulnar axons. The difference in their susceptibility to cooling can be attributed simply to the difference in their anatomical locations; for most of its course the median nerve lies deeper, and closer to blood vessels, and so can be expected to have remained appreciably the warmer.

This differential effect of limb cooling on the two nerves provides the basis for distinguishing between cutaneous and muscular reflexes acting on FDI. A muscular reflex will have both its afferent and efferent limbs in the ulnar nerve; thus, if it is dependent upon fast afferents, it will show the same slowing as the ulnar F wave. A cutaneous reflex evoked from the index finger will normally have its afferent limb in the median nerve and its efferent limb in the ulnar nerve. Thus, if it is mediated by fast afferents its slowing should be the mean of that for the median and ulnar F waves.

That a cutaneous reflex actually behaves in the expected way was readily verified by studying a definite cutaneous reflex, namely that elicited by electrical stimulation of the index finger with ring electrodes. The resulting E_2 reflex then slowed by an amount almost precisely half-way between that shown by the fast motor axons of the two nerves, as assessed by the F waves. A cutaneous reflex that was dependent upon fast afferents was also found to be elicited by tapping the index finger, since in all three subjects a later component of the response to a tap could be separated which showed this intermediate degree of slowing on cooling. It may be noted that its separation from the initial short-latency component of the tap response thus decreased slightly (in contradistinction to the statement of Darton et al., 1985, about their supposed cutaneous reflex). It may be concluded, as occasions no surprise, that mechanical stimuli to the finger may elicit long-latency cutaneous reflexes mediated by fast afferents.

We can now return to the question of the afferents of origin of the response to a ramp stretch; as just noted, this shows the same slowing with cooling as the ulnar motor fibres. It cannot be a cutaneous reflex dependent upon fast afferents, since it would then have shown less slowing than the ulnar motor fibres, as above. It might be suggested to be a cutaneous reflex dependent upon slow afferents; since the median nerve is cooled less than the ulnar nerve, small median afferents might show the same absolute amount of slowing on cooling as large ulnar axons. However, if this were so then a quite different explanation would be required for the observation that the apparently homologous ramp response of ADM also showed the same slowing as the ulnar motor fibres. For this muscle the cutaneous afferents run in the ulnar nerve, and so slow afferents would show more slowing than the large motor axons. Accepting that the responses of the two muscles can be equated it follows, first, that fast afferents must be involved (because of the results with ADM), and second that these must be muscular afferents (because of the results with FDI).

It may be concluded that group I afferents from these two muscles can elicit a distinct long-latency reflex, quite separate from short-latency tendon jerk type responses. In the light of all the previous evidence those responsible seem likely to be Ia afferents from spindles rather than Ib afferents from tendon organs; moreover, it is simplest to believe that long central delay is due to the response being mediated via the motor cortex.

Summing up

What then remains of the hypothesis that spindle group II afferents should be held responsible for the long-latency response? Clearly it is very sick, but it will be understood that the present author is not prepared to see it buried prematurely. In the direct conflict between the conclusions of the two kinds of experiment (vibration and cooling), those using cooling must currently take precedence since the situation is a simpler one and thus the deductions more secure. However, if the group II hypothesis be rejected in toto, then there is no obvious explanation for the different effects of stretch and vibration, especially on their termination.

The first possible let-out, permitting the conclusions of both sets of experiments to be accepted without defying logic, is that different muscles may differ, and that the group II hypothesis is still applicable to forearm muscles for which the vibration experiments were performed. But this would require appreciable supporting evidence before it carried any conviction. The next more plausible possibility is that both mechanisms operate in parallel, with their relative contributions depending upon a variety of additional factors. In the present experiments it proved possible on the basis of an anatomical quirk to separate a cutaneous from a muscular reflex for FDI. However, the recognition of a further reflex of about the same latency, due to slow muscle afferents, is a much more daunting problem; the present experiments can, as yet, certainly not be taken to exclude its existence.

Thus, while the group II hypothesis has certainly been eliminated as the sole mechanism responsible for long-latency responses originating from muscle, nonetheless it should remain sub judice as a subsidiary mechanism. It is enough for the time being that three separate mechanisms have already been shown to be operating in parallel to produce the increased EMG activity on joint rotation, namely group Ia short-latency action, group I (probably Ia) long-latency action, and fast cutaneous long-latency action. Given such plurality, the problem has already shifted away from the falsely simple question "Which pathway is (uniquely) responsible?", to the more complex quantitative question "How much does each of several mechanisms contribute?".

References

Barcroft, H. and Edholm, O.G. (1943) The effect of temperature on blood flow and deep tissue temperature in human forearm. *J. Physiol. (London),* 102: 5 – 20.

Bawa, P. and McKenzie, D.C. (1981) Contribution of joint and cutaneous afferents to longer-latency reflexes in man. *Brain Res.,* 211: 185 – 189.

Chan, C.W.Y., Melvill-Jones, G. and Cutchlove, R.F.A. (1979) The "late" electromyographic response to limb displacement in man. II. Sensory origin. *Electroenceph. Clin. Neurophysiol.,* 46: 182 – 188.

Darton, K., Lippold, O.C.J., Shahani, M. and Shahani, U. (1985) Long-latency spinal reflexes. *J. Neurophysiol.,* 53: 1604 – 1618.

Franz, D.N. and Iggo, A. (1968) Conduction failure in myelinated and non-myelinated axons at low temperatures. *J. Physiol. (London),* 199: 319 – 345.

Gandevia, S.C., Hall, L.A., McCloskey, D.I. and Potter, E.K. (1983) Proprioceptive sensation at the terminal joint of middle finger. *J. Physiol. (London),* 335: 507 – 517.

Hammond, P.H. (1960) An experimental study of servo action in human muscular control. *Proc. III International Conference in Medical Electronics,* Butterworths, London, pp. 190 – 199.

Iles, J.F. (1977) Responses in human pretibial muscles to sudden stretch and to nerve stimulation. *Exp. Brain Res.,* 30: 451 – 470.

Jenner, J.R. and Stephens, J.A. (1982) Cutaneous reflex responses and their central nervous pathways studied in man. *J. Physiol. (London),* 333: 405 – 419.

Loo, C.K.C. and McCloskey, D.I. (1985) Effect of prior instruction and anaesthesia on long-latency responses to stretch in the long flexor of the human thumb. *J. Physiol. (London),* 365: 285 – 296.

Marsden, C.D., Merton, P.A. and Morton, H.B. (1972) Servo action in human voluntary movement. *Nature (London),* 238: 140 – 143.

Marsden, C.D., Merton, P.A. and Morton, H.B. (1976a) Servo action in the human thumb. *J. Physiol. (London),* 257: 1 – 44.

Marsden, C.D., Merton, P.A. and Morton, H.B. (1976b) Stretch reflex and servo action in a variety of human muscles. *J. Physiol. (London),* 259: 531 – 560.

Marsden, C.D., Merton, P.A. and Morton, H.B. (1977) The

sensory mechanism of servo action in human muscle. *J. Physiol. (London),* 265: 521 – 535.

Marsden, C.D., Rothwell, J.C. and Traub, M.M. (1979) Effect of thumb anaesthesia on weight perception, muscle activity and stretch reflex in man. *J. Physiol. (London),* 294: 303 – 315.

Marsden, C.D., Rothwell, J.C. and Day, B.L. (1983) Long-latency automatic responses to muscle stretch in man: origin and function. In J.E. Desmedt (Ed.), *Motor Control Mechanisms in Health and Disease,* Raven, New York, pp. 509 – 539.

Matthews, P.B.C. (1984a) Evidence from the use of vibration that the human long-latency stretch reflex depends upon spindle secondary afferents. *J. Physiol. (London),* 348: 383 – 415.

Matthews, P.B.C. (1984b) The contrasting stretch reflex responses of the long and short flexor muscles of the human thumb. *J. Physiol. (London),* 348: 545 – 558.

Matthews, P.B.C. (1985) Human long-latency stretch reflexes – A new role for the secondary ending of the muscle spindle? In W.J.P. Barnes and M.H. Gladden (Eds.), *Feedback and Motor Control in Invertebrates and Vertebrates,* Croom Helm, London, pp. 431 – 449.

Matthews, P.B.C. (1986a) What are the afferents of origin of the human stretch reflex, and is it a purely spinal reaction? *Prog. Brain Res.,* 64: 55 – 66.

Matthews, P.B.C. (1986b) The effect of cooling the arm on the ''long-latency'' response of the human abductor digiti minimi. *J. Physiol. (London),* 382: 75P.

Matthews, P.B.C. (1987) Effect of arm cooling on long-latency reflex responses from the human first dorsal interosseus muscle – evidence for a group I contribution. *J. Physiol. (London),* 394: 102P.

Matthews, P.B.C. (1988) Is the F wave a valid indicator of the slowing of motor axons on cooling the human arm? *J. Physiol. (London),* 406: 31P.

Matthews, P.B.C. and Miles, T.S. (1988a) Is the ''let go'' response of the human flexor digitorum profundus due to stretch of its antagonists? *J. Physiol. (London),* 401: 49P.

Matthews, P.B.C. and Miles, T.S. (1988b) On the long-latency reflex responses of the human flexor digitorum profundus. *J. Physiol. (London),* 404: 515 – 534.

Paintal, A.S. (1965) Effects of temperature on conduction in single vagal and saphenous myelinated nerve fibres of the cat. *J. Physiol. (London),* 180: 20 – 49.

Wiesendanger, M. (1986) Experimental evidence for the existence of a proprioceptive transcortical loop. *Prog. Brain Res.,* 64: 67 – 74.

J.H.J. Allum and M. Hulliger (Eds.)
Progress in Brain Research, Vol. 80
© 1989 Elsevier Science Publishers B.V. (Biomedical Division)

CHAPTER 10

Eye, head and skeletal muscle spindle feedback in the elaboration of body references*

J.-P. Roll, J.-P. Vedel and R. Roll

Laboratoire de Neurobiologie Humaine, Université de Provence, U.A. CNRS 372, Av. Escadrille Normandie Niemen, 13397 Marseille Cédex 13, France and Unité de Neurosciences du Comportement, CNRS-LNF2, 31 chemin J. Aiguier, B.P.71, 13402 Marseille Cédex 9, France

Evidence is presented to support the notion that the sensory feedback originating in muscles is of major importance in the central elaboration of motor representation. The muscle spindle messages during movement and postural performance may be processed in order to elaborate continuously updated static and dynamic body references. These may then form the basis for the interpretation of retinal information in terms of spatial coordinates. The main arguments supporting this view are as follows. Experimental manipulation of muscle spindle proprioceptive feedback by tendon vibration induced segmental or postural kinaesthetic illusory movements in the direction of stretch of the vibrated muscles. By modifying the spatial distribution (agonists and/or antagonists), the frequency and the duration of the vibratory stimuli it is possible to induce simple or complex kinaesthetic illusions the parameters of which may be predicted. Microneurographic recordings confirmed that vibration rather selectively excited spindle Ia afferents, eliciting 1 : 1 driving up to 80 – 100 Hz. Moreover painless vibration, applied at increasing frequency (from 10 to 80 Hz) to either the medial, lateral, superior or inferior rectus of a subject's eye, was found to induce directional perceptual and motor effects which were closely related to the postural context. Likewise, the subjects reported illusory directional shifts of a visually fixed target in darkness during extraocular muscle vibration. These data suggest that extraocular proprioception contributes to the coding of eye, head and body position in relation to postural and environmental conditions. As with eye muscle stimulation, directional visual and postural effects were induced by vibration of neck and/or ankle postural muscles. These effects were found to summate when vibrations were applied simultaneously to the eye, neck and ankle muscles. The likely involvement of extraocular proprioception in interrelating body space with extrapersonal space in oriented behaviour is discussed.

Key words: Man; Body reference; Kinaesthesia; Extraocular proprioception; Postural control; Visual illusion; Muscle vibration; Microneurography; Muscle spindle feedback; Golgi tendon organ

Introduction

The aim of the present paper is to suggest the existence of a close linkage between the eyes and plantar support via congruent muscle proprioceptive information, and to describe the decisive contribution of this chain to the control of human body posture.

The fact that most of our behavioural activities are based first and foremost on the visual grasping of a target suggests that the direction of gaze might play a decisive role in body and limb orientation (Roll et al. 1987). However, previous studies on the interactions between posture and vision have usually focused on the role of retinal factors, especially on the involvement of the peripheral

---

* This paper is based on presentations given at two different meetings on Posture and Locomotion held in Marseilles (June 1988) and in Rheinfelden (September 1988).

retina in the control of dynamic whole-body posture (Berthoz, 1974; Lee and Lishman, 1975; Dichgans and Brandt, 1978). Few have dealt with the relationship between postural control and eye movements and the associated proprioceptive feedback from extraocular muscles.

Without overlooking the role played by outflowing information (corollary discharge) and visual and vestibular afferent inputs we would like to stress the decisive contribution of muscle proprioception to posture regulation. In particular, this study was intended to demonstrate the fact that extraocular proprioception may, like other proprioceptive inputs from neck or postural muscles, play an important part in the organization of whole-body posture. Furthermore, we propose that the direction of gaze, i.e. the position of the eyes in space, might also be coded on the basis of proprioceptive signals originating from all the body segments involved in a given configuration. These assumptions are based on both psychophysiological and neurophysiological data obtained in our laboratory.

The main experimental argument is the fact that it is possible, in the absence of any actual movement, to induce kinaesthetic illusions and associated motor responses in humans when mechanical vibrations are applied to the distal tendon of a limb muscle (Goodwin et al., 1972; Roll and Vedel, 1982). These effects are frequency dependent and the direction of the low velocity displacements perceived always corresponds to the direction of muscle stretch, which would elicit proprioceptive discharge comparable to that provoked by vibration (Roll et al., 1980). Illusory movements and/or motor responses can extend to the whole-body when vibrations are applied to muscles involved in postural stance (Eklund, 1972; Roll, 1981). For instance, vibration of the two Achilles tendons or the tibialis anterior muscles gives rise to a persistent sensation of forward or backward body movement, respectively. As in the case of a single limb, the perceived speed of whole-body illusory movements depends on the vibration frequency.

The second experimental argument we have provided is that the afferent messages underlying kinaesthetic sensations are almost exclusively of muscle spindle origin (Roll and Vedel, 1982). Indeed, by means of microneurographic recordings from human sensory nerves, we have confirmed that the vibratory stimulus preferentially activates Ia muscle spindle afferents, mainly because in man, the response of most primary endings to vibration within the frequency range of 1 to 100 Hz is nearly proportional to the stimulus frequency. The existence of a one to one stimulus-response linkage within this frequency range means that, by modulating the vibration frequency, it is possible to induce a proportional modulation in the primary afferent discharge frequency. As an example of the sensitivity of muscle spindle primary endings to vibrations in man, Fig. 1 shows the activation of this type of receptor by vibrations applied to the tendon of the receptor bearing muscle.

Fig. 2 illustrates, for different kinds of proprioceptors (primary and secondary muscle spindle endings, Golgi tendon organs), the response of populations of units submitted to low-amplitude

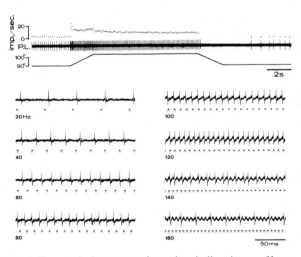

Fig. 1. Top: typical response of muscle spindle primary afferent from tibialis anterior muscle in man to constant velocity trapezoidal movement. Bottom: sensitivity of muscle spindle primary afferent to tendon vibration. Lower trace, period markers indicate frequency of the mechanical stimulus. Upper trace, unitary action potentials (Ia afferent from tibialis anterior). From Roll and Vedel, 1982.

vibrations, 0.2 to 0.5 mm peak to peak, with frequency increasing in steps up to 180 Hz.

Primary endings. The upper diagrams in Fig. 2 show the relationships observed between the vibration frequency and the discharge frequency induced in each of the Ia fibres tested. It can be seen that for all the primary endings tested there was a fre-

quency range in which the response was locked 1 : 1 to the stimulus. With some units the locking occurred up to between 150 and 200 Hz. But generally it was limited to the 80 to 100 Hz frequency range. Increasing the vibration frequency beyond a critical value was found to decrease the afferents' firing rate. This decrease could take place in two ways: the afferent discharged either at

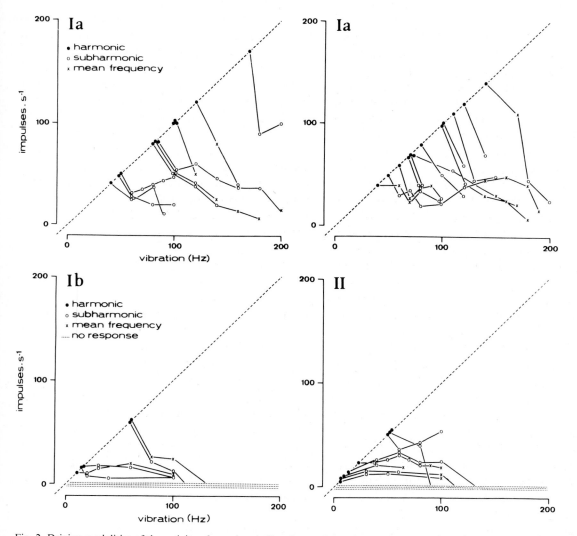

Fig. 2. Driving modalities of the activity of muscle spindle primary (Ia) and secondary (II) endings and of tendon organs (Ib) induced by mechanical vibration applied at various frequencies to the tendon of the receptor-bearing muscles (tibialis anterior, extensor digitorum longus). Black circles indicate for each unit the frequency of 1:1 driving; open circles illustrate sub-harmonic responses and crosses symbolize the mean frequency of the induced sensory activity which was not phase-related to vibratory stimulus. Vibrations were imposed on relaxed muscles (EMG silence), maintained slightly stretched (From Roll et al., 1989).

a sub-harmonic of the vibration frequency or else it fired in a random manner. For the vibratory amplitudes used in our experiments, the stimuli were in all cases no longer able to activate the primary endings at frequencies of about 180 – 200 Hz. It was thus in the 80 to 100 Hz vibration range that it was possible to activate the greatest number of primary muscle spindle endings of one muscle with a 1 : 1 mode of response.

Secondary endings. The sensitivity to vibration of the muscle spindle secondary endings is given in the lower right diagram of Fig. 2. It can be seen that, out of the 11 units studied, 3 did not respond to the stimulus at all, 5 could be driven 1 : 1 up to between 10 to 30 Hz, and only 3 up to 60 Hz. As with the primary endings, beyond a critical frequency at which the units responded 1 : 1, the units showed either a sub-harmonic or a random mode of response. Thus, with the muscle at rest and under an intermediate degree of stretch, the sensitivity of secondary endings to low-amplitude vibration was much lower than that of the primary endings. The majority of the population of units did not respond to frequencies beyond 10 to 20 Hz.

Golgi tendon organs. The lower left diagram of Fig. 2 illustrates the sensitivity of a population of 8 Golgi tendon organs to vibration. No tonic muscle activity was present when these recordings were made. About 30% of the receptors were unresponsive to the stimulus. The majority of receptors was activated by vibrations in a 1 : 1 driving mode, up to a frequency of 10 Hz, and two units fired in the same manner up to 50 Hz.

As with the spindle afferents, beyond a critical frequency which was characteristic of each receptor, the response mode became either sub-harmonic or random. In the absence of tonic activity in the receptor-bearing muscle, the Golgi tendon organs are thus difficult to activate by applying low-amplitude vibrations to the appropriate tendons.

Vibration therefore constitutes an efficient means of generating defined patterns of sensory, especially Ia, inputs. These can then be used to elicit "at will" illusory movements the direction, speed and duration of which can be preselected. Given this tool of selective activation of muscle spindle afferents by vibration and the high density of stretch receptors in extraocular muscles (Cooper et al., 1955; Barker, 1974; Mukuno, 1986), we attempted to selectively activate the eye muscle proprioceptors in man.

Thanks to the great mobility of the eyeball, the eye is constantly exploring the environment and informing the organism so that it can act or react by adopting a postural configuration which is appropriate for an ongoing or forthcoming motor event. Then, since body segments like the head, trunk and legs can connect the eye with the ground, the experimental manipulation of proprioception by vibration of these linked body parts might help to specify their respective contributions to postural regulation in man. Furthermore, under some particular conditions, the central processing of retinal information might also be dependent on the proprioceptive body reference.

Methods

Eye muscle vibration

Mechanical vibration, with an amplitude of 0.1 to 0.2 mm peak to peak, was applied to various points in the periphery of the eyeball by means of mini vibrators which could be fitted with small probes, adapted to each subject's eye morphology. Their length and shape varied depending on whether medial or external muscles were to be vibrated. Vibrators were fixed on a helmet and various kinds of combined stimulation of both eyes could be chosen as indicated in Fig. 3.

The vibration train duration was 2 or 5 s; the frequency could vary from 1 to 100 Hz.

Neck and ankle muscle vibration

Vibrations with an amplitude of 0.2 to 0.4 mm peak to peak were applied to the tendons of neck and ankle muscles by means of excentric DC motor vibrators attached with rubber bands to the

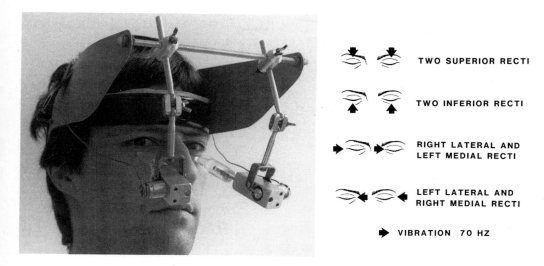

Fig. 3. Left: experimental device. Right: combined stimulation of both eyes. For details see text.

stimulation sites. In the case of co-stimulations of muscle groups, the vibrators were synchronized and the stimulation durations were identical (2 s). Before testing, the stimulation intensity was adjusted for each muscle so that the vibration gave rise to postural sways of about the same amplitude in all cases.

In studies dealing with the postural effects of eye, neck and ankle muscle vibration, the subjects were standing with their eyes closed and the postural sways were recorded from four strain gauges, which were enclosed in the stabilometer, placed under each subject's feet.

In the target viewing situation, the subject was standing in the dark, looking monocularly through a small slot at an electroluminescent diode located 57 cm ahead of him, at eye level. The slot was used to check whether the subject moved his eye during stimulation: if the eye moved the subject had to inform the experimenter that the target had disappeared. Vertical and horizontal eye movement recordings (EOG) were carried out with some subjects in order to ensure that no eye movements occurred during the vibration.

Body movement was prevented by means of a mechanical device fixed at shoulder level.

Results

Postural effects of extraocular muscle vibration
Application of low amplitude mechanical vibration to the extraocular muscles of a standing subject with his eyes closed elicited, within a latency range of 1 to 2 s, whole-body shifts, the direction of which was found to strictly depend on which muscle was vibrated. The main results are illustrated in Fig. 4. The posturograms give two-dimensional plots of lateral (x) and anteroposterior (y) components of postural forces recorded during simultaneous vibration of both eyes. The four different experimental vibration combinations that were used, are illustrated schematically in the inserts (head sketches with arrows marking the eyeball areas which were vibrated).

Simultaneous vibration of the two superior recti resulted in a whole body forward displacement (C), whereas a backward shift was observed during vibration of the two inferior recti (D). When the stimulation was applied simultaneously to the lateral rectus of the right eye and the medial rectus of the left eye (A), a leftward displacement was elicited and vice-versa (B).

The main postural effect, induced by combined

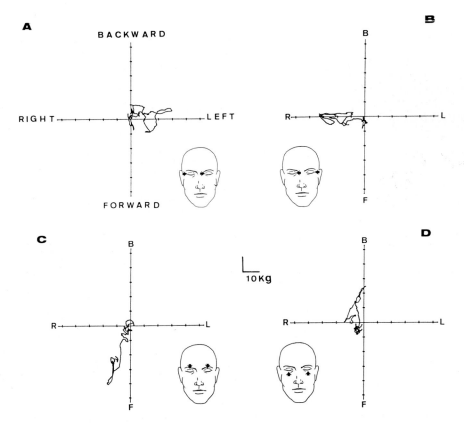

Fig. 4. Directional postural effects of high frequency vibration (70 Hz, 5 s) applied to homonymous extraocular muscles of both eyes. The arrows indicate the muscles stimulated. See also text.

vibrations of extraocular muscles, was that the direction of these body shifts was found to clearly depend on the eye muscle pair which was stimulated. This fact suggests the existence of a close linkage between eye *posture* or movements and the spatial organization of whole-body posture.

Further, the mean amplitude of postural shifts induced by vibrations was frequency dependent. As an example, Fig. 5 shows one subject's increasing backward displacement when vibration, increasing in steps from 20 to 100 Hz, was applied to both inferior recti over a period of 5 s. This relationship between the vibration frequency and the mean amplitude of postural sway is illustrated in the lower part of the diagram. Both the path length

and the maximum amplitude varied as a function of the vibration frequency.

Postural effects of eye, neck and ankle muscle vibration and co-vibration

As with extraocular proprioceptive manipulation, vibration of neck and ankle muscles was capable of giving rise to similar body sways when a relevant stimulus location was chosen; whole-body displacements, whose direction is consistent with the previously described effects on eye muscles, could then easily be obtained. Vibrations applied separately to the inferior recti, sterno-cleido-mastoidus or the soleus muscles induced almost analogous postural effects, i.e. a backward whole-body displacement. Likewise, vibrations applied separately to the superior recti, splenii or tibialis anterior muscles gave rise to a forward body shift. Moreover, it was possible to combine these stimulations in different ways. Co-stimulations of this kind were used in order to determine whether any "additive" postural effect resulted from these different proprioceptive inputs, and to establish whether each input had a differential weight in postural regulation.

Co-vibration of soleus and sterno-cleido mastoidus muscles (S + SCM), soleus and inferior recti (S + IR), or sterno-cleido-mastoidus and inferior recti (SCM + IR) induced postural sways in the backward direction. In all cases, co-stimulation of two muscle groups had a more powerful influence on body posture than isolated vibrations applied separately to each muscle group. The results did not clearly point to the existence of any dominance

of one proprioceptive input over another. Lastly, co-vibration of soleus, sterno-cleido-mastoidus and inferior recti gave rise to the most extensive postural sway.

The mean data on the postural effects of separate and combined vibration situations are given in Fig. 6. The means of the maximum postural forces corresponding to each situation reflect the results just described; that is, they show that the various proprioceptive inputs coming from the body segments linking eye with foot add together in modulating postural control. However, whilst the effects of combined vibration of "synergistic" muscle groups were additive, the summation was not linear, since the combined effects were clearly smaller than the sums of the individual effects (Fig. 6).

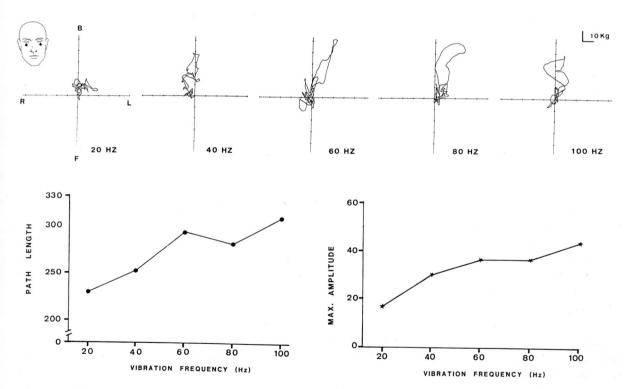

Fig. 5. Effects of the vibration frequency on the amplitude of the postural sway. Upper part: Vibration-induced postural sway of increasing amplitude induced by inferior rectivibration of increasing frequency (20 to 80 Hz). Data from a single subject. Lower part: mean results (*n* = 5). Dependence on frequency of vibration of path length (left) and maximum amplitude (right) of postural sway. B, backward; F, forward; R, right; L, left.

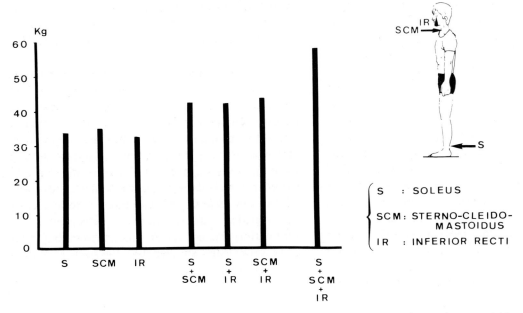

Fig. 6. Mean postural forces provoked by separate and combined vibration of inferior recti, sterno-cleido-mastoidus and soleus muscles. See also text.

Visual effects of extraocular, neck and ankle muscle vibration

Vibration applied to extraocular muscles of a subject looking monocularly at a small luminous target in darkness resulted in an illusory perception of a slow apparent movement of the target in a specific direction. The target displacement direction depended strictly on which eye muscle was vibrated: vibration of the inferior rectus induced an upward target shift and, conversely, a downward shift occurred during superior rectus vibration. External rectus vibration elicited an illusory target displacement in the medial direction and vibration of the medial rectus a displacement in the external direction. Likewise, a directional shift of the visual target was elicited by vibration applied to neck muscles (splenius, sterno-cleido-mastoidus or trapezius) and, more surprisingly, to ankle pustural muscles (soleus, tibialis or peroneus). The most noteworthy findings are summarized in Fig. 7 and concern the directional similarity of the apparent target movement obtained by applying vibration to specific muscles which are often stretched or released together during a given whole-body postural orientation. For example, vibration of either the inferior recti, the sterno-cleido-mastoidus, or the tibialis anterior muscles can induce, in darkness, identical illusory shifts of the target in the upward direction. In this case, since the only available cue is the position of the target on the retina, the vibration-induced proprioceptive pattern simulating either an eye lift, a backward head or whole-body movement, is interpreted by the stationary subject in darkness as if it were an upward displacement of the target.

Discussion and Conclusions

The experimental data presented here support the idea that proprioceptive input contributes to the control of human stance, for at least two reasons.

First it was demonstrated that eye muscle proprioception – and not merely retinal cues as classically assumed – can take part in this regula-

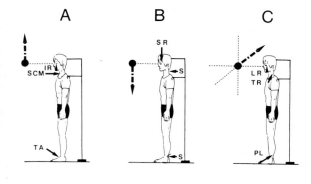

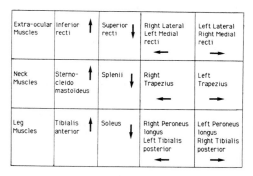

Extra-ocular Muscles	Inferior recti ↑	Superior recti ↓	Right Lateral Left Medial recti ←	Left Lateral Right Medial recti →
Neck Muscles	Sterno-cleido mastoideus ↑	Splenii ↓	Right Trapezius ←	Left Trapezius →
Leg Muscles	Tibialis anterior ↑	Soleus ↓	Right Peroneus longus Left Tibialis posterior ←	Left Peroneus longus Right Tibialis posterior →

Fig. 7. Apparent movement of a visual target induced by muscle vibration (70 Hz). See also text.

tion. Secondly, it was shown that the same directional whole-body displacement, for instance a forward movement, can be obtained by vibrating either a single muscle, or several muscles involved at different levels of postural organization but which contribute together to a given postural synergy.

On the first point, clinical observations have corroborated this view by showing, for example, that alterations of the static or dynamic control or eye movements are often associated with defects in postural control (Martins Da Cunha, 1987; Gagey, 1987; Marruchi and Gagey, 1987). Our results also agree with findings by Baron, in 1955, on the goldfish. In this species, surgical modification of the length of a particular extraocular muscle induced specific changes in axial muscle tone distribution and, consequently, altered the ongoing behaviour. In addition, Gagey et al. (1973) also

observed that, in man, the tonic activity of leg muscles can be modified by directional displacement of the eyeballs.

From other studies, it now emerges that extraocular proprioceptive cues may also be involved in the development of visual perception (Buisseret and Gary-Bobo, 1979; Milleret, 1987) and that, at behavioural level, early suppression of these afferents in kittens alters the development of visually guided activity (Hein and Diamond, 1982).

The second point suggests that the extraocular proprioceptive input might add its postural regulatory influence to that of other inputs coming from various body segments. This may be intuitively acceptable, since the legs, like the trunk and head, are also carriers of the eyes in space. This suggests that integrative processing of all these sources of muscular feedback subserves postural adjustment and that these feedback channels participate in conjoint elaboration of a body reference. This proposal may contribute to further specifying the body scheme concept in terms of its proprioceptive content. Moreover, the centrally elaborated postural scheme, built up from simultaneously collected proprioceptive cues, might be used in the spatial processing of retinal information as shown by the fact that vibration of eye, neck or leg muscles gives rise to apparent movements of a visual target in a specific direction (Roll and Roll, 1987; Biguer et al., 1988).

In conclusion, we suggest that the muscular proprioceptive chain linking eye to foot may be of major importance in inter-relating body space with extrapersonal space.

Reply to P.H. Ellaway's critique

This criticism of the paper is based on a cybernetic approach to the results, which interprets the visual and postural effects of eye, neck and ankle muscle vibration like compensatory responses to eye or head movements, where it is attempted to extend the VOR model to the whole body.

We disagree with this kind of interpretation and since we prefer to assume that the observed responses might correspond to whole-body orienting reactions, depending heavily on eye position and movements via proprioceptive extraretinal messages. Some methodological and experimental arguments can be put forward to support this view.

First, it seems necessary to recall that the vibration-induced postural effects were recorded with the subject's eye closed, and that the visual effects (apparent movement of a target) were obtained in standing subjects with the body restrained.

Secondly, both the EOG recordings and the experiment where the target was presented in the foveal area showed that the eye was stationary during vibratory stimulation. In the case of limited vision, the subject looked at the target through a small slot; if the eye actually moved, the subject could no longer see the target. This paradigm has also been described and used by others (Biguer et al. 1988) .

Furthermore, directional illusory displacements of an after-image induced by a flash-light on the retina are observed when extraocular muscle vibration is applied. In this case, the "retinal locus" stimulated cannot change and the target is bound up with the eye. From the behavioural point of view, this kind of situation might correspond to a smooth pursuit of a moving target with the eye, head and, when appropriate, the whole body.

Finally, Lackner and Levine (1978) reported that in darkness, a small target light fixed to the index tip was perceived as moving by subjects when vibration was applied to their biceps or triceps brachii, without any actual movement of the arm or the target having occurred.

Acknowledgements

This work was supported by CNRS (UA 372) and Ministère de l'Environnement grants. English revision was carried out by Dr Jessica Blanc.

References

Barker, D. (1974) The morphology of muscle receptors. In C.C. Hunt (Ed.), *Handbook of Sensory Physiology,* Vol. 3, part 2, Springer Verlag, New York, pp. 1 – 190.

Baron, J.B. (1955) Muscles moteurs oculaires, attitudes et comportements des vertébrés. *Thèse Faculté des Sciences,* Paris.

Berthoz, A. (1974) Oculomotricité et proprioception. *Rev. EEG et Neurophysiol.,* 4: 569 – 586.

Biguer, B., Donaldson, I.M.L., Hein, A. and Jeannerod. M. (1988) Neck muscle vibration modifies the representation of visual motion and direction in man. *Brain,* 111: 1405 – 1424.

Buisseret, P. and Gary-Bobo, E. (1979) Development of visual cortical orientation specificity after dark rearing. *Neurosci. Lett.,* 13: 259 – 263.

Cooper, S., Daniel P.M. and Whitteridge, D. (1955) Muscle spindles and other sensory endings in the extrinsic eye muscles. *Brain,* 78: 564 – 583.

Dichgans, J. and Brandt, T. (1978) Visual-vestibular interaction: effects on self-motion perception and postural control. In R. Held, H.W. Leibowitz and H.L. Teuber (Eds.), *Handbook of Sensory Physiology: Perception, VIII,* pp. 756 – 804.

Eklund, G. (1972) Position sense and state of contraction; the effects of vibrations. *J. Neurol. Neurosurg. Psychiat.,* 35: 606 – 611.

Gagey, P.M. (1987) L'oculomotricité comme endo-entrée du système postural. *Agressologie,* 28: 899 – 903.

Gagey, P.M., Baron, J.B. Lespargot, J. and Poli, J.P. (1973) Variations de l'activité tonique posturale et activité des muscles oculocéphalogyres en cathédrostatisme. *Agressologie,* 14: 87 – 96.

Goodwin, G.M., McCloskey, D.I. and Matthews, P.B.C. (1972) The contribution of muscle afferents to kinaesthesia shown by vibration induced illusions of movement and by the effects of paralysing joint afferents. *Brain,* 95: 705 – 748.

Hein, A. and Diamond, R. (1982) Contribution of eye movement to representation of space. In A. Hein and M. Jeannerod M (Eds), *Spatially Oriented Behavior,* Springer Verlag, New York, pp. 119 – 133.

Lackner, J.R. and Levine, M.S. (1978) Visual direction depends on the operation of spatial constancy mechanisms: the oculobrachial illusion. *Neurosci. Lett.,* 7: 207 – 212.

Lee, D.N. and Lishman, J.R. (1975) Visual proprioceptive control of stance. *J. Hum. Movem. Studies,* 1: 87 – 95.

Martins Da Cunha, H.M. (1987) Le syndrome de deficience posturale (SDP). *Agressologie,* 28: 941 – 943.

Marucchi, C. and Gagey, P.M. (1987) Cécité posturale. *Agressologie,* 28: 947 – 948.

Milleret, C. (1987) Projections centrales des afférences proprioceptives issues des muscles extraoculaires chez les vertébrés. Quelques rôles fonctionnels possibles dans le contrôle de l'oculomotricité, la perception visuelle et l'orientation corporelle. *Agressologie,* 28: 917 – 924.

Mukuno, K. (1986) Morphological demonstration of ocular muscle proprioception in the human extraocular muscles. *Proceedings of International Workshop on Proprioception of Ocular Muscles,* Hakone-Matsuyama, Japan, 1:1.

Roll, J.P. (1981) Contribution de la proprioception musculaire à la perception et au contrôle du mouvement chez l'homme. *Thèse Faculté des Sciences,* Marseille.

Roll, J.P. and Roll, R. (1987) La proprioception extraoculaire comme élément de référence posturale et de lecture spatiale des données rétiniennes. *Agressologie,* 28: 905 – 912.

Roll, J.P. and Vedel, J.P. (1982) Kinaesthetic role of muscle afferents in man studied by tendon vibration and microneurography. *Exp. Brain Res.,* 47: 177 – 190.

Roll, J.P., Gilhodes, J.C. and Tardy-gervet, M.F. (1980) Effets perceptifs et moteurs des vibrations musculaires chez l'homme normal; mise en évidence d'une réponse des muscles antagonistes. *Arch. Ital. Biol.,* 118: 51 – 71.

Roll, J.P., Vedel, J.P. and Ribot, E. (1989) Alteration of proprioceptive messages induced by tendon vibration in man: a microneurographic study. *Exp. Brain Res.,* 76: 213 – 222.

Roll, R., Bard, C. and Paillard, J. (1987) Head orienting contributes to the directional accuracy of aiming at distant targets. *Hum. Movement Sci.,* 5: 359 – 371.

Control and Actions of Vestibular and Visual Inputs

J.H.J. Allum and M. Hulliger (Eds.)
Progress in Brain Research, Vol. 80
© 1989 Elsevier Science Publishers B.V. (Biomedical Division)

Overview and critique of Chapters 11 – 14

V. Henn

Zürich, Switzerland

At first sight, the presentations of this group of papers have little in common. From a functional point of view, however, the one common theme was geometry and how it determines a vestibular response. We observe a directional specificity at the level of the hair cells and can follow it through the orientation of the otoliths and semicircular canals right through to the arrangement of extraocular muscles.

Hudspeth presents details about the mechanical – electrical coupling at the level of the hair cells. With the preparation he introduced, he can now answer such basic questions of how sound or acceleration is transduced. Specifically, the significance of different anatomical details of hair cells can be explored. It is still not clear how specificity is achieved for high frequency sound detection, where hair cells are expected to act as a high pass filter, or for gravity detection where we expect a non-adapting low pass filter characteristic. What is clear is that this type of research already affects clinical thinking as it could be shown that certain classes of antibiotics such as streptomycin directly block receptor currents. One possible consequence is a loss of hearing and vestibular function.

Shinoda et al. discuss the specific branching patterns of vestibulo-spinal neurones distributed over several levels in the spinal cord suggesting that each neurone activates a certain set of motoneurones. This poses the question of how specialized second order vestibular neurones are. Do they preserve directions imposed by the different semicircular canals, or are the directions of second order neurones already specifically adapted towards pulling directions of motoneurones they innervate? Are there certain sets of activity patterns dependent on the context of the motor behaviour? To answer these questions one would like to know the physiological characteristics of both the vestibular neurones as well as of the motoneurones involved. Such an experimental design is at present unrealistic, but still the problem should be kept in mind when creating realistic models reflecting such three-dimensional complexity.

Graf and Wilson address the question of three-dimensional transformations from a physiological and anatomical point of view. Although clinicians have for more than 100 years been accustomed to separate eye movements into horizontal, vertical, and torsional movement components, there is no reason to assume that the nervous system uses the same Cartesian coordinates. There are natural, or intrinsic, frames of reference, like the geometry of the labyrinths, or the geometrical arrangement of the eye muscles. For the muscles which move the head, the frame of reference is less obvious. Graf stresses that there are consistent deviations between the geometry of the labyrinth and the eye muscles which require a neuronal interface to make the necessary transformations. There is clear experimental evidence that other transformations, similar in concept, are necessary for the control of neck muscles. Clearly, the three-dimensional space around us has to be represented in multi-dimensional internal maps, and we would like to know the coordinate systems employed in these maps and the algorithms of their transformations.

Grantyn specifically addresses the question of how collicular output interfaces to the ocular and cervical motor system to generate appropriate output. With his paradigm of head and eye movements he faces all the complexities of the systems involved. The tecto-reticulo-spinal and the reticulo-spinal systems, the focus of his investigation, probably trigger and synchronize motor activity at different bulbar and spinal levels. This is reflected in the fact that activity in these systems might differ depending on whether the cat tries to look at a moving target or not in a particular experiment. This behaviour is different from neuronal systems in the brainstem or spinal cord which generate exactly patterned output for amplitude, velocity and direction of motor activity. We should not be surprised to find neuronal systems with such different direct or conditional connections to motor output. In evolutionary terms, the basic connections for the vestibulo-ocular reflex and orienting head movements are probably hard-wired brainstem connections present in all animals which can move their eyes and head. The one major addition for higher species is the ability to override or cancel such reflexes. This requires networks which are conditionally activated.

To conclude, these presentations at first sight have not much more in common than the word vestibular. However, we can conclude that there is a strong interdependence and design principle to be found in the hair cell, in the geometry of the labyrinths and eye muscles, in the hard-wiring of the basic vestibulo-ocular reflex, and probably also

for the vestibulo-collic and cervico-ocular reflexes. What we see when experiments are done in the alert animal is no more and nothing less of what we know from behaviour: reflexes can be adapted, habituated, plastically changed, or compensated for after lesions.

The ability to modify the VOR is addressed by Dr Collewijn (see Chapter 17, this volume), who questioned whether one should actually call it a reflex. In the ensuing discussion it was questioned whether one should further try to isolate small behavioural units and characterize neurone populations, or whether one should rather consider the behaviour of brainstem networks as a functional unit with certain 'emerging properties'. This view was opposed by Grüsser. In his opinion decisive progress has been made by studying subunits of behaviour, determining their anatomy, doing single unit studies, and contrasting this with the behaviour of the intact animal. If one were to study only the phenomenology of such a complex behaviour, one could not hope to arrive at an understanding of neuronal mechanisms. This is a point I would especially like to stress. As a clinician one is faced with the problem that a patient complains about a symptom, e.g. dizziness. Examination will then reveal pathological nystagmus. The possible causes for such symptoms are virtually infinite in terms of location of pathology and its etiology. Only with a clear understanding of pathophysiology, the logical description of functional elements, and the knowledge about possibilities of compensation after focal lesions, can we ever hope to understand the complexity of brainstem disease.

J.H.J. Allum and M. Hulliger (Eds.)
Progress in Brain Research, Vol. 80
© 1989 Elsevier Science Publishers B.V. (Biomedical Division)

CHAPTER 11

Mechanoelectrical transduction by hair cells of the bullfrog's sacculus

A.J. Hudspeth

Department of Cell Biology and Neuroscience, University of Texas Southwestern Medical Center, Dallas, TX 75235-9039, U.S.A.

Hair cells of the internal ear respond to excitatory mechanical stimulation of their hair bundles by the rapid opening of poorly cation-selective transduction channels. These channels, which are located near the bundles' tips, may be gated by forces applied through elastic linkages between adjacent stereocilia.

Key words: Vestibular receptor; Hair cell; Bullfrog

Introduction

The sense of equilibrium and the capacity for locomotion require the normal operation of the vestibular end organs; these organs, in turn, depend crucially on the function of hair cells, the sensory receptors of the internal ear. Despite differences in the organs in which they occur, it seems probable that all vertebrate hair cells function in fundamentally the same way (for reviews, see Howard et al., 1988; Roberts et al., 1988; Hudspeth, 1989). Much can therefore be learned from the study of various model systems whose simplicity makes them more amenable to modern biophysical approaches than are hair cells in the mammalian internal ear. The present review summarizes experimental approaches to the study of hair cells in vitro and our present understanding of the way in which these cells operate.

Materials and Methods

For the investigation of transduction in vitro, our group has developed three experimental prepara-tions employing hair cells from the sacculus of the bullfrog *(Rana catesbeiana)*. This frog's sacculus, an oblate ellipsoid about 3 mm in greatest length in an adult animal, is a receptor for ground-borne vibration. The saccular macula, a discoidal structure approximately 1 mm across, contains some 3000 hair cells disposed among about twice as many supporting cells. A hair cell from the sacculus is typical in its structure and innervation; because the hair bundle is of a relatively simple form and resembles those of many other hair cells in its size, number of constituent processes, and geometrical arrangement (Hillman, 1969), it can be taken as a model for bundles in other organs and species.

The saccular macula is thin and transparent enough that individual hair cells are readily visible with differential-interference-contrast optics; as a consequence, one may perform experiments that depend upon the manipulation of hair bundles or of their constituent processes. The organ is hardy enough to survive for several hours at room temperature in a simple saline solution; with appropriate attention to the medium, to oxygen tension, and to temperature, one can maintain the cells in a functional state for days. Finally, the sacculus lends itself to electrical recording techniques in several ways that are useful for answering different experimental questions.

The original preparation of the frog's sacculus (Hudspeth and Corey, 1977) involves stretching the macula flat against a coverslip that forms the bottom of an experimental chamber. Hair cells are viewed at a total magnification of 800× through a water-immersion objective lens; for convenient placement under a 1.6-mm-working-distance lens, stimulus probes and recording electrodes are bent near their tips (Hudspeth and Corey, 1978). With this preparation, it is possible to record from an in-

dividual hair cell with one or two microelectrodes while moving its hair bundle in a controlled fashion with a glass microprobe (Fig. 1). The simplest probes push against the elastic hair bundles (Hudspeth, 1982); for firmer coupling, a hair bundle may be made to adhere to a clean probe surface or held with the aid of suction (Holton and Hudspeth, 1986). The probes are in turn moved by calibrated piezoelectrical micromanipulators (Corey and Hudspeth, 1980) that may be modified for special functions such as operating along two or three mutually orthogonal axes (Shotwell et al., 1981) or moving with risetimes as short as 100 μs (Corey and Hudspeth, 1983b). In addition to serving in the recording of receptor potentials, this

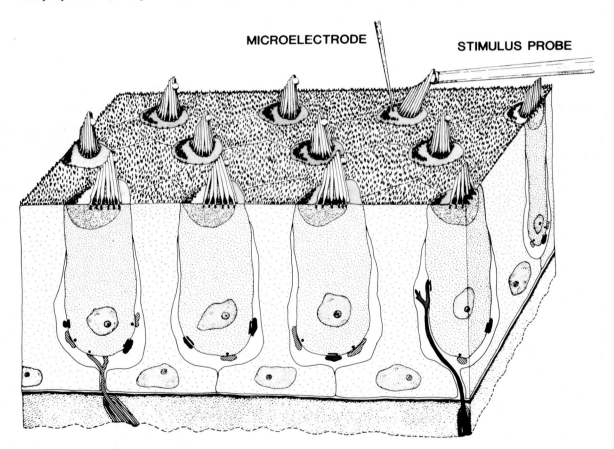

MICROELECTRODE   **STIMULUS PROBE**

Fig. 1. Technique for recording receptor potentials from a hair cell in vitro. While the receptor potential is monitored through a conventional microelectrode inserted through the apical plasma membrane, the mechanoreceptive hair bundle is displaced with a glass stimulus probe attached to the bundle's tip. (From Hudspeth, 1989.)

preparation suffices for the measurement of field potentials around activated hair bundles (Hudspeth, 1982) and may be used with tight-seal electrodes for cell-attached-patch or for whole-cell recordings (Holton and Hudspeth, 1986).

A second way of recording from the saccular macula is to mount it in a chamber so that it forms a barrier between two fluid-filled compartments. To hold the macula firmly in place and to prevent leakage of fluid or current around the preparation, we glue the isolated macula onto a plastic diaphragm with surgical adhesive (Holton and Hudspeth, 1983). When the otolithic membrane, to which almost all the hair bundles in the frog's sacculus are attached, is moved with a stimulus probe, transduction currents flow through many of the hair cells. The transepithelial potential changes caused by these currents can then be monitored, or one may voltage-clamp the epithelium and measure the transduction current itself (Corey and Hudspeth, 1979a, 1983a, b).

The third preparation for recording from hair cells of the bullfrog's sacculus involves enzymatically dissociated cells (Hudspeth and Lewis, 1988). The principal virtue of this method is that the basolateral cellular surfaces exposed upon isolation provide an admirable substrate for patch or whole-cell recording with tight-seal electrodes. These recording techniques in turn confer the advantages of a broad bandwidth and relatively low electrical noise, the capacity readily to voltage-clamp cells, and the ability to substitute for cytoplasm an ionic solution of the experimenter's choosing.

The use of glass stimulus probes and micromanipulators, instead of natural stimulation of hair cells, confers a substantial advantage in that the experimenter may disregard the complex transfer properties of the vestibular accessory structures. At the same time, however, direct stimulation of hair cells introduces technical problems which one must consider. It is necessary to establish a stable environment in which to conduct experiments; modern vibration-isolation tables, particularly those with internal damping, provide such an ex-

perimental condition. It is important to position the recording electrodes and stimulating probes with accuracy and especially with stability; a drift in the position of a stimulus probe through only 10 nm, well below notice by microscopic observation and without significant consequence in ordinary recording circumstances, amounts to a stimulus at least tenfold above threshold for hair cells! The experimenter must also ascertain that there is tight coupling between the stimulus probe and the hair bundle, for example by stroboscopic observation of the moving bundle (Holton and Hudspeth, 1983).

Results

When the hair bundle of a hair cell in the bullfrog's sacculus is driven back and forth with a stimulus probe, the cell produces a receptor potential whose peak-to-peak amplitude ranges from a fraction of a millivolt to more than 30 mV, depending on the quality of the electrode penetration, the resting potential of the cell, and the amplitude, orientation, and frequency of the stimulus. In typical recordings from cells in standard saline solution and at a resting potential near -60 mV, the response to large stimuli is a somewhat asymmetrical waveform that shows saturation in both the depolarizing and the hyperpolarizing directions (Hudspeth and Corey, 1977; Shotwell et al., 1981).

The relation between mechanical stimulation of a hair cell and the ensuing response is conveniently summarized in a plot of the relevant response against hair-bundle displacement or a related parameter. Such displacement-response relationships have been obtained for the frog's sacculus (Corey and Hudspeth, 1977, 1983b; Shotwell et al., 1981), the turtle's and chick's basilar papillae (Crawford and Fettiplace, 1981; Ohmori, 1987), and the guinea pig's cochlea (Russell et al., 1986). All are sigmoidal curves; most show relatively sharp saturation in the negative stimulus direction and asymptotic behaviour, without abrupt or complete saturation, for positive stimuli. There is a pronounced asymmetry between the depolarizing and hyperpolarizing phases of the receptor potential; large, oscillatory stimuli depolarize the membrane considerably more than they hyperpolarize it.

One of the most remarkable features of the hair cell's response is its directionality. The hypothesis that the excitatory component of the receptor potential corresponds to movement of the hair bundle's tip in the positive direction (Lowenstein and Wersäll, 1959) was verified by micromanipulation of saccular hair cells from the bullfrog (Shotwell et al., 1981). Direct stimulation of hair bundles also confirmed the suggestion (Flock, 1965) that response amplitude scales with the cosine of the angle by which a stimulus deviates from the the hair cell's axis of bilateral symmetry (Shotwell et al., 1981).

The receptor potential arises as the result of a stimulus-induced change in membrane conductance (Hudspeth and Corey, 1977); the depolarizing phase of the receptor potential corresponds with an increase in membrane conductance, while the hyperpolarizing component reflects a decrease in conductance from the value at rest. Voltage-clamp studies indicate that the transduction channels opened by mechanical stimuli are relatively non-selective; in addition to the K^+ normally present at a high concentration in endolymph, they also pass Na^+, Ca^{2+}, and many other small cations (Corey and Hudspeth, 1979b; Ohmori, 1985).

The geometrical complexity of the hair bundle and the associated structures at the apical end of the hair cell is such that it is not obvious where the actual mechanoelectrical transduction event occurs. Because there is as yet no molecular probe for the transduction molecule, the unequivocal localization of the transducer is not presently feasible. The site of transduction does have one unambiguous signature, however: the flow of current across the hair-cell membrane in response to mechanical stimulation. Recordings with extracellular microelectrodes reveal signals of the expected size (Hudspeth, 1982). Because the strongest current sink is at the top end of the hair

bundle (Fig. 2), the experiment suggests that the transduction channels occur within the hair bundle, near the tips of the stereocilia, rather than on the flattened apical surface of the hair cell.

There is now morphological evidence for a specialized structure at the stereociliary tips that could be involved in transduction: the tip of each stereocilium is joined by a thin, extracellular filament to the side of the longest adjacent stereocilium (Pickles et al., 1984). These links could be stretched by shear between the stereocilia when a bundle is displaced in the excitatory direction. This mechanism would explain the directional sensitivity of the hair bundle; because they occur only between adjacent stereocilia in a given file, rather than between processes in the same rank, the links should be distorted solely by stimulus components along the cell's axis of bilateral symmetry (Shotwell et al., 1981).

When a hair bundle is abruptly deflected, the rate of rise of the subsequent response depends upon the amplitude of the stimulus (Fig. 3). This result, which suggests that mechanical stimuli act by altering the free-energy difference between the open and closed states of a transduction molecule, leads to a simple model for transduction (Corey and Hudspeth, 1983b). The transducer is posited to be coupled to an elastic linkage, the gating spring, upon which stimuli exert a force. If the stereociliary tip links are the elastic elements, the

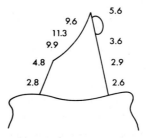

Fig. 2. Localization of transduction in a hair bundle. While the bundle is continuously stimulated, an extracellular microelectrode measures the potential at various positions around the bundle. The average values of the peak-to-peak response (in μV), shown at the sites of recording, suggest that transduction occurs near the bundle's tip. (From Hudspeth, 1989.)

resultant model (Fig. 4) accounts for most of the properties of the transduction process (Howard and Hudspeth, 1988; Howard et al., 1988; Roberts et al., 1988).

Mechanical displacement of the hair bundle is thought to influence a channel's probability of adopting its open configuration by doing work on the transduction linkage. By the use of minute, flexible glass fibres attached to a hair bundle, it is possible to demonstrate that the bundle's stiffness decreases over the range of bundle positions in which the channels are gated (Howard and Hudspeth, 1988). Analysis of this gating compliance indicates that opening a channel requires a force of about 2 pN acting through a distance of approximately 4 nm.

If hair cells of the frog's sacculus are presented with a step stimulus that persists for some time, the ensuing response does not maintain a constant amplitude indefinitely, but instead gradually returns toward its resting level (Corey and Hudspeth, 1983a; Eatock et al., 1987). The same phenomenon also manifests itself in recordings of

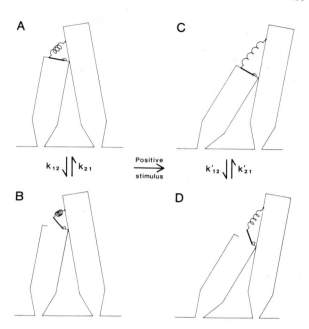

Fig. 4. A model for mechanoelectrical transduction in hair cells. The transduction-channel molecule is posited to possess a gate that regulates the flow of ionic current and that can exist in either of two states, closed or open. The free-energy difference between the states is affected by stretching an elastic filament, the gating spring, which may be an inter-stereociliary tip link. When the hair bundle's distal tip is displaced in the positive direction (right), the linkage is stretched by an amount proportional to the bundle's displacement. This motion makes the open configuration of the channel energetically more favourable than the closed, and thus leads to a redistribution of the channels to a condition in which more are open.

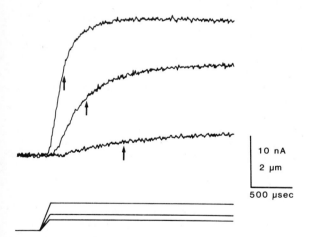

Fig. 3. Kinetics of transduction by the bullfrog's saccular hair cells. As the stimuli (lower traces) applied to an epithelial preparation increase in amplitude, the resultant responses (upper traces) not only become larger, but also rise more swiftly to their final levels. The arrows, which are situated at the times when the traces reach 63% of their final values, indicate the time constants of the three responses.

the receptor potential or transduction current in response to an oscillatory stimulus, when the hair bundle experiences an additional, static offset (Fig. 5). The alteration in the response in both instances is not due to slippage of the stimulus probe or drift in the micromanipulator, but is indicative of an adaptation process intrinsic to the hair cell's transduction mechanism.

Mechanical measurements indicate that, while adaptation is taking place, the stiffness of a hair bundle from the frog's sacculus declines (Howard and Hudspeth, 1987a, b): adaptation involves a relaxation of the tension in an elastic element of the hair bundle, the gating spring. How this comes

134

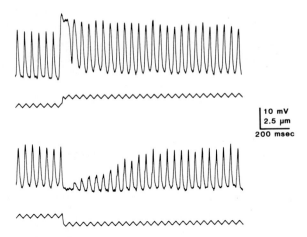

| 10 mV |
| 2.5 μm |
| 200 msec |

Fig. 5. Adaptation of the receptor potential of a saccular hair cell. While the response to a continuous, triangle-wave stimulus is measured, the hair bundle is abruptly offset in the excitatory (upper two traces) or the inhibitory (lower traces) direction. After transient saturation of the response in each instance, the adaptation process restores the bundle's sensitivity over a period of a few hundred milliseconds.

about remains unknown; it is possible, however, that the tension in elements such as the tip links is adjusted by rearrangements in the stereociliary cytoskeleton (Howard and Hudspeth, 1987a, b) or cuticular plate.

Adaptation likely serves the frog's sacculus by rejecting large, relatively constant gravitational stimuli; the organ can consequently detect transient accelerations only one millionth as large (Eatock et al., 1987). Although adaptation has not yet been directly demonstrated in other preparations, it may account for time-dependent changes in the responses of other vestibular receptors.

Acknowledgements

For fiscal support of the original research discussed herein, the author is grateful to the National Institutes of Health (grants NS-13154, NS-20429, and NS-22389) and to System Development Foundation. I am indebted to a number of colleagues for their aid during the conduct of the research and especially to Mr R. Jacobs, who produced the specialized apparatus that made the experiments possible.

References

Corey, D.P. and Hudspeth, A.J. (1979a) Response latency of vertebrate hair cells. *Biophys. J.*, 26: 499–506.

Corey, D.P. and Hudspeth, A.J. (1979b) Ionic basis of the receptor potential in a vertebrate hair cell. *Nature (London)*, 281: 675–677.

Corey, D.P. and Hudspeth, A.J. (1980) Mechanical stimulation and micromanipulation with piezoelectric bimorph elements. *J. Neurosci. Methods*, 3: 183–202.

Corey, D.P. and Hudspeth, A.J. (1983a) Analysis of the microphonic potential of the bullfrog's sacculus. *J. Neurosci.*, 3: 942–961.

Corey, D.P. and Hudspeth, A.J. (1983b) Kinetics of the receptor current in bullfrog saccular hair cells. *J. Neurosci.*, 3: 962–976.

Crawford, A.C. and Fettiplace, R. (1981) Non-linearities in the responses of turtle hair cells. *J. Physiol. (London)*, 315: 317–338.

Eatock, R.A., Corey, D.P. and Hudspeth, A.J. (1987) Adaptation of mechanoeletrical transduction in hair cells of the bullfrog's sacculus. *J. Neurosci.*, 7: 2821–2836.

Flock, Å. (1965) Transducing mechanisms in the lateral line canal organ receptors. *Cold Spring Harbor Symp. Quant. Biol.*, 30: 133–145.

Hillman, D.E. (1969) New ultrastructural findings regarding a vestibular ciliary apparatus and its possible functional significance. *Brain Res.*, 13: 407–412.

Holton, T. and Hudspeth, A.J. (1983) A micromechanical contribution to cochlear tuning and tonotopic organization. *Science*, 222: 508–510.

Holton, T. and Hudspeth, A.J. (1986) The transduction channel of hair cells from the bull-frog characterized by noise analysis. *J. Physiol. (London)*, 375: 195–227.

Howard, J. and Hudspeth, A.J. (1987a) Mechanical relaxation of the hair bundle mediates adaptation in mechanoelectrical transduction by the bullfrog's saccular hair cell. *Proc. Natl. Acad. Sci. USA*, 84: 3064–3068.

Howard, J. and Hudspeth, A.J. (1987b) Adaptation of mechanoelectrical transduction in hair cells. In A.J. Hudspeth, P.R. MacLeish, F.L. Margolis and T.N. Wiesel (Eds.), *Sensory Transduction, Discussions in Neurosciences, Volume IV, No. 3*, Fondation pour l'Etude de Système Nerveux Central et Périphérique, Geneva, pp. 138–145.

Howard, J. and Hudspeth, A.J. (1988) Compliance of the hair bundle associated with gating of mechanoelectrical transduction channels in the bullfrog's saccular hair cell. *Neuron*, 1: 189–199.

Howard, J., Roberts, W.M. and Hudspeth, A.J. (1988) Mechanoelectrical transduction by hair cells. *Ann. Rev.*

Biophys. Biophys. Chem., 17: 99 – 124.

Hudspeth, A.J. (1982) Extracellular current flow and the site of transduction by vertebrate hair cells. *J. Neurosci.,* 2: 1 – 10.

Hudspeth, A.J. (1989) How the ear's works work. *Nature (London),* 341: 397 – 404.

Hudspeth, A.J. and Corey, D.P. (1977) Sensitivity, polarity, and conductance change in the response of vertebrate hair cells to controlled mechanical stimuli. *Proc. Natl. Acad. Sci. USA,* 74: 2407 – 2411.

Hudspeth, A.J. and Corey, D.P. (1978) Controlled bending of high-resistance glass microelectrodes. *Am. J. Physiol.,* 234: C56 – C57.

Hudspeth, A.J. and Lewis, R.S. (1988) Kinetic analysis of voltage- and ion-dependent conductances in saccular hair cells of the bull-frog, *Rana catesbeiana. J. Physiol. (London),* 400: 237 – 274.

Lowenstein, O. and Wersäll, J. (1959) A functional interpretation of the electron-microscopic structure of the sensory hairs in the cristae of the elasmobranch *Raja clavata* in terms of directional sensitivity. *Nature (London),* 184: 1807 – 1808.

Ohmori, H. (1985) Mechano-electrical transduction currents in isolated vestibular hair cells of the chick. *J. Physiol. (London),* 359: 189 – 217.

Ohmori, H. (1987) Gating properties of the mechano-electrical transducer channel in the dissociated vestibular hair cell of the chick. *J. Physiol. (London),* 387: 589 – 609.

Pickles, J.O., Comis, S.D. and Osborne, M.P. (1984) Crosslinks between stereocilia in the guinea pig organ of Corti, and their possible relation to sensory transduction. *Hearing Res.,* 15: 103 – 112.

Roberts, W.M., Howard, J. and Hudspeth, A.J. (1988) Mechanoelectrical transduction, frequency tuning, and synaptic transmission by hair cells. *Ann. Rev. Cell Biol.,* 4: 63 – 92.

Russell, I.J., Richardson, G.P. and Cody, A.R. (1986) Mechanosensitivity of mammalian auditory hair cells in vitro. *Nature (London),* 321: 517 – 519.

Shotwell, S.L., Jacobs, R. and Hudspeth, A.J. (1981) Directional sensitivity of individual vertebrate hair cells to controlled deflection of their hair bundles. *Ann. New York Acad. Sci.,* 374: 1 – 10.

J.H.J. Allum and M. Hulliger (Eds.)
Progress in Brain Research, Vol. 80
© 1989 Elsevier Science Publishers B.V. (Biomedical Division)

CHAPTER 12

Comparison of the branching patterns of lateral and medial vestibulospinal tract axons in the cervical spinal cord

Y. Shinoda, T. Ohgaki, Y. Sugiuchi and T. Futami

*Department of Physiology and Department of Otolaryngology, School of Medicine, Tokyo Medical and Dental University,
1 – 5 – 45, Yushima, Bunkyo-ku, Tokyo 113, Japan*

The morphology of single physiologically-identified lateral and medial vestibulospinal tract (LVST and MVST) axons was analysed, using intracellular staining with horseradish peroxidase (HRP) and three-dimensional reconstruction of axonal trajectories in the cat. Axons were penetrated in the cervical cord at C1 – C8 with a microelectrode filled with 7% HRP. These axons were identified as vestibulospinal axons by their monosynaptic responses to stimulation of the vestibular nerve and further classified as either LVST or MVST axons by their responses to stimulation of the LVST and MVST. The stained axons could be traced over distances of 3 – 16 mm rostrocaudally. Within these lengths, both LVST and MVST axons were found to have multiple axon collaterals at different segments in the cervical cord. Up to seven collaterals were given off from the stems of MVST axons and LVST axons. The LVST axons included both neurones terminating at the cervical cord and those projecting further caudally to the thoracic or lumbar cord. Each collateral of these LVST axons, after entering into the gray matter, ramified successively in a δ-like fashion and terminated mainly in lamina VIII and in the medial part of lamina VII. Many boutons of both terminal and en passant types seemed to make contact with the cell bodies and proximal dendrites of neurones in the ventromedial nucleus (VM). Each collateral had a narrow rostrocaudal extension (0.2 – 1.6 mm, average 0.8 mm) in the gray matter in contrast to a much wider intercollateral interval (average 1.5 mm), so that there were gaps free from terminal boutons between adjacent collateral arborizations. The morphology of axon collaterals of MVST axons was very similar to that of LVST axons. The rostrocaudal extent of single axon collaterals was very restricted (0.3 – 2.1 mm) in contrast to the wide spread in a mediolateral or a dorsoventral direction. MVST axons had intensive projections to the upper cervical cord with multiple axon collaterals. One to seven collaterals of single MVST axons were found at C1 – C3. Terminals of MVST axons were distributed in laminae VII, VIII and IX, including the VM, the nucleus spinalis n. accessorii (SA), and the commissural nucleus. Many terminals seemed to make contact with retrogradely-labelled motoneurones of neck muscles. Both axosomatic and axodendritic contacts were observed on motoneurones in various sizes. Some collaterals gave rise to terminal arborizations in both the VM and the SA. These results suggest that single LVST and MVST axons may control excitability of multiple dorsal axial muscles concurrently with their multiple axon collaterals at multisegmental levels.

Key words: Vestibulocollic reflex; Spinal cord; Cat; Intracellular recording; Neuroanatomical technique

Introduction

Vestibular nucleus neurons give rise to three separate vestibulospinal tracts (VST): the lateral vestibulospinal tract (LVST), the medial vestibulo-spinal tract (MVST), and the caudal vestibulospinal tract (CVST; Peterson and Coulter, 1977). The LVST arises mainly in the lateral nucleus and descends ipsilaterally all the way to sacral levels (Brodal, 1974). LVST axons terminate in the medial portion of the ventral horn and have an excitatory action on all target neurons (Wilson and Yoshida, 1969; Grillner et al., 1970; Akaike et al., 1973). The MVST originates in the medial, descending and lateral nuclei. MVST axons descend bilaterally as far as the thoracic cord (Nyberg-Hansen, 1964). They terminate medially in the ventral horn; some of them are excitatory and others are inhibitory in action (Wilson and Yoshida, 1969). In spite of considerable knowledge compiled about the neural connections linking between the labyrinth and spinal motoneurons, the intraspinal morphology of VST axons has not yet been described. It has been tacitly assumed that VST axons like other long descending motor tract axons project to a localized region of the spinal cord. Recent electrophysiological studies, however, showed that about 50% of the LVST neurones sending terminal branches to the cervical enlargement also have axon branches extending to lumbar levels (Abzug et al., 1974) and that the axons of 62% of ipsilateral lateral nucleus neurones not only give off a collateral to C3, but also extend as far as the cervical enlargement (Rapoport et al., 1977). More detailed branching patterns of single LVST axons could not be determined using electrophysiological techniques, nor with Golgi impregnation methods. Recently, the parent axons and their collaterals of corticospinal and rubrospinal axons have been successfully visualized in the spinal cord with an intracellular staining method (Futami et al., 1979; Shinoda et al., 1981, 1982).

The present study was aimed at analysing the morphology of single electrophysiologically-identified VST axons, using the same intracellular staining method with horseradish peroxidase (HRP) as used for analysis of other long tract axons. This paper will summarize the morphological evidence concerning the branching patterns and terminal arborizations of LVST and MVST axons in the cervical cord of the cat.

Methods

Experiments were performed in cats anaesthetized with pentobarbital sodium (initial dose of 35 mg/kg and supplemented as required). Details of the experimental procedures and the staining method have been fully described previously and will not be repeated here (Shinoda and Yoshida, 1974; Shinoda et al., 1986; Shinoda et al., 1988). In short, single MVST and LVST axons were penetrated in the ventral funiculus of the cervical cord with glass micropipettes filled with 7% HRP (Toyobo Co., Osaka, Japan). After electrophysiological identification, the axons were injected with HRP iontophoretically through the recording microelectrode. After survival time of 5 – 36 h, the cats were perfused and the serial sections of the spinal cord (100 μm thick) were treated for HRP with the diaminobenzidine method (Graham and Karnovsky, 1966). Drawings were prepared with an Olympus microscope equipped with a camera lucida drawing attachment. The axonal trajectory reconstructed in the transverse plane was converted to that in the horizontal or sagittal plane.

Results

I. Identification of VST axons

MVST axons were penetrated in the mediodorsal portion of the ventral funiculus at a depth of 3.5 – 5.0 mm from the dorsal cord surface and LVST axons in the ventral funiculus at a depth of 4.0 – 6.6 mm. Since only vestibular nucleus neurones can be activated monosynaptically from vestibular primary afferents (Wilson and Melvil-Jones, 1979; Precht and Shimazu, 1965), axons activated monosynaptically from vestibular primary afferents were identified as VST axons (Fig. 1). When the difference between the latencies of the vestibular-nerve-induced spikes and of the nucleus-induced or tract-induced spikes was shorter than 1.3 ms (the longest value for monosynaptic activation (1.4 ms) minus a latent period for spike generation after stimulus onset (0.1 ms)) (Wilson and Melvil-Jones, 1979; Precht and Shimazu, 1965), the axons were considered to be activated monosynaptically from the vestibular nerve. The axons were identified as LVST axons when they were activated directly from the ipsilateral LVST at a medullary level at a much lower stimulus intensity than from the MLF, whereas they were identified as MVST axons when they were directly activated from the MLF at a medullary level at a lower intensity (Shinoda et al., 1986, 1988).

II. The morphology of single LVST axons

The stem axons of LVST axons ran in the ipsilateral ventral funiculus or ventrolateral funiculus. The stained distances of the stem axons ranged from 3.4 to 16.3 mm with a mean of 8.5 mm. Over their course, most LVST axons terminating in the cervical cord gave off at least one axon collateral (Fig. 2). Up to 7 collaterals per axon were observed, mean 3.2 (Fig. 5A). Some LVST axons (4/11) projecting to the thoracic or lumbar spinal cord also had axon collaterals in the cervical cord. The maximum number of their cervical collaterals per

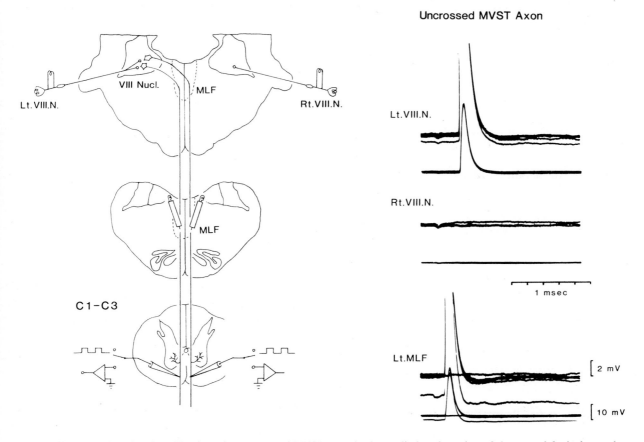

Fig. 1. Electrophysiological identification of an uncrossed MVST axon in the mediodorsal portion of the ventral funiculus at the upper cervical spinal cord. Left: schematic diagram of the experimental set-up. Upper right: monosynaptic response to stimulation of the ipsilateral vestibular nerve (500 μA). Middle right: no response to stimulation of the contralateral vestibular nerve. Lower right: direct response to stimulation of the ipsilateral MLF in the medulla in an all or none manner at threshold of 40 μA. This axon was not activated from the ipsilateral LVST at an intensity of 500 μA (unpublished data).

axon was two. This was in contrast to the finding that 22 out of 23 axons terminating in the cervical cord had 1 to 7 collaterals. The collaterals were given off at right angles from the stem axons and ran dorsally into the ventral horn. At the entrance into the gray matter, the primary collaterals ramified into a few thick branches in a delta-like or a Y-shaped fashion. These branches extended further dorsally through lamina VIII to lamina VII. The branches to the dorsomedial portion of lamina VII gave off thin side branchlets intensively to lamina VIII including the ventromedial nucleus (VM) of lamina IX of Rexed (Rexed, 1954), and the nucleus commissuralis (CO) as shown in the upper middle drawing of Fig. 2. The branches in

their further extensions gave rise to terminal arborizations in lamina VII adjacent to the dorsal boder of lamina VIII. Terminal branches were thin (0.2 – 0.8 μm) and bore boutons en passant along their length and one bouton at each terminus, or bore only one terminal bouton. Up to 6 en passant boutons were strung out along the last 25 – 50 μm of a terminal branch. The total number of boutons per collateral varied from 38 to 262 with a mean of 161. This distribution of terminal boutons is in good agreement with the results of previous degeneration studies (Nyberg-Hansen, 1969; Nyberg-Hansen and Mascitti, 1964). According to a previous degeneration study (Nyberg-Hansen and Mascitti, 1964), terminations of LVST axons

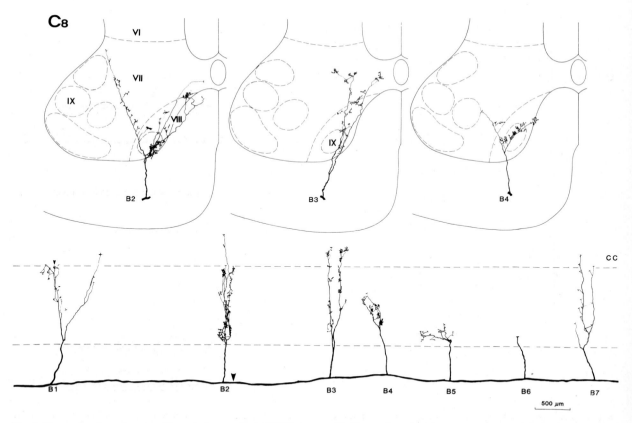

Fig. 2. Reconstruction of axon collaterals from a single LVST axon at C8. Upper three drawings are reconstructions in the transverse plane of B2 – B4 axon collaterals shown in the sagittal plane in the lower drawing. The lower border of the central canal (CC) and the lower border of the ventral horn are indicated by the dashed lines. The arrowhead indicates an injection site of HRP. The stem axon extended further rostrally by 5.9 mm from B1 and caudally by 2.7 mm from B7 (from Fig. 2 in Shinoda et al., 1986.)

were not found on motoneurones in the VM in the spinal enlargements, although a few terminations could be observed on this group of motoneurones of the thoracic cord. In the present study, terminal boutons appeared to make contact on not only small, and medium-sized neurones but also large neurones in the VM, which are presumably motoneurones to axial muscles. These included both apparent axosomatic and axodendritic contacts. The CO is a well-defined cell group lying close to the medial border of the ventral horn and towards its base, where commissural cells exist sending their axons across the midline in the anterior commissure (Szenthágothai, 1951). Some of these commissural interneurones terminate on contralateral motoneurones (Harrison et al., 1986; Scheibel et al., 1969). A large number of terminal boutons of LVST axons were found in this nucleus. Contralateral effects following unilateral vestibular nucleus stimulation are probably exerted by way of these commissural cells (Bruggencate et al., 1969; Hongo et al., 1975). Some other branches extended dorsally or dorsolaterally in lamina VII, giving off thin branchlets with en passant boutons and terminating in the middle portion of the dorsal lamina VII. Many boutons were observed in lamina VII adjacent to lamina IX in the lateral ventral horn. An LVST projection to this area has not been reported before, however this projection is important in view of inhibition evoked disynaptically from Deiters nucleus (Grillner et al., 1970). It has been shown that the LVST inhibits some flexor motoneurones via Ia inhibitory interneurones in the segmental reciprocal inhibitory pathway (Hultborn and Udo, 1972; Hultborn et al., 1976). These Ia inhibitory interneurones are located in lamina VII adjacent to lamina IX (Jankowska and Lindström, 1972). The present finding of terminal boutons in this area gives morphological support for this electrophysiological result.

In contrast to the wide spread of axon collaterals in a transverse plane of the cord, the rostrocaudal extent of single axon collaterals was very restricted (see the lower drawing of Fig. 2), ranging from 230 to 1560 μm, average 760 μm ($n = 16$). There were usually gaps free from terminal boutons between terminal fields of adjacent axon collaterals, since intercollateral intervals (mean = 1490 μm) were much longer than the rostrocaudal extent of each terminal field. The MVST axons described so far sent terminal branches to the medial portion of the ventral horn. But about one-fourth of the stained axons had a main projection to lamina IX in the lateral ventral horn. These axons had common branching patterns and terminal arborizations to those axons projecting to the more medial portion of the ventral horn (Shinoda et al., 1986). Terminal boutons of these axons were mainly distributed in lamina IX in the lateral ventral horn and its adjacent lamina VII.

III. Morphology of single MVST axons

MVST axons were classified into two groups: crossed and uncrossed MVST axons. Crossed and uncrossed MVST axons descend in the spinal cord contralateral and ipsilateral to their cell bodies, respectively. Both MVST axons were activated directly from the ipsilateral MLF at a medullary level rostral to the recording site at C2 and C3. This indicated that crossed MVST axons cross the midline at a level of the vestibular nucleus or at its caudal vicinity and then descend in the spinal cord. This short report will describe only the morphology of uncrossed MVST axons. The stem axons of uncrossed MVST axons ran along the medial side of the ventral horn in the mediodorsal portion of the ventral funiculus. They were stained over distances from 2.5 to 14.4 mm (average 8.6 mm, $n = 10$) at C1 – C4. Typical branching patterns of an uncrossed MVST axon are illustrated in Fig. 3. In the axon of this figure, three axon collaterals arose from the stem axon at right angles. The primary collaterals ran laterally and entered into the ventral horn at its medial boder. They divided into several thick branches immediately after the entrance to the ventral horn and spread in a delta-like fashion in a transverse plane. Three groups of branches were separable in terms of their course and destination. A typical example is seen

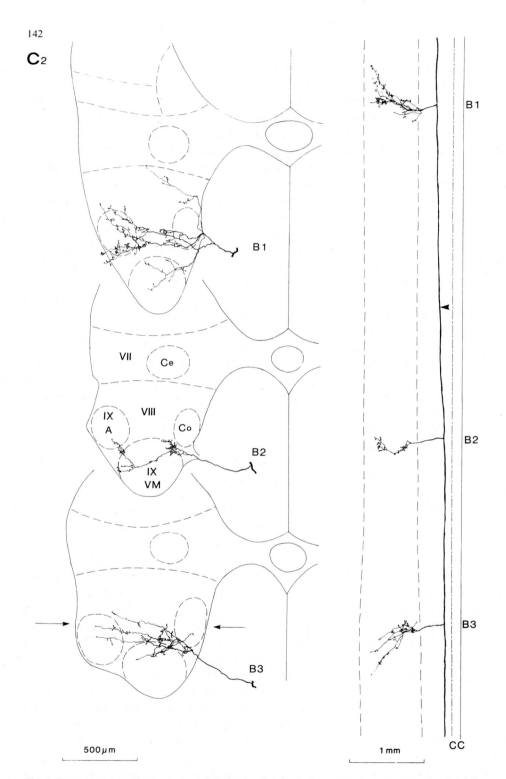

C₂

VII Ce

IX VIII
A

Co

IX
VM

B1

B2

B3

B1

B2

B3

CC

500 μm

1 mm

Fig. 3. Reconstruction of an uncrossed MVST axon in the upper cervical cord. Dorsal view of the axon is shown on the right (broken lines show the borders of the ventral horn at a level indicated by two arrows). An arrowhead indicates an injection site of HRP. Ce, nucleus cervicalis centralis; Co, nucleus commissuralis; Cc, central canal; VM, nucleus ventromedialis; A, nucleus spinalis n. accessorii (from Fig. 5 in Shinoda et al., 1988).

in the collateral B1 of Fig. 3. One group of branches ran ventrolaterally into the VM and gave rise to extensive terminal arborizations there. Some of them extended further into the nucleus spinalis n. accessorii (SA). A second group of branches ran almost horizontally or laterally to the SA or its adjacent lamina VIII. Over their course, thin branchlets were given off to lamina VIII dorsal to the VM. A third group of branches ran dorsolaterally, emitting thin branchlets and terminating in the medial portion of the dorsal lamina VIII and its adjacent lamina VII. These three groups of branches did not always exist and usually one or two groups were lacking; an example is shown on the right in Fig. 4. This collateral projected extensively to the dorsal portion of the medial ventral horn and only a small number of branchlets were sent to the VM. In contrast to the wide spread of terminal arborizations in a transverse plane, the rostrocaudal extent of single axon collaterals was very restricted (Fig. 3, right, ranging from 300 to 2100

μm (mean 620 μm), $n = 19$). The average distance between adjacent primary collaterals was 1870 μm. Since the intercollateral intervals were much wider than the rostrocaudal extent of single axon collaterals, there were usually gaps free from terminal boutons between the terminal fields of adjacent axon collaterals. One of the most important characteristics of branching patterns was the existence of multiple axon collaterals. One to 7 axon collaterals were seen for individual uncrossed MVST axons ($n = 10$) that were well stained. Six of them are shown as an example in Fig. 5B.

Although we do not describe the morphology of crossed MVST axons in this report, both uncrossed and crossed MVST axons had many common features of branching patterns and terminal distributions. The terminal area of uncrossed MVST axons occupied lamina IX including both the VM and the SA, lamina VIII including the CO, and lamina VII. Terminal boutons were most predominant in lamina IX, especially in the VM.

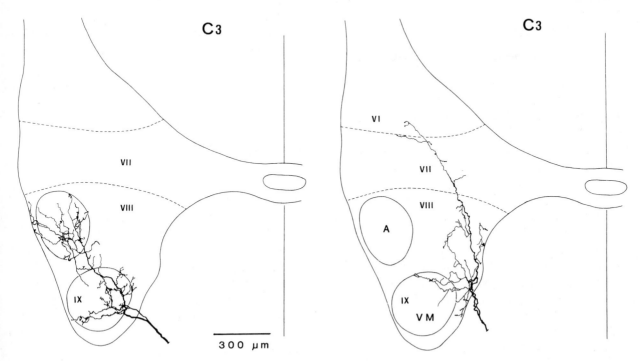

Fig. 4, Reconstruction of two uncrossed MVST axons in the transverse plane at C3 (Shinoda, Ohgaki and Sugiuchi, unpublished data).

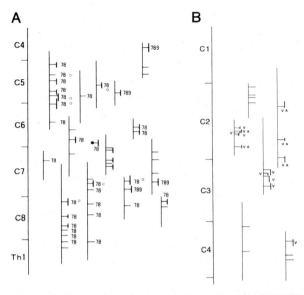

Fig. 5. Spinal distribution of axon collaterals of single LVST axons (A) and MVST axons (B). Thin vertical lines indicate stem axons and dark thick bars indicate terminal fields of single axon collaterals in a rostrocaudal direction. The numbers beside each collateral in A indicate the laminae of Rexed where the collaterals terminate. The letters, V and A, in B indicate the locations of terminal arborizations in the nucleus ventromedialis and the nucleus spinalis n. accessorii, respectively.

Boutons were irregular (elliptical rather than round) and the average size was 2.8 × 1.8 μm (longer × shorter diameter, n = 100). Both en passant and terminal boutons were seen and the percentage of boutons en passant was 48%. In lamina IX, many boutons appeared to make contact with cell bodies and proximal dendrites of the counter-stained cells. Apparent axosomatic and axodendritic contacts were observed on large, medium-sized and even small-sized cells. By an axodendritic contact is meant a contact with a proximal dendrite, since distal dendrites could not be identified in preparations counterstained with Cresyl violet. The neurones in the VM and the SA, some of which were very large, were most likely motoneurones innervating neck muscles (Richmond et al., 1987). To confirm that MVST axons make apparent contact with motoneurones in lamina IX, motoneurones of different neck muscles were retrogradely labelled with HRP. Some boutons of MVST axons were observed on the cell bodies or proximal dendrites of the retrogradely-labelled motoneurones. Moreover, other terminal boutons of the same axon seemed to make contact with the cell bodies or proximal dendrites of the unlabelled counter-stained large cells in a different portion of the VM. This finding strongly suggests that single MVST axons innervate multiple motor nuclei of different neck muscles. This idea was further supported by the following finding. Three axon collaterals of the MVST axon in Fig. 3 projected to both the VM and the SA. The VM contains motor nuclei of neck extensors (m. dorsi proprii) and the SA contains motor nuclei of neck flexors (Reighard and Jennings, 1951; Crouch, 1969). About one-third of the examined MVST axons projected to both the VM and the SA. In such axons as the axon in Fig. 3, one set of terminal arborizations in either the VM or the SA usually tended to be more intensive. However, some MVST axons like the one shown in Fig. 4 gave rise to extensive terminal arborizations in both the VM and the SA and apparent axodendritic contacts were observed on large neurones in each nucleus. This finding gives more morphological support to multiple innervation of single VST axons on different paravertebral muscles.

Discussion

The vestibular receptors providing inputs to uncrossed MVST axons can only be determined by further investigation, using natural stimulation or selective electrical stimulation of individual afferent nerves (Shinoda and Yoshida, 1974; Suzuki and Cohen, 1964). It is also impossible to speculate on whether uncrossed MVST axons are excitatory or inhibitory (Wilson and Yoshida, 1969), without further appropriate examination. We have evidence only that all the examined MVST axons run ipsilaterally in the MLF to axial muscles. This evidence, however, provides an important suggestion on the synaptic nature of uncrossed MVST axons. The pattern of disynaptic excitation and inhibition between individual semicircular canals and neck motoneurones has been extensively analysed by Wilson and his colleagues (Wilson and Maeda, 1974; Fukushima et al., 1979). MVST neurons receive mainly canal inputs, although some are also influenced by otolith inputs (Wilson and Peterson, 1978; Wilson et al., 1977). All semicircular canal ampullae, with the exception of that of the ipsilateral anterior canal, have disynaptic connections with neck extensor motoneurones via the MVST. Stimulation of anterior and posterior canal nerves on both sides gives disynaptic excitation and inhibition, respectively; stimulation of the ipsilateral horizontal canal nerve evokes disynaptic inhibition and that of the contralateral horizontal canal nerve evokes disynaptic excitation. Neck flexor motoneurones receive disynaptic excitatory inputs from the contralateral three semicircular canals and disynaptic inhibitory inputs from the ipsilateral three semicircular canals via the MVST. Based on these electrophysiological data, all uncrossed MVST axons to neck motoneurones are most likely considered to be inhibitory in nature, but further experiments are required to provide direct evidence about their synaptic nature.

Abzug et al. (1974) demonstrated electrophysiologically that many axons of the LVST give off axon collaterals to the cervical cord before they terminate in the lumbar cord. Our data have confirmed this electrophysiological observation and further provide additional evidence of the existence of multiple axon collaterals from single LVST and MVST axons at different segments of the cervical cord. Since LVST axons appear to make contact with motoneurones innervating axial muscles at different segments, this finding strongly suggests that single LVST axons may control the excitability of different axial muscles concurrently at multisegmental levels, even at widely separate levels between the cervical and the lumbar regions. Multiple branching of single LVST axons might function to coordinate properly widespread activation of the muscles of the neck, trunk and limbs.

MVST axons have extensive terminals in the cervical cord and innervate mainly neck motoneurones with their multiple axon collaterals. They give off collaterals over up to three segments. This rostrocaudal extension is, of course, underestimated due to technical limitation. A single MVST axon probably has multiple collaterals over a much wider length of its stem axon. In addition to this wide multisegmental spread, axon collaterals seem to innervate more than one motor nuclei of neck muscles even at the same segment. Accordingly, this result suggests that a single MVST axon receiving input from a particular semicircular canal may diverge onto multiple motor nuclei of neck muscles, creating a functional set of muscles for a particular postural movement, thereby producing a compensatory head movement in an appropriate direction. Further study on functional sets of muscles innervated by single VST axons, in other words, what combination of axial muscles are innervated by a single VST axon receiving a particular vestibular input, will provide important clues to our understanding of the neural mechanisms underlying postural control.

Acknowledgements

This research was supported by grants from the Japanese Ministry of Education, Science and Culture for Scientific Research (62221011, 63870008).

References

Abzug, C., Maeda, M., Peterson, B.W., and Wilson, V.J. (1974) Cervical branching of lumbar vestibulospinal axons. *J. Physiol. (London),* 243: 499 – 522.

Akaike, T., Fanardjian, V.V., Ito, M. and Ohno, T. (1973) Electrophysiological analysis of the vestibulospinal reflex pathway of rabbit. II. Synaptic actions upon spinal neurones. *Exp. Brain Res.,* 17: 497 – 515.

Brodal, A. (1974) Anatomy of the vestibular nuclei and their connections. In H.H. Kornbuber (Ed.), *Handbook of Sensory Physiology, Vol. 6, Vestibular System,* Berlin, Springer, pp. 239 – 352.

Bruggencate, G. Ten, Burke, R., Lundberg, A. and Udo, M. (1969) Interaction between the vestibulospinal tract, contralateral flexor reflex afferents and Ia afferents. *Brain Res.,* 14: 529 – 532.

Crouch, J.E. (1969) *Text-Atlas of Cat Anatomy,* Lea and Febiger, Philadelphia,

Fukushima, K., Peterson, B.W. and Wilson, V.J. (1979) Vestibulospinal, reticulospinal and interstitiospinal pathways in the cat. In R. Granit and O. Pompeiano (Eds.), *Prog. Brain Res., Vol. 50, Reflex Control of Posture and Movement,* Elsevier, Amsterdam, pp. 121 – 136.

Futami, T., Shinoda, Y. and Yokota, J. (1979) Spinal axon collaterals of corticospinal neurons identified by intracellular injection of horseradish peroxidase. *Brain Res.,* 164: 279 – 284.

Graham, R.C., Jr. and Karnovsky, M.J. (1966) The early stages of absorption of injected horseradish peroxidase in the proximal tubules of mouse kidney: Ultrastructural cytochemistry by a new technique. *J. Histochem. Cytochem.,* 14: 291 – 302.

Grillner, S., Hongo, T. and Lund, S. (1970) The vestibulospinal tract. Effects on alpha-motoneurones in the lumbosacral spinal cord in the cat. *Exp. Brain Res.,* 10: 94 – 120.

Harrison, P.J., Jankowska, E. and Zytnick, D. (1986) Lamina VIII interneurones interposed in crossed reflex pathways in the cat. *J. Physiol. (London),* 371: 147 – 166.

Hongo, T., Kudo, N. and Tanaka, R. (1975) The vestibulospinal tract: Crossed and uncrossed effects on hindlimb motoneurones in the cat. *Exp. Brain Res.,* 24: 37 – 55.

Hultborn, H. and Udo, M. (1972) Convergence in the reciprocal Ia inhibitory pathway of excitation from descending pathways and inhibition from motor axon collaterals. *Acta Physiol. Scand.,* 84: 95 – 108.

Hultborn, H., Illert, M., and Santini, M. (1976) Convergence on interneurones mediating the reciprocal Ia inhibition of motoneurones. III. Effects from supraspinal pathways. *Acta Physiol. Scand.,* 96: 368 – 391.

Jankowska, E., and Lindström, S. (1972) Morphology of interneurones mediating Ia reciprocal inhibition of motoneurones in the spinal cord of the cat. *J. Physiol (London),* 266: 805 – 823.

Nyberg-Hansen, R. (1964) Origin and termination of fibers from the vestibular nuclei descending in the medial longitudinal fasciculus. An experimental study with silver impregnation methods in the cat. *J. Neurol.,* 122: 355 – 367.

Nyberg – Hansen, R. (1969) Do cat spinal motoneurones receive direct supra-spinal fiber connection? A supplementary silver study. *Arch. Ital. Biol.,* 107: 67 – 78.

Nyberg-Hansen, R. and Mascitti, T.A. (1964) Sites and mode of termination of fibers of the vestibulospinal tract in the cat. An experimental study with silver impregnation methods. *J. Comp. Neurol.,* 122: 369 – 388.

Peterson, B.W. and Coulter, J.D. (1977) A new long spinal projection from the vestibular nuclei in the cat. *Brain Res.,* 122: 351 – 356.

Precht, W. and Shimazu, H. (1965) Functional connections of tonic and kinetic vestibular neurons with primary vestibular afferents. *J. Neurophysiol.,* 28: 1014 – 1028.

Rapoport, S., Susswein, A., Uchino, Y. and Wilson, V.J. (1977) Properties of vestibular neurons projecting to neck segments of the cat spinal cord. *J. Physiol. (London),* 268: 493 – 510.

Reighard, J. and Jennings, H.S. (1951) *Anatomy of The Cat,* Henry Holt and Company, New York.

Rexed, B. (1954) A cytoarchitectonic atlas of spinal cord in the cat. *J. Comp. Neurol.,* 100: 297 – 379.

Richmond, F.J.R., Scott, D.A. and Abrahams, V.C. (1978) Distribution of motoneurones to the neck muscles, biventer cervicis, splenius and complexus in the cat. *J. Comp. Neurol.,* 181: 451 – 464.

Scheibel, M.E. and Scheibel, A.B. (1969) A structural analysis of spinal interneurons and Renshow cells. In M.A.B. Brazier (Ed.), *The Interneuron,* University of California Press, Berkeley and Los Angeles, pp. 159 – 208.

Shinoda, Y., Ohgaki, T. and Futami, T. (1986) The morphology of single lateral vestibulospinal tract axons in the lower cervical cord of the cat. *J. Comp. Neurol.,* 249: 226 – 241.

Shinoda, Y., Ohgaki, T., Futami, T. and Sugiuchi, Y. (1988) Vestibular projections to the spinal cord: The morphology of single vestibulospinal axons. In O. Pompeiano and J.H.J. Allum (Eds.), *Prog. Brain Res., Vol. 76, Vestibulospinal Control of Posture and Movement,* Elsevier, Amsterdam, pp. 121 – 136.

Shinoda, Y., Yokota, J. and Futami, T. (1981) Divergent projection of individual corticospinal axons to motoneurons of multiple muscles in the monkey. *Neurosci. Lett.,* 23: 7 – 12.

Shinoda, Y., Yokota, J. and Futami, T. (1982) Morphology of physiologically identified rubrospinal axons in the spinal cord of the cat. *Brain Res.,* 242: 321 – 325.

Shinoda, Y. and Yoshida, K. (1974) Dynamic characteristics of responses to horizontal head angular acceleration in the vestibulo-ocular pathway in the cat. *J. Neurophysiol.,* 37: 653 – 673.

Suzuki, J.-I. and Cohen, B. (1964) Head, eye, body and limb movements from semicircular canal nerves. *Exp. Neurol.,* 10: 393 – 405.

Szenthágothai, J. (1951) Short propriospinal neurons and intrinsic connections of the spinal grey matter. *Acta Morph. Acad. Sci. Hung.,* 1: 81 – 94.

Wilson, V.J. and Maeda, M. (1974) Connection between semicircular canals and neck motoneurons in the cat. *J. Neurophysiol.,* 37: 346 – 357.

Wilson, V.J. and Melvil-Jones, G. (1979) *Mammalian Vestibular Physiology,* Plenum Press, New York, pp. 130.

Wilson, V.J. and Peterson, B.W. (1978) Peripheral and central substrates of vestibulospinal reflexes. *Physiol. Rev.,* 58: 80 – 105.

Wilson, V.J. and Yoshida, M. (1969) Comparison of effects of stimulation of Deiters' nucleus and medial longitudinal fasciculus on neck, forelimb, and hindlimb motoneurons. *J.*

Neurophysiol., 32: 743 – 758.

Wilson, V.J., Yoshida, M., and Schor, R.H. (1970) Supraspinal monosynaptic excitation and inhibition of thoracic back motoneurones. *Exp. Brain Res.*, 11: 282 – 295.

Wilson, V.J., Gacek, P.R., Maeda, M. and Uchino, Y. (1977) Saccular and Utricular input to cat neck motoneurons. *J. Neurophysiol.*, 40: 63 – 73.

J.H.J. Allum and M. Hulliger (Eds.)
Progress in Brain Research, Vol. 80
© 1989 Elsevier Science Publishers B.V. (Biomedical Division)

CHAPTER 13

Afferents and efferents of the vestibular nuclei: the necessity of context-specific interpretation

W. Graf and V.J. Wilson

The Rockefeller University, 1230 York Ave., New York, NY 10021, U.S.A.

A synopsis of physiological and anatomical results is presented that leads to the conclusion that experimental data have to be interpreted in a context meaningful for the system investigated. For example, since there is an obvious spatial relationship between semicircular canals and extraocular muscles, the interdependence between the three-neurone-arc circuitry, and vestibular and visual signals follows quite naturally from a common geometry inherent in the sensory and motor periphery. It is emphasized that signals related to compensatory eye movements have to be interpreted within a vestibular/eye muscle frame of reference. By the same argument, when dealing with the head-neck movement system, the appropriate reference frame will have to be applied to arrive at a meaningful interpretation of related sensorimotor functions. Thus, in general terms, each system has to be interpreted within its own meaningful biological context.

Key words: Vestibulo-ocular reflex; Visuo-ocular reflex; Vestibulo-spinal reflex; Eye movement; Eye-head coordination; Intrinsic coordinate system; Semicircular canal plane

Introduction

An animal in its normal habitat will utilize eye and head movements in a temporally and spatially coordinated manner for orienting responses. This behaviour results from different sensory inputs that produce a response involving a number of motor systems (eye, neck, ear, etc). At issue is, how these different inputs are efficiently integrated and transformed into meaningful behaviour. In this presentation we will consider spatial coordination of orienting behaviour, with a focus on input – output systems of the vestibular nuclei.

The labyrinth as an intrinsic reference frame

Spatial coordination of eye and head movements has to be addressed within the conceptual framework of intrinsic reference frame systems (Pellionisz and Llinás, 1980; Simpson and Graf, 1985). One such framework is exemplified in the three-dimensional geometry of the semicircular canals of the labyrinth. The three canals of one labyrinth (anterior, posterior and horizontal) are approximately orthogonal to each other and form a functional entity with a mirror-symmetrical system on the other side of the head. The vertical canals are oriented diagonally in the head, i.e. one co-planar anterior-posterior canal pair forms an angle of approximately 45° with the midsagittal plane. The extraocular muscle orientations have a similar geometrical arrangement (Fig. 1). By contrast, the architecture of the head-neck movement system, with its many muscles, is much more complex, although there is a considerable reduction in degrees of freedom for head movement control (see below).

Afferents to the vestibular nuclei

The signals arising from vestibular endorgans are transmitted to the vestibular nuclear complex via primary vestibular afferents. Naturally, spatial information on primary vestibular afferents coming from the semicircular canals is coded in canal coordinates (Goldberg and Fernández, 1971; Estes et al., 1975; Reisine et al., 1988). In the vestibular nuclei, one synapse away from the vestibular endorgan, the directional coding of second-order vestibular neurones receiving canal input no longer necessarily reflects the geometry of the semicircular canals (Baker et al., 1984; Kasper et al., 1988a): because of convergence of afferents from different canals, quite a number of vestibular neurones have their best response plane shifted away from true canal plane orientations. Instead, sensitivity vectors of these neurones can be found orientated in many directions of three-dimensional space, although a clustering around canal planes is noticeable (Fig. 2). Neurones with these diverse sensitivity vectors presumably include vestibulo-ocular and vestibulo-spinal neurones, although only the latter were identified in the experiments of Kasper et al. (1988a).

Is semicircular canal geometry reflected in the behavior of neurones receiving otolith or otolith plus canal input? This would not be a frequently expected response, because no such coding is seen for otolith afferents (Fernández and Goldberg, 1976). To some extent the spatial tuning of otolith

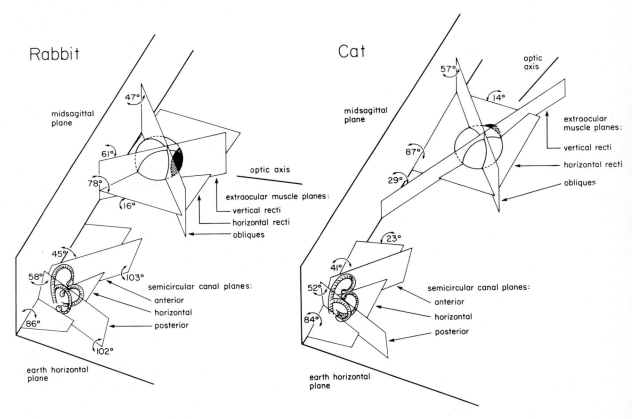

Fig. 1. Spatial orientation of semicircular canal and paired extraocular muscle planes in rabbit and cat. In the rabbit, the horizontal semicircular canal is set to earth horizontal; in the cat all angles are calculated in reference to stereotaxic coordinates. Note slight mismatch of respective canal and extraocular muscle planes necessitating coordinate transformation between the two reference frames (from Ezure and Graf, 1984a).

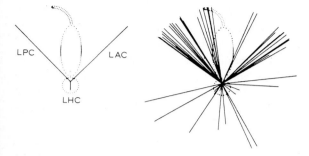

Fig. 2. Normalized vestibular neurone vectors representing the best axes orientations as projected onto the horizontal plane. On the left, the response axes of the left semicircular canal system are depicted for comparison (LAC, left anterior canal; LPC, left posterior canal; LHC, left horizontal canal) (modified after Baker et al., 1984).

responses shows variability depending on the laboratory investigating the system. Daunton and Melvill Jones (1982) did find otolith responses reflecting semicircular canal geometry in central vestibular neurones; a substantial majority of neurones responded better to transverse rather than fore-aft accelerations (N. Daunton, personal communication). Schor et al. (1984, 1985) and Kasper et al. (1988a) described a broad distribution of response vector orientations, with many neurones, especially in the lateral vestibular nucleus, responding best to stimuli near roll. The majority of the neurones of Chan et al. (1985, 1987), on the other hand, were more sensitive to pitch than to roll. Whatever the reason for these differences, the fact remains that the best response vector orientations of the majority of sampled neurones receiving otolith or otolith-plus-canal input are only remotely reminiscent of semicircular canal geometry.

Another important source of afferents to the vestibular nuclei is from receptors in the neck (e.g. Boyle and Pompeiano, 1980). These receptors most likely include spindle afferents from perivertebral and other neck muscles (Chan et al., 1987). Only a restricted population of such spindle afferents, recorded in the C2 dorsal root ganglion, has been studied so far. The response vector orien-

tations of these afferents presumably reflect the best pulling directions of the muscles in which they are located, and it is therefore not surprising that, whether studied with head rotations in two or in three dimensions, they bear no relation to semicircular canal planes (Chan et al., 1987; Kasper et al., 1988c). The same is true for the response of vestibular neurones following neck rotation. Kasper et al. (1988b) showed that sensitivity to neck rotation is found in neurones with a variety of input patterns from vestibular receptors. Activation by neck rotation occurs most frequently in neurones with otolith-plus-canal convergence, or convergence from the ipsilateral anterior and posterior canals, but is also present in neurones with input only from the otoliths or a single canal. The response vector orientations of a population of neurones in the lateral and descending vestibular nuclei, determined with stimuli combining roll and pitch is illustrated in Fig. 3. It is evident that most neck vectors lie near roll and that few are in the planes of the vertical semicircular canals.

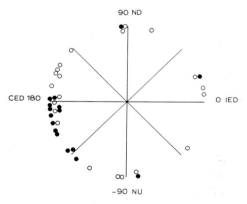

Fig. 3. Response vector orientations of responses to neck rotation of 37 vestibular neurones, determined with stimuli combining roll and pitch. Although the stimulus consisted of body rotation on a stationary head, vector orientations are treated as though the head was moved. ND and NU, nose up and nose down; IED and CED, ipsilateral and contralateral ear down. Diagonal lines, which divide diagram into "roll" and "pitch" quadrants, are approximately in the planes of the vertical canals. Filled circles, neurones identified as projecting to the spinal cord (from Kasper et al., 1988b).

Vestibular nuclei and the vestibulospinal system

As pointed out in the preceding section, there is a roll bias in the responses of vestibular neurones to two-dimensional stimulation of vestibular and neck receptors. This bias is consistent with the spatial organization of vestibular reflexes acting on the limbs, which, at least in the forelimb, are themselves preferentially tuned to roll (Wilson et al., 1986). Similarly, the presence of vestibular neurones with response vectors near canal planes is consistent with the observation that electric (and presumably natural) stimulation of individual canals produces head movements in the plane of the stimulated canal (Suzuki and Cohen, 1964). These canal-driven vestibular neurones make excitatory and inhibitory connections with the neck motoneurones innervating the muscles required to produce head movements in the correct plane; such connections may be via disynaptic (Wilson and Maeda, 1974) or more complex (e.g. Bilotto et al., 1982) pathways. Attempts have been made to model the sensorimotor transformations required to produce the appropriate head movements in response to vestibular stimulation (Pellionisz and Peterson, 1988), but our understanding of the spatial qualities of various afferents to the vestibular nuclei in relation to their significance for head-neck movements is still at a very early stage.

The reference frame of the vestibulo-oculomotor system

A much clearer example of intrinsic geometry in regard to spatial coordination and sensorimotor transformation can be presented for the ascending vestibular reflex pathways to the extraocular muscles.

The most direct neuronal network between the semicircular canals and the eye muscles in vertebrates is the three-neurone vestibulo-ocular reflex arc, which can transmit information rapidly and provide a motor reaction as soon as 14 ms after a vestibular stimulus (e.g. a head movement) has occurred (Lisberger, 1981). Via this connectivi-ty, the anterior canal excites the ipsilateral superior rectus and the contralateral inferior oblique muscles. The posterior canal excites the ipsilateral superior oblique and the contralateral inferior rectus. Horizontal canal stimulation results in contraction of the contralateral lateral rectus and the ipsilateral medial rectus muscle. Inhibitory connections link the antagonists of the above muscles with the same semicircular canals (Szentágothai, 1943, 1950; see also Highstein, 1971, 1973; Ito et al., 1973a,b, 1976a,b). The specific connectivity of the three-neurone-arc reflects the three-dimensional geometry of the semicircular canal and extraocular muscle systems by linking a given canal to a particular set of extraocular muscles, so-called yoke muscles, which move each eye close to the respective canal plane. The principal three-neurone-arc connectivity is the same in all vertebrates studied thus far, whether lateral-eyed or frontal-eyed. This conservative neuronal network can only be preserved because extraocular muscles which receive their principal input from one particular canal share this canal's spatial orientation. However, it should be stated at this point that the above constitutes an idealized situation. In reality, canal planes and extraocular muscle planes are not exactly coplanar (Ezure and Graf, 1984a) (Fig. 1), and, in order for eye movements to be compensatory, additional connections are necessary to perform the appropriate sensorimotor transformation from vestibular into eye muscle coordinates (Pellionisz and Llinás, 1980; Robinson, 1982; Ezure and Graf, 1984b; Pellionisz and Graf, 1987).

When selectively recording from second-order vestibulo-oculomotor neurones, a distinct signal content in regard to extraocular muscle and vestibular semicircular canal coordinates becomes obvious in neurones that show either single-canal responses or have multiple-canal convergent signals (Graf et al., 1986a; Peterson et al., 1987). Multiple-canal convergence can shift the response of vertical canal neurones into the plane of oblique eye muscles (Fig. 4). Thus, in the anterior canal system, some neurones have their best responses in

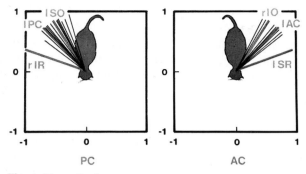

Fig. 4. Normalized vector orientations as projected onto the horizontal plane of maximal activation directions of excitatory posterior (PC) and anterior canal (AC) neurones (indicated by thin lines) in the cat. The respective canal and their principal muscle motor axes are illustrated by thick lines. Note cluster of neurones connected to the left posterior canal (lPC) around the canal axis and the left superior oblique axis (lSO), but not for the right inferior rectus muscle. A similar scenario can be observed for left anterior canal (lAC) neurones which are grouped around the canal axis and the right inferior oblique (rIO) motor axis. Not a single response axis is found for the left superior rectus (lSR) activation direction (data from Graf et al., 1986; Peterson et al., 1987).

the canal plane, and some neurones in the inferior oblique plane. Similarly, for posterior canal neurones, responses of single-canal nature are found, as are signals that receive sufficient convergent-canal input to shift the response to the superior oblique plane. However, there is a conspicuous absence of neurones responding to stimulation in the plane of the vertical recti. Nevertheless, in the vestibulo-oculomotor system the response properties regarding spatial tuning of second-order vestibular neurones can be clearly interpreted in terms of canal coordinates or extraocular muscle coordinates.

The visual input to vestibular neurones participating in the production of compensatory eye movements via a visuo-vestibulo-ocular reflex can also be interpreted within the conceptual framework of intrinsic reference frames. Vision plays an important role for orientation and posture since most vertebrates tend to move with their eyes open. This visual input is expressed in an 'optokinetic' reference frame which is also

geometrically closely related to that of the canal and the extraocular muscle arrangement. In the rabbit, recordings from identified vertical second-order vestibulo-oculomotor neurones have revealed that neurone responses group around the anterior or the posterior canal planes (McGurk and Graf, 1987a,b). In these experiments, receptive field properties and the axes of visual field rotation producing a best response were established. For the latter part, a planetarium projector was utilized whose rotation axis could be oriented in any direction in space via a gimbal system.

All recorded neurones received binocular visual input. Excitatory anterior canal neurones were excited by upward and backward movement of visual increments in the anterior three quadrants of the ipsilateral hemifield, and by downward and backward movement in the posterior three quadrants of the contralateral hemifield. This response is consistent with rotation of the entire visual world about an axis passing from approximately 135° ipsilateral (average: 138°; $n = 7$) to 45° contralateral (0° represents an axis pointing rostrally). Excitatory posterior canal neurones were recruited by upward and forward movement in the ipsilateral posterior three quadrants, and by downward and forward movement in the contralateral anterior three quadrants of the visual field. This response is consistent with rotation about an axis passing from 45° ipsilateral (average: 41°; $n = 8$) to 135° contralateral. Ipsilateral projecting neurones could be driven from any portion of the visual field consistent with rotation about their respective canal axes. These results demonstrate that the optokinetic input to second-order vestibular neurones is also coded in coordinates comparable to the vestibular and/or extraocular muscle sensory and motor axes (Fig. 5).

Head-neck movements

When further elaborating on orienting behaviour, we will also have to consider head movements and eye-head coordination. Higher vertebrates display an almost identical head-neck geometry, with a

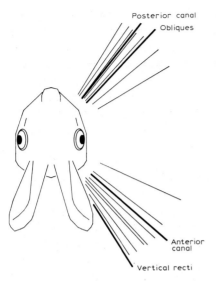

Fig. 5. Best axis orientations of vertical second-order vestibular neurones following optokinetic stimulation with the planetarium projector and their correspondence to related anterior canal, posterior canal, and extraocular muscle axes (data from McGurk and Graf, 1987a,b).

vertically oriented cervical vertebral column and distinct mechanical constraints within the head-neck ensemble (Graf et al., 1986b; Vidal et al., 1986, 1988). Although different strategies for head movement control are employed by different vertebrate species regarding the differential utilization of the various head-neck articulations, these differences are only quantitative (de Waele et al., 1987; Graf et al., 1988).

The apparent complexity of the head-neck movement system, however, may not be as great as it appears at first sight. Mechanical constraints limit the number of degrees of freedom of the head movement system with horizontal movement largely possible only in the atlanto-axial articulation. Movement in the sagittal plane is only possible in the atlanto-occipital articulation and at the cervico-thoracic junction. Side tilt of the entire head-neck ensemble occurs via rotation of upper thoracic vertebrae. During all these movements, the entire cervical vertebral column retains its original intrinsic configuration (Graf et al., 1986b;

Vidal et al., 1988). Although the geometrical frameworks of the head-neck movement systems are not as tidy as those of the eye movement system, there may nevertheless be an avenue to arrive at a generalized concept about the former.

Eye-head coordination

For coordinated eye and head movements, a meaningful spatial and temporal relationship between eye movers and head-neck movers has to be established. In this context we have to consider the synchrony between eye movements in a given direction and activation of particular neck muscles (Vidal et al., 1982, 1983). Vestibular nucleus neurones may be involved in mediating the co-contraction of eye and neck muscles since they have multi-target termination patterns with axons collateralizing not only into oculomotor but also into spinalmotor areas (McCrea et al., 1981; Graf et al., 1983; Uchino and Hirai, 1984; Graf and Ezure, 1986; Isu et al. 1988; Uchino et al., 1988). Thus, these neurones could simultaneously participate in the control of vestibulo-ocular and vestibulo-neck reflexes, or when taking into account the entire eye-head movement system, control the full scope of visuo-vestibulo-ocular-neck reflexes. Via their extensive axon collaterals, a given motor control signal would be economically distributed to multiple target sites which have the same functional context (e.g. orienting behaviour involving eye and head movements) (Fig. 6). The distribution of one control signal to different motor systems calls for the above-mentioned common, although system-specific, geometrical organization of involved motor systems.

Functional considerations

The introduction of constraints establishing intrinsic reference frames and thereby reducing the degrees of freedom of sensory and motor systems points to an important principle of brain function. Intrinsic reference frames simplify neuronal operations and economize brain function by establishing a common geometry at the sensory and motor periphery, thus obviating large scale sensorimotor transformations, at least, in the vestibulo-oculo-motor system. Similarly, the relevant visual input is coded within the same geometrical framework.

Furthermore, the spatial orientation of the semicircular canals in the head provides an optimal resolution for the detection of head movements in three-dimensional space (Robinson, 1982). Although, a priori, there is no necessity to assume that the brain could not calculate or reconstruct a

movement vector from any minimally required or even overcomplete number of sensors arranged at random, we have to assume that calculations mean connections, and consequently require more nerve fibres and synapses. Thus, aspects of timing have to be contemplated (e.g. the 14 ms latency for the onset of the vestibulo-ocular reflex; Lisberger, 1981). Furthermore, since there is a narrow window of optimal brain-to-body ratio, the aspect of animal economy also has to be taken into consideration (Gould, 1977; Grüsser and Weiss, 1985). Besides the mechanical issues and speed and volume-to-weight aspects, embryological criteria also will have to be considered, in particular, the question of establishing bilateral symmetry as a necessary prerequisite for vertebrate ontogenesis.

As a general operational principle of sensorimotor function, we observe that peripheral mechanisms are largely utilized to take care of spatial coordination of orienting behaviour in particular, and presumably also of movement control in general.

Whether a similar arrangement can be demonstrated for the head-neck movement system as clearly as it was possible for the vestibulo-oculomotor system remains to be seen. However, the distinct reduction of degrees of freedom across vertebrate species points to such a possibility. In this context, we again have to take into consideration the vestibular neurones that send axon collaterals to extraocular muscle and spinal motor centres. Thus, the same signal which is meaningful for the oculomotor system presumably fulfils a function at the neck motoneurone level. The extent to which this information is utilized, however, remains open to discussion.

In conclusion, vertebrates possess an organizational blueprint for eye-head coordination and orienting responses which includes a uniform architecture of the sensory and motor systems involved, shared neuronal networks and common control signals (Fig. 6). However, a meaningful interpretation of brain function can come only within a context of system specificity, animal economy, ontogeny and phylogeny.

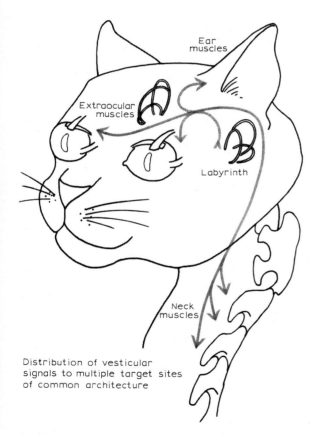

Distribution of vesticular signals to multiple target sites of common architecture

Fig. 6. Schematic of vestibular neurone connectivity to motor centres of related architecture and common behavioural context. The shared neuronal pathway (shown in grey) would provide an economical distribution of motor control signals to motoneurone pools involved in orienting behaviour.

156

Acknowledgements

This work was supported by grants from the NIH (EY-04613, NS-02619) and from NASA (NSG 2380).

References

Baker, J., Goldberg, J., Hermann, G. and Peterson, B. (1984) Optimal response planes and canal convergence in secondary neurons in vestibular nuclei of alert cats. *Brain Res., 294*: 133 – 137.

Bilotto, G., Goldberg, J., Peterson, B.W. and Wilson, V.J. (1982) Dynamic properties of vestibular reflexes in the decerebrate cat. *Exp. Brain Res., 47*: 343 – 352.

Boyle, R. and Pompeiano, O. (1980) Responses of vestibulospinal neurons to sinusoidal rotation of neck. *J. Neurophysiol., 44*: 633 – 649.

Chan, Y.S., Cheung, Y.M. and Hwang, J.C. (1985) Effect of tilt on the response of neuronal activity within the cat vestibular nuclei during slow and constant velocity rotation. *Brain Res., 345*: 271 – 278.

Chan, Y.S., Cheung, Y.M. and Hwang, J.C. (1987a) Response characteristics of neurons in the cat vestibular nuclei during slow and constant velocity off-vertical axes rotations in the clockwise and counterclockwise rotations. *Brain Res., 406*: 294 – 301.

Chan, Y.S., Kasper, J. and Wilson, V.J. (1987b) Dynamics and directional sensitivity of neck muscle spindle response to head rotation. *J. Neurophysiol., 57*: 1716 – 1729.

Daunton, N. and Melvill Jones, G. (1982) Distribution of sensitivity vectors in central vestibular units responding to linear acceleration. *Soc. Neurosci. Abstr., 8*: 16 – 15.

de Waele, C., Graf, W. and Vidal, P.P. (1987) Biomechanical constraints limit the number of degrees of freedom of the vertebrate head-neck ensemble: Its consequences for the postural syndrome following hemilabyrinthectomy. *Soc. Neurosci. Abstr., 13*: 338.7.

Estes, M.S., Blanks, R.H.S. and Markham, C.H. (1975) Physiologic characteristics of vestibular first-order canal neurons in the cat. I. Response plane determination and resting discharge characteristics. *J. Neurophysiol., 38*: 1232 – 1249.

Ezure, K. and Graf, W. (1984a) A quantitative analysis of the spatial organization of the vestibulo-ocular reflexes in lateral- and frontal-eyed animals. I. Orientation of semicircular canals and extraocular muscles. *Neuroscience, 12*: 85 – 93.

Ezure, K. and Graf, W. (1984b) A quantitative analysis of the spatial organization of the vestibulo-ocular reflexes in lateral- and frontal-eyed animals. II. Neuronal networks underlying vestibulo-oculomotor coordination. *Neuro-science, 12*: 95 – 109.

Fernández, C. and Goldberg, J.M. (1976) Physiology of peripheral neurons innervating otolith organs of the squirrel monkey. I. Response to static tilts and to long-duration centrifugal force. *J. Neurophysiol., 39*: 970 – 984.

Goldberg, J.M. and Fernández, C. (1971) Physiology of peripheral neurons innervating semicircular canals of the squirrel monkey. I. Resting discharge and response to constant angular accelerations. *J. Neurophysiol., 34*: 634 – 660.

Gould, S.J. (1977) Size and shape, from churches to brains to planets. In S.J. Gould (Ed.), *Ever Since Darwin,* W.W. Norton, New York, pp. 169 – 198.

Graf, W. and Ezure, K. (1986) Morphology of vertical canal related second order vestibular neurons in the cat. *Exp. Brain Res., 63*: 35 – 48.

Graf, W., McCrea, R.A. and Baker, R. (1983) Morphology of posterior canal related secondary vestibular neurons in rabbit and cat. *Exp. Brain Res., 52*: 125 – 138.

Graf, W., Baker, J.F., Peterson, B.W. and Wickland, C.R. (1986a) Differential canal-canal convergence in second-order vestibulo-oculomotor neurons in the cat. *Soc. Neurosci. Abstr., 12*, Part 2: 214.11.

Graf, W., Vidal, P.P. and Evinger, L.C. (1986b) How animals move their heads. *Proc. Int. Union Physiol. Sci., 16*: 394, P411.08.

Graf, W., Vidal, P.P., de Waele, C. and Evinger, L.C. (1988) Biomechanics of the head-neck articulations and head movement strategies in monkey. *Soc. Neurosci. Abstr., 14*: 74.10.

Grüsser, O.J. and Weiss. L.R. (1985) Quantitative models on phylogenetic growth of the hominid brain. In Ph. V. Tobias (Ed.), *Hominid Evolution: Past, Present and Future,* Alan R. Liss, Inc. New York, pp. 457 – 464.

Highstein, S.M. (1971) Organization of the inhibitory and excitatory vestibulo-ocular reflex pathways to the third and fourth nuclei in the rabbit. *Brain Res., 32*: 218 – 234.

Highstein, S.M. (1973) The organization of the vestibulo-oculomotor and trochlear reflex pathways in the rabbit. *Brain Res., 17*: 285 – 300.

Isu, N., Uchino, Y., Nakashima, H., Satoh, S. Ichikawa, T. and Watanabe, S. (1988) Axonal trajectories of posterior canal-activated secondary vestibular neurons and their coactivation of extraocular and neck flexor motoneurons in the cat. *Exp. Brain Res., 70*: 181 – 191.

Ito, M., Nisimaru, N. and Yamamoto, M. (1973a) The neural pathways mediating reflex contraction of extraocular muscles during semicircular canal stimulation in rabbits. *Brain Res., 55*: 183 – 188.

Ito, M., Nisimaru, N. and Yamamoto, M. (1973b) The neural pathways relaying reflex inhibition from semicircular canals to extraocular muscles of the rabbits. *Brain Res., 55*: 189 – 193.

Ito. M., Nisimaru, N. and Yamamoto, M. (1976a) Pathways for the vestibulo-ocular reflex excitation arising from semicircular canals of rabbits. *Exp. Brain Res.,* 24: 257 – 271.

Ito, M., Nisimaru, N. and Yamamoto, M. (1976b) Postsynaptic inhibition of oculomotor neurons involved in vestibulo-ocular reflexes arising from semicircular canals of rabbits. *Exp. Brain Res.,* 24: 273 – 283.

Kasper, J., Schor, R.H. and Wilson V.J. (1988a) Response of vestibular neurons to head rotations in vertical planes. I. Response to vestibular stimulation. *J. Neurophysiol.,* 60: 1753 – 1764.

Kasper, J., Schor, R.H. and Wilson, V.J. (1988b) Response of vestibular neurons to head rotations in vertical planes. II. Response to neck stimulation and vestibular-neck interaction. *J. Neurophysiol.,* 60: 1765 – 1778.

Kasper, J., Schor, R.H., Yates, B.J. and Wilson, V.J. (1988c) Three-dimensional sensitivity and caudal projection of neck spindle afferents. *J. Neurophysiol.,* 59: 1497 – 1509.

Lisberger, S.G. (1981) The latency of pathways containing the site of motor learning in the monkey vestibulo-ocular reflex. *Science,* 225: 74 – 76.

McCrea, R.A., Yoshida, K., Evinger, C. and Berthoz, A. (1981) The location, axonal arborization, and termination sites of eye-movement-related secondary vestibular neurons demonstrated by intra-axonal HRP injection in the alert cat. In A. Fuchs and W. Becker (Eds.), *Developments in Neuroscience, Vol. 12, Progress in Oculomotor Research,* Elsevier/North Holland Biomed. Press, Amsterdam, pp. 379 – 386.

McGurk, J.F. and Graf, W. (1987a) Spatial tuning of second-order vestibular neurons of the vertical system to optokinetic stimulation in the rabbit. *Neuroscience,* 22 Suppl.: S736, 2201P.

McGurk, J.F. and Graf, W. (1987b) Optokinetic responses of second-order vestibular neurons in the rabbit. *Soc. Neurosci. Abstr.,* 13: 338.5.

Pellionisz, A. and Llinás, R. (1980) Tensorial approach to the geometry of brain function. Cerebellar coordination via a metric tensor. *Neurscience,* 5: 1125 – 1136.

Pellionisz, A. and Graf, W. (1987) Tensor network model of the three-neuron vestibulo-ocular reflex-arc in cat. *J. Theor. Neurobiol.,* 5: 127 – 151.

Pellionisz, A, and Peterson, B.W. (1988) A tensorial model of neck motor activation. In B.W. Peterson and F.J. Richmond (Eds.), *Control of Head Movement,* Oxford Univ. Press, Oxford and New York, pp. 178 – 186.

Peterson, B.W., Graf, W. and Baker, J.F. (1987) Spatial properties of signals carried by second order vestibuloocular relay neurons in the cat. *Soc. Neurosci. Abstr.,* 13: 303.16.

Reisine, H., Simpson, J.I. and Henn, V. (1988) A geometric analysis of semicircular canals and induced activity in their peripheral afferents in the Rhesus monkey. *Ann. NY Acad. Sci.,* 545: 10 – 20.

Robinson, D.A. (1982) The use of matrices in analyzing the three-dimensional behavior of the vestibulo-ocular reflex. *Biol. Cybern.* 46: 53 – 66.

Schor, J., Miller, A.D., and Tomko, D.L. (1984) Responses to head tilt in cat central vestibular neurons. I. Direction of maximum sensitivity. *J. Neurophysiol.,* 51: 136 – 146.

Schor, H., Miller, A.D., Timerick, S.J.B. and Tomko, D.L. (1985) Responses to head tilt in cat central vestibular neurons. II. Frequency dependence of neural response vectors. *J. Neurophysiol.,* 53: 1444 – 1452.

Simpson, J.I. and Graf, W. (1985) The selection of reference frames by nature and its investigators. In A. Berthoz and G. Melvill Jones (Eds.), *Reviews of Oculomotor Research, Vol. I, Adaptive Mechanisms in Gaze Control,* Elsevier/North-Holland Biomed. Press, Amsterdam, pp. 3 – 16.

Suzuki, J.-I. and Cohen, B. (1964) Head, eye, body and limb movements from semicircular canal nerves. *Exp. Neurol.,* 10: 393 – 405.

Szentágothai, J. (1943) Die zentrale Innervation der Augenbewegungen. *Arch. Psychiatr. Nervenkr.,* 116: 721 – 760.

Szentágothai, J. (1950) The elementary vestibulo-ocular reflex arc. *J. Neurophysiol.,* 13: 395 – 407.

Uchino, Y. and Hirai, N. (1984) Axon collaterals of anterior semicircular canal-activated vestibular neurons and their coactivation of extraocular and neck motoneurons in the cat. *Neurosci. Res.,* 1: 309 – 325.

Uchino, Y., Isu, N., Ichikawa, T., Satoh, S. and Watanabe, S. (1988) Properties and localization of the anterior semicircular canal-activated vestibulocollic neurons in the cat. *Exp. Brain Res.,* 71: 345 – 352.

Vidal, P.P., Roucoux, A. and Berthoz, A. (1982) Horizontal eye position related activity in neck muscles of the alert cat. *Exp. Brain Res.,* 46: 448 – 453.

Vidal, P.P., Corvisier, J. and Berthoz, A. (1983) Eye and neck motor signals in periabducens reticular neurons of the alert cat. *Exp. Brain Res.,* 53: 16 – 28.

Vidal, P.P., Graf, W. and Berthoz, A. (1986) The orientation of the cervical vertebral column in unrestrained awake animals. I. Resting position. *Exp. Brain Res.,* 61: 549 – 559.

Vidal, P.P., De Waele, C., Graf W. and Berthoz, A. (1988) Skeletal geometry underlying head movements. *Ann. NY Acad Sci.,* 545: 228 – 238.

Wilson, V.J. and Maeda, M. (1974) Connections between semicircular canals and neck motoneurons in the cat. *J. Neurophysiol.,* 37: 346 – 357.

Wilson, V.J., Schor, R.H., Suzuki, I., and Park, B.R. (1986) Spatial organization of neck and vestibular reflexes acting on the forelimb of the decerebrate cat. *J. Neurophysiol.,* 55: 514 – 526.

J.H.J. Allum and M. Hulliger (Eds.)
Progress in Brain Research, Vol. 80
© 1989 Elsevier Science Publishers B.V. (Biomedical Division)

CHAPTER 14

How visual inputs to the ponto-bulbar reticular formation are used in the synthesis of premotor signals during orienting

A. Grantyn

Laboratoire de Physiologie Neurosensorielle du C.N.R.S., 15, rue de l'Ecole de Médecine, 75270 Paris Cedex 06, France

The primate superior colliculus (SC) is known as a structure subserving the transformation of visual information into "commands" for orienting eye movements. Collicular burst neurons discharging with short lead times in relation to visually triggered or spontaneous saccades are supposed to be the output elements linking the SC to immediately premotor pattern generators.

In this paper we summarize some data available for the cat's SC neurones, identified as tecto-reticulo-spinal projection cells (TRSN), and reticulospinal neurones (RSN), identified as receiving excitatory collicular input. Some TRSNs respond to visual stimuli in the absence of orienting movements and, hence, their signals cannot be regarded as motor "commands", in spite of their proven connections with premotor pools in the brain stem and with the spinal cord. Moreover, a small fraction of RSNs belonging to polysynaptic descending collicular pathways also displays visual responses dissociated from movement, in addition to discharges related to the performance of orienting eye-head synergies. The processes of visual to motor transformation, assumed by current models as being definitively accomplished in the SC, appear thus to be partially performed in the reticular network incorporating the overlapping collaterals of tectal projection cells and their target neurons in the reticular core. It is concluded that, at least as for visuomotor transformations underlying orienting movements in the cat, the deep division of the SC and the brain stem reticular formation represent an ensemble, rather than a sequence of hierarchically arranged levels of processing.

Key words: Superior colliculus; Reticular formation; Reticulospinal neuron; Axonal branching; Visuomotor transformation; Orienting reaction; Eye movement; Head movement

Introduction

Orienting reaction towards visual targets appears to represent a relatively simple behavioural model of visuo-motor transformations. Contribution of the superior colliculus (SC) to the control of orienting eye and head movements has been firmly established by Hess et al. (1946). Modern views on its function, derived from the studies in monkeys, have been summarized by Wurtz and Albano (1980) and Sparks (1986). An exhaustive review of this topic is beyond the scope of this article which is limited to the organization of the tectal efferent system.

It should suffice to recall that some neurones of the intermediate and deep SC layers discharge with short lead time before saccades whose direction is characterized by a particular vector. Such neurones are usually considered as output elements of the SC, connected to the saccadic generator (Robinson, 1975) in the brain stem reticular formation. Although experimental data documenting this assumption are sparse (Keller, 1979), it is believed that the signals leaving the SC along its descending pathways are essentially motor, i.e., represent a "command for control of saccadic eye movements" (Sparks, 1986). There is a general agreement, however, that additional transformations of spatially coded ouput activity of the SC into the spatio-temporal pattern of excitation and inhibition of motor pools occurs in the reticular formation (RF) (Keller, 1979; Hepp and Henn, 1983). Until recently, the question remained open whether the signals transmitted by the descending

tectal pathways to the reticular circuits are functionally homogeneous and "motor" in the strict sense, i.e., related exclusively to an immediate execution of the movement. This uncertainty was due to the lack of behavioural data on tectal neurones, unequivocally identified as projecting to the lower brain stem. Such data have now been obtained in cats (Grantyn and Berthoz, 1985; Munoz and Guitton, 1985, 1986; Berthoz et al., 1986). In the following we shall summarize some of our obser-

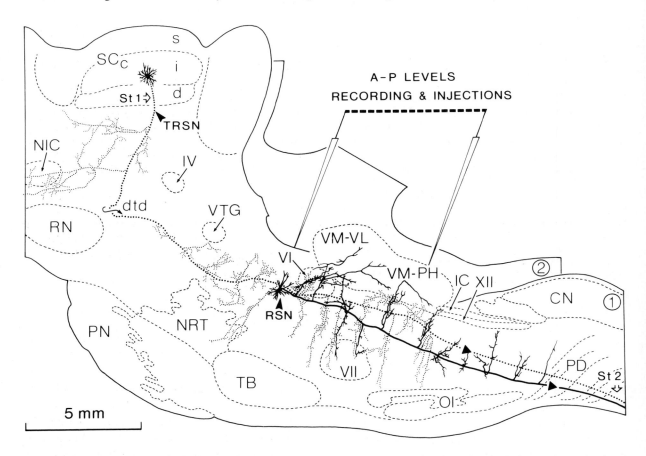

Fig. 1. Anatomical connectivity in the tecto-reticulo-spinal system. Drawing in projection on parasagittal planes 1.2 mm (section 1) and 3.2 mm (section 2) from the midline. Dotted lines: axonal branching of a representative TRSN, reconstructed from three neurones injected with HRP at different rostro-caudal levels. Solid lines: same for representative EN-RSN (see text), based on data from two neurones. Black triangles on caudal portions of main axons delimit the levels for which intracellular HRP data are available. St 1, St 2: positions of stimulating electrodes for orthodromic and antidromic identification of impaled axons. Abbreviations: CN, n. cuneatus; dtd, dorsal tegmental decussation; IC, n. intercalatus; NIC, n. interstitialis of Cajal; NRT, n. reticularis tegmenti pontis; OI, inferior olive; PN, pontine nuclei; SCc, contralateral superior colliculus (s = superficial, i = intermediate, d = deep layers); TB, trapezoid body; VM-VL, medial and lateral vestibular nuclei; VM-PH, medial vestibular and prepositus hypoglossi nuclei; VTG, ventral tegmental nucleus of Gudden; IV, VI, VII, XII, trochlear, abducens, facial and hypoglossal nuclei, respectively.

vations on tectal neurones and then extend the topic to transformation processes in the reticular core.

Methods

Experiments were conducted on untrained alert cats, under a "head fixed" condition. Orienting reactions were induced by presenting a moving visual target whose velocity was controlled by a servomotor and the direction could be changed manually. Due to the absence of reinforcement, cats often did not track the target by eye movements, which allowed for comparisons of neuronal activity accompanied by or dissociated from the motor components of orienting (Fig. 2). During preparatory surgery, a scleral coil was implanted on one eye, and chronic electromyographic (EMG) electrodes were inserted in the obliquus capitis cranialis and longissimus capitis muscles. This enabled monitoring of two components of motor orienting: eye movement and attempted head movements.

Neuronal activity was recorded intra-axonally in the caudal pons and rostral medulla, as indicated in Fig. 1. This type of recording is preferred to conventional extracellular recordings, since it permits intracellular HRP injections and subsequent morphological reconstruction of recorded neurones. Tectal axons descending in the predorsal bundle were identified by direct orthodromic spike responses to stimulation of the contralateral SC (Fig. 1, St 1). The same stimulation electrodes served to search for reticular neurones activated transsynaptically by collicular stimulation (Fig. 6, A). Tectal and reticular axons descending in the spinal cord were identified by antidromic invasion from the C1 or C2 segments (Fig. 1, St 2).

Results

Some morphological features of the tecto-reticular system

According to the studies with anterograde tracing techniques, the terminations of the crossed tecto-bulbo-spinal tract extend through the entire reticular core, showing somewhat increased density at midpontine level and in the rostral medulla (Kawamura et al., 1974; Graham, 1977; Huerta and Harting, 1982). Intracellular staining with HRP (Grantyn and Grantyn, 1982) revealed, somewhat unexpectedly, that virtually all tegmental target areas of the SC are contacted by collaterals of a single tectal efferent neurone projecting to the spinal cord as well. The abundance of collaterals in the RF led us to call them "tecto-reticulo-spinal neurones" – TRSNs. As can be seen in Fig. 1, collateral connections are established not only with the well known "preoculomotor" structures (medial pontine RF, n. prepositus hypoglossi, rostral mesencephalic RF) but also with abducens and facial nuclei, and with the sites of origin of ascending and descending reticular projections. Among the latter are the regions of the RF which project specifically to the upper cervical segments, containing motoneurones of neck muscles (Peterson, 1977; Huerta and Harting, 1982). Apparently, any individual TRSN, giving origin to a long descending axon, can distribute the same signal to functionally different structures.

Axonal morphology of TRSNs suggests that signals generated by TRSNs are processed by parallel pathways originating in the RF. Indeed, monosynaptic effects of tectal stimulation recorded in motoneurones are much weaker than disynaptic, transmitted through the medial pontobulbar RF (Anderson et al., 1971; Grantyn and Grantyn, 1976; Vidal et al., 1988). Fig. 1 illustrates the morphological relationships between a representative TRSN and a reticulospinal neurone (RSN) receiving monosynaptic excitatory input from the SC and discharging in relation to ipsiversive orienting eye-head synergies (Grantyn et al., 1987). The overlap of termination zones is obvious in the region for which complete intracellular labelling was obtained for both TRSNs and RSNs, i.e., in the caudal pons and rostral medulla. Therefore, RSNs receiving monosynaptic collicular input are not just "relay neurones" but rather the elements of a network incorporating parallel and, most likely, re-entrant connections (Scheibel and Scheibel, 1958). Connectivity patterns of this network are established by collaterals of both TRSNs and their target neurones in the RF. The "tecto-reticulo-spinal network" is a more appropriate term to describe the interface between the collicular output and motor nuclei.

Activity of TRSNs during visually triggered orienting

Identification of movement related signals is not enough to describe the operation of such a network, if the location and connectivity of its neurones are unknown. This point is well illustrated by the diversity of signals recorded in the SC of the cat when visual stimuli are presented and when, eventually, these stimuli evoke targeting eye movements. For example, according to Peck et al. (1980), among units located in the deep subdivision of the SC, only about 20% discharge before and during saccadic eye movements. Still less (about 10%) do so in the absence of a visual stimulus, when spontaneous saccades are made in darkness. By contrast, 76% of units show different types of responses to visual stimuli in the absence of movement. It might be tempting to assume that presaccadic units discharging independently of visual stimulus are the output neurones projecting to the saccadic generator. "Pure" visual cells could be candidates for ascending diencephalic connections or, together with visual-motor group, conceived as elements of local intracollicular circuits. The uncertainty of such assumptions is obvious.

Observations relating discharge patterns to orienting behaviour are now available for tectal efferent neurones with axons descending at least to the caudal pons and eventually as far as the cervical spinal cord (TRSNs, as defined above). The sample studied in our experiments (Grantyn and Berthoz, 1985; Berthoz et al., 1986) consists of large neurones, with axonal conduction velocities of 50–90 m/s. These TRSNs share a common pro-

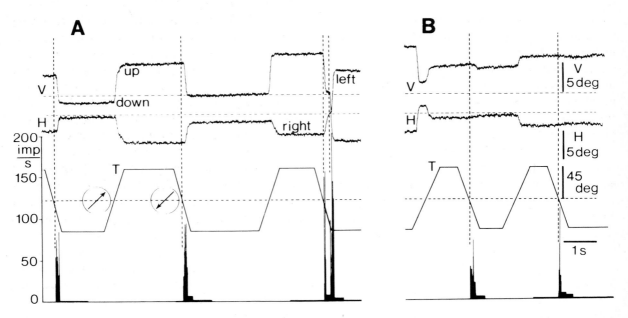

Fig. 2. Burst activity of an identified TRSN axon originating in the right SC. A: discharges associated with tracking saccades. B: in the absence of orienting to a moving target. From top to bottom: vertical (V) and horizontal (H) eye position; target position (T) on the horizontal meridian inclined by 45° (direction of target movement shown in the insets); firing rate obtained by averaging in 6.5 ms bins.

perty: they do not discharge with spontaneous saccades in darkness or in front of a homogeneously illuminated visual field. Hence, they are different from purely "motor" saccade related burst neurones observed in extracellular recordings in cats (Peck et al., 1980) and monkeys (cf. Sparks, 1986). According to the type of activity, revealed by our behavioural tests, TRSNs can be roughly separated into two groups, "visuomotor" and "visual" TRSNs.

"Visuomotor" TRSNs

This group includes all TRSNs with discharges correlated to saccadic eye movements. Typical recordings are shown in Fig. 2 for a TRSN axon originating in the right SC. It generated bursts preceding oblique saccades with leftward horizontal component (Fig. 2A) when the cat attempted to track the moving target. The presaccadic activity was directionally selective for a sector of 60° off-vertical, with maximum activity for movement directions close to 45°. Average lead time with respect to saccades in this preferred direction was 60 ms. Burst durations of this TRSN (range 40 – 360 ms) are representative of a vast majority of TRSNs whose activity can be characterized as "phasic".

Trials on which the passage of target did not induce tracking eye movements clearly revealed the "pure" visual responsiveness of the neurone. We use the term "pure" visual to denote the activity evoked by a visual stimulus in the absence of detectable motor components of orienting. This term is operational and bears no implications concerning either the mechanisms of formation of such signals or their possible role in motor control. As can be seen in Fig. 2B, burst discharges were observed each time the target crossed the centre of the visual field and entered the lower left quadrant. Directional selectivity is demonstrated by the absence of response to the opposite direction of target movement (Fig. 2 A,B) or to horizontal and orthogonal directions. Hence, there is a close correspondence between the directional tuning of both visual and saccade related activity. This is a general feature of "visuomotor" TRSNs, with the exception of a small fraction of omnidirectional neurones. Firing rates of saccade related bursts are always higher than those of "pure" visual responses, this being a criterion to classify a neurone as "visuomotor". However, as shown in Fig. 2, firing rates in the absence of movement are not negligible, and the excitatory effects of visual stimulus per se can make an important contribution to the build-up of movement related discharges.

"Visual" TRSNs

This group includes about one-third of identified TRSNs, for which no difference could be demonstrated between the bursts generated in the absence or in the presence of tracking saccades. Most of these neurones are directionally selective, although the sharpness of tuning varies considerably from cell to cell. Preferred directions usually contain a centrifugal horizontal component, contralateral with respect to the SC. However, no clear directional bias can be demonstrated for the whole sample. An example of a TRSN with a downward vertical directional selectivity is shown in Fig. 3. The border of the receptive field, as defined by target position at burst onset, could not be precisely defined. The earliest activation was observed when the target reached 15° above the horizontal meridian, the latest −20° below. On many occasions (not shown), the passage of the target was accompanied by tracking saccades in preferred (downward) direction. No statistically significant difference was found between "visual" responses and bursts associated with saccades with respect to the number of spikes and mean or maximal frequencies.

It can be concluded that visual information on target movement can reach the lower brain stem through TRSN axons without being used for execution of orienting movements. This might depend on some specific features of collateral connections established by "visual" TRSNs, as opposed to "visuomotor". Systematic comparisons cannot yet be made but, as shown by intra-axonal

HRP labelling (Grantyn and Ong-Meang-Jaques, unpublished data), the overall pattern of terminations is closely similar for the two groups, in particular, within the medial pontine and rostral bulbar RF. Hence, "pure" visual signals can converge with presaccadic discharges of "visuomotor" TRSNs to reticular neurones belonging to the saccadic generator and to RSNs participating in the control of eye-head synergies. Unfortunately, such a convergence cannot be proven at single neurone level with the available methods.

Activity of reticulo-spinal neurones (RSNs) involved in the orienting behaviour

Bearing in mind the morphological organization of tecto-motoneuronal interface (Fig. 1), it is natural to enquire what kind of transformations do the tectal efferent signals undergo at the level of reticular neurones to which they project. We reported recently on the behavioural properties of RSNs receiving monosynaptic input from the contralateral SC (Grantyn and Berthoz, 1987; Grantyn et al., 1987). This work was limited to the so called "eye-neck" RSN (EN-RSN), showing a combination of phasic and decaying tonic components of firing rate modulation during ipsiversive orienting eye-neck synergies. Signals generated by EN-RSNs are strongly correlated with the saccades and/or transient components of neck muscle activity but they cannot be brought in relation to a prolonged maintenance of eccentric eye positions or to tonic neck muscle activity.

The most obvious functional differences between EN-RSNs and their presynaptic "input" neurones, TRSNs, are the following. (1) Burst activity of TRSN does not critically depend on eye position. EN-RSNs, by contrast, do not discharge at all when gaze shifts of appropriate (ipsilateral) direction are made within the contralateral half of

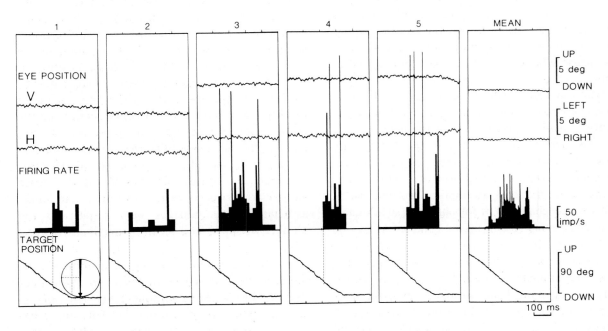

Fig. 3. Responses of a "visual" TRSN axon originating from the left SC to a vertically moving target in the absence of orienting saccades. From top to bottom: vertical (V) and horizontal (H) eye position; instantaneous firing rate; target position on the vertical trajectory (inset). Columns 1 – 5: individual trials; right column: peri-event time histogram aligned on the beginning of target movement from up to down.

the oculomotor range. Apparently, EN-RSNs receive an inhibitory gating input of extracollicular origin. (2) With rare exceptions, TRSNs generate bursts of short duration. Prolonged firing of EN-RSNs must then depend on other input, derived, probably, from medullary circuits underlying the elaboration of eye position signals. (3) TRSNs discharge only with visually triggered gaze shifts, whereas EN-RSNs are active also in the absence of discrete visual targets. (4) Finally, responses to visual stimuli in the absence of orienting movements have not been observed in the EN-RSN population. These latter two observations suggest that "visuomotor" TRSNs probably participate in the build-up of the phasic component of EN-RSN bursts, provided the eye position-related "gate" is open. On the other hand, activity of "visual" TRSNs, as well as non-enhanced, "pure" visual responses of "visuomotor" TRSNs seems not to be reflected at all at the level of EN-RSNs.

However, our preliminary observations on a larger sample (Grantyn, Hardy, Berthoz, unpublished) indicate that some RSNs generate predominantly bursts lasting no longer than 500 ms, well in the range of typical values for TRSNs. It is in this group of "phasic" RSNs that visual responses have been detected in dissociation from the motor components of orienting. The axon of the cell illustrated in Figs. 4 and 5 has been penetrated in the rostral medulla, at the level of the facial nucleus (Fig. 4A). The latency of attenuated EPSP (1.5–1.7 ms) indicated a disynaptic excitatory input from the contralateral SC and the intra-axonal HRP injection revealed a retrogradely labelled cell body in a paramedian location, just anterior to the abducens nucleus (Fig. 4B). The first collateral of this cell passed through the abducens nucleus, branched there, and continued into the rostral pole of the medial vestibular nucleus (Fig. 2B). Boutons could not be detected due to a weak staining. The second, completely labelled collateral (Fig. 4B,C), gave origin to a total of 179 boutons in the dorsal RF, n. prepositus hypoglossi and ventral part of the medial vestibular nucleus. These collaterals are similar to rostral collaterals of

EN-RSNs (Fig. 1). However, the main axon passed from the level of the facial nucleus to the bulbospinal junction without additional collaterals (Fig. 4A). A less extensive branching in the brain stem has been observed also in other completely stained RSNs of predominantly phasic type.

Specimen recordings from the same neurone during presentations of a horizontally moving target are shown in Fig. 4D,E. Leftward target movement induced a burst whose maximal frequency was augmented, if the cat made a tracking saccade in the same direction. Such a behaviour obviously resembles that of "visuomotor" TRSNs. Cell activity illustrated in Fig. 4F was induced by presenting a hand held three-dimensional object to the left. The burst appears to consist of two parts: a presumably visual response beginning 0.7 s before the orienting movement and a later component which precedes the saccade by 45 ms and coincides with the burst in the ipsilateral EMG. Qualitatively similar patterns have been previously reported both for TRSNs (Munoz and Guitton, 1986) and for unidentified deep collicular units (Peck et al., 1980). On the other hand, the movement related burst of Fig. 4F corresponds to a typical pattern of EN-RSNs.

A more detailed analysis of the same RSN is presented in Fig. 5. Rasters of Fig. 5A represent the spike activity, as a circular target subtending 5° traversed the visual field from right to left. The structure of the receptive field appears to be complex, since the initial activation at target positions between 20 and 30° on the right is followed by a suppression, until the target approaches the midline. A weak visual response was observed also with leftward target movement (Fig. 5B). A suppression during passage of the target from about 30° on the left to the midline suggests a strong directional selectivity in this part of the visual field. Rasters labelled with small letters correspond to the activity in trials with leftward saccades whose vectors and time course are shown in C and D. It can be seen that when saccades (a, d) are made in the direction of target movement, visual response can merge with later portion of the

166

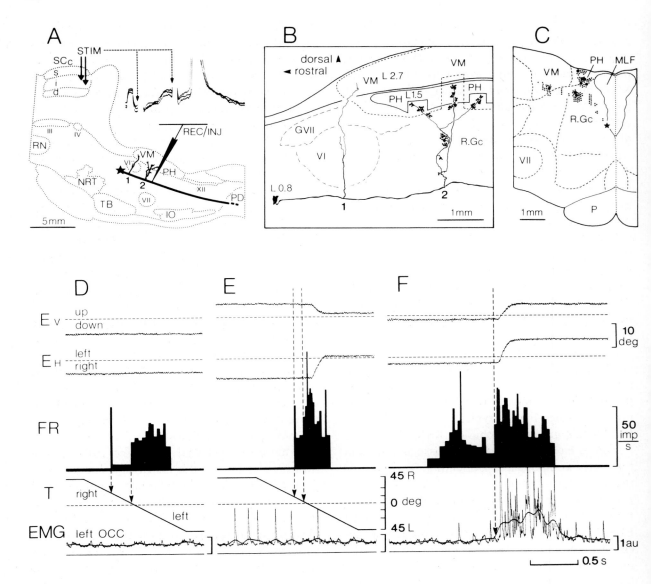

Fig. 4. Morphology and activity patterns of a predominantly phasic RSN. A: scheme of experimental arrangement indicating site of recording and injection (REC/INJ) and position of the neurone reconstructed after HRP injection. Inset: EPSP and spike response to contralateral SC stimulation (calibration pulse: 0.5 mV, 0.5 ms). B: enlarged drawing of axon collaterals projected on parasagittal planes 1.5 and 2.7 mm from the midline. C: plot of all synaptic boutons from collateral N° 2 on frontal plane about 1.5 mm posterior to the abducens nucleus. Large dots correspond to 10, small dots to 1 bouton. Location of the main axon indicated by star. Note that terminals of two tertiary branches in VM and PH, separated rostro-caudally by up to 1.5 mm, innervate homologous parts of the nuclei. Abbreviations as in Fig. 1 and: GVII, genu of the facial nerve; P, pyramid; PD, pyramidal decussation; R.Gc, n. reticularis gigantocellularis; RN, red nucleus. D, E: burst activity during horizontal passage of target from right to left in the absence (D) and in the presence (E) of tracking saccade. From top to bottom: vertical (E_v) and horizontal (E_H) eye position; instantaneous firing rate (FR); horizontal target position (T); EMG from left m. obliquus capitis cranialis: superposition of traces obtained by integration (time constant 5 ms) and by digital filtering (cutoff at 4 Hz) of raw rectified EMG. F: same as D, E, but during presentation of hand-held three-dimensional object from the left.

enhanced perisaccadic discharge. With "spontaneous" leftward saccades (e, c, b), the timing of visual activity precludes its participation in the high frequency part of saccade related bursts, but it matches well its prelude. Finally, by aligning the rasters on saccade onset (Fig. 5E,F) one obtains a perisaccadic time histogram resembling those of long lead bursters (Kaneko et al., 1981). During recording from this RSN, tests with automatically moved standard target rendered no examples of at-

tempted head movements. However, orienting eye-neck synergies were induced when using novel objects (Fig. 4F), in which case a partial correlation of neuronal discharge with the EMG pattern was evident. Hence, RSNs of this type appear to contribute to the execution of both eye and head movements and, in addition, transmit visual information to the lower brain stem and to the spinal cord.

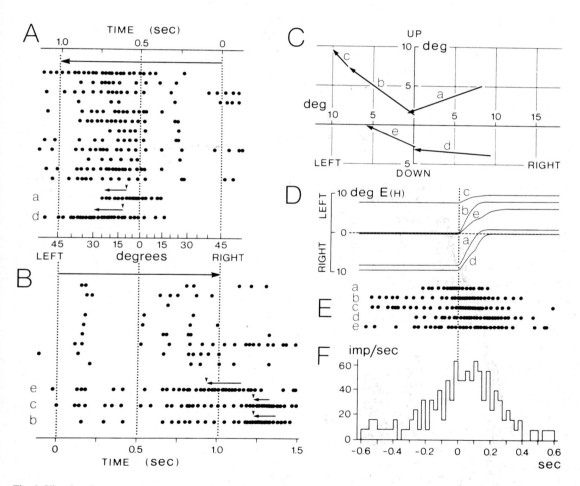

Fig. 5. Visual and saccade related activity of a predominantly phasic RSN (same cell as in Fig. 4). A: rasters of spikes during horizontal passage of target from right to left. Tracking saccades occurred on trials (a) and (d) only. Onset of saccades at vertical arrowheads. Length of horizontal arrows corresponds to saccade duration. Note that time runs from right to left. Lower scale, target position as function of time. B: same as A but for rightward target movement. Spontaneous leftward saccades on trials (e, c, b) only. C: vectors of saccades during correspondingly labelled trials, represented in craniocentric coordinates. D – F: horizontal eye position records, spike rasters and cumulative time histogram of spike activity, aligned on saccade onset.

Discussion

We have presented morphological and functional data suggesting that a modification of generally accepted views on the organization of the tectal efferent system is necessary, at least, concerning the crossed ''tecto-bulbo-spinal'' component in the cat. The conception of uniform output signals coding contraversive movements in spatial coordinates and forwarding them to premotor pattern generators is unsatisfactory in view of qualitative differences between activity patterns of individual TRSNs during a standard visuo-motor task. ''Pure'' visual signals dissociated from movement are definitely transmitted by tectal projection neurones (TRSNs) and even, though less frequently, by reticulo-spinal neurones. Hence, the formation of the final premotor signal is a distributed property of the tecto-reticular network. This view is close to the idea of a progressive transformation of the collicular signals by the reticular neurones (Hepp and Henn, 1983), but it puts more emphasis on the parallel transmission and multiple convergence of partially processed signals.

It appears probable that the processes of visuomotor transformations usually reserved for the deep subdivision of the SC could also be performed simultaneously within the medial reticular formation. These processing networks extend down to the medullary levels, although functional gradients do exist. It has been demonstrated that the formation of presaccadic burst activity in the monkey SC depends on extracollicular sources, such as, e.g., facilitatory inputs from the frontal eye fields (FEF) (Mohler et al., 1973; Wurtz and Mohler, 1976) and disinhibitory effect of nigral afferents (Hikosaka and Wurtz, 1983). However, these effects may also gain access to the lower brain stem independently, since projections from the FEF (Leichnetz et al., 1987) and the substantia nigra pars reticulata (Schneider et al., 1985; Perciavalle, 1987) to the medial rhombencephalic RF do exist. Therefore, from the point of view of anatomical connectivity, the processes of target selection and of enhancement of appropriate visual information can be partly accomplished in the reticular core. Supporting physiological evidence is furnished, to quote only one example, by observations on reticular neurones during visually triggered hand movements in monkeys (Ray et al., 1982). It was shown that some mesencephalic and pontine reticular units respond weakly to indifferent visual stimuli, but such responses are considerably enhanced for stimuli serving as a cue in the Go – No Go paradigm.

Visual responsiveness of units in the reticular formation is a well known phenomenon. Initially, this property was ascribed to the mesencephalic RF because of its relation to afferents from the superior colliculus (Bell et al., 1964; Horn and Hill, 1966). Interpretations of visually evoked activity tended to emphasize its relationship to ascending functions of the mesencephalic RF regulating wakefulness and transmission through the specific sensory nuclei (cf. McGinty and Szymusiak, 1988). Although visual responses have also been observed in the medial pontine RF (Groves et al., 1973), this did not lead to a reinterpretation, since, in the absence of appropriate identification, an ascending projection could have been ascribed to the recorded units. It is only recently that a substantial fraction (32%) of identified reticulospinal neurones located in the dorsal bulbar RF and projecting in the ventral funiculus have been shown to respond to visual stimuli (Yen and Blum, 1984). Our present data obtained in alert cats confirm this result and extend it by showing that a visual signal is present on RSNs whose activity is correlated with the performance of orienting movements.

As to the question posed in the title, *how* visual inputs are used in motor performance during orienting, it must be admitted that a clear-cut answer cannot be given yet. To assume that ''pure'' visual responses are too weak to be of any functional significance is obviously unsatisfactory. A more positive view consists in ascribing to such responses a role in both preparation and execution of specific movements. This role can be conceived as a facilitatory modulation by visual volleys of approximately the same set of neurones, as those more intensely activated during eventual execution of the movement. For this scheme to work, the primarily visual signals coding the location and velocity vector of the target and signals responsible for motor enhancement must be topographically matched within the efferent network. The question has not been examined in sufficient detail for the reticular components of the descending pathways. The often observed lack of temporal coincidence between "visual" and "motor" components of neuronal activity is not in contradiction with the idea of topographically matched facilitatory interaction. A convincing example is the observation by Munoz and Guitton (1985, 1986) on identified TRSNs. They have described a tonic discharge which developed when gaze was still deviated ipsilaterally and persisted until the execution of a contraversive orienting movement. In the presence of a visible target, the latter was preceded by a usual phasic burst. The tonic activity conducted through the crossed projection should facilitate the contralateral ponto-bulbar reticular neurones, including those described in the present paper. Such a facilitation should counteract the suppression of EN-RSNs which acts on these neurones when gaze is deviated in OFF-direction. Hence, signals representing the actual or memorized target position can represent a part of gating mechanisms operating within the tecto-reticulo-spinal network.

Acknowledgements

The author wishes to express his deep gratitude to all who collaborated with him in the tecto-reticular research and, in particular, to R. Grantyn, A. Berthoz and O. Hardy.

References

Anderson, M.E., Yoshida, M. and Wilson, V.J. (1971) Influence of superior colliculus on cat neck motoneurones. *J. Neurophysiol.*, 34: 898 – 907.

Bell, C., Sierra, G., Buendia, N. and Segundo, J. (1964) Sensory properties of neurons in the mesencephalic reticular formation *J. Neurophysiol.*, 27: 961 – 987.

Berthoz, A., Grantyn, A. and Droulez, J. (1986) Some collicular neurons code saccadic eye velocity. *Neurosci. Lett.*, 72: 289 – 294.

Graham, J. (1977) An autoradiographic study of the efferent connections of the superior colliculus in the cat. *J. Comp. Neurol.*, 173: 629 – 654.

Grantyn, A. and Berthoz, A. (1985) Burst activity of identified tecto-reticulo-spinal neurons in the alert cat. *Exp. Brain. Res.*, 57: 417 – 421.

Grantyn, A. and Berthoz, A. (1987) Reticulo-spinal neurons participating in the control of synergic eye and head movements during orienting in the cat. I. Behavioral properties. *Exp. Brain Res.*, 66: 339 – 354.

Grantyn, A. and Grantyn, R. (1976) Synaptic actions of tectofugal pathways on abducens motoneurons in the cat. *Brain Res.*, 105: 269 – 285.

Grantyn, A. and Grantyn, R. (1982) Axonal patterns and sites of termination of cat superior colliculus neurons projecting in the tecto-bulbo-spinal tract. *Exp. Brain Res.*, 46: 243 – 256.

Grantyn, A., Ong-Meang Jacques, V. and Berthoz, A. (1987) Reticulo-spinal neurons participating in the control of synergic eye and head movements during orienting in the cat. II. Morphological properties as revealed by intra-axonal injections of horseradish peroxidase. *Exp. Brain Res.*, 66: 355 – 377.

Groves, P.M., Miller, S.W., Parker, M.V. and Rebec, G.V. (1973) Organization by sensory modality in the reticular formation of the rat. *Brain Res.*, 54: 207 – 224.

Hepp, K. and Henn, V. (1983) Spatio-temporal recording of rapid eye movement signals in the monkey paramedian pontine reticular formation (PPRF). *Exp. Brain Res.*, 52: 105 – 120.

Hess, W.R., Bürgi, S. and Bucher, V. (1946) Motorische Funktion des Tectal- und Tegmentalgebietes. *Mschr. Psychiat. Neurol.*, 112: 1 – 52.

Hikosaka, O. and Wurtz, R.H. (1983) Visual and oculomotor functions of monkey substantia nigra pars reticulata. IV. Relation of substantia nigra to superior colliculus. *J. Neurophysiol.*, 49: 1285 – 1301.

Horn, G. and Hill, R.M. (1966) Responsiveness to sensory stimulation of units in the superior colliculus and subjacent tectotegmental region in the rabbit. *Exp. Neurol.*, 14: 199 – 223.

Huerta, M.F. and Harting, J.K. (1982) Tectal control of spinal cord activity: Neuroanatomical demonstration of pathways connecting the superior colliculus with the cervical spinal cord grey. In H.G.J.M. Kuypers and G.F. Martin (Eds.), *Descending Pathways to the Spinal Cord., Prog. Brain Res., Vol. 57*, Elsevier Biomedical Press, Amsterdam, pp. 293 – 328.

Kaneko, C.R.S., Evinger, C. and Fuchs, A.F. (1981) The role of cat pontine burst neurons in the generation of saccadic eye movements. *J. Neurophysiol.,* 46: 387–408.

Kawamura, K., Brodal, A. and Hoddevik, G. (1974) The projection of the superior colliculus onto the reticular formation of the brain stem. An experimental anatomical study in the cat. *Exp. Brain Res.,* 19: 1–19.

Keller, E.L. (1979) Colliculoreticular organization in the oculomotor system. In R. Granit and O. Pompeiano (Eds.), *Reflex Control of Posture and Movement, Progr. Brain Res., Vol. 50,* Elsevier Biomedical Press, Amsterdam, pp. 725–734.

Leichnetz, G.R., Gonzalo-Ruiz, A., DeSalles, A.A.F. and Hayes, R.L. (1987) The frontal eye field and prefrontal cortex project to the paramedian pontine reticular formation in the cat. *Brain Res.,* 416: 195–199.

McGinty, D. and Szymusiak, R. (1988) Neuronal unit activity patterns in behaving animals: brainstem and limbic system. *Ann. Rev. Psychol.,* 39: 135–168.

Mohler, C.W., Goldberg, M.E. and Wurtz, R.H. (1973) Visual receptive fields of frontal eye field neurons. *Brain Res.,* 61: 385–389.

Munoz, D.P. and Guitton, D. (1985) Tectospinal neurons in the cat have discharges coding gaze position error. *Brain Res.,* 341: 184–188.

Munoz, D.P. and Guitton, D. (1986) Presaccadic burst discharges of tecto-reticulo-spinal neurons in the alert head-free and -fixed cat. *Brain Res.,* 398: 185–190.

Peck, C.K., Schlag-Rey, M. and Schlag, J. (1980) Visuo-oculomotor properties of cells in the superior colliculus of the alert cat. *J. Comp. Neurol.,* 194: 97–116.

Perciavalle, V. (1987) Substantia nigra influence on the reticulospinal neurons: an electrophysiological and ionophoretic study in cats and rats. *Neuroscience,* 23: 243–251.

Peterson, B.W. (1977) Identification of reticulospinal projections that may participate in gaze control. In R. Baker and A. Berthoz (Eds.), *Control of Gaze by Brain Stem Neurons,* Elsevier, Amsterdam, pp. 143–152.

Ray, C.L., Mirsky, A.F. and Pragay, E.B. (1982) Functional analysis of attention-related unit activity in the reticular formation of the monkey. *Exp. Neurol.,* 77: 544–562.

Robinson, D.A. (1975) Oculomotor control signals. In G. Lennerstrand and P. Bach-y-Rita (Eds.), *Basic Mechanisms of Ocular Motility and their Clinical Implications,* Pergamon Press, Oxford, New York, Toronto, pp. 337–374.

Scheibel, M.E. and Scheibel, A.B. (1985) Structural substrates for integrative patterns in the brain stem reticular core. In H.H. Jasper, L.D. Proctor, R.S. Knighton, W.C. Noshay and R.T. Costello (Eds.), *Reticular Formation of the Brain,* Little, Brown and Comp., Boston, pp. 31–55.

Schneider, J.S., Maneto, C. and Lidsky, T.I. (1985) Substantia nigra projection to medullary reticular formation: Relevance to oculomotor and related motor functions in the cat. *Neurosci. Lett.,* 62: 1–6.

Sparks, D.L. (1986) Translation of sensory signals into commands for control of saccadic eye movements: role of primate superior colliculus. *Physiol. Rev.,* 66: 118–171.

Vidal, P.-P., May, P.J. and Baker, R. (1988) Synaptic organization of tectal-facial pathways in the cat. I. Synaptic potentials following collicular stimulation. *J. Neurophysiol.,* 60: 769–797.

Wurtz, R.H. and Albano, J.E. (1980) Visual-motor function of the primate superior colliculus. *Ann. Rev. Neurosci.,* 3: 189–226.

Wurtz, R.H. and Mohler, C.W. (1976) Enhancement of visual responses in monkey striate cortex and frontal eye fields. *J. Neurophysiol.,* 39: 766–772.

Yen, C.-T. and Blum, P.S. (1984) Response properties and functional organization of neurons in midline region of medullary reticular formation of cats. *J. Neurophysiol.,* 52: 961–979.

J.H.J. Allum and M. Hulliger (Eds.)
Progress in Brain Research, Vol. 80
© 1989 Elsevier Science Publishers B.V. (Biomedical Division)

Overview and critique of Chapters 15 – 17

J.I. Simpson

New York City, U.S.A.

Collewijn presents a position paper cautioning against slipping into the belief that the vestibulo-ocular reflex (VOR) identifies a distinct, separable entity in the brain. He is concerned that some colleagues treat the VOR, a sometime useful abstraction, as if it had an independent material existence. In arguing against reification of the VOR and, by extension, the optokinetic reflex, Collewijn reminds us of the shortcomings imposed by the simplifications that have been used. In pushing for greater realism in our models and representations, he stresses that the nervous system uses all relevant signals, both of peripheral and central origin, in making eye movements to optimize vision. While there is no difficulty in agreeing with the view that the brain uses all relevant information in carrying out processes of target selection, spatial localization and gaze control, it is quite a challenge to the investigator to manage all of the requisite variables in conducting an experiment, particularly at the neurophysiological level. Even so, the recent increase in the number of behavioural studies of gaze control that incorporate head movement on the body represents a move in the advocated direction. Pointing out the deficiencies in the present "subsystems" approach is the first step in effecting change toward the holistic view, but suggestions as to how this shift is to be accomplished in practice would be welcomed, especially at the neuronal level. How far can the imposed constraints be relaxed to obtain more realistic behavioural contexts and still permit extraction and interpretation of neuronal measures? Perhaps, just perhaps, neural network models with their hidden units and back-propagation will suggest new views of how the nervous system processes multidimensional inputs, in conjunction with varying internal representations, to achieve effective gaze control.

The two other papers in this section offer two different avenues toward understanding optokinetic performance in primates. *Hoffmann* takes the neurophysiological route, while *Behrens et al.* take the behavioural route. Hoffmann's characterization of the visual response properties of neurones in the nucleus of the optic tract (NOT) and dorsal terminal nucleus (DTN) of the accessory optic system in anaesthetized macaque monkeys continues his long-standing interest in the neuronal activity underlying optokinetic nystagmus in cat and monkey. Several of the findings distinguish the response properties of NOT-DTN neurones in monkey from those in non-primates, but one of them is particularly noteworthy. In the monkey, NOT-DTN neurones responded not only to large textured patterns in a speed- and direction-selective manner, but they also respond with similar speed and direction selectivity to small spots (on the order of 1 degree) moved in the neighbourhood of the fovea. This additional feature of primate NOT-DTN neurones led Hoffmann to conclude that they may contribute not only to optokinetic nystagmus, but also to smooth pursuit, in parallel with cortical-pontine-cerebellar circuits. The specifics of this contribution are not spelled out, but the interactive effects found when a large textured background and a spot were moved in opposite directions suggest that the NOT-DTN could contribute to smooth pursuit by overriding, or at least reducing the competing effects that exist during pursuit of a small object moving relative to a patterned background. In light of the finding by Behrens et al. that stimulation of the temporal and nasal parts of the retina results in different open loop optokinetic responses, it would be of interest to know the contributions of the temporal and nasal retina to the responses of NOT-DTN neurones. Another remaining question is whether the sensitivity to small objects moving at low speeds is conferred by cortical projections to the NOT-DTN. Hoffmann's study leads directly to the question of whether eye movement signals are present on NOT-DTN neurones in the alert monkey. Addressing this point is clearly the next step in his study of the neural underpinnings of optokinetic responses. In the process, information necessary to resolve the continuing debate about distinctions between optokinetic responses and smooth pursuit may be forthcoming.

The study by Behrens et al. on open and closed loop optokinetic nystagmus in squirrel monkeys (and in a man) updates and extends a related study of the rhesus monkey (Körner and Schiller, 1972). The findings from the squirrel monkey are qualitatively in line with those from the rhesus monkey, although some quantitative differences apparently exist with regard to the retinal slip speeds at which the open loop gain and eye velocity are largest. The fact that the maximum open loop eye velocity in the squirrel monkey occurred at retinal slip speeds of 20 – 40 deg/s should be compared with the finding of Hoffmann in macaque monkeys that the maximum response of the NOT-DTN neurone population occurred over a broad range of slip speeds, from 3 to 30 deg/s. Retrobulbar injection of botulinum toxin to reversibly immobilize an eye for the open loop measurements is a novel procedure of general interest. The variation in the human subject's open loop performance with different states of attention and with different attempted tracking strategies is revealing because it shows that the performance of humans is in several ways different from that of squirrel monkeys and because it reinforces Collewijn's emphasis on the importance of target selection in determining gaze control performance.

Reference

Körner, F. and Schiller, P.H. (1972) The optokinetic response under open and closed loop conditions in the monkey. *Exp. Brain Res.,* 14: 318 – 330.

J.H.J. Allum and M. Hulliger (Eds.)
Progress in Brain Research, Vol. 80
© 1989 Elsevier Science Publishers B.V. (Biomedical Division)

CHAPTER 15

Control of the optokinetic reflex by the nucleus of the optic tract in primates

K.-P. Hoffmann

Allgemeine Zoologie and Neurobiologie, Ruhr-Universitaet Bochum, P.O. Box 10 21 48, D-4630 Bochum, F.R.G.

Physiological and anatomical experiments clearly established the existence of a pretectal relay of visual information to the ipsilateral inferior olive in the macaque monkey. Horseradish peroxidase injected into the inferior olivary nucleus retrogradely labelled neurons in the nucleus of the optic tract (NOT) and the dorsal terminal nucleus of the accessory optic tract (DTN). The response characteristics of NOT-DTN neurones are described in this chapter. The visual receptive fields of neurones in NOT and DTN in anaesthetized and paralysed macaque monkeys prefer horizontal ipsiversive movements of single objects or whole field random dot patterns, i.e. neurones in the left NOT-DTN prefer leftward movements and vice versa. The directional tuning widths of NOT-DTN neurones are very broad. Directions withing a mean range of $127 \pm 25°$ visual angle elicit response strengths greater than 50% of the maximal response. Visual latencies to reversals in directions of stimulus movement are in a range from 40 to 80 ms (mean 61 ± 13 ms). Combining two visual stimuli by moving a random dot pattern and a single bar of light simultaneously but in opposite directions causes NOT-DTN neurones to respond to each stimulus as soon as it moves in the cell's preferred direction. The reduced overall response strengths indicate additional inhibitory interactions. All NOT-DTN neurones can be activated from each eye. Interactions between the two eyes are modest and unspecific. Optical speeds of stimulus movement vary for different NOT-DTN neurones (4 – 60 deg/s). The effective range of speeds is broad (0.1 – 400 deg/s for the total population). With oscillating horizontal stimulation NOT-DTN neurones follow repetition rates up to 4 Hz. Receptive fields are mostly large (20 – 40° visual angle), include the fovea, and extend up to 20° into the ipsilateral hemifield. The sensitivity to moving stimuli is highest near the fovea. Our results thus indicate that direction selective cells in the NOT and DTN have all the properties and connections which are necessary and sufficient to control the stability of the image on the retina by supplying retinal slip information to the velocity storage integrator in the brainstem (Raphan et al., 1979).

Key words: Optokinetic reflex; Nucleus of the optic tract; Vision; Monkey

Introduction

The visuomotor system of monkey or man can produce smooth eye movements fast enough to catch up with stimuli moving at velocities well above 100 deg/s (Cohen et al., 1977; Meyer et al., 1985). This is especially true when the stimulus covers some 10° of the central retina (Cheng and Outerbridge, 1975; Dubois and Collewijn, 1979). A typical example of high velocity ocular following due to continuous stimulation is optokinetic nystagmus (OKN) (Ter Braak, 1936; van Die and Collewijn, 1982). Slow phase velocities during OKN in primates can reach 180 deg/s with monocular stimulation in either horizontal direction. In addition, monocular OKN is almost completely symmetrical at all horizontal velocities tested, i.e. the eye velocity during monocular OKN reaches the same values with either temporo-nasal or naso-temporal stimulus movements (Körner and Schiller, 1972).

The nucleus of the optic tract (NOT) and the

dorsal terminal nucleus of the accessory optic tract (DTN) have been identified to contain the neurones essential for eliciting OKN in non-primate mammals (Collewijn, 1975; Cazin et al., 1980; Hoffmann and Schoppmann, 1981). In monkeys NOT and DTN also play an important role in the generation of continuous and high velocity OKN (Kato et al., 1986; Hoffmann et al., 1988; Schiff et al., 1988). In this review we shall document that the properties of neurones in these structures are ideally suited to transmit the sensory information about retinal image slip, necessary for compensatory eye movements, into the optokinetic circuitry.

It has been proposed that the NOT in monkeys is part of the indirect pathway which excites the velocity storage mechanisms in the vestibular system to enhance the slow component of OKN as well as to support the vestibulo-ocular reflex at low velocities (Schiff et al., 1988). A prediction of this suggestion would be that the NOT cells are the source of the visual modulation of the horizontal canal related neurones in the vestibular system (Precht and Strata, 1980). To test this hypothesis we compared the latencies and response characteristics of NOT cells to the visual response characteristics of vestibular neurones (Henn et al., 1974; Boyle et al., 1985).

Supported by our results we conclude quantitatively that all the properties measured in NOT neurones fit perfectly to the characteristics of OKN, and therefore the NOT could provide a powerful visual input to the OKN circuitry in monkey as well as in man.

Methods

Visual responses of NOT and DTN neurones could be elicited by large area random dot patterns as well as by single dots and slits of light. Neutral density filters were used to adjust the intensity of the two stimuli for good visibility of both when they were presented simultaneously. These stimuli were moved by a galvanometer system under computer control on a tangential screen in front of the

animal in order to accumulate peri-stimulus – time histograms (PSTH) from the responses of individual neurones. The PSTHs could be displayed in linear and polar coordinates and provided the data base for further analysis. The following properties of NOT and DTN neurones were analysed quantitatively: (1) specificity and tuning width for direction of stimulus movement; (2) latency to visual stimuli; (3) sensitivity to different visual stimuli and their interactions; (4) ocular dominance and binocular interactions; (5) responses to different stimulus velocities; (6) location and extent of the receptive fields.

Results

Direction specificity

As in other mammals, NOT and DTN neurones in monkeys respond direction specifically to large area random dot patterns. This provides a convenient way of testing their direction specificity by moving the pattern along a circular path on the screen. In this way the direction of movement is continuously changed through 360° and responses to all possible directions can be deduced if response latencies are taken into account.

All NOT and DTN neurones prefer ipsiversive movements, i.e. neurones in the left nuclei prefer movements from right to left in the visual world and vice versa. In many cases, the directions of stimulus movement yielding the strongest responses deviate somewhat from the horizon (Fig. 1). The directional tuning width of monkey NOT-DTN neurones appears very broad. It is expressed as half-width which is calculated as the range of directions of movement yielding response strengths greater than 50% of the maximal response. The range of half-widths is from 80 to 180°, the mean is 127°.

Visual latency

For this analysis, only PSTHs with high temporal resolution (2 ms – 4 ms/bin) were used. The visual latency is defined as the delay between the reversal in horizontal direction of stimulus movement and the completion of the corresponding change in discharge rate. When the direction of movement reverses from preferred to non-preferred (or from non-preferred to preferred) neurones decrease (or increase) their discharge rate

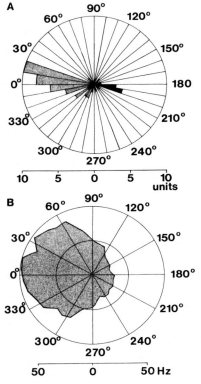

Fig. 1. Preferred directions of visual stimulus motion (A) and directional tuning curve (B) of neurones recorded in the nucleus of the optic tract (NOT) and dorsal terminal nucleus DTN of macaque monkeys. A: the preferred directions of 39 neurones from 7 animals are plotted in 10 degree-wide sectors of a polar histogram. 27 neurones from the left NOT preferring movements to the left are presented by shaded sectors, 12 neurones from the right NOT preferring movements to the right by black sectors. Most neurones prefer movements along the horizon. B: continous mapping of direction specificity was carried out by moving an extensive random dot pattern along a circular path and accumulating average response histograms. The average responses measured for individual cells in spikes/s were then averaged for all 7 cells investigated in the left NOT of one animal and displayed in polar coordinates. The central circle represents spontaneous activity (30 spikes/s), the outer circle maximal activation (67 spikes/s). The activity is clearly reduced below spontaneous activity when the stimulus moves in the direction opposite to the preferred one.

within 45 – 80 ms. The changes in discharge rate are mostly completed within 10 – 20 ms. During these very short intervals the neurones' alter their discharge frequency by approximately 100 – 200 Hz. The mean visual latency for all 29 neurones analysed is 60.9 ± 12.9 ms.

Interactions of different visual stimuli

As already reported (Hoffmann et al., 1988), monkey NOT and DTN neurones respond not only to large area random dot patterns, but also to small moving objects like spots or bars of light. The preferred direction is equal for both kinds of visual stimuli, i.e. the neurones prefer ipsiversive movement of spots or bars, as well as of large area random dot patterns. Although the neurones' sensitivity for one or the other stimulus can vary considerably, the quantitative measures of direction specificity, tuning width, latencies, ocular dominance and velocity tuning agree very well. Due to its spatial extent a random dot pattern will elicit a constant discharge frequency as long as it moves in a given direction (Fig. 2A). Single objects, however, reveal the neurone sensitivity profile across the receptive fields (Fig. 2B). In all neurones tested the sensitivity to single moving objects is highest near the fovea (see also Fig. 5).

Combining the two visual stimuli by moving a random dot pattern in one direction and a slit of light in the opposite direction, the neurones will respond to each stimulus as soon as it moves in the cells' preferred direction (Fig. 2C). The response strength, however, can be significantly reduced when compared to the neurones' response to one of the stimuli alone. This inhibitory effect can also be shown by the antiphase movement of two random dot patterns. The data from these tests are summarized in Table 1.

Columns 2 and 3 in Table 1 give the neuronal response strengths to the movement in the preferred direction of one of the two stimuli alone. Column 4 gives the response to the random dot pattern moving in the preferred direction while the spot crosses the fovea in the non-preferred direction. Column 5 shows the responses for the reversed

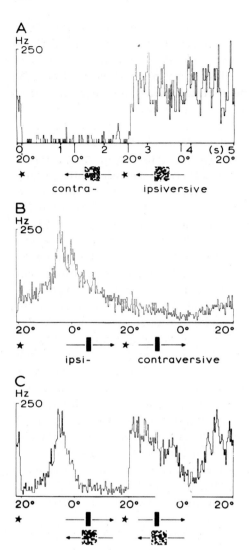

Fig. 2. The direction-specific response of a NOT neurone to a large area random dot pattern (A), to a bar of light (B) and the interaction of the two stimuli (C). The reversal of stimulus movement at the beginning and in the middle of the histogram is marked by a star (*). Note that the movement of the bar (B) is 180° out of phase to that of the random dot pattern (A). In C, both stimuli are moved simultaneously, but in opposite directions. The neurone responds to both stimuli as soon as they move in ipsiversive direction (to the bar in the first half, to the random dot pattern in the second half of the histogram). The response strength to the random dot pattern, however, is significantly reduced when the bar moves across the fovea in the non-preferred direction. Ordinate: discharge frequency (Hz), abscissa: position of stimulus, and in A, time in seconds.

directions. Columns 6 and 7 express the percentage of reduction in response strength when values in columns 4 and 5 are compared to the corresponding values in columns 2 and 3.

Ocular dominance (OD) and binocular interactions

During the recording sessions, we never noticed any neurone exclusively driven by one or the other eye, i.e. all neurones are binocular. In 16 neurones, we measured quantitatively the relative influence of both eyes upon the neurones' discharge frequency. The resulting ocular dominance distribution is shown in Fig. 3. In most of the neurones (82%) no eye dominates over the other by more than a factor of 1.5 (OD 3). Only 2 neurones are dominated by the contralateral eye (OD 2) and one by the ipsilateral eye (OD 4).

Velocity tuning

Monkey NOT and DTN neurones respond to a very broad spectrum of stimulus velocities reaching from less than 0.1 deg/s to several hundred degrees per second. For the quantitative analysis of this paper only responses to random dot patterns oscillating horizontally are taken into account. To change speed we altered the frequency (in the high velocity range) or the amplitude (in the low velocity range) of the triangular waveform

TABLE 1

Interactions of different visual stimuli

1	2	3	4	5	6	7
Cell	Random dot	Spot/bar	Random dot + spot/bar interaction		Reduction	
N 0	53 Hz	63 Hz	20 Hz	28 Hz	62.3%	55.6%
F39	91 Hz	49 Hz	42 Hz	9 Hz	53.8%	81.6%
D 8	61 Hz	54 Hz	44 Hz	46 Hz	25.1%	14.8%
A 1	104 Hz	91 Hz	55 Hz	28 Hz	47.1%	69.2%
A 2	142 Hz	183 Hz	70 Hz	116 Hz	50.7%	36.6%
D 8	54 Hz	31 Hz*	54 Hz	15 Hz*		51.6%
A 2	213 Hz	205 Hz*	132 Hz	78 Hz*	38.0%	62.0%

* Instead of a spot a second random dot pattern was used.

driving the galvanometer. All velocities were presented for a more or less constant time and the mean responses in the preferred and the null-direction were read from the PSTHs. According to the most effective or cut-off velocities, we subdivided the neurones into 3 groups with peak sensitivities at about 4 deg/s, 20 deg/s, and 60 deg/s (Fig. 4A – C). If the responses to different stimulus velocities are pooled over all NOT and DTN neurones, discharge rate increases or stays at its maximal level with increasing velocities up to about 20 – 30 deg/s (Fig. 4D). Another measure for the sensitivity of the neurones with respect to different stimulus velocities is their discharge rate modulation between preferred and non-preferred directions. These values are plotted by open symbols in Fig. 4. The overall shapes and peaks of these curves correspond very well with the curves presenting the responses to the preferred direction. Repetition rates of the oscillating movement of the

random dot pattern below 2 Hz had little if any influence on the neurones' discharge rate or modulation. We could test the neurones quantitatively only up to 4 Hz but up to this frequency a clear direction specific modulation could be detected in the response.

In 10 neurones the reaction to very high stimulus velocities of more than 1500 deg/s, occurring during saccadic image displacements, was tested. Half of the cells tested do not respond at all to this kind

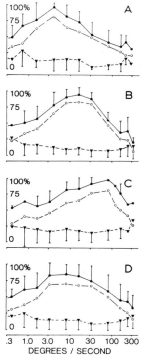

Fig. 4. The response of NOT-DTN neurones in monkeys to different stimulus velocities. Abscissa: stimulus velocity (deg/s); ordinate: relative response strength (%). Response to movement in the preferred direction (V) is indicated by solid lines, response to movement in the opposite (null-) direction (N) by dotted lines, the directional modulation (V − N) by broken lines and open symbols. According to their preferred stimulus velocity, the neurones can be subdivided into 3 groups with low (A), medium (B) and high preferred stimulus velocities (C). The maximal response of each neurone was set at 100%, and the responses of 9 (A, B) and 7 cells (C), respectively, are averaged for these tuning curves. The averaged response of all neurones (25) is presented in D. One standard deviation is indicated (vertical bars).

OCULAR DOMINANCE

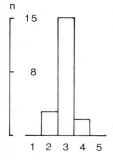

Fig. 3. Ocular dominance distribution of monkey NOT-DTN neurones. Ocular dominance values (OD) of the neurones were assessed quantitatively by comparing the response strength during monocular stimulation of the contralateral (co) and ipsilateral eye (ip).

$$OD = (co - ip)/(co + ip).$$

Group 1 neurones are exclusively activated by the contralateral eye, group 5 neurones by the ipsilateral eye. Neurones forming group 3 are nearly equally influenced by both eyes (OD < 0.2). If a neurone's activity during monocular stimulation of the contralateral (ipsilateral) eye was 1.5-times higher than during stimulation of the ipsilateral (contralateral) eye, it was assigned to group 2 (4) (OD > 0.2). Ordinate: number of cells.

of stimulus. The remainder reduced their ongoing activity almost to zero in response to the saccade-like stimulus movement. This reduction of activity is independent of the direction of stimulus movement.

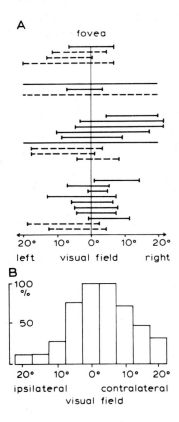

Fig. 5. A: location and horizontal extent of receptive fields in NOT-DTN in relation to the fovea (0°). Abscissa: positions in the visual field (degrees of visual angle). Neurones recorded in the left NOT-DTN are marked by solid lines, neurones recorded in the right NOT-DTN are marked by broken lines. Data from 4 individual animals are presented separately. The receptive fields mostly include the fovea, large parts of the contralateral and also considerable parts of the ipsilateral hemifield. The horizontal extent of the receptive fields reaches 10° − > 40°. B: to show the sensitivity of the NOT-DTN for visual stimuli appearing in different parts of the visual field, the percentage of neurones (ordinate) activated from defined parts of the visual field (abscissa) is indicated. Again it is very evident that the central visual field is represented best.

Location and extent of the receptive fields

The location and the extent of the receptive fields of monkey NOT-DTN neurones were judged by evaluation of PSTHs measured during stimulation with a spot or bar of light. Fig. 5 shows the accumulated receptive fields of all animals tested. As can be seen clearly, the activity can be influenced from a very large area (40 degrees or more horizontal extent). This area includes the fovea and extends substantially (up to 20° visual angle) into the ipsilateral visual hemifield. The extent into the contralateral visual field is sometimes well beyond 20°.

The vertical extent of the receptive fields was estimated by presenting moving spots of light at different vertical positions. With these stimuli, the receptive fields extend 8 − 12° above and below the horizon. With larger random dot stimuli responses can be elicited also from locations beyond 20° above or below the horizon. To judge the relative contribution of central and peripheral parts of the visual field to a neurone's activity we compared the neurone's response during stimulation of the whole visual field and during exclusive stimulation of certain parts of the visual field with a random dot pattern (Fig. 6). Visual stimulation which excludes the fovea often leads to a severe reduction of the cell's activity and directional modulation when compared to whole field stimulation. This can also occur with exclusive stimulation of the foveal region. Exclusive stimulation of the ipsilateral hemifield leads to a reduction of the directional modulation of a cell by 50% − 90%. The strength of the contribution of different parts of the receptive fields can vary a lot. But in all cases it seems that increasing the stimulated area of the receptive field increases the response strength and that the highest sensitivity is near the fovea.

Discussion

The NOT and DTN clearly are areas concerned with the evaluation of direction and speed of stimulus movement. Therefore it may be interesting to compare the movement sensitivity of

NOT-DTN neurones with this property to neurones of area MT — the middle temporal area in the extrastriate cortex of primates, unequivocally identified as a movement processing area (Zeki,

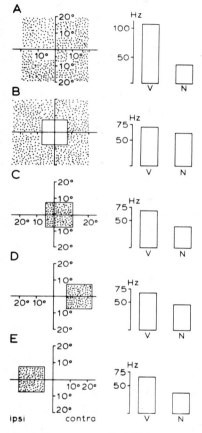

Fig. 6. The response of a NOT neurone to visual stimulation of different parts of the visual field with a restricted random dot pattern. In the left part of the diagram the different conditions of visual stimulation are indicated. The right part of the diagram shows the neuronal response strength (Hz) to stimulus movement in the preferred (V) and non-preferred (N) direction as vertical columns. A: whole field stimulation of the central 40°; B: whole field stimulation without stimulation of the foveal region (central 16°); C: exclusive stimulation of the fovea; D: exclusive stimulation of a 16° field in the contralateral hemifield; E: exclusive stimulation of a 16° field in the ipsilateral hemifield. Neuronal modulation, i.e. the difference of neuronal response to stimulus movement in the preferred and non-preferred direction is greatest during full field stimulation, and smallest when the fovea is excluded from stimulation. It is clear that all parts of the receptive field add up to the neurone's response.

1974; Newsome et al., 1985). MT-neurones, like NOT-DTN neurones, are direction selective irrespective of the type of moving stimuli like slits, single spots, or random dot fields. Preferred direction and directional tuning width is independent of the speed at which the stimuli move. The optimal speed for NOT-DTN neurones is in the same range as that of MT-neurones. In MT all directions, in NOT-DTN only ipsiversive directions are represented. Directional tuning width in NOT-DTN neurones is much broader than in MT (127° in NOT-DTN versus 90° in MT) (Albright, 1984).

Interactions between two stimuli moving in opposite directions seem to be very simple in the NOT-DTN. Any stimulus moving in the preferred direction will activate the cells. A single stimulus (spot or bar, 1 degree wide) moving in the non-preferred direction across the fovea can strongly suppress the response to whole field stimulation in the preferred direction. In MT, these interactions are much more diverse and sophisticated. The response to a moving bar is facilitated by background movement in the opposite direction or suppressed by background movement in the same direction. In addition, these effects are velocity dependent (Allman et al., 1985).

There are, however, important properties of NOT and DTN neurones which cannot be found in MT. First, there is a strong bias for horizontal ipsiversive object motion in NOT-DTN cells, whereas all directions are effective in driving neurones in MT (Albright, 1984). A second difference is the representation of the ipsilateral visual field in NOT-DTN neurones. Comparing the visual field representations in areas MT, MST and FST as provided by Desimone and Ungerleider (1986) and van Essen et al. (1981) and with the visual field representation in NOT and DTN as measured in this study, it becomes evident that only area FST consistently contains neurones with an ipsilateral field representation as large as that found in NOT-DTN. Receptive fields in MT are much smaller and more localized and only some extend more than a few degrees into the ipsilateral hemifield. The ipsilateral visual field representation in NOT is dependent on cortico-cortical connections across the corpus callosum. After callosotectomy no receptive field recorded in the NOT-DTN extended into the ipsilateral hemifield (Hoffmann et al. in preparation). Thus some of the receptive field properties of different areas surrounding the superior temporal sulcus, e.g. area MT and area FST, influence those found in NOT-DTN and therefore these areas may provide a parallel input to the neurones studied in this investigation. Electrical stimulation of these areas surrounding the superior temporal sulcus clearly give rise to orthodromic responses in NOT-DTN cells (Hoffmann et al., 1987). Further anatomical analysis of the stimulation sites is needed to clarify the exact origins of these projections.

The asymmetry of directional preference of the NOT-DTN neurones is particularly striking. It consists of a clear segregation of preferred directions for NOT-DTN neurones on each side of the brain for ipsiversive movement. There are many reports of asymmetries in the slow phase of optokinetic nystagmus as well as in smooth pursuit after cortical damage in humans (Leigh and Thurston, 1986) or monkeys (Lynch and McLaren, 1983; Zee et al., 1987) or strabismus in humans (Tychsen and Lisberger, 1986). It is obvious that the destruction of cortical areas surrounding the superior temporal sulcus would reduce the highly motion specific input to the ipsilateral NOT. Because of the receptive fields extending into the ipsilateral hemifield and because all NOT-DTN neurones are binocular, a directional deficit should be identical within the central 20° for the visual field ipsilateral as well as contralateral to the lesioned side. The assumption is that we have seen in the NOT the changes which must occur also at other subcortical sites − probably in the pontine nuclei − to the same degree which then could explain the deficits in smooth pursuit. After total occipital cortical lesions the optokinetic response in primates becomes very poor (Ter Braak and Van Vliet, 1963; Zee et al., 1987). So far we have no data on NOT-DTN responses after decortication but inferring from our results in the cat (Hoff-

mann, 1983) it can be suggested that binocularity and responses to high velocities are lost after decortication. The consequence would be the highly asymmetric optokinetic nystagmus, elicited only by low stimulus velocities directed towards the lesioned hemisphere (Zee et al., 1987).

When comparing the responses of the primate's NOT-DTN neurones with those found in other mammals important distinctions can be seen. First, in no other species are neurones in the NOT-DTN able to respond to such high velocities as in primates (well above 200 deg/s). Optimal response velocities in cats are about 1 − 10 deg/s (Hoffmann and Schoppmann, 1981), in rats and rabbits these are even lower (Collewijn, 1975; Cazin et al., 1980; Maekawa et al., 1984). The optimal speed reported in this study for primates ranges from 5 to 60 deg/s with the mean for the total population of about 30 deg/s. The optimal velocity of 30 deg/s for NOT-DTN neurones is exactly the value predicted as the most effective slip velocity to charge the velocity storage integrator in a model of Raphan et al. (Raphan et al., 1979). It is interesting to note that the human sensitivity to visual motion as measured by differential speed detection thresholds is best at values of 4 − 32 deg/s (Orban et al., 1984). This seems to indicate that the motor system is provided with the same information about the speed of visual motion as higher visual centres leading to perception. The same conclusion was reached by Tychsen and Lisberger (1986) by comparing smooth pursuit performance and velocity judgement in strabismic persons. Second, equal sensitivity to single objects (spots and lines) and to full field stimulation as shown in this study was never reported in the studies of rabbits and cats. Again, we believe that the strong projection from specialized motion analysing areas in the primate cortex to the NOT and DTN are responsible for these unique responses.

Another striking feature of NOT-DTN neurones is their brisk and short latency response to the reversal of direction of stimulus movement. This is specifically interesting with respect to possible sites in the brainstem receiving this information. One hypothesis argues that the visual modulation of the vestibular neurones comes via the NOT output to the nucleus prepositus hypoglossi (NPPH) (Magnin et al., 1983). The latencies and the rise time to maximal discharge frequencies in vestibular neurones in response to a velocity step are much slower than those measured for the NOT-DTN neurones (Waespe and Henn, 1977). The average latency between start of drum rotation and first sign of frequency change in vestibular neurones was 240 ms. In the NOT-DTN it is less than 60 ms. This is true for activation as well as for inhibition. Also with sinusoidal oscillation of the visual stimulus clear differences between NOT-DTN neurones and vestibular neurones can be seen. Boyle et al. (1985) report that vestibular neurones almost cease to respond to stimulus oscillations above 0.2 Hz whereas the optokinetic response in the same animal continues well above 2 Hz. Clearly the response to stimulus steps and stimulus reversals seen in the NOT-DTN neurones could provide an input for the optokinetic reflex at all frequencies the reflex is able to follow. Vestibular neurones could also receive this input but have a velocity saturating output. The latter clearly represents only the 'slow' component of OKN (Cohen et al., 1977; Lisberger et al., 1981). A lesion of the NOT-DTN completely abolishes the optokinetic response when the stimulus moves towards the lesioned side (Kato et al., 1986). The structure in the brainstem receiving the output of the NOT-DTN neurones in order to drive the optokinetic reflex without the involvement of neurones in the vestibular nuclei at frequencies above 1 Hz is not known. A candidate for the high velocity high frequency optokinetic response could be the visual projection to the cerebellar flocculus via the inferior olive and a, so far unspecified, mossy fibre projection from pontine nuclei.

In conclusion we would like to suggest that the NOT-DTN is a mirror for the whole cortical motion analysing system concerned with horizontal movements. The information flow from most cortical areas to the midbrain passes by the NOT-DTN cells and can influence them. Their activity then reflects all the information on motion processing which is made available for the velocity storage integrator and possibly to other structures generating, more directly, visuomotor responses.

Acknowledgements

This study was supported by DFG grant Ho 450/17. I gratefully acknowledge the cooperation of C. Distler, R. Erickson and W. Mader.

References

Albright, T.D. (1984) Direction and orientation selectivity of neurons in visual area MT of the macaque. *J. Neurophysiol.*, 52: 1106 – 1130.

Allman, J., Miezin, F. and McGuinness, E. (1985) Stimulus specific responses from beyond the classical receptive field: Neurophysiological mechanisms for local-global comparisons in visual neurons. *Ann. Rev. Neurosci.*, 8: 407 – 430.

Boyle, R., Büttner, U. and Markert, G. (1985) Vestibular nuclei activity and eye movements in the alert monkey during sinusoidal optokinetic stimulation. *Exp. Brain Res.*, 57: 362 – 369.

Cazin, L., Precht, W. and Lannou, J. (1980) Pathway mediating optokinetic responses of vestibular nucleus neurons in the rat. *Pfluegers Arch.*, 384: 19 – 29.

Cheng, M. and Outerbridge, J.M. (1975) Optokinetic nystagmus during selective retinal stimulation. *Exp. Brain Res.*, 23: 129 – 139.

Cohen, B., Suzuki, J. and Raphan, T. (1977) Quantitative analysis of the velocity characteristics of optokinetic nystagmus and optokinetic after-nystagmus. *J. Physiol. (London)*, 270: 321 – 344.

Collewijn, H. (1975) Direction-Selective units in the rabbit's nucleus of the optic tract. *Brain Res.*, 100: 489 – 508.

Desimone, R. and Ungerleider, L.G. (1986) Multiple visual areas in the caudal superior temporal sulcus of the macaque. *J. Comp. Neurol.*, 248: 164 – 189.

Dubois, M.F.W. and Collewijn, H. (1979) Optokinetic reactions in man elicited by localized retinal motion stimuli. *Vision Res.*, 19: 1105 – 1115.

Henn, V., Young, L.R. and Finley, C. (1974) Vestibular nucleus units in alert monkeys are also influenced by moving visual fields. *Brain Res.*, 71: 144 – 149.

Hoffmann, K.-P. (1983) Control of the optokinetic reflex by the nucleus of the optic tract in the cat. In A. Hein and M. Jeannerod (Eds.), *Spatially Oriented Behavior*, Springer, New York, pp. 135 – 153.

Hoffmann, K.-P. and Schoppmann, A. (1981) A quantitative

analysis of the direction-specific response of neurons in the cat's nucleus of the optic tract. *Exp. Brain Res.*, 42: 146–157.

Hoffmann, K.-P., Erickson, R. and Distler, C. (1987) Retinal and cortical projections to the nucleus of the optic tract and dorsal terminal nucleus in macaque monkeys. *Soc. Neurosci. Abstr.*, 13: 1436.

Hoffmann, K.-P., Distler, C., Erickson, R.G. and Mader, W. (1988) Physiological and anatomical identification of the nucleus of the optic tract and dorsal terminal nucleus of the accessory optic tract in monkeys. *Exp. Brain Res.*, 69: 635–644.

Kato, I., Harada, K., Hasegawa, T., Igarashi, T., Koike, Y. and Kawasaki, T. (1986) Role of the nucleus of the optic tract in monkeys in relation to optokinetic nystagmus. *Brain Res.*, 364: 12–22.

Körner, F. and Schiller, P. (1972) The optokinetic response under open and closed loop conditions in the monkey. *Exp. Brain Res.*, 14: 318–330.

Leigh, R.J. and Thurston, S.E. (1986) Recovery of ocular motor function in humans with cerebral lesions. In E.L. Keller and D.S. Zee (Eds.), *Adaptive Processes in Visual and Oculomotor Systems, Advances in the Biosciences, Vol. 57*, Pergamon, Oxford, pp. 231–238.

Lisberger, S.G., Miles, F.A., Optican, L.M. and Eighmy, B.B. (1981) Optokinetic response in monkey: Underlying mechanisms and their sensitivity to long term adaptive changes in vestibulo-ocular reflex. *J. Neurophysiol.*, 45: 869–890.

Lynch, J.C. and McLaren, J.W. (1983) Optokinetic nystagmus deficits following parieto-occipital cortex lesions in monkeys. *Exp. Brain Res.*, 49: 125–130.

Maekawa, K., Takeda, T., and Kimura, M. (1984) Responses of the nucleus of the optic tract neurons projecting to the nucleus reticularis tegmenti pontis upon optokinetic stimulation in the rabbit. *Neurosci. Res.*, 2: 1–25.

Magnin, M., Courjon, J.H. and Flandrin, J.M. (1983) Possible visual pathways to the cat vestibular nuclei involving the nucleus prepositus hypoglossi. *Exp. Brain Res.*, 51: 298–303.

Meyer, C.H., Lasker, A.G. and Robinson, D.A. (1985) The upper limit of human smooth pursuit. *Vision Res.*, 25: 561–563.

Newsome, W.T., Wurtz, R.H., Dursteler, M.R. and Mikami, A. (1985) Deficits in visual motion processing following ibotenic acid lesions of the middle temporal visual area of the macaque monkey. *J. Neurosci.*, 5: 825–840.

Orban, G.A., DeWolf, J. and Maes, H. (1984) Factors influencing velocity coding in the human visual system. *Vision Res.*, 24: 33–37.

Precht, W. and Strata, P. (1980) On the pathway mediating optokinetic responses in vestibular nuclear neurons. *Neuroscience*, 5: 777–787.

Raphan, T., Matsuo, V. and Cohen, B. (1979) Velocity storage in the vestibulo-ocular reflex arc (VOR). *Exp. Brain Res.*, 35: 229–248.

Schiff, D., Cohen, B. and Raphan, T. (1988) Nystagmus induced by stimulation of the nucleus of the optic tract in the monkey. *Exp. Brain Res.*, 70: 1–14.

Ter Braak, J.W.G. (1936) Untersuchungen über optokinetischen Nystagmus. *Arch. Neerl. Physiol.*, 21: 309–376.

Ter Braak, J.W.G. and Van Vliet, A.G.M. (1963) Subcortical optokinetic nystagmus in the monkey. *Psychiatr. Neurol. Neurochir.*, 66: 277–283.

Tychsen, L. and Lisberger, S.G. (1986) Maldevelopment of visual motion processing in humans who had strabismus with onset in infancy. *J. Neurosci.*, 6: 2495–2508.

Van Die, G. and Collewijn, H. (1982) Optokinetic nystagmus in man. *Human Neurobiol.*, 1: 111–119.

Van Essen, D.C., Maunsell, J.H.R. and Bixby, J.L. (1981) The middle temporal visual area in the macaque: Myeloarchitecture, connections, functional properties, and topographic representation. *J. Comp. Neurol.*, 199: 293–326.

Waespe, W. and Henn, V. (1977) Neuronal activity in the vestibular nuclei of the alert monkey during vestibular and optokinetic stimulation. *Exp. Brain Res.*, 27: 523–538.

Zee, D.S., Tusa, R.J., Herdman, S.J., Butler, P.H. and Gücer, G. (1987) Effects of occipital lobectomy upon eye movements in primate. *J. Neurophysiol.* 58: 883–907.

Zeki, S.M. (1974) Functional organization of a visual area in the posterior bank of the superior temporal sulcus of the rhesus monkey. *J. Physiol. (London)*, 236: 549–573.

J.H.J. Allum and M. Hulliger (Eds.)
Progress in Brain Research, Vol. 80
© 1989 Elsevier Science Publishers B.V. (Biomedical Division)

CHAPTER 16

Open-loop and closed-loop optokinetic nystagmus in Squirrel monkeys (*Saimiri sciureus)* and in man*

F. Behrens, O.-J. Grüsser and P. Roggenkämper

Department of Physiology, Freie Universität, Arnimallee 22, 1 Berlin 33, F.R.G.

Horizontal optokinetic nystagmus (OKN) was measured in 3 normal Squirrel monkeys by means of the electromagnetic search coil technique. Binocular and monocular stimulation of each eye to the left and the right by moving vertical stripe patterns of 2.37 or 15 degree period were applied at angular velocities of 0.5 to 400 deg/s. After measurement of horizontal OKN under normal conditions, open-loop OKN gain was determined by monocular stimulation of an eyeball immobilized by means of retrobulbar injections of 11 units botulinum toxin (BoTx type A) and compared with the pre-injection data or with monocular stimulation of the other eye, which remained mobile. In normal Squirrel monkeys gain of optokinetic nystagmus reached values between 0.8 and 0.97 at angular velocities below 1.5 deg/s. Gain under these conditions was related to stimulus angular velocities V_s, i.e. $G_e = V_e/V_s$. A slightly higher gain was found for binocular than for monocular stimulation. No significant differences were found in OKN when monocular stimulation in the naso-temporal and in the temporo-nasal direction was applied. The upper cut-off angular velocity (-3 dB-point) reached values of $180-230$ deg/s, significantly above those observed in man under similar stimulus conditions. Monocular optokinetic stimulation of an immobilized eye led to vigorous optokinetic nystagmus and OKAN of the other eye, whereby maximum gain ($G_i = V_e/V_r$) was found to be between 20 and 30 at lower retinal stimulus velocities ($2-5$ deg/s). Gain was related to retinal stimulus velocity V_r. Increase in V_r above 10 deg/s led to a decrease in gain with a slope of about 20 dB per decade. Measurement of gain of closed-loop OKN related to retinal stimulus velocity V_r (which was determined by the difference between V_s and V_e) led to a similar dependence of OKN as in closed-loop stimulus conditions. Differences in sensitivity between the temporal and the nasal visual hemifield stimulation evoking horizontal open-loop OKN are described. Directional selectivity appeared in these experiments. Open-loop OKN data from a human subject are reported. With highly attentive horizontal optokinetic gaze nystagmus, V_e depended on the duration of the pursuit phases of OKN. V_e accelerated with the duration of the individual slow phase of OKN and was reset by each backward saccade (of the covered mobile eye). OKN gain was considerably smaller when the subject intentionally pursued as many stripes as possible of the 1.15 degree period stripe pattern (gain related to V_r about $1.5-3$). With inattentive optokinetic stare nystagmus, gain was also less than with attentive prolonged pursuit-OKN, but reached values of 5 and more.

Key words: Optokinetic reflex; Retinal slip velocity; Binocular and monocular stimulation; Closed and open loop gain; Monkey; Man

Introduction

The main purpose of the optokinetic reflex (OKR) is to minimize retinal image movement during head

---

*This paper was presented by O.-J. Grüsser.

or body movements. This gaze stabilization is induced by foveal and extrafoveal retinal movement signals. It supports the foveal fixation mechanism operating by saccades and by the "foveal" attentive gaze pursuit. At moderate head velocities the OKR acts in cooperation with the compensatory eye movements evoked by the vestibulo-ocular reflex (VOR). Both mechanisms seem to use, at least in part, the same gaze motor control structures of the brainstem.

It is well known that, as in man, the optokinetic stimulation of untrained monkeys by means of a large continuously rotating visual pattern (e.g. an optokinetic drum) activates the extrafoveal OKR and evokes conjugate optokinetic stare-nystagmus (OKN) (Ohm, 1921, 1927, 1934, 1943; ter Braak, 1936). During the last years many laboratories have contributed to the knowledge that the optokinetic pathway responsible for OKN also consists of direct neuronal connections between retina and brainstem. Movement-sensitive and direction-selective ganglion cells, having rather large receptive fields, project from the retina to the pretectal nuclei of the accessory optic tract, which in turn are connected with the vestibular nuclei (Collewijn 1976, 1981; Hoffmann and Schoppmann, 1975; Hoffmann, 1979, 1982; Grasse and Cynader, 1984; Hoffmann and Distler, 1986; Kato et al., 1986; Simpson, 1984; Hutchins and Weber, 1985; Weber, 1985). Restricting the experiments to horizontal OKN, the nucleus of the optic tract (NOT) and the dorsal terminal nucleus (DTN) of the accessory optic tract are the predominant subcortical visual structures which mediate visual movement signals controlling OKN. These structures are target areas of ganglion cells located in the nasal half of the contralateral retina. The cells of the NOT respond preferentially to horizontal pattern movements through the visual field in the temporo-nasal direction (Hoffmann, 1987). In addition to the direct input from the contralateral retina, corticofugal axons originating from cells in the striate visual cortex (area V1) and in the movement-sensitive cortical areas MT and MST, located around the supratemporal sulcus, contact NOT cells. Thus cortical visual structures control the activity of nerve cells in the NOT which mediate retinal velocity error signals to the vestibular nuclei in the gaze motor system of the brainstem. By means of these cortical loops, NOT- and DTN-neurones can be activated by the con-

tralateral and the ipsilateral eye. Most of the corticofugal axons from area V1 originate from binocularly driven pyramidal cells of cytoarchitectonic layer 3. Thus the corticofugal input conveys information from both eyes to the NOT on nasotemporal and temporo-nasal movements.

As Hoffmann and Distler (1986) have demonstrated in cats and monkeys, the nerve cells of the NOT and DTN have large receptive fields of more than 30° diameter, always including the fovea. They respond best to ipsilaterally moving visual stimuli in a velocity range of 10 to 80 deg/s. The axons of the NOT terminate on nerve cells of the dorsal cap of the inferior olive. These nerve cells in the inferior olive form part of the climbing fibres within the cerebellum and provide visual movement inputs to the "oculomotor" and "vestibular" structures of the cerebellum (Fig. 1). Axon collaterals of NOT and DTN nerve cells project to the nucleus prepositus hypoglossi (NPH), from which connections also reach the oculomotor regions of the cerebellum via mossy fibres (Baker and Berthoz, 1975). Finally the nucleus reticularis tegmenti pontis (NRTP) seems to be another target area of NOT and DTN axon collaterals (Keller and Crandall, 1983). From NRTP and perhaps also from NPH, visual movement signals are transmitted to the brainstem vestibular nuclei, which in turn are connected with the horizontal gaze centres of the paramedian pontine reticular formation (PPRF) and the oculomotor nuclei (OMN, Fig. 1). These structures also receive input signals from the oculomotor cerebellum via the brainstem vestibular nuclei (VN, Boyle et al., 1985). The structures mentioned are part of the brainstem horizontal OKR-network which was recently reviewed by Waespe and Henn (1987, Fig. 1).

It is evident that OKN depends not only on retinal error signals but also on internal feedback mechanisms ("efference copy"), by which the gaze pursuit control system is informed about neuronal commands finally reaching the oculomotor nuclei during slow gaze movements. These efference copy signals are added to the retinal error signals in controlling the gaze motor commands. Efference copy signals may originate at different levels including the cortical structures involved in gaze movement and space perception (Collewijn et al., 1982) and the brainstem. In addition to the velocity error signals, retinal position error signals (distance of a given part of the moving visual field from the fovia centre) can be applied in controlling slow-phase angular velocity of OKN. This mechanism strongly depends on spatially directed attention and operates only during attentive optokinetic gaze

nystagmus (ter Braak, 1936; Collewijn et al., 1982; Grüsser, 1986 in Berthoz, 1986). In general, OKN-gain increases when a human subject augments his attention towards the moving visual pattern. This attention characterizes the transition from optokinetic stare nystagmus to gaze nytagmus (ter Braak, 1936). In animal experiments, however, except under special training conditions, one usually investigates the reflex-type optokinetic stare nystagmus.

A simple method to explore the efficacy of retinal velocity signals on OKN is an experiment under open-loop conditions. Such experiments are possible in human patients suffering from a sudden complete palsy of the extraocular muscles of one eye (e.g. Ohm, 1926, 1943), a fairly rare symptom in neurological diseases. In the laboratory setting, open-loop OKN can be studied when all extraocular muscles have been immobilized by retrobulbar injection of a local anaesthetic (Kornmüller, 1931; Grüsser et al., 1981). In monkeys, in addition to the short-term retrobulbar injection of a local anaesthetic, two methods can be employed to immobilize one eye: (a) transection of all oculomotor nerves (Körner and Schiller, 1972), or (b) transient immobilization of extraocular eye muscles by retrobulbar injection of Botulinum toxin (BoTx).

In the following we will describe experimental data obtained in Squirrel monkeys with the latter method and will compare these data with those obtained in a human observer whose extraocular eye muscles were immobilized by retrobulbar injection of a local anaesthetic.

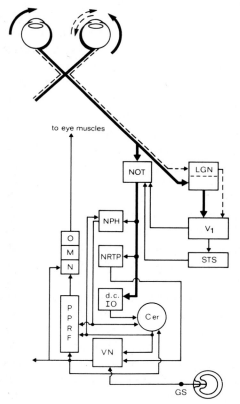

Fig. 1. Scheme of the optokinetic reflex and OKN system of the right half of the brain. The connections of the nasal retina of the left eye and the temporal retina of the right eye are shown. NOT, nucleus of the optic tract; LGN, lateral geniculate nucleus; V1, primary visual cortex; STS, movement sensitive areas MT and MST in the cortex around the supratemporal sulcus; NPH, nucleus praepositus hypoglossi; NRTP, nucleus reticularis tegmenti pontis; dcIO, dorsal cap of inferior olive; Cer, cerebellum; VN, complex of the brainstem vestibular nuclei; GS, ganglion Scarpae; PPRF, paramedian pontine reticular formation; OMN, ocular motor nuclei (Behrens and Grüsser, 1988).

Methods

The experiments were performed during the last three years in 3 normal adult Squirrel monkeys raised in the monkey colony of our institute.

Implantation of the scleral search coil and the headholder

After the monkeys were adapted to the experimental chair, a scleral search coil was implanted in one eye outside the corneal limbus behind the conjunctiva (Robinson, 1963; Collewijn, 1981). No postoperative complications were observed and the coil and the skull implants (socket and fixation device) were tolerated up to 36 months. In one monkey (M 71) a second search coil was implanted on the other eye several months later.

Eye movement recordings

The animals which had become accustomed to the monkey chair tolerated mechanical immobilization of the head without difficulty for recording periods of 60 to 90 min per day. They received 0.2 to 1 mg DL-amphetamine i.m. before recording and were rewarded for cooperation during the experiments with small amounts of juice. Without amphetamine the OKN was rather variable and the monkeys became drowsy and fell asleep 10 to 15 min after the experiment had commenced.

The eye with the scleral search coil was placed in the centre of two pairs (one vertical, one horizontal) of Helmholtz coils, 58 cm in diameter and 20 to 30 kHz electromagnetic fields, which were fixed on four sides of a cube of 64 cm side length. Eye position could be measured by this method with an error of less than 0.5%, provided one took into consideration that a deviation in the position of the scleral search coil from the parallel to the vertical or horizontal plane determined by the Helmholtz coils led to an error in the position signals. This could be easily compensated by taking into account the signals induced from the other pair of Helmholtz coils (Behrens, 1988).

Monocular immobilization

One eye was immobilized by a retrobulbar injection of 11 units Botulinum toxin A (BoTx, Oculinum, Dr. A. Scott, Smith Kettlewell Institute, San Francisco, kindly provided by Prof. G. Kommerell from the Freiburg University Eye Clinic and one of the authors, P.R., Bonn University Eye Clinic) or BoTx produced at the Department of Pharmacology, University of Giessen, donated to us by Prof. G. Habermann. The BoTx was dissolved in 10 ml Ringer solution. BoTx uptake in the external eye muscles and the m. levator palpebrae was completed after about 72 h. In three experiments neither vertical nor horizontal eye movements could be seen under the 24 × binocular microscope. In one animal very small eye movements, smaller than 10% of the normal eye, remained visible in the recordings (for details see Behrens and Grüsser, 1989). The pupil diameter of the immobilized eye was about 30% larger than that of the right eye. The full BoTx effects lasted about 10 – 12 days and diminished slowly within the following three weeks. A general systemic spill-over was observed in one monkey which showed a mild general muscular weakness, but no signs of impairment in the extraocular muscles of the other eye. In another monkey a small amount of BoTx seemed to have reached the other orbita by diffusion through the nasal septum. This led to a mild palsy of the m. rectus medialis of the normal eye lasting about two weeks. It should be mentioned that the nasal part of the orbita in Squirrel monkeys is not completely closed by the bones of the skull. General effects other than those mentioned were not observed, in particular a disturbance in intestinal function, typical for botulism (Kerner 1820, 1822).

During the experiments the upper eyelid of the immobilized eye was held open by a small piece of tape and lubricated with artifical tears (60% Ringer solution, 40% water). During monocular stimulation the eye not stimulated was always covered by an eye patch applied carefully so as not to hinder eye movements. In general, the immobilization of the eyeball by BoTx provided a simple and efficient tool for research of open-loop oculomotor responses.

Optokinetic stimulation

The monkey was placed in a plastic monkey chair built by Mr. J. Lerch and surrounded by a vertically striped drum of 58 cm diameter and 60 cm height. The drum was moved inside of the Helmholtz coils and constructed exclusively of plastic and fibreglass. A thin piece of cardboard with precise, silk-screen-printed, vertical black and white stripes of equal widths (2.37 degree-periods) covered the inside of the cylinder (white-black luminance modulation about 0.7). In a few experiments stripes of 15 degree-periods were used. Continuous rotation of the drum at different speeds to the left or right at 0.5 – 400 deg/s was achieved by means of a servomotor with homogeneous illumination from a light source placed above the head of the monkey. The light reached this secondary source through an optical system and was projected through the tube-shaped axis around which the cylinder was rotated. The illumination could be turned on and off within less than 20 ms by an electromagnetic shutter. The average illumination of the striped cylinder was in the lower photopic range (about 15 lux).

Data analysis

Horizontal and vertical eye position, drum speed and drum illumination were continuously monitored and simultaneously stored after AD-conversion on the disk of a digital computer (HP1000) and later transferred to digital tape. By computer programs, the average speed of individual slow nystagmus periods was measured and printed out numerically or graphically. Algebraic means and standard error were usually computed from more than 10 successive slow OKN-periods. By means of digital differentiation the eye angular velocity could be continuously monitored (Figs. 4, 7 etc.). The computer programs applied are described in detail in Behrens, Grüsser and Weiss (1989).

Experiments in man

Two successful experiments were performed in human subjects; data from the one with the senior author (O.-J. G.) are reported. His left eye was immobilized by a retrobulbar injection of 5 ml 1.5% Scandicaine solution (with noradrenaline). The injection was kindly performed by Professor J. Wollensak from the Eye Clinic of the Freie Universität. A complete paresis of the extraocular muscles was obtained. The horizontal electrooculogram (EOG) was recorded from the immobile and the mobile eye before and after the injection of Scandicaine, and the angular velocity V_e of the OKN of the mobile eye was determined from the recordings on a paper oscilloscope ($0 – 100$ Hz frequency limits). The subject sat with the head fixed in the centre of an optokinetic drum with vertical black-white stripes of 1.15 degree-periods which was illuminated continuously and moved horizontally at different angular velocities V_s (Grüsser et al., 1981).

Results

Optokinetic nystagmus in normal Squirrel monkeys (N-animals)

Fig. 2 illustrates recording examples of Squirrel monkey horizontal OKN at different stimulus velocities. The high regularity of the OKN is evident. Fig. 3a – c show gain vs stimulus-velocity curves obtained in such experiments for monocular and binocular stimulation. The maximum speed of horizontal OKN slow phases varied between 160 and 180 deg/s and was significantly higher than in man. Differences between OKN evoked by monocular stimulation in the ipsilateral and nasal directions were marginal. As a rule, binocular stimulation led to a somewhat higher gain at stimulus angular velocities above 150 deg/s. As a consequence the -3 dB point in the gain re stimulus-velocity curves was reached with binocular stimulation at somewhat higher angular velocities than with monocular stimulation (Fig. 3a – c). When the monkey was sitting in total darkness and the light was suddenly turned on while the drum rotated at a constant angular velocity, a steady state of OKN was reached within 3 to 5 s. When stimulus velocity was above 40 deg/s, an early fast increase and later slow increase in slow-phase angular velocity characterized the responses (Fig. 4b), but this difference was not as pronounced as in the Rhesus monkey (Raphan et al., 1977). When the light illuminating the rotating drum was suddenly turned off, the OKN slow-phase angular velocity slowly decreased with an exponential time function and a time constant of about 8 – 12 s (optokinetic after-nystagmus, OKAN I). In a few experiments slight differences between the OKN-gain evoked by stimuli of the left and the right eye were present.

Retinal slip velocity in closed-loop OKN

The ongoing OKN is controlled predominantly by three mechanisms: (a) the retinal slip velocity V_r during the OKN slow phase, i.e. the difference between stimulus velocity V_s and eye velocity V_e; (b) the internally generated efference copy signals;

and (c) a slow storage mechanism responsible for OKAN I.

We tried to separate these components experimentally by computing V_r of closed-loop OKN. Retinal slip velocity V_r increased slowly with increasing stimulus angular velocity V_s up to about 120 deg/s. Above this value up to V_s of 400 deg/s the slope of V_r/V_s was near 1 (Fig. 5a). From this data one could plot the dependence of eye angular velocity V_e on retinal slip velocity V_r (Fig. 5b): V_e increased with V_r, reached a maximum at V_r values of about 30 to 40 deg/s and decreased slowly thereafter with a further increase in V_r.

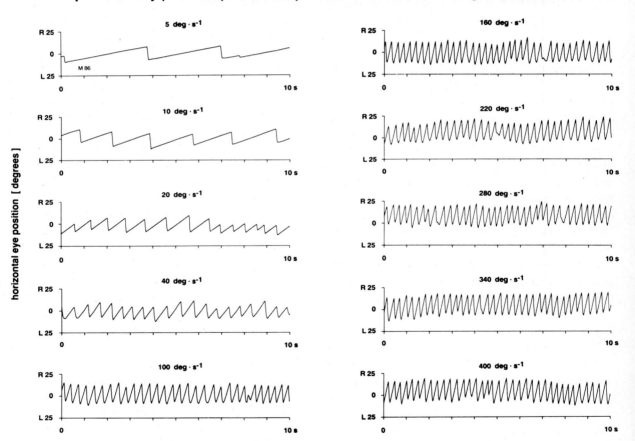

Squirrel monkey (N-animal) binocular optokinetic stimulation, 2.37 deg. stripe pattern period

Fig. 2. Selected examples of horizontal optokinetic nystagmus recorded in a normal Squirrel monkey from the right eye during binocular stimulation. Stimulus angular velocities as indicated: 5, 10, 20, 40, 100, 160, 220, 280, 320 and 400 deg/s.

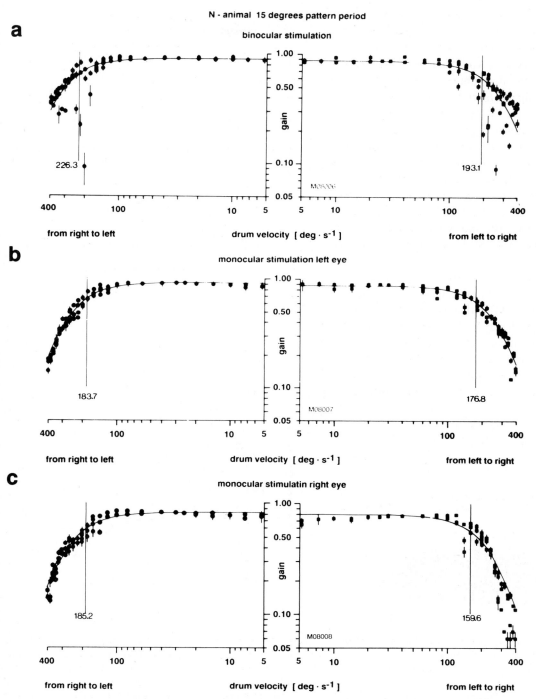

Fig. 3. Gain (ordinate) re stimulus velocity curves of the OKN in a normal monkey. Gain defined as V_e/V_s. The individual data are average values obtained from at least 10 successive slow phases of the OKN. The drawn curves are Bessel filter functions of the third order fitted to the experimental data. For the Bessel filter the following function was used:

$$\text{Gain}_B = \text{Gain}_{Bo} (1 + K_2 V_n^2 + K_4 V_n^4 + K_6 V_n^6)^{-1/2}$$

$$V_n = V_s/V_{s\,(-3\,\text{dB})}; \quad K_2 = 0.618; \quad K_4 = 0.252; \quad K_6 = 0.130$$

Retinal stimulus velocity and open-loop OKN

Stimulating the immobilized eye and recording horizontal OKN from the other eye, which was covered by a dark eye patch, the relationship between the OKN slow-phase angular velocity V_e and retinal slip velocity V_r could be measured directly. With the sudden onset of constant-speed stimuli, this relationship depended on the duration of the stimulus (Fig. 4): When the optokinetic drum, rotating for example at 10 deg/s, was suddenly illuminated, the OKN-gain reached a time constant of about 15 – 18 s per plateau, which was maintained during the stimulation, provided the attentive state of the animal remained constant. When, however, the animal became drowsy during OKN, V_e decreased again, despite constant V_s, and finally OKN was replaced by pendular eye movements. Since the animal could not close the "taped" eyelids (cf. Methods), this change in OKN during lowered levels of wakefulness was clearly caused by a change in the central neuronal state. In the gain-plots only data from OKN during maintained states of wakefulness were used. When the light was turned off after 60 s stimulation, the time

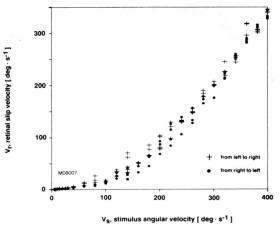

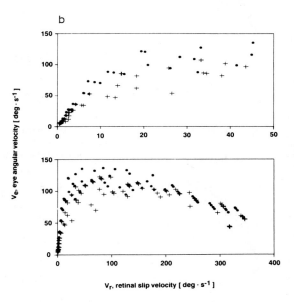

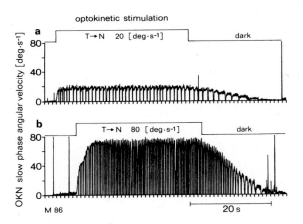

Fig. 4. OKN slow-phase angular velocity (ordinate) of horizontal OKN in normal Squirrel monkey evoked by monocular stimulation of the left eye. Data obtained by digital differentiation of eye position signals. Stimulus angular velocities V_s were in (a) 20 deg/s and in (b) 80 deg/s; 2.37 degree-period stripe pattern. Note the different time course of increase in OKN speed and in decrease, after the light illuminating the rotating drum turned off (OKAN I) (from Behrens and Grüsser, 1988).

Fig. 5. Data from normal Squirrel monkey horizontal OKN. a: horizontal monocular optokinetic stimulation of the left eye. The retinal slip velocity V_r (ordinate) was computed from the difference between stimulus angular velocity V_s (abscissa) and horizontal OKN slow phase velocity V_e and is plotted as a function of V_s. b: relationship between V_r (abscissa) and V_e (ordinate). In the upper part of the graph a different scale is applied for V_r than in the lower graph.

constant of the V_e decrease during OKAN I was always shorter (5 – 7 s) than the time constant of its increase when the stimulus was turned on. From the dependence of OKN-gain on duration of open-loop stimulation, it was clear that when one plots the open-loop OKN-gain as a function of stimulus angular velocity, one has to regard the time after

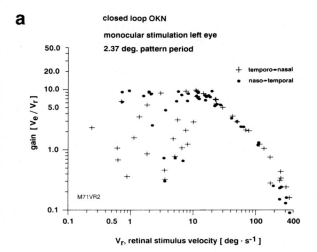

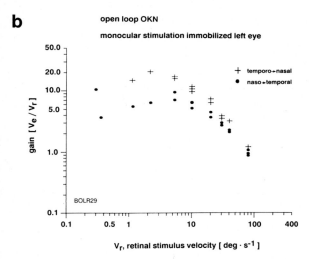

Fig. 6. Monocular horizontal internal gain G_i under closed-loop (a) and open-loop (b) stimulus conditions plotted as a function of retinal slip velocity V_r (abscissa). Note that in these graphs gain is defined as the quotient V_e/V_r. The V_e values were measured after the slow-phase angular velocity curves had reached a plateau, i.e., about 45 s after onset of stimulation; 2.37 degree-period stripe pattern.

the onset of optokinetic stimulation as a parameter. Otherwise a fairly large variability in the data will result (Körner, 1972; Körner and Schiller, 1972). The time-dependent increase in V_e during open-loop OKN showed no uniform time constant for different stimulus conditions. The time constant was considerably longer with retinal slip velocities below 2 deg/s than with higher V_r values. In order to obtain meaningful data, it was necessary therefore to measure open-loop gain either for constant plateau values maintained during the last third of the 60-s-stimulation period or to take the gain after a defined time of optokinetic stimulation, e.g., 10 s after stimulus onset.

Examples of the relationship of OKN-gain (V_e/V_r) to retinal stimulus angular velocity V_r obtained under closed-loop stimulus conditions are shown in Fig. 6a. Comparing open-loop gain to closed-loop OKN-gain, the efficacy of retinal pattern movement reached a maximum under both conditions at rather low V_r values, namely 2 – 3 deg/s for open-loop conditions and 4 – 8 deg/s for closed-loop conditions, but the maximum open-loop gain was about 5-times higher than the closed-loop gain. In general, above V_r values of 10 deg/s, the attenuation of OKN-gain with increasing V_r was very similar for closed-loop and open-loop OKN and the attenuation was in both cases about 20 dB per decade (Figs. 6a, b).

Different contributions of the nasal and temporal visual hemifields

Open-loop optokinetic stimulation provided a relatively simple tool for measuring the efficacy of optokinetic stimulation for the nasal and temporal visual hemifields separately as well as for testing whether the effectiveness of naso-temporal and temporo-nasal movement in the visual field differed. Fig. 7a, b illustrates data from such an experiment. In general, stimulation of the temporal visual hemifield led to a somewhat higher OKN-gain than stimulation of the nasal visual hemifield. Furthermore, in the nasal visual hemifield naso-temporal stimulus movement was more effective than temporo-nasal movement. The time course of

a

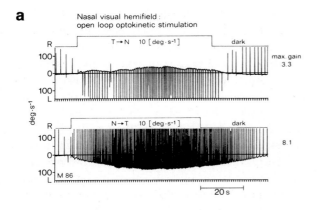

b

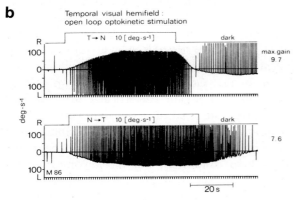

Fig. 7. Time course of open-loop, horizontal, OKN, slow-phase, angular velocity V_e. Stimulation of the nasal (a) or the temporal (b) visual hemifield of the immobilized left eye. OKN was recorded from the mobile right eye, covered by a dark eye patch. Stimulus angular velocities ($V_s = V_r$) were 10 deg/s for all recordings. Note the strong directional difference in OKN-gain for temporo-nasal and naso-temporal stimulation in the nasal visual hemifield (a), but not in the temporal field (b). 2.37 degree vertical stripe pattern (from Behrens and Grüsser, 1988).

Binocular summation of open-loop and closed-loop optokinetic effects

As seen from Fig. 3, the gain of closed-loop OKN below 120 deg/s was near 1. With open-loop stimulation, however, gain was above 1 when stimulus velocity was below 80 deg/s. In a few experiments we tested what type of OKN is obtained when both eyes are stimulated simultaneously. If the overall OKN-gain was above 1 under such stimulus conditions, the optokinetic input to the moving eye would constitute a stimulus which should drive the eyes in the opposite direction to that of the moving stripe pattern, since the mobile eye is faster than the stimulus. Simultaneously, the open-loop stimulation of the immobile eye should drive the eye in the direction of the moving stimulus pattern. When both inputs are summed within the neuronal gaze control system, the OKN-gain with binocular stimulation is expected to be below the values obtained with monocular stimulation of the immobile eye. As Fig. 8 illustrates for selected examples, this was indeed the case and dependent on stimulus angular velocity V_s. Thus binocular stimulation with different angular velocities provides a tool of indirect "titration" of the efficacy of the two separate "channels" from the left and the right eye driving OKN.

The time course of BoTx eyeball immobilization

The palsy of the extraocular eye muscles caused

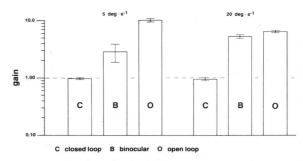

Fig. 8. Average gain of horizontal OKN at two different stimulus angular velocities (5 and 20 deg/s) for closed-loop monocular stimulation (c), open-loop monocular stimulation (o) and binocular (b) stimulation of the mobile and immobile eye.

the slow increase in OKN-gain after sudden onset of the optokinetic stimulus was about the same for both hemifields and directions. The decrease in V_e during OKAN I, however, was dependent in both hemifields on the stimulus direction and was shorter for temporo-nasal optokinetic stimulation than for naso-temporal (Behrens and Grüsser, 1988).

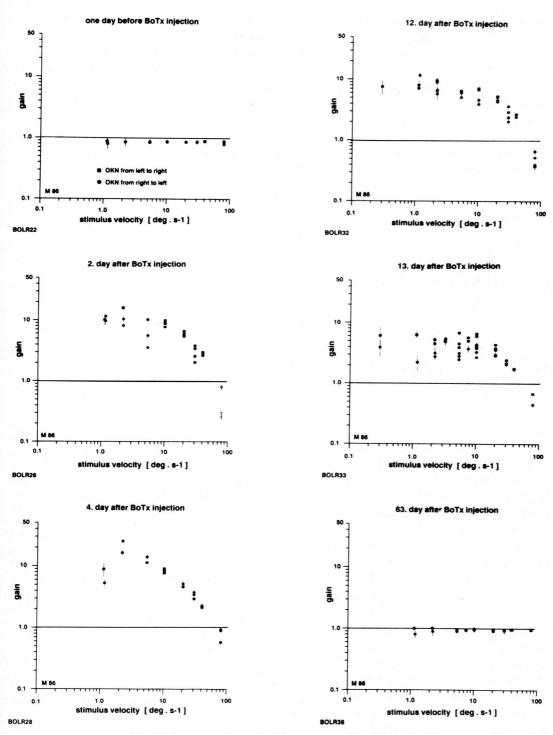

Fig. 9. OKN open-loop gain V_e/V_r as a function of time elapsed since injection of 11 units of BoTx, type A. Six selected time delays since BoTx was injected.

by the blockage in the synaptic transmission at the motor endplates by BoTx was mirrored by the changes in OKN open-loop gain. The latter was maximal when the eyeball was totally immobilized. This state was reached after about 48 to 72 h and maintained for 10 to 15 days. Thereafter mobility of the BoTx-treated eye slowly returned and consequently the "open-loop"-gain decreased with time. About 6 weeks after the BoTx immobilization normal eye-movement conditions were again attained. Measurement 63 days after BoTx injection yielded normal data not significantly different from pre-injection responses (Fig. 9).

Optokinetic stimulation of an immobilized eye in man

As described in the Methods, monocular immobilization in two human voluntary subjects was obtained by a retrobulbar injection of a local anaesthetic. For technical reasons useable OKN recordings by means of DC-electrooculography were obtained in only one subject. Within a few minutes the eye of the subject was totally immobilized, the pupil dilated and accommodation interrupted. When the subject observed the world with free head movements monocularly through the immobilized eye, every intended saccade, which could not be performed due to the palsy, led to an apparent shift in the visual world in the direction of the purposed eye movement (cf. Graefe, 1854; Kornmüller, 1931). Furthermore, head movements also evoked an apparent shift in the visual world, but in the opposite direction to the head movement. The EOG-recordings of the mobile eye also indicated significantly different states of OKN, depending on the pursuit strategies applied vis-a-vis the optokinetic stripe pattern. When the subject tried to pursue the moving pattern as long as possible, eye velocity increased during a single OKN slow phase according to a parabolic time function (Fig. 10). V_e was reset by each backward saccade and the angular velocity during the slow phase of OKN again started at low values. The course of the individual OKN-periods was fairly repetitive, provided the same pursuit

strategy was applied. However when the subject tried to pursue every stripe moving across the centre of his visual field, small-amplitude OKN was evoked and OKN-gain under such conditions did not exceed $2-3$ (Fig. 10).

Depending on the self-instruction of the subject,

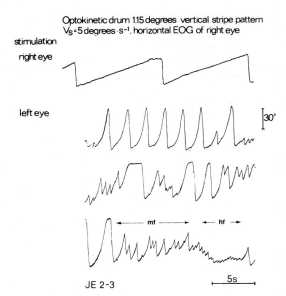

Fig. 10. Horizontal OKN in man. Monocular stimulation trace of the mobile right eye is shown at top at 5 deg/s by a 1.15 degree stripe pattern moving towards the right; attentive gaze nystagmus. Left eye stimulation: the open-loop horizontal OKN is depicted at different states of self-instruction of the subject (O.-J. G.). Upper row: high-attention-pursuit OKN. Middle row: medium attention. Lower row: attentive pursuit OKN fixating every 5 th to 10 th stripe (mf) or as many moving stripes as possible (hf). The time-course of the slow phase in the open-loop optokinetic gaze nystagmus demonstrates that eye angular velocity accelerated in time when attentive prolonged pursuit of the optokinetic striped pattern was intended. The backward saccades led to a reset of eye angular velocity recorded from the covered mobile right eye. This reset was correlated with the reduction in the perceived speed of the continuously moving stripe pattern. When the subject, however, intended to pursue every single stripe of the moving vertical stripe pattern (hf), slow-phase OKN speed did not exceed gain $2-3$. When the subject only stared at the moving stripe pattern without any special intention (but highly attentive to his own percepts), the increase in open-loop gain was also at a medium level and rather variable. Eye immobilization by a retrobulbar injection of 5 ml 1.5% Scandicaine (from unpublished data of Grüsser, Kulikowski, Pause and Wollensak, 1981).

all intermediate responses between these two types of open-loop OKN could be obtained (Fig. 10). When he just stared at the moving stripe pattern, a steady-state OKN-gain was reached within $1-2$ s, i.e. much faster than in the monkeys, the nystagmus frequency increased and V_e was considerably smaller than in the case of the attentive pursuit mode. The OKN-gain was still higher than 1 (Fig. 10). V_e dropped to values near 1 when the subject fixated every stripe moving across the visual field as carefully as possible. It is evident from the EOG-recordings shown in Fig. 10 that the increase in V_e above gain 1 was "reset" by each backward saccade. In contrast to the findings in monkeys, V_e was not constant during the slow nystagmus phases when the latter lasted longer than $0.8-1.2$ s. We think that these differences between man and monkey are due to two components: firstly, the human subject was highly attentive to the perceptual phenomena, which he had to report during or immediately after the individual tests, and secondly, the brainstem "velocity storage mechanisms" responsible for horizontal OKN (Raphan et al., 1977) differ in man and monkey.

Acknowledgements

This work was supported in part by a grant of the Deutsche Forschungsgemeinschaft (Gr 161). We thank Mr. J. Lerch for his active role in the skilful construction of part of the experimental equipment, Dipl.-Ing. L.-R. Weiss for his help in computer programming, Mrs. Ch. Dreykluft for technical assistance and Mrs. J. Dames for her help in the English translation of the manuscript. We are indebted to Prof. J. Wollensak, Universitätsaugenklinik Berlin-Charlottenburg, for his cooperation in the experiment with human subjects. The senior author (O.-J.G.) was supported by an Akademie-Stipendium from the Stiftung Volkswagen-Werk.

References

Baker, R. and Berthoz, A. (1975) Is the prepositus hypoglossi nucleus the source of another vestibular ocular pathway? *Brain Res.*, 86: 121–127.

Behrens, F. and Grüsser, O.-J. (1988) The effect of monocular pattern deprivation and open-loop stimulation on optokinetic nystagmus in squirrel monkeys (Saimiri sciureus). In H. Flohr (Ed.), *Post-Lesion Plasticity,* Springer, Berlin, pp. 453–472.

Behrens, F., and Grüsser, O.-J. (1989) Open-loop optokinetic nystagmus in squirrel monkeys (in preparation).

Behrens, F., Grüsser, O.-J. and Weiss, L.-R. (1989) The optokinetic nystagmus of squirrel monkeys (in preparation).

Berthoz, A. (1986) Discussion. In H.-J. Freund, U. Büttner, B. Cohen and J. Noth (Eds.), *Progress in Brain Research, Vol 64,* Elsevier, Amsterdam, pp. 405–408.

Boyle, R., Büttner, U. and Markert, G. (1985) Vestibular nuclei activity and eye movements in the alert monkey during sinusoidal optokinetic stimulation. *Exp. Brain Res.,* 57: 362–369.

Collewijn, H. (1976) Direction-selective units in the rabbit's nucleus of the optic tract. *Brain Res.,* 100: 489–508.

Collewijn, H. (1981) The oculomotor system of the rabbit and its plasticity. In Braitenberg et al. (Eds.), *Studies in Brain Function,* Springer, Berlin Heidelberg New York. pp.

Collewijn, H, Curio, G., Grüsser, O.-J. (1982) Spatially selective visual attention and generation of eye pursuit movements. *Hum. Neurobiol.,* 1: 129–139.

Graefe, A. von (1854) Beiträge zur Physiologie und Pathologie der schiefen Augenmuskeln. *Arch. f. Ophthalm.,* I (1.) 1–81.

Grasse, K.L. and Cynader, M.S. (1984) Electrophysiology of lateral and dorsal terminal nuclei of the cat accessory optic system. *J. Neurophysiol.,* 51: 276–293.

Grüsser, O.-J., Kulikowski, J., Pause, M., and Wollensak, J. (1981) Optokinetic nystagmus, Sigmaoptokinetic nystagmus and eye pursuit movements elicited by stimulation of an immobilized human eye. *J. Physiol. (London),* 320: 21–22.

Hoffman, K.-P. (1979) Optokinetic nystagmus and single-cell responses in the nucleus tractus opticus after early monocular deprivation in the cat. In R.D. Freemann (Ed.), *Developmental Neurobiology of Vision.* Plenum Press, New York, pp. 63–72.

Hoffmann, K.-P. (1982) Cortical versus subcortical contributions to the optokinetic reflex in the cat. In G. Lennerstrand (Ed.), *Functional Basis of Ocular Motility Disorders,* Pergamon Press, Oxford, pp. 303–310.

Hoffmann, K.-P. (1986) Visual inputs relevant for the optokinetic nystagmus in mammals. In H.J. Freund, U. Büttner, B. Cohen and J. Noth (Eds.), *Progress in Brain Research Vol. 64*, Elsevier, Amsterdam, pp. 75 – 84.

Hoffmann, K.-P. (1987) The influence of visual experience on the ontogony of the optokinetic reflex in mammals. In J. Rauschecker and P. Marler (Eds.), *Imprinting and Cortical Plasticity*, John Wiley, New York, pp. 267 – 286.

Hoffmann, K.-P. (1988) Neural basis for changes of the optokinetic reflex in animals and man with strabismus and amblyopia. In O. Lennerstrand (Ed.), *Strabismus and Amblyopia — Experimental Basis for Advances in Clinical Management*, MacMillan, London, pp. 89 – 98.

Hoffmann, K.-P. and Distler, D.S. (1986) The role of direction selective cells in the nucleus of the optic tract of cat and monkey during optokinetic nystagmus. In E.L. Keller and D.S. Zee (Eds.), *Adaptive Processes in Visual and Oculomotor System,* Pergamon Press, Oxford, pp. 261 – 266.

Hoffmann, K.-P. and Schoppmann, A. (1975) Retinal input to direction selective cells in the nucleus tractus opticus of the cat. *Brain Res.,* 99: 359 – 366.

Hutchins, B. and Weber, J.T. (1985) The pretectal complex of the monkey: a reinvestigation of the morphology and retinal terminations. *J. Comp. Neurol.,* 232: 425 – 442.

Kato, I., Harada, K., Hasegawa, T., Igarashi, T., Koike, Y. and Kawasaki, T. (1986) Role of the nucleus of the optic tract in monkeys in relation to optokinetic nystagmus. *Brain Res.,* 364: 12 – 22.

Keller, E.L. and Crandall, W.F. (1983) Neuronal responses to optokinetic stimuli in pontine nuclei of behaving monkey. *J. Neurophysiol.,* 49: 169 – 187.

Kerner, J. (1820) *Neue Beobachtungen über die in Würtemberg so häufig vorfallenden tödlichen Vergiftungen durch den Genuss geräucherter Würste.* Osiander, Tübingen, 120 pp.

Kerner, J. (1822) *Das Fettgift oder die Fettsäure und ihre Wirkungen auf den thierischen Organismus, ein Beytrag zur Untersuchung des in verdorbenen Würsten giftig wirkenden Stoffes.* Cotta, Stuttgart und Tübingen, 368 pp.

Körner, F. (1972) Optokinetic stimulation of an immobilized eye. *Bibl. Ophthal.,* 82: 298 – 307.

Körner, F. and Schiller, P.H. (1972) The optokinetic response under open and closed loop conditions in the monkey. *Exp.*

Brain Res., 14: 318 – 330.

Kornmüller, A.W. (1931) Eine experimentelle Anästhesie der äußeren Augenmuskeln am Menschen und ihre Auswirkungen. *J. Psychol. Neurol (Lpz.),* 41: 354 – 366.

Ohm, J. (1921) Über Registrierung des optischen Drehnystagmus. *Münch. med. Wochschr.,* 45: 1451 – 1452.

Ohm, J. (1926) Ist der optische Drehnystagmus von einem unbeweglichen Auge auslösbar? *Klin. Monatsbl. Augenhlk.,* 77: 330 – 336.

Ohm, J. (1927) Zur Augenzitterkunde. 7. Mitteilung der optische drehnystagmus. *Graefes Arch. Ophthalm.,* 118: 103 – 117.

Ohm, J. (1934) Zur Augenzitternkunde. 34. Mitteilung. Die Auslösung des optokinetischen Nystagmus mittels des Konzentrisches Drehzylinders beim Gesunde. *Graefes Arch. Ophthal.,* 131: 401 – 409.

Ohm, J. (1943) *Die Mikroneurologie des Auges und seiner Bewegung.* Enke, Stuttgart, 308 pp.

Raphan, T., Cohen, B. and Matsuo, V. (1977) A velocity-storage mechanism responsible for optokinetic nystagmus (OKN), optokinetic afternystagmus (OKAN) and vestibular nystagmus. In R. Baker and A. Berthoz (Eds.), *Control of Gaze by Brainstem Neurons, Development. Neurosci. Vol. I,* Elsevier, Amsterdam, pp. 37 – 47.

Robinson, D.A. (1963) A method of measuring eye movement using a scleral search coil in a magnetic field. *IEEE Trans. Biomed. Electron.,* 10: 137 – 145.

Simpson, J.I. (1984) The accessory optic system. *Ann. Rev. Neurosci,* 7: 13 – 41.

Ter Braak, J.W.G. (1936) Untersuchungen über den optokinetischen Nystagmus. *Arch. Neerl. Physiol.,* 21: 309 – 376. (Translated "Investigations on optokinetic nystagmus". In H. Collewijn (1981) *The Oculomotor System of the Rabbit and its Plasticity. Studies in Brain Function, Vol 5,* Springer, Berlin, Heidelberg, New York).

Waespe, W. and Henn, V. (1987) Gaze stabilization in the primate. The interaction of the vestibuloocular reflex, optokinetic nystagmus, and smooth pursuit. *Rev. Physiol. Biochem. Pharmacol.,* 106: 37 – 125.

Weber, J.T. (1985) Pretectal complex and accessory optic system of primates. *Brain Behav. Evol.,* 26: 117 – 140.

J.H.J. Allum and M. Hulliger (Eds.)
Progress in Brain Research, Vol. 80
© 1989 Elsevier Science Publishers B.V. (Biomedical Division)

CHAPTER 17

The vestibulo-ocular reflex: an outdated concept?

H. Collewijn

Department of Physiology I, Faculty of Medicine, Erasmus University Rotterdam, P.O. Box 1738, NL 3000 DR Rotterdam, The Netherlands

Traditionally, the vestibulo-ocular reflex (VOR) is described as a distinct, phylogenetically old oculomotor subsystem, which serves to stabilize gaze direction. It is supposed to act as a stereotyped reflex with definite input – output relations, which can be measured by rotating a subject passively in darkness, and which are kept at an ideal level by adaptive, parametric adjustments. This paper argues that such a view is not realistic: (1) the VOR in darkness does not have an ideal, or even well defined, gain; (2) a fixed, automatic VOR is not appropriate in most behavioural situations, and would need continuous conditioning by other subsystems. As there is no compelling phylogene-

tic, physiological or anatomical evidence for an independent VOR subsystem, a more fruitful hypothesis may be that vestibular signals are just one of many inputs to a spatial localization process, which computes the relative position (and motion) between the subject and a target of his choice. The VOR in darkness may represent no more than a default operation, based on incomplete information, of this larger, multiple input gaze control system. Likewise, adaptation phenomena of the VOR in darkness may be merely an epiphenomenon of adaptation of gaze control with vision active.

Key words: Vestibulo-ocular reflex; Eye movement; Head movement; Vestibular nucleus; Ocular control model; Optokinetic reflex

Introduction

The vestibulo-ocular reflex (VOR), and specifically the canal-ocular reflex, which is addressed in this paper, has a special status in current concepts of the structure of the oculomotor control system. It is usually considered as the most primitive and phylogenetically oldest subsystem, upon which other oculomotor subsystems have been built. This view is succinctly expressed in Fig. 1, after Robinson (1987). The special function of the VOR is assumed to be the stabilization of gaze during head rotation. Such stabilization appears to be necessary for maintaining good visual acuity. In man, visual acuity is degraded when retinal image velocities exceed 2.5 deg/s (Westheimer and McKee, 1975; Murphy, 1978), while naturally occurring head velocities reach several hundreds of

deg/s. To be effective, such a stabilizing system should be fast and accurate. The VOR is thought to have these properties. Due to its simple connections it has a very short latency, and it would basically act as an automatic system, not requiring any elaborate data processing or decision making. Furthermore, its accuracy would be maintained over a life-time by adaptive recalibration, achieved through parametric adjustments made on the basis of long-term retinal image slip or some related parameter. Adaptive changes in the VOR have become extremely popular in recent years as a model of motor learning (see e.g. Berthoz and Melvill Jones, 1985; Lisberger, 1988).

Attractive as this concept of the VOR as a fast, automatic, well-calibrated and independent subsystem may seem, it deserves some scrutiny, along with the theoretical framework of the structure of

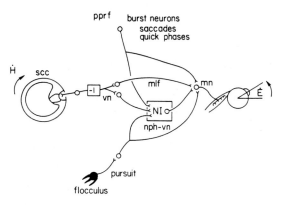

Fig. 1. Functional organization of the vestibulo-ocular reflex and the final common integrator, after Robinson (1987). The semicircular canals (scc) transduce head velocity, $\dot{H}$, into the discharge rates of primary vestibular afferents going to the vestibular nucleus (vn). This signal is sent directly to the motoneurones via the medial longitudinal fasciculus (mlf). To produce the appropriate compensatory eye velocity, $\dot{E}$, the motoneurones must also receive an eye position signal from the neural integrator (NI), located in the nucleus prepositus hypoglossi (nph) and the vn. The saccadic eye velocity command originates from burst neurones in the paramedian pontine reticular formation (pprf). The pursuit command originates in part of the flocculus. All three systems share the integrator.

the oculomotor control system as a whole. The specific purpose of this paper is to examine the origins and foundations of the VOR as a subsystem, and to see whether its special status as a cornerstone in the structure of oculomotor control is fruitful, justifiable, or even tenable. A more general purpose is to question the traditional approach to the oculomotor system as an assembly of, more or less independently functioning, subsystems. For an earlier critical evaluation of the systems approach to oculomotor function, see the inspiring article by Steinman (1986).

Historical roots of the VOR

The history of the VOR starts about a century ago, when serious studies began of the physics of the labyrinth, as well as the psychophysical and (oculo)motor responses of animals and people to rotation (for reviews see Cohen, 1971, 1974). In

the absence of suitable recording techniques, strong rotatory accelerations were usually applied to obtain responses that could be visually observed. The responses appeared to be stereotyped and involuntary. Moreover, the Sherringtonian "reflex" concept was considered a powerful explanatory principle at that time. Thus, the identification of a vestibulo-ocular "reflex" followed naturally.

The compensatory nature of vestibulo-ocular reactions was perceived early. Quantitative verification of the adequacy of the compensation was impossible until the work of Dodge, a pioneer in developing objective recording techniques as well as of profound ideas with respect to eye movements. In a landmark paper Dodge (1903) described compensatory eye movements, generated by an actively moving and viewing subject, as one of the basic types of eye movements, maintaining fixation of a stationary object. However, Dodge considered such eye movements as the result of central coordination, and not as controlled by a peripheral stimulus as such. He considered the eye movements elicited by passive rotation in darkness as another type, different in nature from compensatory eye movements in a normally viewing and moving subject. Further types of eye movements described by Dodge (1903) were (in modern terms) saccades, smooth pursuit and vergence. In a later paper, Dodge (1923) concluded: "All of our records agree that the vestibule is not a quantitatively exact regulator of action. It reflexly initiates with very low reaction latency a useful compensation of the eyes which is occasionally entirely adequate but whose adequacy depends on the subsequent control of vision". Thus, Dodge recognized clearly the advantages, as well as the limitations, of vestibular gaze control.

In the years after Dodge the VOR assumed a kind of independence as a research topic. For a number of years it attracted in particular biophysically oriented researchers, who emphasized the mechanical properties of the motions of the cupula (e.g. Steinhausen, 1933). Eye movements such as postrotatory nystagmus were largely treated as a convenient parameter for measuring cupular time constants (Van Egmond et al., 1949), and central nervous operations were, by and large, ignored.

One important conclusion from mechanical analyses was that canal signals basically represent the integral of head acceleration, i.e. head velocity, at least over a middle frequency range, but that for head rotations at low frequencies, or for constant velocities, the canals provide incorrect or no information (for review see e.g. Wilson and Melvill Jones, 1979). This made it clear, once again, that by itself the VOR could not maintain gaze stability over the full range of natural head movements. Ter Braak (1936) was probably the first to recognize that, at least in the rabbit, the deficient dynamics of the VOR at low frequencies were ideally complemented by the properties of optokinetic nystagmus (OKN). OKN in the rabbit is built up slowly, but shows a sustained response to steady stimulus velocities and to motion at low frequencies. As a result a rabbit, rotated in steady visual surroundings, shows adequate stabilization of gaze in the sense that compensatory eye movements start quickly and show no inappropriate after-phenomena.

The modular concept of oculomotor control

With the advent of the systems-analytical approach (e.g. Robinson 1975, 1977, 1981, 1986, 1987), such ideas as expressed by Ter Braak (1936) were more formally modelled. Fig. 2 shows the idea of a synthesis between optokinetic and vestibulo-ocular responses as first proposed by Robinson (1977). Essential elements of the model are the exact complementarity of OKN and VOR velocity responses as a function of time after stimulation with a velocity step, and the presence of a positive feedback loop carrying an efference-copy of eye-in-head position. This efference-copy signal is summed with a retinal image-slip signal, which represents the eye movement relative to space. The sum represents the visual equivalent of head rotation in space, which is directly compati-

ble with the vestibular signal. In addition, the positive feedback loop could account theoretically for the phenomenon of velocity storage, common to OKN and VOR (Robinson, 1977). The synthesis of vestibular and visual signals in the vestibular nuclei is well supported by neurophysiological evidence (e.g. Waespe and Henn, 1979).

A further essential element in the model is the neural integrator, which serves to transform the vestibular (and visual) velocity-coded signals into a position-coded signal. The concept of this integrator is central to all current models of oculomotor control. It would function not only in the VOR, but also in smooth pursuit and the generation of saccades (Skavenski and Robinson, 1973; Robinson, 1975, 1987).

The problem with this kind of explanation is not in the synthetic view, but in the preceding dissection of the oculomotor system into a number of subsystems. A basic assumption in current systems-descriptions of the oculomotor system is, that it can be broken down functionally into a few

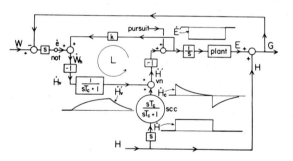

Fig. 2. Robinson's (1977) model of the optokinetic and vestibulo-ocular subsystems. Head velocity $\dot{H}$ is tranduced by the semicircular canals, scc, into $\dot{H}_c$, the canals' best estimate of head velocity which is correct only transiently. This signal is integrated in the integrator (1/s) and then reaches the motoneurones to create eye position in the head, E. Eye position in space, gaze G, is the sum of E and head position H. The visual system extracts the relative motion $\dot{e}$ of gaze relative to the world W. This signal is found in the nucleus of the optic tract, not. An efference copy of eye velocity $\dot{E}'$ is added to $\dot{e}$ to reconstruct $\dot{H}_v$, the visual system's estimate of head velocity in space. The high frequencies are filtered out and the low frequency version $\dot{H}'_v$ is added to $\dot{H}_c$ in the vestibular nucleus vn, to obtain the brain stem's best estimate $\dot{H}'$ of the velocity of self-rotation.

subsystems, each of which serves a specific purpose (e.g. Robinson, 1981). I shall call this the ''modular'' approach to oculomotor control. How does one identify the basic modules? The modern systems-approach has not attempted to make an analysis of the structure of oculomotor control, without starting from preconceived notions. Instead, systems-analysts have taken the traditional classifications of eye movement types (e.g. Dodge, 1903) and reflexes more or less for granted. In this process, particular stimulus – response relations, obtained under certain laboratory conditions, have more or less silently obtained the status of subsystems with a certain amount of autonomy. Actually, the conventional distinction of vestibulo-ocular, optokinetic, smooth-pursuit, saccadic, vergence (and maybe fixation) subsystems is based on a vague mixture of historical, teleological, phylogenetic and neurobiological arguments.

Take for instance the VOR and OKN. They are based on the assumption that passive rotation in darkness isolates a vestibulo-ocular subsystem, while rotation of the whole visual surroundings around a stationary subject isolates an optokinetic system. The problem is that in the first situation the response is functionally meaningless, because there is nothing to be seen, while the type of stimulus used in the second situation never occurs naturally. Why would nature have bothered to develop such unlikely subsystems independently, only to synthesize them later?

Phylogenetic considerations

The origin of the tendency to consider the VOR as the phylogenetically oldest, primaeval oculomotor control system goes back, at least, to Walls (1962), who propagated this view rather emphatically. Some of his arguments were the organization of the eye muscles in a similar coordinate system as the canals, and the short anatomical connections between canals and muscles. Walls described the function of the archaic VOR as a crude field-holding reflex, and assumed that it was supplemented and refined early in fish evolution by an

optokinetic system. These evolutionary arguments are, however, not terribly convincing. Eyes undoubtedly conveyed visual information from the beginning, and OKN has been found in all animals (vertebrate or invertebrate) with mobile eyes; optomotor orienting responses (of the body) are well developed even in insects, in which the eyes are immobile in the head. In the accessory optic system, inferior olive and flocculus of the rabbit, ''optokinetic'' visual motion information is coded in similar coordinates as the canals and eye muscles (Simpson and Graf, 1985). Thus, there is no compelling reason for supposing that vestibulo-ocular responses are any older than optokinetic responses.

The exclusive role of vestibular signals in the stabilization of gaze in fish is relativized even further by a judicious look at the limited literature on compensatory eye movements in primitive vertebrates. The physiological control of such movements is studied most appropriately in relation to natural movement, i.e. swimming. In this behaviour the axis of head rotation is usually eccentric to the head, on the side towards which the fish is turning. During swimming, compensatory eye movements in the dogfish (Harris, 1965) and goldfish (Easter et al., 1974) tend to have a gain smaller than unity; due to the geometrical relations, this results in retinal stabilization of objects that are fairly close to the fish. The point of interest is, that these compensatory eye movements are controlled by no means exclusively or even predominantly by the labyrinths. After bilateral destruction of the horizontal canals, the gain of compensatory eye movements in goldfish was diminished from the normal value of about 0.95 only to about 0.80 (Easter and Johns, 1974). Blinding alone diminished the gain to about 0.50. Combined blinding and canal-lesioning left the gain still at about 0.41 during active swimming, although the combined lesions did completely abolish compensatory eye movements in response to passive rotation of the fish. Obviously, active compensatory eye movements were controlled to a large part by non-visual, non-vestibular signals, the nature of which could not be identified by Easter and Johns (1974). Graf and Meyer (1978) described oculomotor responses associated with tail bending in fishes. The eye movements were larger when the tail was bent actively by the fish than when it was bent passively by the experimenter. Thus, central commands might be involved, in addition to somato-sensory inputs. Recent work by Stehouwer (1987) on isolated nervous systems of tadpoles, which show activity patterns corresponding to "fictive swimming", strongly suggests that a good part of the compensatory oculomotor activity during active swimming is internally generated by the brain, independent of any sensory inflow. In the dogfish, "swimming eye movements" depend on signals of spinal origin (Harris, 1965) and it seems likely that proprioceptive signals play a role.

Observations such as these strongly suggest that the idea, that the hard core of oculomotor control in primitive vertebrates is formed by a vestibulo-ocular subsystem, is incorrect. A more appropriate model seems to be that compensatory eye movements are generated by a multi-input system, in which vestibular, visual, proprioceptive, corollary motor and probably also other behaviourally relevant signals are used in various combinations.

Neuroanatomical and neurophysiological identity of the VOR

A major factor promoting the concept of the VOR as a distinct subsystem has been the identification of the three-neurone arc, i.e. the connection between primary vestibular afferents and oculomotor neurones through a single interneurone in the vestibular nuclei. The physiological reality of these short-latency connections, which had been correctly inferred by Cajal, Lorente de Nó and Szentagothai, was finally proven by intracellular recording and tracing techniques (for recent reports see Goldberg et al., 1987; Highstein et al., 1987; McCrea et al., 1987a,b). The interneurones, described as position-vestibular-pause (PVP) cells, carry signals related to head velocity, eye velocity

and eye position, and pause during all types of saccades. It is clear that such disynaptic connections form the shortest possible vestibulo-ocular route. They are probably responsible for the vestibulo-ocular responses with the shortest latency (about 14 ms according to Lisberger, 1984). However, by themselves these disynaptic connections can account for no more than a quick start of the eye in the correct direction. As the signals carried by PVP neurones are not simple copies of the signals on the canal afferents, signal processing in secondary circuits must have a major impact on PVP neurones. Moreover, the PVP cells carry too little position information to account for the behaviour of ocular motoneurones (Tomlinson and Robinson, 1984). Thus, motoneurones must receive other inputs as well to generate compensatory eye movements. One obvious source is the nucleus prepositus hypoglossi.

Without going into further details, it should be clear that the network, supporting vestibulo-ocular responses more elaborate than a short-latency start in the right direction, is infinitely more complex than the three-neurone arc. It involves multisynaptic loops through vestibular nuclei, prepositus nuclei, cerebellar circuits and probably many other stations. All of these deal not only with vestibular information, but also with visual, proprioceptive and motor-activity related signals. Therefore, it seems to be fruitless to even try to demarcate a VOR subsystem neurophysiologically or neuroanatomically.

Behavioural considerations

One of the teleological arguments for the VOR as a subsystem is that it would be advantageous to have an automatic, fast and well calibrated stabilization system. Three types of objections can be made to this idea: (1) a fixed-gain VOR would, under natural circumstances, be more a problem than a help; (2) it is not clear that the gain of the VOR, measured in darkness, has some ideal value; and (3) the input-output relations of the VOR are extremely labile, and can be easily changed even by mental imagery.

The ideal gain of the VOR

It is often supposed that the ideal gain of compensatory eye movements is unity. Such movements would stabilize the retinal image of distant targets during head rotations. However, if this were a rigid reflex, it would already become a handicap during a change in gaze between distant targets with a substantial angular separation. During the coordinated eye-head movement which would be probably used for such a change of gaze, a hard-wired VOR would slow down gaze velocity. Actually, there is evidence that the VOR does not operate during gaze shifts with large amplitude (Tomlinson and Bahra, 1986; Laurutis and Robinson, 1986; Guitton and Volle, 1987; Pelisson et al., 1988).

For relatively close targets, the geometrical relations of head and eye rotational axes during natural head rotations in most mammals demand compensatory eye movements with a gain larger than unity. This effect can be exaggerated by rotating a subject around an eccentric axis, lying posterior to the head. In all these cases, eye movements with the appropriate calibration for continued fixation are made, and part of this distance-adaptation is even maintained in darkness, with the target removed (see e.g. Viirre et al., 1986; Gresty and Bronstein, 1986).

Finally, a gain smaller than unity is required for targets moving in the same direction as the head. Head-fixed targets are a bit unusual, but the same applies for pursuit of moving objects with combined eye and head movements. This class of movements is often described as "cancellation of the VOR".

It is of course possible to consider all these examples as special cases, in which a basic VOR with a fixed (e.g. unity) gain is modified. One can also argue, however, that compensatory eye movements with unity gain are the special case (for distant targets) of a more general goal. The general goal of the oculomotor system is to orient each of the eyes, at any moment, in such a way as is optimal for vision. It is clear that such control requires the specification of a target, in addition to signals relevant to spatial localization.

Gain of the VOR in darkness

The gain of the VOR, measured with passive oscillation in darkness, is almost invariably lower than unity. Only for the rhesus monkey have gains of about unity been reported (e.g. Miles and Eighmy, 1980; frequency range 0.1 – 1 Hz). In goldfish, mean gain is about 0.71 ± 0.24 (S.D.) at 0.125 Hz (Schairer and Bennett, 1986a). Similar, and often lower, values are found in rabbits (Baarsma and Collewijn, 1974). Typical values for humans, kept alert by mental arithmetic but left without special instructions with regard to spatial references, are on the order of 0.65 (e.g. Barr et al., 1976). Moreover, VOR gain in darkness shows great variability among subjects and over time. Gain tends to be higher for active head oscillation in darkness (Collewijn et al., 1983). The poor compensation in darkness markedly contrasts with the performance in the presence of a visible target, which is accurate to about 2.5% on the horizontal and vertical meridians (Ferman et al., 1987). If the human VOR would have indeed a gain of something like 0.65, about one-third of the compensatory movements would have to be supplemented by visual control (smooth pursuit, OKN). Apart from the extra delays involved, this situation appears to defeat the concept of the VOR as an automatic, well-calibrated system.

Voluntary control of VOR gain

The fact that the VOR in darkness does not behave as a calibrated feed-forward system, with (at least at any moment) a fixed input – output relation, was proven by Barr et al. (1976). They reported that humans could change their VOR gain momentarily from 0.65 (the value obtained during mental arithmetic) to either about 0.95 or 0.35, simply by "looking" in darkness at an imagined target, which was fancied as either stationary in space or fixed to the head. These findings, which have been replicated by many other groups, can be related to the earlier finding of Yasui and Young (1975) that a retinal afterimage (providing a visual target, but no retinal image slip information) improved the gain of VOR in darkness. Recently, we found that a foveally stabilized target has a similar effect (Lemij and Collewijn, in preparation). Briefly, subjects oscillated their heads while fixating a light spot, shown at (apparent) optical infinity in a stationary position. After about 13 s of viewing, the spot was either extinguished or foveally stabilized while the subjects continued to oscillate the head, and look at the position of the target. In either of the two conditions visual motion information was discontinued after 13 s, but in the second case the target remained visible. Remarkably, when the target was switched to the stabilized condition, the subjects did not notice any change in the stimulus situation, and gaze continued to be stabilized equally well as in the preceding episode with normal viewing. This effect was consistently present over the tested frequency range (0.25 − 1.5 Hz). Extinction of the spot, however, resulted in a decline of the gain of the compensatory eye movements to the levels which are usually measured for the VOR gain in darkness. Interestingly, this decline was not instan-

taneous at the onset of darkness, but gradual over a period of a few seconds.

Results such as discussed above strongly suggest (1) that the VOR cannot be interpreted as a subsystem with a definite input − output relation; (2) that one does not need additional, non-vestibular signals carrying real motion information (retinal image slip, otolith signals etc.) in order to change VOR gain significantly; and (3) that eye-head coordination is not governed by vestibular input as such, but by an internal reconstruction of the spatial relations between subject and target, based on an interpretation of the peripheral signals.

The gain of the VOR in darkness is not a hard number, but some rather arbitrary default setting of a gaze-control system which does not get sufficient information to operate properly. The system needs a target, albeit an imaginary or stabilized one, and some understanding of how this target is supposed to move. The importance of separating complex central factors from underlying reflex mechanisms was stressed by Steinman (1986) in his recent evaluation of the "systems approach" in the study of the oculomotor system.

We are only beginning to understand how higher cerebral levels could exert an effective control on vestibular responses. Recent work has supported a role of the parietal cortical area 7 in this respect. Lesions of this area cause a decrease in gain of the VOR in monkeys (Ventre and Faugier-Grimaud, 1986). Interestingly, tracing experiments have revealed a direct projection of area 7 to the vestibular nuclei (Faugier-Grimaud and Ventre, 1989).

The VOR and other subsystems: are they real?

In a conservative approach, one might maintain the concept of a hard-wired VOR as a basically independent and automatic system. If such a system is to function properly in natural behaviour, it can almost never be left alone. Changes in gaze by coordinated eye and head movements require the VOR to be turned off and on again. VOR gain has to be continuously adjusted for the distance of

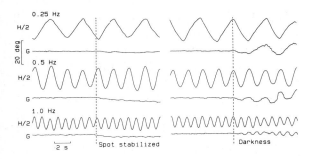

Fig. 3. Compensatory eye movements elicited during active head oscillation at 0.25, 0.5 or 1.0 Hz while viewing a point target at infinity. During the first half of each record the target was normally viewed. At the time marked by the vertical interrupted line, the target was either foveally stabilized (left column) or extinguished (right columns). G: gaze position (eye relative to target; a flat line represents perfect compensation). H: head position, shown reduced by a factor 2. See text.

(selected) objects and the effective site of the axis of head rotation. Monitoring of VOR gain by otolith signals or vergence-related signals has been invoked for this purpose (Viirre et al., 1986; Gresty et al., 1986, 1987; Hine and Thorn, 1987). When targets move along with the head, the VOR has to be cancelled by smooth pursuit or signals related to intended head motion (Robinson, 1982). Furthermore, long-term adjustment of VOR gain has to be made by adaptive processes. The VOR has apparently become so dependent on these secondary controls, that it cannot work properly without at least some rudimentary visual target; its apparent teleological elegance and simplicity are lost in the process.

The alternative approach, which I like to propose, is to discard the VOR as a "subsystem", along with a number of other ill-defined "subsystems" such as the optokinetic, smooth pursuit, and even the saccadic and vergence subsystems. The basic, and only, oculomotor function required by vision is that each eye be oriented optimally with respect to the object of current interest. To achieve this, the following steps are required: (1) selection of a target among many potential targets; (2) computation of the spatial localization (position, trajectory of motion) of the selected target, relative to the subject; and (3) generation of oculomotor commands to direct gaze to the computed, fixed or moving target position. It seems attractive to hypothesize that, throughout evolution, such gaze control has evolved as a holistic system, not as a bunch of subsystems with partial, and often conflicting, goals.

The importance of stimulus selection, quite independently of retinal localization, in controlling oculomotor responses has been demonstrated previously for pursuit by Collewijn et al. (1982) and by Kowler et al. (1984b), who should be consulted for further details. The role of selective spatial attention was recently also demonstrated for the control of vergence (Erkelens, 1989).

Vestibular signals are undoubtedly used in the computation of the relative spatial localization of a target, but the experiments as done first by Barr

et al. (1976) make it clear that they are used to generate eye movements only to the degree that the subject decides that compensatory eye movements are relevant in the present context. If this is the case, the vestibular signals are especially useful in generating a very rapid, initial phase of the response. However, in natural head movements, proprioceptive and efference-copy signals may also be very early sources of information. Evolutionary pressure will have undoubtedly favoured the use of all relevant signals in computing spatial localization and motion of objects of interest; such information is crucial to the programming of all motor activity, not only eye movements, and indeed to meaningful interaction of a subject with the surrounding world in general. In some very simplified conditions, the system may masquerade as a simple VOR. However, it seems illusory to isolate a VOR by passive rotation in darkness, because the spatial localization system will continue to act, albeit in an unspecified and somewhat unpredictable way. Vestibulo-ocular responses in darkness reflect some (labile) default status of a complex spatial localization system, not the status of a hard-wired VOR.

Spatial localization as a basis for gaze control

The hypothesis of a neural process computing spatial localization is, of course, not new at all, and has been invoked in different forms in previous models of oculomotor control (e.g. Barr et al., 1976; Young, 1977; Guitton and Volle, 1987). Barr et al. (1976) thought of such a process as being superimposed upon a "normal VOR"; they did not take the step of channelling all oculomotor programming through the spatial localization process. This step was, however, taken by Young (1977) who proposed, in the context of a "perceptual feedback" hypothesis, a "target velocity regenerator", driving all forms of smooth eye movement. Interestingly, Young saw no fundamental reason for distinguishing between smooth pursuit movements tracking a visible target, and the slow phase vestibular compensatory eye movements involved in attempting to stabilize an imagined target.

Fig. 4, which resembles Young's (1977) diagram, summarizes the hypothesis of a holistic gaze control system. It is not a model in any formal sense and just indicates that a unitary, multi-input process of relative spatial localization may control all oculomotor activity. In this concept there is no place for a separate VOR, although vestibular signals may be among the first to initiate compensatory eye movements.

If labyrinth-function is lost, the spatial localization system will (after a period of disorganization) continue to compute relative target localization on the basis of the remaining inputs. Properties that are specific for vestibular signals cannot be substituted by other information, but on the whole the ability to recover functions of gaze control, including some compensatory eye movements in the dark, is remarkable (Kasai and Zee, 1978; Baloh et al., 1984; Leigh et al., 1987). On the other hand, loss or maldevelopment of visual function is reflected by subnormal or absent vestibulo-ocular responses (Collewijn, 1977; Sherman and Keller, 1986). Apparently, vestibulo-ocular responses are not developed or maintained without a meaningful context of visual function. Even an acute loss of vision, due to intra-vitreal injection of tetrodotoxine, leads to an immediate reduction, followed by a slow progressive further decline of the VOR of the rabbit in the dark (Collewijn and Van der Steen, 1987).

The process of interaction between the multiple inputs into the spatial localization process, and the neural structures involved, will have to be investigated. It is likely that the interaction will involve more than a simple addition of the various signals. Probably, some parallel processing is involved, in which the computation of target localization and motion becomes more accurate as more information is available and congruent. If a continuous flow of position and/or motion information is available, relative position and motion of the target may be estimated with great accuracy and precision in place and time. Accordingly, eye movements may be programmed which track the target smoothly and accurately. Smooth eye movements are usually emphasized in the analysis of vestibulo-ocular responses. There is, however, evidence that saccades that contribute to gaze control can also be programmed on the basis of vestibular information (Berthoz et al., 1987; Segal

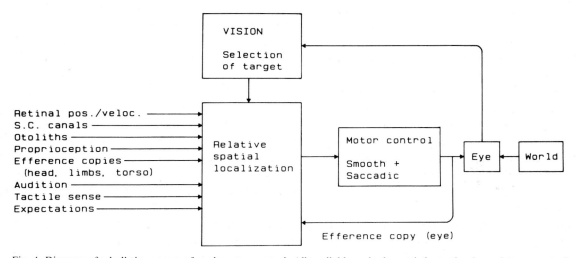

Fig. 4. Diagram of a holistic concept of oculomotor control. All available and relevant information is used to compute the position and motion of a selected target, relative to the subject. This spatial representation is then used to control all types of eye movements. There is no separate subdivision forming a VOR.

and Katsarkas, 1988).

The effective gaze stabilization of a retinally stabilized target, shown in Fig. 3, could be accounted for as follows. During the first part of the trial, the subject sees a stable target at infinity while he oscillates his head. This is a very common situation, and we may suppose that the spatial localization process will recognize this on the basis of the combination of vestibular, proprioceptive, visual and motor signals. Accordingly, compensatory eye movements with a unity eye/head gain will be programmed. The subsequent elimination of retinal image slip by stabilization will not disrupt this tracking, because the non-visual signals continue to report the same head motion, while visual signals suggest the continued tracking of the same target with no error. (A similar tendency to continue ongoing eye movements after the stabilization of a target was demonstrated for smooth pursuit by Van den Berg, 1988.) When the visual target is eliminated by darkness, the spatial localization apparently loses its accuracy, although not instantly (Fig. 3).

Apart from sensory and efference-copy signals, memorized information of target positions and trajectories is likely to be used in the spatial localization process. A clear example, although not directly related to the VOR, of such a process is the smooth anticipatory eye movement preceding the expected motion of a target, as described extensively by Kowler and colleagues (see e.g. Kowler et al., 1984a). A very different example is formed by the spontaneous sinusoidal eye movements which sometimes follow, and apparently mimic, preceding oscillatory vestibular or optokinetic stimulation of relatively long duration, in rabbits (Collewijn and Grootendorst, 1979) as well as in goldfish (Schairer and Bennett, 1986a, b).

Adaptation of the VOR: an epiphenomenon?

Numerous experiments in the last 15 years have shown that the gain of vestibulo-ocular responses in darkness can be changed in magnitude or direction when the habitual relations between head movements and the appropriate compensatory eye movements are systematically changed by inverting prisms, magnifying spectacles and similar devices. Adaptive changes in vestibulo-ocular responses are undoubtedly real, but what do they reflect? In the view of the VOR as an independent, automatic subsystem, the need for continuous recalibration is obvious, as no biological feed-forward system could conceivably operate accurately over a lifetime in the absence of some system for readjustment. "Parametric adjustment" (Robinson, 1975) would be one way to retain the speed of a feed-forward system, and yet use a form of visual feedback to optimize its setting.

Elegant as this hypothesis may be, it is somewhat hard to reconcile with the generally very imperfect performance of the VOR in darkness. Apparently, life-long training is not sufficient to achieve an ideal VOR. The same tendency is seen in most adaptation experiments: the VOR in darkness adapts only partially to the changed condition. In the light, however, adaptation is usually relatively fast and complete; this is obviously the situation that really matters.

If we accept the holistic view, then the study of "VOR adaptation", using vestibulo-ocular responses in darkness as a parameter, may be an awkward and indirect way to look at the adaptability of the spatial localization process. When confronted with unusual combinations of signals, the spatial localization process will undoubtedly learn to re-interpret these signals, until appropriate (oculo)motor coordination is achieved once more. These changes are relevant, and therefore fully expressed, only in the presence of a visible target. Aspects of these changes transferred to eye movements in darkness may represent an epiphenomenon of adaptation, not adaptation itself. Such a view is also more compatible with exotic, posture-contingent forms of "VOR adaptation" such as described recently by Baker et al. (1987a, b), in which compensatory eye movements assume features of complex, conditioned behaviour rather than of an automatic reflex.

References

Baarsma, E.A. and Collewijn, H. (1974) Vestibulo-ocular and optokinetic reactions to rotation and their interaction in the rabbit. *J. Physiol. (London),* 238: 603 – 625.

Baker, J.F., Perlmutter, S.I., Peterson, B.W., Rude, S.A., and Robinson, F.R. (1987) Simultaneous opposing adaptive changes in cat vestibulo-ocular reflex direction for two body orientations. *Exp. Brain Res.,* 69: 220 – 224.

Baker, J., Wickland, C., and Peterson, B. (1987) Dependence of cat vestibulo-ocular reflex direction adaptation on animal orientation during adaptation and rotation in darkness. *Brain Res.,* 408: 339 – 343.

Baloh, R.W., Honrubia, V., Yee, R.D., and Hess, K. (1984) Changes in the human vestibulo-ocular reflex after loss of peripheral sensitivity. *Ann. Neurol.,* 16: 222 – 228.

Barr, C.C., Schultheis, L.W., and Robinson, D.A. (1976) Voluntary, non-visual control of the human vestibulo-ocular reflex. *Acta Otolaryngol.,* 81: 365 – 375.

Berthoz, A. and Melvill Jones, G. (1985) *Adaptive Mechanisms in Gaze Control,* Elsevier, Amsterdam.

Berthoz, A., Israel, I., Vieville, T., and Zee, D. (1987) Linear head displacement measured by the otoliths can be reproduced through the saccadic system. *Neurosci. Lett.,* 82: 285 – 290.

Cohen, B. (1971) Vestibulo-ocular relations. In P. Bach-y-Rita, C.C. Collins, and E. Hyde (Eds.), *The Control of Eye Movements,* Academic Press, New York, pp. 105 – 148.

Cohen, B. (1974) The Vestibulo-ocular reflex arc. In H. Autrum et al. (Eds.), *Handbook of Sensory Physiology,* Springer, Berlin, pp. 477 – 540.

Collewijn, H. (1977) Optokinetic and vestibulo-ocular reflexes in dark-reared rabbits. *Exp. Brain Res.,* 27: 287 – 300.

Collewijn, H. and Grootendorst, A.F. (1979) Adaptation of optokinetic and vestibulo-ocular reflexes to modified visual input in the rabbit. In R. Granit and O. Pompeiano (Eds.), *Reflex Control of Posture and Movement,* Elsevier, Amsterdam, pp. 771 – 781.

Collewijn, H. and Van der Steen, J. (1987) Visual control of the vestibulo-ocular reflex in the rabbit: a multi-level interaction. In M. Glickstein, C. Yeo and J. Stein (Eds.), *Cerebellum and Neuronal Plasticity. NATO ASI Series A, Vol. 148,* Plenum, New York, pp. 277 – 291.

Collewijn, H., Curio, G., and Grusser, O.J. (1982) Spatially selective visual attention and generation of eye pursuit movements. Experiments with sigma-movement. *Human Neurobiol.,* 1: 129 – 139.

Collewijn, H., Martins, A.J., and Steinman, R.M. (1983) Compensatory eye movements during active and passive head movements: fast adaptation to changes in visual magnification. *J. Physiol. (London),* 340: 259 – 286.

Dodge, R. (1903) Five types of eye movement in the horizontal meridian plane of the field of regard. *Am. J. Physiol.,* 8: 307 – 329.

Dodge, R. (1923) Adequacy of reflex compensatory eye movements including the effects of neural rivalry and competition. *J. Exp. Psychol.,* 6: 169 – 181.

Easter, S.S. and Johns, P.R. (1974) Horizontal compensatory eye movements in goldfish (*Carassius auratus*). II. A comparison of normal and deafferented animals. *J. Comp. Physiol.,* 92: 37 – 57.

Easter, S.S., Johns, P.R., and Heckenlively, D. (1974) Horizontal compensatory eye movements in goldfish (*Carassius auratus*). I. The normal animal. *J. Comp. Physiol.,* 92: 23 – 35.

Erkelens, C.J. (1989) Ocular vergence induced by changes in spatially selective visual attention (abstract of presentation at 11th ECVP meeting, Bristol, 1988). *Perception,* 17: A8.

Faugier-Grimaud, S. and Ventre, J. (1989) Anatomical connections in inferior parietal cortex (area 7) with subcortical structures related to vestibulo-ocular function in a monkey *(Macaca fascicularis)*. *J. Comp. Neurol.,* 280: 1 – 15.

Ferman, L., Collewijn, H., Jansen, T.C., and Van den Berg, A.V. (1987) Human gaze stability in horizontal, vertical and torsional direction during voluntary head movements, evaluated with a three-dimensional scleral induction coil technique. *Vision Res.,* 27: 811 – 828.

Goldberg, J.M., Highstein, S.M., Moschovakis, A.K., and Fernandez, C. (1987) Inputs from regularly and irregularly discharging vestibular nerve afferents to secondary neurons in the vestibular nuclei of the squirrel monkey. I. An electrophysiological analysis. *J. Neurophysiol.,* 58: 700 – 718.

Graf, W. and Meyer, D.L. (1978) Eye positions in fishes suggest different modes of interaction between commands and reflexes. *J. Comp. Physiol.,* 128: 241 – 250.

Gresty, M.A. and Bronstein, A.M. (1986) Otolith stimulation evokes compensatory reflex eye movements of high velocity when linear motion of the head is combined with concurrent angular rotation. *Neurosci. Lett.,* 65: 149 – 154.

Gresty, M., Bronstein, A.M., and Barratt, H. (1987) Eye movement responses to combined linear and angular head movement. *Exp. Brain Res.,* 65: 377 – 384.

Guitton, D. and Volle, M. (1987) Gaze control in humans: eye-head coordination during orienting movements to targets within and beyond the oculomotor range. *J. Neurophysiol.,* 58: 427 – 459.

Harris, A.J. (1965) Eye movements of the dogfish *Squalus acanthias* L. *J. Exp. Biol.,* 43: 107 – 130.

Highstein, S.M., Goldberg, J.M., Moschovakis, A.K., and Fernandez, C. (1987) Inputs from regularly and irregularly discharging vestibular nerve afferents to secondary neurons in the vestibular nuclei of the squirrel monkey. II. Correlation with output pathways of secondary neurons. *J. Neurophysiol.,* 58: 719 – 738.

Hine, T. and Thorn, F. (1987) Compensatory eye movements during active head rotation for near targets: effects of imagination, rapid head oscillation and vergence. *Vision Res.,* 27: 1639 – 1657.

208

Kasai, T. and Zee, D.S. (1978) Eye-head coordination in labyrinthine-defective human beings. *Brain Res.,* 144: 123 – 141.

Kowler, E., Martins, A.J., and Pavel, M. (1984a) The effect of expectations on slow oculomotor control-IV. Anticipatory smooth eye movements depend on prior target motions. *Vision Res.,* 24: 197 – 210.

Kowler, E., Van der Steen, J., Tamminga, E.P., and Collewijn, H. (1984b) Voluntary selection of the target for smooth eye movement in the presence of superimposed, full-field stationary and moving stimuli. *Vision Res.,* 24: 1789 – 1798.

Laurutis, V.P. and Robinson, D.A. (1986) The vestibulo-ocular reflex during human saccadic eye movements. *J. Physiol. (London),* 373: 209 – 233.

Leigh, R.J., Sharpe, J.A., Ranaili, P.J., Thurston, S.E., and Hamid, M.A. (1987) Comparison of smooth pursuit and combined eye-head tracking in human subjects with deficient labyrinthine function. *Exp. Brain Res.,* 66: 458 – 464.

Lisberger, S. (1984) The latency of pathways containing the site of motor learning in the monkey vestibulo-ocular reflex. *Science,* 225: 74 – 76.

Lisberger, S.G. (1988) The neural basis for motor learning in the vestibulo-ocular reflex in monkeys. *Trends Neurosci.,* 11: 147 – 152.

McCrea, R.A., Strassman, A., and Highstein, S.M. (1987) Anatomical and physiological characteristics of vestibular neurons mediating the vertical vestibulo-ocular reflexes of the squirrell monkey. *J. Comp. Neurol.,* 264: 571 – 594.

McCrea, R.A., Strassman, A., May, E., and Highstein, S.M. (1987) Anatomical and physiological characteristics of vestibular neurons mediating the horizontal vestibulo-ocular reflex of the squirrel monkey. *J. Comp. Neurol.,* 264: 547 – 570.

Miles, F.A. and Eighmy, B.B. (1980) Long-term adaptive changes in primate vestibuloocular reflex. I. Behavioral observations. *J. Neurophysiol.,* 43: 1406 – 1425.

Murphy, B.J. (1978) Pattern thresholds for moving and stationary gratings during smooth eye movement. *Vision Res.,* 18: 521 – 530.

Pelisson, D., Prablanc, C., and Urquizar, C. (1988) Vestibuloocular reflex inhibition and gaze saccade control characteristics during eye-head orientation in humans. *J. Neurophysiol.,* 59: 997 – 1013.

Robinson, D.A. (1975) Oculomotor control signals. In G. Lennerstrand and P. Bach-y-Rita (Eds.), *Basic Mechanisms of Ocular Motility and their Clinical Implications,* Pergamon Press, Oxford, pp. 337 – 374.

Robinson, D.A. (1977) Vestibular and optokinetic symbiosis: an example of explaining by modelling. In R. Baker and A. Berthoz (Eds.), *Control of Gaze by Brain Stem Neurons,* Elsevier, Amsterdam, pp. 49 – 58.

Robinson, D.A. (1981) Control of eye movements. In V.B. Brooks (Ed.), *Handbook of Physiology – The Nervous System,* Williams and Wilkins, Baltimore, pp. 1275 – 1320.

Robinson, D.A. (1982) A model of cancellation of the vestibulo-ocular reflex. In G. Lennerstrand, D.S. Zee and E.L. Keller (Eds.), *Functional Basis of Ocular Motility Disorders,* Pergamon Press, Oxford, pp. 5 – 13.

Robinson, D.A. (1986) The systems approach to the oculomotor system. *Vision Res.,* 26: 91 – 99.

Robinson, D.A. (1987) The windfalls of technology in the oculomotor system. *Invest. Ophthal. Vis. Sci.,* 28: 1912 – 1925.

Schairer, J.O. and Bennett, M.V.L. (1986a) Changes in gain of the vestibulo-ocular reflex induced by combined visual and vestibular stimulation in goldfish. *Brain Res.,* 373: 164 – 176.

Schairer, J.O. and Bennett, M.V.L. (1986b) Changes in gain of the vestibulo-ocular reflex induced by sinusoidal visual stimulation in goldfish. *Brain Res.,* 373: 177 – 181.

Segal, B.N. and Katsarkas, A. (1988) Goal-directed vestibulo-ocular function in man: gaze stabilization by slow-phase and saccadic eye movements. *Exp. Brain Res.,* 70: 26 – 32.

Sherman, K.R. and Keller, E.L. (1986) Vestibulo-ocular reflexes of adventitiously and congenitally blind adults. *Invest. Opthalmol. Vis. Sci.,* 27: 1154 – 1159.

Simpson, J.I. and Graf, W. (1985) The selection of reference frames by nature and its investigators. In A. Berthoz and G. Melvill Jones (Eds.), *Adaptive Mechanisms in Gaze Control,* Elsevier, Amsterdam, pp. 3 – 16.

Skavenski, A. and Robinson, D.A. (1973) Role of abducens neurons in vestibuloocular reflex. *J. Neurophysiol.,* 36: 724 – 738.

Stehouwer, D.J. (1987) Compensatory eye movements produced during fictive swimming of a deafferented, reduced preparation in vitro. *Brain Res.,* 410: 264 – 268.

Steinhausen, W. (1933) Ueber die Beobachtung der Cupula in den Bogengangsampullen des Labyrinths des lebenden Hechts. *Pflügers Arch.,* 232: 500 – 512.

Steinman, R.M. (1986) The need for an eclectic, rather than systems, approach to the study of the primate oculomotor system. *Vision Res.,* 26: 101 – 112.

Ter Braak, J.W.G. (1936) Untersuchungen ueber optokinetischen Nystagmus. *Arch. Neerl. Physiol.,* 21: 309 – 376.

Tomlinson, R.D. and Bahra, P.S. (1986) Combined eye-head gaze shifts in the primate. II. Interactions between saccades and the vestibuloocular reflex. *J. Neurophysiol.,* 56: 1558 – 1570.

Tomlinson, R.D. and Robinson, D.A. (1984) Signals in vestibular nucleus mediating vertical eye movements in the monkey. *J. Neurophysiol.,* 51: 1121 – 1136.

Van den Berg, A.V. (1988) Human smooth pursuit during transient perturbations of predictable and unpredictable target movement. *Exp. Brain Res.,* 72: 95 – 108.

Van Egmond, A.A.J., Groen, J.J., and Jongkees, L.B.W. (1949) The mechanics of the semicircular canal. *J. Physiol. (London),* 110: 1 – 17.

Ventre, J. and Faugier-Grimaud, S. (1986) Effects of posterior parietal lesions (area 7) on VOR in monkeys. *Exp. Brain*

Res., 62: 654 – 658.

Viirre, E., Tweed, D., Milner, K., and Vilis, T. (1986) A reexamination of the gain of the vestibulo-ocular reflex. *J. Neurophysiol.,* 56: 439 – 450.

Waespe, W. and Henn, V. (1979) The velocity response of vestibular nucleus neurons during vestibular, visual, and combined angular acceleration. *Exp. Brain Res.,* 37: 337 – 347.

Walls, G.L. (1962) The evolutionary history of eye movements. *Vision Res.,* 2: 69 – 80.

Westheimer, G. and McKee, S.P. (1975) Visual acuity in the presence of retinal-image motion. *J. Opt. Soc. Am.,* 65: 847 – 850.

Wilson, V.J., and Melvill Jones, G. (1979) *Mammalian Vestibular Physiology,* Plenum Press, New York, London.

Yasui, S. and Young, L.R. (1975) Perceived visual motion as effective stimulus to pursuit eye movement system. *Science,* 190: 906 – 908.

Young, L.R. (1977) Pursuit eye movement – What is being pursued? In R. Baker and A. Berthoz (Eds.), *Control of Gaze by Brain Stem Neurons,* Elsevier, Amsterdam, pp. 29 – 36.

J.H.J. Allum and M. Hulliger (Eds.)
Progress in Brain Research, Vol. 80
© 1989 Elsevier Science Publishers B.V. (Biomedical Divison)

Overview and critique of Chapters 18 and 19

K.-P. Hoffmann

Bochum, F.R.G.

The paper by *Simpson et al.* brings together two related representations of three-dimensional eye movements in the rabbit flocculus: (1) The sensory representation of rotational optical flow as reflected in the modulation of climbing fibre activity and (2) the motor representation of eye movements as revealed by electrical stimulation.

In a series of elegant studies Simpson and collaborators have provided convincing evidence that the climbing fibre activity in the flocculus represents retinal image movements in a reference frame whose axes have spatial orientations similar those of the best-response axes of the vestibular semicircular canals as well as those of the eye rotation axes of the extraocular muscles. Electrical microstimulation in the flocculus in most cases led to slow eye movements which are consonant with the orientations of the preferred visual climbing fibre axes. Of the 12 possibilities (2 eyes) (3 axes) (clockwise-counterclockwise) 2 of them accounted for 80% of the responses: (1) a counter-clockwise rotation of the ipsilateral (left) eye about its 135° axis and (2) leftward rotation of the left eye about its vertical axis. From some stimulation sites a clear counterclockwise rotation of the contralateral (right) eye about its 135° axis was evoked. This response is at variance with the orientations of the preferred climbing fibre axes. However the latencies of this component were greater than those consonant with the climbing fibre axes. It is suggested that the longer latency may indicate stimulation of neurones other than Purkinje cells. The best stimulation sites were, in fact, in the deep

granular layer or white matter and not in the Purkinje layer.

Here seems to be the important question. Stimulation of which neuronal element causes the motor behaviour? One would expect that electrical stimulation works more easily on the output axons (i.e. Purkinje cell axons) than in activating specific intracerebellar circuitries (i.e. via input fibres). It would be revealing to remove the Purkinje cells by a chemical lesion and repeat the stimulation studies to see what eye movements might still be evoked. There is a straightforward mapping between the classes of short latency evoked eye movements and the anatomical compartments revealed in the flocculus white matter by the acetylcholinesterase stain, as shown in a Poster by Tan et al. at the Rheinfelden meeting. If each anatomical compartment can be assorted with a particular set of extraocular muscles then, in a motor behavioural context, the meaning of the grid formed by the climbing fibre input running perpendicular to the parallel fibres might be understood. After years of cerebellar research there is still no functional — not to mention behavioural — interpretation of this anatomical arrangement, which is fundamental to the cerebellar cortex.

Waespe et al. state in their introduction that ''Purkinje-cells (of the cerebellum) may carry information which cannot directly be correlated to single parameters of the stimulus or the motor act, but rather to signals (probably not known to the examiner) within extracerebellar neuronal circuitries.'' Is the oculomotor system or more precisely the vestibulo-optokinetic system an exception to this problem? The authors suggest it is, however their review does not give strong support to this view.

According to Ito's hypothesis neurones in the vestibular nuclei which are premotor cells for the ocular motoneurones are modulated by an input from floccular Purkinje-cells by (dis)inhibition. Against this seemingly simple scheme several inconsistencies and questions are raised for the monkey vestibulo-oculomotor system. In short, activity of floccular Purkinje-cells can be related directly to the oculomotor output (eye or gaze velocity) for certain stimulus conditions (smooth pursuit and VOR suppression) but not for other conditions (OKN). Modulation during OKN is complementary to the so-called eye velocity storage component of vestibular neuronal activity thereby extending the range of adequate slow eye velocity responses for gaze stabilization. The authors therefore raise the question where the target cells of floccular Purkinje cells involved in the regulation of horizontal eye movements are located and what their characteristics are.

To answer this question the major input to vestibular nuclei neurones was abolished by bilateral vestibular neurectomy. It was expected by the authors (1) to find a severe loss of neuronal activity within the vestibular nuclei and (2) to be able to identify more easily neurones which could be target cells of floccular Purkinje cells. What did they find?

(a) There is still a rich neuronal activity in the vestibular nuclei. Surprisingly all classes of neurons defined in normal monkeys are present. The number of inactivated "central" (secondary) vestibular neurones is too small to be detectable by population studies.

(b) According to the proposed model of Purkinje cells influence on vestibular neurones only about 10 – 15% of all neurones could be target cells of floccular "gaze velocity" or "eye movement only" Purkinje cells.

(c) The authors failed to find cells in the medial vestibular nucleus which were responsive to retinal slip. Neuronal activity was strictly related to parameters to the oculomotor response (i.e. eye velocity).

Here is the dilemma: There is a histologically demonstrated dense projection of the flocculus to the vestibular nuclei. Despite this, only a seemingly low number of vestibular nuclei neurones express the clear oculomotor control functions exerted onto them by floccular Purkinje cells.

Two possible explanations are suggested: (1) Some floccular Purkinje cells could also exert an excitatory action upon their target cells, and (2) previous single cell studies also included a region which according to newer anatomical studies belongs to the ventral paraflocculus. The authors draw the conclusion that horizontal "gaze velocity" Purkinje cells could have been recorded in the paraflocculus and therefore project to other structures than the vestibular complex.

After an extensive and elaborate review we are left in a deep puzzle. Have so many investigatiors mislocated or not verified their recording sites? Or do we have to accept that although the Purkinje cell activity in the flocculus can be interpreted by the examiner and correlated to single parameters of the oculomotor act, we do not understand so far their modulatory influence upon extracerebellar neuronal circuitries. The advice to be drawn from the article then seems to be straightforward: verify the recording sites and projections of Purkinje cells precisely before putting them into your model.

J.H.J. Allum and M. Hulliger (Eds.)
Progress in Brain Research, Vol. 80
© 1989 Elsevier Science Publishers B.V. (Biomedical Division)

CHAPTER 18

Representations of ocular rotations in the cerebellar flocculus of the rabbit

J.I. Simpson[1], J. Van der Steen [2], J. Tan[3], W. Graf[4] and C.S. Leonard[1]

[1]*Dept. of Physiology and Biophysics, New York University, Medical Center, New York, NY 10016, U.S.A; [2]Dept. of Physiology I, [3]Dept. of Anatomy, Faculty of Medicine, Erasmus University, 3000 DR Rotterdam, The Netherlands; and [4]The Rockefeller University, New York, NY 10021, U.S.A.*

The climbing fibres (CFs) of the rabbit flocculus that respond in a speed- and direction-selective manner to retinal image slip produced by eye rotations can be divided into three classes on the basis of the orientation of the rotation axis associated with their greatest modulation (the preferred axis). The similarity of the orientations of these axes to those of the eye rotation axes of the extraocular muscles suggests that a simple geometrical correspondence may exist between the eye rotation associated with the preferred axis of a given class of CFs and the eye rotation produced by activation of the Purkinje cells upon which that class of CFs synapse. To pursue this possibility, the axes of the eye rotations evoked by electrical microstimulation of the alert rabbit's flocculus were determined simultaneously for both eyes in three dimensions using two orthogonal search coils on each eye. A limited number of slow eye movement response patterns were found, and of these, two predominated. The most common response was a counterclockwise (CCW) rotation of the ipsilateral (left) eye around an axis close to the horizontal plane and at about 140° posterior to the nose. The other predominant response was abduction of the ipsilateral eye. These two response patterns, together with the smaller conjugate components for the contralateral eye, are consonant with the orientations of the preferred CF axes. In addition, a clear CCW rotation of the contralateral (right) eye about its 135° axis was also evoked from some stimulation sites. This response, which occurred either alone or as a component of an upward rotation about the nasal-occipital (roll) axis, is at variance with the orientations of the preferred CF axes. However, the latencies of the CCW contralateral 135° component (80–140 ms) were greater than those of the CW contralateral 45° component, the CCW ipsilateral 135° component and the ipsilateral abduction component (8–48 ms). These latency differences may distinguish stimulation of Purkinje cells from stimulation of other neurones.

Key words: Visual response; Cerebellum; Flocculus; Purkinje cell; Rabbit; Eye muscle; Semicircular canal response plane; Retinal image slip; Micro-electrical stimulation

Introduction

The contributions of the flocculus to compensatory eye movement control provide a useful model for studying cerebellar operations in a behavioural context. Since compensatory eye movements occur with three degrees of rotational freedom, the spatial organization of the sensory and motor representations of these eye movements is an important aspect of sensorimotor integration in the flocculus. This paper brings together two related studies of representations of three-dimensional eye movements in the rabbit flocculus. One part treats the sensory representation of rotational optical flow as reflected in the modulation of climbing fibre (CF) activity (Simpson et al., 1981; Graf et al., 1988; Leonard et al., 1988), while the other part presents work in progress on the motor representation of eye movements as revealed by electrical stimulation.

In both the anaesthetized and alert rabbit, floccular CF activity is modulated in relation to the speed and direction of movement of large, textured visual patterns (Simpson and Alley, 1974; Leonard, 1986). The pathways underlying the visual CF responses pass from the retina to the accessory optic system and then to the dorsal cap of the inferior olive (Meakawa and Simpson, 1973; Mizuno et al., 1973; Alley et al., 1975; Soodak and Simpson, 1988; Simpson et al., 1988). Recordings from neurones in the dorsal cap of the inferior olive (Simpson et al., 1981; Leonard et al., 1988) have shown that the visual CF modulation can be divided into three classes according to the axes about which rotation of the visual world evokes the greatest modulation (the preferred axes). For one class of CFs the preferred axis is vertical; for the other two classes the preferred axes lie close to the horizontal plane at about 45° or 135° to the midsagittal plane. The CFs dominated by the ipsilateral eye have preferred axes that are either vertical or close to 135° azimuth; the floccular CFs dominated by the contralateral eye have preferred axes close to 45° azimuth. These findings support the idea that retinal image movement is represented by visual CF activity in a reference frame whose axes have spatial orientations similar to those of the best-response axes of the vestibular semicircular canals (Simpson and Hess, 1977; Simpson et al., 1979) as well as to those of the eye rotation axes of the extraocular muscles (Simpson et al., 1981; Leonard et al., 1988; Graf et al., 1988). These geometrical similarities suggest that neural operations in the flocculus are organized in relation to such reference frames. To pursue this notion, precise measurements of the spatial orientation of the visual CF reference frame were obtained by recording from floccular Purkinje cells in the rabbit (Graf et al., 1988). Part of that study is summarized here and related to a second study in which the axes of the eye rotations elicited by electrical microstimulation of the rabbit flocculus were determined for both eyes in three dimensions.

Methods

Extracellular recordings of Purkinje cell CF activity were made in the *left* flocculus of 24 pigmented rabbits anaesthetized initially with a mixture of Nembutal (10 – 15 mg/kg) and α-chloralose (60 mg/kg) injected into an ear vein. During the recording session anaesthesia was infused intravenously at a constant rate of 5% of the initial dose per hour, and the animals were immobilized with gallamine triethiodide (Flaxedil) and artificially respirated. All pressure points and incisions were infiltrated with long-lasting local anaesthesia. The rabbit's head was positioned with the nasal bone at 57° to the horizontal, which put the plane of the horizontal semicircular canal within a few degrees of earth horizontal.

Visual stimuli were presented using a planetarium projector (Simpson et al., 1981; 1988) that provided a virtually full-field random dot pattern rotating at constant speed about selectable axes. The modulation of Purkinje cell CF activity, recorded using conventional methods, was usually studied with the planetarium axis positioned either vertically or in the earth-horizontal plane. The planetarium was rotated at a constant speed in the midrange of retinal image speeds that produce the greatest modulation of CFs (Simpson and Alley, 1974; Barmack and Hess, 1980), and the sense of rotation (clockwise (CW) or counterclockwise (CCW)) was reversed every 5 s. The modulation was assessed using peristimulus histograms compiled on-line. For each position of the planetarium axis, the average firing rates during the periods of CW and CCW rotation were computed off-line and spatial tuning curves were plotted. Because the tuning curves are approximately sinusoidal, the location of the axis for maximal modulation (the preferred axis) was determined from the best-fit sine curve.

In a separate study, the oculomotor responses to electrical microstimulation in the flocculus were recorded in 12 awake pigmented rabbits. During the experiment, the animals were restrained in a hammock and the head was held with the nasal bone at 57° to the horizontal. There were no pressure points and no signs of discomfort. One to three days prior to the experiment, the rabbit was anaesthetized, the bone above the paramedian lobe of the cerebellum on the *left* side was removed and the opening was surrounded by a chamber made of dental acrylic. The dura was covered with an antibiotic gel and a thin sheet of silicone rubber and then the chamber was filled with bone wax and paraffin. On the day of the experiment, the dura was opened under local anaesthesia. The flocculus was identified by recording the modulation of Purkinje cell CF activity in response to movement of hand-held visual patterns. With the animal in darkness, the glass or metal recording microelectrode was then used to deliver monopolar electrical stimuli at 200 μm intervals during withdrawal along those tracks having visually responsive Purkinje cells. The standard stimulus was a one second train of 0.2 ms pulses at 200 Hz and -20 μA. Some of the more effective locations for evoking eye movements were marked by electrolytic lesions. After termination of the experiment the animals were deeply anaesthetized and perfused. Frozen sections were examined to find the lesions and to reconstruct the electrode tracks.

A recording technique using two orthogonal coils attached to each eye was used to measure the movements of both eyes simultaneously in three dimensions (Van der Steen and Collewijn, 1984). At least five days prior to the experiment, two search coils, one horizontal on top of the superior rectus muscle and one vertical following the limbus, were implanted under the conjunctiva of each eye with the rabbit anaesthetized. The orthogonal coordinate system used to measure the angular displacements consisted of a vertical axis and two horizontal axes oriented at azimuths of 45° and 135°. The 0° reference was rostral in the midsagittal plane and the azimuthal coordinate was taken to increase to each side of the reference direction. The components of the evoked eye movements were named after their respective axes (vertical axis, 45° axis and 135° axis) referenced to the ipsilateral (left) or the contralateral (right) eye. The sense of the rotation components about the horizontal axes was defined as CW or CCW according to how they would be seen by an observer looking along each axis *towards* the rabbit's eye. With these conventions the 135° axis of one eye is parallel to the 45° axis of the other eye and a CW rotation of one eye is conjugate to a CCW rotation of the other eye. The sense of the rotation components about the vertical axis was described for each eye as leftward or rightward. The vertical axis (horizontal) component of rotation was measured with the vertical coil using the phase-angle detection technique (Collewijn, 1977), while the rotation components about the 45° and 135° axes were measured with the horizontal coil using the amplitude detection technique (Robinson, 1963; Van der Steen and Collewijn, 1984). The vertical coils had absolute calibration, whereas the horizontal coils were calibrated prior to implantation. The three eye position components for each eye were charted on a pen recorder and stored on magnetic tape. In the off-line computer analysis each position component was digitized at 125 Hz with a resolution of 10 seconds of arc.

Results

Visual modulation of climbing fibres

The depth of modulation of Purkinje cell CF activity depends upon the orientation of the rotation axis of the visual stimulus and upon which eye is stimulated. The responses can be divided into three main classes according to eye dominance taken in conjunction with the orientation of the stimulus axis for which the modulation is greatest (the preferred axis orientation). The names of the classes — vertical axis, anterior (45°) axis and posterior (135°) axis — are derived from the orientation of the preferred axis referenced to the eye whose stimulation produced the greater CF modulation.

Vertical axis Purkinje cells

The greatest modulation of vertical axis Purkinje cells occurred with stimulation of the ipsilateral eye with the planetarium axis oriented vertically. Vertical axis Purkinje cells were divided into two subclasses according to whether the receptive field of their visual CFs was monocular (93%) or binocular (7%). The CFs of monocular vertical axis Purkinje cells were modulated only by stimulation of the eye ipsilateral to the flocculus. In all cases, the firing rate increased with movement of the external visual world from temporal to nasal and decreased with movement from nasal to temporal. The CFs of vertical axis Purkinje cells showed little or no modulation to rotation of the visual world about axes in the horizontal plane.

For the binocular version of the vertical axis Purkinje cell, stimulation of the contralateral (nondominant) eye increased CF activity when the external visual world moved from nasal to temporal, while movement from temporal to nasal decreased activity. Thus, the direction preferences for the two monocular receptive fields are jointly satisfied by rotation about a vertical axis.

Anterior (45°) axis Purkinje cells

Purkinje cells that receive a CF input whose

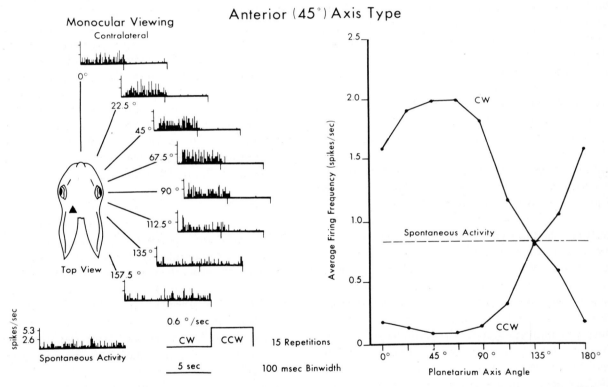

Fig. 1. Climbing fibre responses of an anterior (45°) axis Purkinje cell to monocular stimulation presented to the contralateral (dominant) eye. The tested axes were in the horizontal plane and the orientation with respect to the midsagittal plane was varied in 22.5° steps. In this and the subsequent figure, the solid triangle on the top view of the rabbit's head indicates recording from the *left* flocculus. The peristimulus histograms, next to their respective stimulus axes, depict the firing rate during clockwise (CW) and counterclockwise (CCW) constant speed rotation. CW and CCW indicate the sense of visual world rotation when viewed *from* the rabbit along the axis directed toward the respective histogram. With this convention, CCW rotation about the posterior 135° axis on one side of the head is the same as CW rotation about the anterior 45° axis on the other side of the head. The ordinate scale on the spontaneous activity histogram also applies to the other histograms. The relation between average firing rate for CW and CCW rotation and the orientation of the planetarium axis is graphed at the right. In this case the preferred axis determined from the best-fit sine curve was at 49° contralateral azimuth. (Modified from Graf et al., 1988.)

modulation is dominated by visual stimuli presented to the contralateral eye constitute the anterior (45°) axis class. This name is derived from the fact that the greatest modulation for monocular stimulation occurred for rotation of the visual world about an axis oriented in the horizontal plane and close to 45° contralateral azimuth (Fig. 1). Anterior (45°) axis Purkinje cells could be divided into two subclasses according to whether the receptive field of their visual CFs was monocular (34%) or binocular (66%). The CFs of the monocular members of this class were

modulated only by visual stimuli presented to the contralateral eye. The relation between the orientation of the stimulus axis in the horizontal plane and CF modulation was obtained for ten anterior (45°) axis cells for the contralateral (dominant) eye. The preferred axis, determined by summing the modulations of the ten cells and then calculating the best-fit sine curve, was located at 47° contralateral azimuth (Fig. 3). For all anterior (45°) axis cells the sense of visual world rotation that resulted in excitation for contralateral (dominant) eye stimulation was CW as viewed from the

Posterior (135°) Axis Type

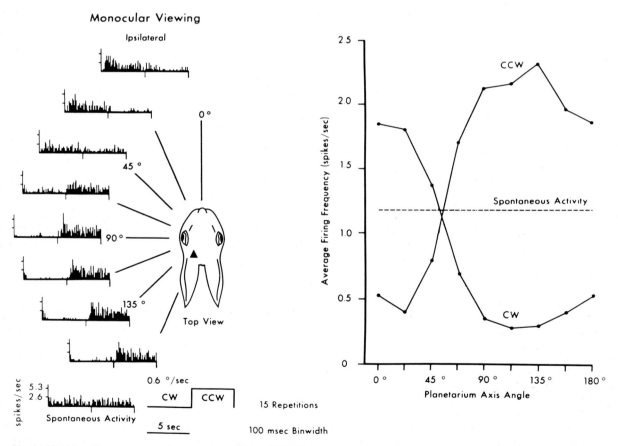

Fig. 2. Climbing fibre responses of a posterior (135°) axis Purkinje cell to monocular stimulation presented to the ipsilateral (dominant) eye. The format is that described for Fig. 1. The variation of the average firing rate with planetarium axis orientation is plotted on the right. In this case the preferred axis determined from the best-fit sine curve was at 138° ipsilateral azimuth. (Modified from Graf et al., 1988.)

along the preferred axis.

With binocular stimulation, the modulation of binocular anterior (45°) axis Purkinje cells was less pronounced than for stimulation of only the contralateral eye. This decrease can be explained qualitatively by the fact that the spatial organizations of the two monocular receptive fields tended to be bilaterally (axially) symmetric and, therefore, the preferences found for each eye alone cannot be jointly satisfied by binocular stimulation.

Posterior (135°) axis Purkinje cells

Posterior (135°) axis Purkinje cells showed a substantial modulation for rotation of the visual world about an axis whose spatial orientation was similar to that of the preferred axis of the anterior

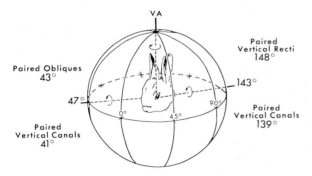

Rotation Axes—Visual Climbing Fibers
(Re: Left Flocculus; Dominant Eye)

Fig. 3. Spatial organization of the visual CF, semicircular canal and extraocular muscle reference frames. The orientations of the three preferred axes of the visual CFs of the *left* flocculus are shown by dashed lines. The numbers next to the two axes in the horizontal plane are the azimuths of the preferred axes determined with monocular stimulation of the respective dominant eye and are, strictly speaking, the angles between the mid-sagittal plane and the projection of the preferred axes into the horizontal plane. The azimuths of the anatomically determined best-response axis of the vertical canal pair that is spatially closely related to the visual CFs are also given, as are the azimuths of the rotation axes of the paired oblique muscles and the paired vertical recti muscles (Simpson, 1983; Ezure and Graf, 1984). The azimuth values are for the projections into the horizontal plane. The axes of the vertical axis CFs, the paired horizontal canals, and the paired horizontal recti are indicated approximately by a single axis (VA) (from Simpson et al., 1989.)

(45°) axis Purkinje cells. However, in contrast to those cells, the posterior (135°) axis cells were dominated by the ipsilateral eye, they always had a binocular receptive field and the difference in modulation strength between the two eyes was not often as large as that for the binocular anterior (45°) axis Purkinje cells. The name posterior (135°) axis is derived from the fact that for visual world rotations about axes in the horizontal plane, the greatest modulation for monocular stimulation occurred for rotation about an axis oriented close to 135° ipsilateral azimuth (Fig. 2). The relation between the orientation of the stimulus axis in the horizontal plane and CF modulation was obtained for ten posterior (135°) axis cells for the ipsilateral (dominant) eye. The preferred axis, determined by summing the modulations of the ten cells and then calculating the best-fit sine curve, was located at 143° ipsilateral azimuth (Fig. 3). For all posterior (135°) axis cells the sense of visual world rotation that resulted in excitation for ipsilateral (dominant) eye stimulation was CCW as viewed from the rabbit along the preferred axis.

With binocular stimulation, the modulation of posterior (135°) axis Purkinje cells was greater than with stimulation of the ipsilateral eye alone. This increase can be explained qualitatively by the fact that the spatial organizations of the two monocular receptive fields are close to being centrally symmetric and, therefore, the preferences found for each eye alone can be jointly satisfied by binocular stimulation.

Eye movements evoked by electrical stimulation

In the electrical stimulation study, an effective site was defined as a site at which the standard stimulus (a 1-s train of 0.2 ms pulses at 200 Hz and −20 μA) evoked an eye movement of at least 0.5° about at least one of the six recorded axes. The amplitude of the slow evoked eye movements was typically 1−5°, but occasionally amplitudes of up to 20° were observed. Eye movements were more readily produced by stimulation in the deep granular layer and white matter than from the Purkinje cell or molecular layers. Usually they had a latency of 8–48 ms. The peak speed (maximum 20°/s) occurred 100–200 ms after movement onset. During the stimulation period the movements were unidirectional and in most instances the eye returned to the initial position within 4–10 s after stimulus offset. The eye movements were classified according to the largest recorded component of the response. Of the 12 possible classes (2 eyes) (3 axes) (2 senses of rotation), two of them alone accounted for nearly 80% of the responses.

For 54% of the effective stimulation sites, the largest component was a CCW rotation of the ipsilateral (left) eye about its 135° axis (Fig. 4). In about half of these cases the response was conjugate in that the largest component of the contralateral (right) eye was a CW rotation about its 45° axis. In a few instances, however, the component of conjugacy of the contralateral eye was essentially absent. The azimuthal orientation of the average rotation axis, which lay close to the horizontal plane, was estimated for each eye by "vector" summation of the 45° and 135° components. Although angular displacements are not vector components, compounding the small displacements involved provides a reasonable indication of the orientation of the rotation axis. For the ipsilateral (left) eye the axis of rotation, projected into the horizontal plane, was located at 139.6° azimuth. For those cases in which the component of conjugacy was the largest component of the accompanying movement of the contralateral (right) eye, the similarly computed rotation axis was located at 31.0° azimuth.

For 24% of the effective stimulation sites, the largest response component was abduction of the ipsilateral eye — that is, a leftward rotation of the

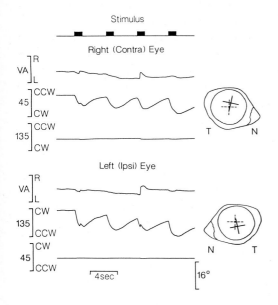

Fig. 4. Example of the class of evoked eye movements for which the largest component was a CCW rotation of the ipsilateral (left) eye about its 135° axis. The largest component of the contralateral (right) eye movement was in this case a conjugate rotation about its 45° axis. In this and the following figures the three traces for each eye show the angular displacement about the indicated axes (L, leftward; R, rightward; CW, clockwise; CCW, counterclockwise). The one second periods of electrical stimulation (0.2 ms pulses, 200 Hz, −20 μA) in the *left* flocculus are indicated at the top. The schematic drawings on the right show how the eye movements would appear if a cross had been placed on the cornea. The dashed cross indicates the initial position and the solid cross shows the position at the end of the stimulation. T, temporal; N, nasal. Note that neither eye movement was "vertical". The downward and temporal movement of the ipsilateral eye is due largely to the actions of the vertical recti while the upward and nasal movement of the contralateral eye is due largely to the actions of the obliques.

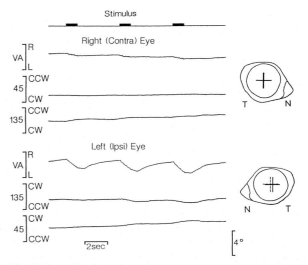

Fig. 5. Example of the class of evoked eye movements for which the largest component was abduction of the ipsilateral (left) eye. The format is the same as that of Fig. 4.

left eye about its vertical axis (Fig. 5). The vertical axis component of the accompanying movement of the right eye was nearly always conjugate – that is, leftward (adducting). The example shown in Fig. 5 had nearly only vertical axis components, but not infrequently a modest CCW component about the ipsilateral (left) 135° axis was also present.

While the two classes of evoked eye movements described above can be related directly to the spatial organization of the preferred axes of the visual CFs, as well as to present knowledge about the influence of the flocculus on particular vestibular ocular reflex pathways (see Discussion), the responses evoked from the remaining 22% of the effective stimulation sites cannot be so explained. Of these responses, one that was often found was a CCW rotation about the contralateral (right)

135° axis that was larger than or comparable to an accompanying CW rotation about the contralateral (right) 45° axis (Fig. 6A). In the latter case, the net result of the two components about the 45° and 135° axes of the contralateral eye was essentially an upward rotation about the roll (nasal-occipital) axis (Fig. 6A). However, the component about the 135° axis had longer latencies than the component about the 45° axis (Fig. 6B). For the contralateral 135° component the latencies ranged from 80 – 140 ms as compared to 8 – 48 ms for the contralateral 45° component. When the response of the contralateral eye was "vertically" upward, the ipsilateral eye did not have a conjugate "vertically" downward movement. Rather, the accompanying response of the ipsilateral (left) eye was predominantly a CCW rotation about its 135° axis (Fig. 6A).

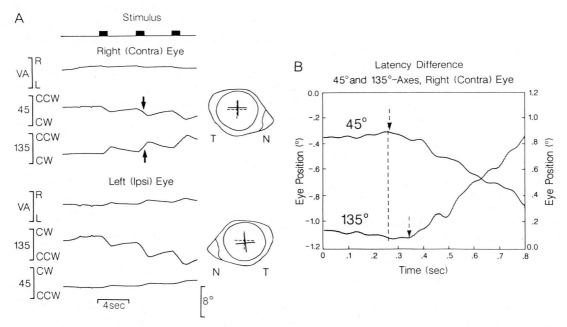

Fig. 6. Latency difference between eye movement components. A: electrical stimulation of the left flocculus produced a CCW rotation of the ipsilateral (left) eye about its 135° axis along with a much smaller CW rotation about its 45° axis. In contrast, the rotation of the contralateral (right) eye had nearly equal, but opposite components about its 45° and 135° axes. The net movement of the contralateral eye was an upward movement about the roll (nasal-occipital) axis, while the net movement of the ipsilateral eye corresponded closely to a rotation about the axis of the paired vertical recti (see Figs. 3 and 4). B: difference in latency between the 45° and 135° components of the contralateral eye movement shown in A (arrows). Stimulus onset is indicated by the dashed line; movement onset is indicated by the arrows.

Discussion

Quantification of the modulation of Purkinje cell CF activity as a function of the orientation of the axis of visual world rotation indicates that this visual measure of self-motion is achieved using an intrinsic reference frame whose spatial orientation is similar to that of the reference frame established by the structure of the vestibular semicircular canals. The visual CF reference frame is also spatially similar to the reference frame composed of the axes about which the three pairs of extraocular muscles rotate the eye. The spatial organizations of these three reference frames are compared in Fig. 3. The three preferred axes for modulating CF activity in the flocculus on one side of the head establish a reference frame, as do the three vestibular canals on one side. Although three axes are present in each case, a striking difference exists with regard to the mutual spatial relations within each set of axes. In the case of the canals, the three axes are widely separated from each other. In the case of the CF reference frame, the two preferred axes lying close to the horizontal plane are only modestly divergent. Both of them are close to the best-response axis of the anterior canal ipsilateral to the recorded flocculus. The absence of a class of CFs that respond preferentially to rotation about an axis at the 45° ipsilateral azimuth is conspicuous. Such an axis would be closely aligned to the best-response axis of the ipsilateral posterior canal. However, the presence of two axes closely related to the orientation of the ipsilateral anterior canal and the absence of an axis related to the ipsilateral posterior canal are consonant with the finding in the rabbit that the flocculus does not act directly on the VOR pathways arising from the ipsilateral posterior canal (Ito et al., 1973, 1977, 1982).

Consideration of the geometry of the preferred axes of the visual CFs in relation to present and previous findings (Dufossé et al., 1977; Nagao et al., 1985) on the eye movements produced by electrical stimulation in the rabbit flocculus must be prefaced by a review of the effects of flocculus stimulation on the various vestibular ocular reflex (VOR) pathways. Purkinje cells of the flocculus monosynaptically inhibit vestibular nuclei neurones in the three-neurone arc of the VOR (Ito et al., 1970; Fukuda et al., 1972; Baker et al., 1972; Highstein, 1973; Kawaguchi, 1985). The selectivity of this inhibition for particular VOR pathways was shown in the rabbit by recording the influence of flocculus stimulation on extraocular muscle activity produced by vestibular nerve stimulation (Ito et al., 1973, 1977, 1982). Of the six pathways influenced, three are inhibitory and three are excitatory. Two of them link the horizontal canal with the ipsilateral medial and lateral recti, and increased flocculus output results in increased activity of the lateral rectus muscle and decreased activity of the medial rectus muscle. The other four pathways under direct floccular control are the anterior canal pathways that excite the ipsilateral superior rectus and contralateral inferior oblique muscles, and inhibit the ipsilateral inferior rectus and contralateral superior oblique muscles.

In the previous attempts to classify the eye movements evoked by electrical stimulation in the rabbit's flocculus the movements were classified as either horizontal, rotatory or vertical (Dufossé et al., 1977; Nagao et al., 1985). As discussed below, the eye rotation axes of the horizontal and rotatory classes correspond to the preferred axes of the visual CFs. However, the vertical class of eye movements consists of rotations about the roll (nasal-occipital) axis, which is not a preferred axis of the visual CFs.

For one of the two predominant classes of eye movements found in the present study abduction of the ipsilateral eye was the largest component. This class, which can be spatially associated with the vertical axis CFs, corresponds to the horizontal class found previously. The vertical axis (horizontal) responses are understandable in terms of the known influence of the flocculus on the lateral and medial recti.

For the class of oculomotor responses most frequently encountered in the present study the largest component was a CCW rotation of the ipsilateral eye about its 135° axis; this response was often accompanied by a smaller CW rotation of the contralateral eye about its 45° axis. This class, which can be spatially associated with the posterior (135°) axis CFs and the anterior (45°) axis CFs, is similar to the rotatory class reported in both previous studies. There are, however, some differences. The rotatory class of Dufossé et al. (1977) contained only contralateral eye movements, and while the rotatory class of Nagao et al. (1985) also included a conjugate movement of the ipsilateral eye, it was smaller than that of the contralateral eye. In these studies, the rotatory movements of the contralateral eye were considered to be due to the inhibitory influence of the flocculus on the pathways from the ipsilateral anterior canal to the contralateral oblique muscles, but a satisfactory explanation was not given for the rotatory movement of the ipsilateral eye. In the present study, the rotation axis of the ipsilateral eye movements in the rotatory class was located at about 140° azimuth, which is very close to the location (148° azimuth) of the rotation axis of the paired vertical recti (Fig. 3). This similarity indicates that the ipsilateral "rotatory" eye movements are essentially the result of floccular inhibition of the pathways from the ipsilateral anterior canal to the ipsilateral superior and inferior recti.

The vertical eye movement class, comprised of rotations of both eyes about the roll axis, is inconsistent with the eye movements predicted by combining the results of the electromyographic studies (Ito et al., 1973, 1977, 1982) with measurements of the kinematic effects of individual extraocular muscles in the rabbit (Graf and Simpson, 1981; Simpson and Graf, 1981, 1985). The inconsistency follows from the fact that the geometrical arrangements of the vertical recti and the obliques are incompatible with producing an eye movement about the roll axis by inhibition of only the pathways from the ipsilateral anterior canal. The contralateral "vertical" eye movements found in this study (shown in Fig. 6 as nearly equal, but opposite rotations of the contralateral eye about its

45° and 135° axes) are apparently the same as the contralateral eye movements in the vertical class of Dufossé et al. (1977) and Nagao et al. (1985). The presence of "vertical" eye movements indicates that the flocculus stimulation influenced both anterior and posterior canal pathways. However, the latencies of the 135° axis component were longer than those of the 45° axis component. This difference implies that the effect on the posterior canal pathways was less direct and possibly not the result of stimulation of Purkinje cells. In the present study, the accompanying ipsilateral eye movement was not "vertical", but rather it was predominantly a CCW rotation about the 135° axis, which places it in the rotatory class. In the previous studies, the ipsilateral "vertical" eye movements were considered to be due to the influence of the flocculus on the pathways from the ipsilateral anterior canal to the ipsilateral vertical recti. However, this conclusion is not in agreement with anatomical and physiological measurements of the actions of these muscles (Graf and Simpson, 1981; Simpson and Graf, 1981; Simpson, 1983; Ezure and Graf, 1984). From those measurements it can be concluded that "rotatory" movements of the ipsilateral eye are due to the action of the vertical recti and that a combined action of the obliques and vertical recti is required to produce "vertical" movements.

Acknowledgements

Supported by National Institutes of Health grants NS-13742 and EY-04613, the Deutsche Forschungsgemeinschaft (Gr 688/1), the Irma T. Hirschl Trust, and Medigon grant 900-550.092.

References

Alley, K.E., Baker, R., and Simpson, J.I. (1975) Afferents to the vestibulo-cerebellum and the origin of the visual climbing fibers in the rabbit. *Brain Res.,* 98: 582 – 589.

Baker, R.G., Precht, W., and Llinas, R. (1972) Cerebellar modulatory action on the vestibulo-trochlear pathway in the cat. *Exp. Brain Res.,* 15: 364 – 385.

Barmack, N.H. and Hess, D.T. (1980) Multiple-unit activity

evoked in dorsal cap of inferior olive of the rabbit by visual stimulation. *J. Neurophysiol.,* 43: 151 – 164.

Collewijn, H. (1977) Eye- and head movements in freely moving rabbits. *J. Physiol. (London),* 266: 471 – 498.

Dufossé, M., Ito, M., and Miyashita, Y. (1977) Functional localization in the rabbit's cerebellar flocculus determined in relationship with eye movements. *Neurosci. Lett.,* 5; 273 – 277.

Ezure, K. and Graf, W. (1984) A quantitative analysis of the spatial organization of the vestibulo-ocular reflexes in lateral and frontal eyed animals. I. Orientation of semicircular canals and extraocular muscles. *Neuroscience,* 12: 85 – 93.

Fukuda, J., Highstein, S.M., and Ito, M. (1972) Cerebellar inhibitory control of the vestibulo-ocular reflex investigated in rabbit IIIrd nucleus. *Exp. Brain Res.,* 14: 511 – 526.

Graf, W. and Simpson, J.I. (1981) The relations between the semicircular canals, the optic axis, and the extraocular muscles in lateral-eyed and frontal-eyed animals. In A. Fuchs and W. Becker (Eds.), *Progress in Oculomotor Research, Developments in Neuroscience,* Elsevier, Amsterdam, pp. 411 – 420.

Graf, W., Simpson, J.I., and Leonard, C.S. (1988) The spatial organization of visual messages in the flocculus of the rabbit's cerebellum. II. Complex and simple spike responses of Purkinje cells. *J. Neurophysiol.,* 60: 2091 – 2121.

Highstein, S.M. (1973) Synaptic linkage in the vestibulo-ocular and cerebello-vestibular pathways to the VIth nucleus in the rabbit. *Exp. Brain Res.,* 17: 301 – 314.

Ito, M., Highstein, S.M., and Fukuda, J. (1970) Cerebellar inhibition of the vestibulo-ocular reflex in rabbit and cat and its blockage by picrotoxin. *Brain Res.,* 17: 524 – 526.

Ito, M., Nisimaru, N., and Yamamoto, M. (1973) Specific neural connections for the cerebellar control of vestibulo-ocular reflexes. *Brain Res.,* 60: 238 – 243.

Ito, M., Nisimura, N., and Yamamoto, M. (1977) Specific patterns of neuronal connexions involved in the control of rabbit's vestibulo-ocular reflexes by the cerebellar flocculus. *J. Physiol. (London),* 265: 833 – 854.

Ito, M., Orlov, I., and Yamamoto, M. (1982) Topographical representation of vestibulo-ocular reflexes in rabbit cerebellar flocculus. *Neuroscience,* 7: 1657 – 1664.

Kawaguchi, Y. (1985) Two groups of secondary vestibular neurons mediating horizontal canal signals, probably to the ipsilateral medial rectus muscle, under inhibitory influences from the cerebellar flocculus in rabbits. *Neurosci. Res.,* 2: 434 – 446.

Leonard, C.S. (1986) Signal characteristics of cerebellar Purkinje cells in the rabbit flocculus during compensatory eye movements. PhD Dissertation, New York University.

Leonard, C.S., Simpson, J.I., and Graf, W. (1988) The spatial organization of visual messages in the flocculus of the rabbit's cerebellum. I. Typology of inferior olive neurons of the dorsal cap of Kooy. *J. Neurophysiol.,* 60: 2073 – 2090.

Maekawa, K. and Simpson, J.I. (1973) Climbing fiber responses evoked in vestibulocerebellum of rabbit from visual system. *J. Neurophysiol.,* 36: 649 – 666.

Mizuno, N., Mochizuki, K., Akimoto, C., and Matsushima, R. (1973) Pretectal projections to the inferior olive in the rabbit. *Exp. Neurol.,* 39: 498 – 506.

Nagao, S., Ito, M., and Karachot, L. (1985) Eye field in the cerebellar flocculus of pigmented rabbits determined with local electrical stimulation. *Neurosci. Res.,* 3: 39 – 51.

Robinson, D.A. (1963) A method of measuring eye movement using a scleral search coil in a magnetic field. *IEEE Trans. Biomed. Electron.,* BME-10: 137 – 145.

Simpson, J.I. (1983) Transformations of coordinates intrinsic to the vestibulo-ocular reflex. *Soc. Neurosci. Abstr.,* 9: 315.

Simpson, J.I. and Alley, K.E. (1974) Visual climbing fiber input to rabbit vestibulo-cerebellum: a source of direction-specific information. *Brain Res.,* 82: 302 – 308.

Simpson, J.I. and Graf, W. (1981) Eye muscle geometry and compensatory eye movements in lateral-eyed and frontal-eyed animals. *Ann. N.Y. Acad. Sci.,* 374: 20 – 30.

Simpson, J.I. and Graf, W. (1985) The selection of reference frames by nature and its investigators. In A. Berthoz and G. Melvill Jones (Eds.), *Adaptive Mechanisms in Gaze Control,* Elsevier, Amsterdam, pp. 3 – 16.

Simpson, J.I. and Hess, R. (1977) Complex and simple visual messages in the flocculus. In R. Baker and A. Berthoz (Eds.), *Control of Gaze by Brain Stem Neurons,* Elsevier/North Holland, Amsterdam, pp. 351 – 360.

Simpson, J.I., Soodak, R.E., and Hess, R. (1979) The accessory optic system and its relation to the vestibulocerebellum. In R. Granit and O. Pompeiano (Eds.), *Reflex Control of Posture and Movement,* Elsevier, Amsterdam, pp. 715 – 725.

Simpson, J.I., Graf, W., and Leonard, C. (1981) The coordinate system of visual climbing fibers to the flocculus. In A. Fuchs and W. Becker (Eds.), *Progress in Oculomotor Research, Developments in Neuroscience,* Elsevier/North Holland, Amsterdam, pp. 475 – 484.

Simpson, J.I., Leonard, C.S., and Soodak, R.E. (1988) The accessory optic system of rabbit. II. Spatial organization of direction selectivity. *J. Neurophysiol.,* 60: 2055 – 2072.

Simpson, J.I., Graf, W., and Leonard, C.S. (1989) Three-dimensional representation of retinal image movement by climbing fiber activity. In P. Strata (Ed.), *The Olivocerebellar System in Motor Control, Exp. Brain Res. Suppl. 17,* Springer, pp. 323 – 327.

Soodak, R.E. and Simpson, J.I. (1988) The accessory optic system of rabbit. I. Basic visual response properties. *J. Neurophysiol.,* 60: 2037 – 2054.

Van der Steen, J. and Collewijn, H. (1984) Ocular stability in the horizontal, frontal and sagittal planes in the rabbit. *Exp. Brain Res.,* 56: 263 – 274.

J.H.J. Allum and M. Hulliger (Eds.)
Progress in Brain Research, Vol. 80
© 1989 Elsevier Science Publishers B.V. (Biomedical Division)

CHAPTER 19

Oculomotor functions of the flocculus and the vestibular nuclei after bilateral vestibular neurectomy

W. Waespe[1], U. Schwarz[3] and M. Wolfensberger[2]

Departments of [1]Neurology and [2]Otorhinolaryngology, University Hospital, 8091 Zürich, Switzerland; and [3]NIH, Bethesda, MD 20892, U.S.A.

Ito's hypothesis of an important role of the flocculus of the vestibulocerebellum in the immediate visual control of the VOR during visual-vestibular interaction has received substantial support. Nevertheless, several parts in this hypothesis are unclear, at least in primates. In normal monkey, vestibularly driven neurones in the vestibular nuclei do not carry signals which are adequate to account for the full range of eye movement responses during optokinetic tracking (OKN) and different situations of visual-vestibular interaction (especially VOR-suppression). Thus these neurones seem not to be located at the final stage where floccular "gaze-velocity" Purkinje cells (PCs) exert their control function on the three-neurone-reflex arc. The signals of these "central" vestibular neurones (if relevant for the oculomotor output) must further be processed. After bilateral vestibular neurectomy (BVN) only a small number of vestibular nuclei neurones were found with eye velocity sensitivities during smooth pursuit tracking (SP) and OKN in the range of those of floccular PCs (also after BVN), and with the appropriate polarity of modulation. Our difficulties in finding neurones in the vestibular nuclei which, according to their neurophysiological behaviour, could be main target cells of floccular PCs, either in normal or in BVN monkeys, are discussed.

Key words: Cerebellum; Vestibular nucleus; Neurectomy; Integrator; Oculomotor; Interaction; Smooth pursuit; Optokinetics; Velocity storage; Flocculus

Introduction

The cerebellum participates in a wide variety of functions, particularly motor acts and "learning" (Holmes, 1939; Ito, 1984). Several lines of evidence suggest that cerebellar structures are involved in the initiation of movements, and in the control of smooth pursuing and rapidly alternating movements. If the "cerebellum functions as an accessory system adjusting the gains of control loops, which are mediated by extracerebellar centers, for the efficient attainment of motor purposes under a great variety of conditions" (MacKay and Murphy, 1979), Purkinje cells (PCs)

may carry information which cannot directly be correlated to single parameters of the stimulus or the motor act, but rather to signals (probably not known to the examiner) within extracerebellar neuronal circuitries. Although our knowledge about the intrinsic connections and electrophysiology of the cerebellum has greatly increased (Eccles et al., 1967; Ito, 1984), it is difficult to assign motor functions to specific cerebellar structures, and to quantify the contribution of each of the various elements within interconnected neuronal circuitries to the elaboration of motor command signals.

An exception to this seems to be the oculomotor

system, more precisely the vestibulo-optokinetic system. Here a synthesis is under way to correlate functional deficits, neuronal activity and anatomy (Ito, 1982). The vestibulo-ocular reflex (VOR) is an open-loop reflex and its basic layout is a three-neuronal arc. The input – output relationship is described in terms of head and eye velocity. The VOR is susceptible to internal and external disturbances by lesions and by changes in the visual surround. Ito (1972, 1982) put forward the important hypothesis that shortcomings in the VOR may be complemented, instantaneously or adaptively, by visual information via the flocculus of the vestibulo-cerebellum. The flocculus constitutes a "side-path" of the VOR-arc, it receives vestibular signals directly from primary vestibular neurones and visual signals from mossy fibres (MFs) of brainstem nuclei and from climbing fibres (CFs) of the inferior olive. Floccular Purkinje cells (PCs) project to the vestibular nuclei and modulate the activity of secondary vestibular neurones of the three neuronal reflex arc by (dis)inhibition (Fig. 1A). A crucial assumption is that these secondary vestibular neurones are *premotor* cells for the ocular motoneurones. For example, during visual suppression of the VOR, the head velocity signal of primary vestibular neurones is nullified at the level of these secondary vestibular neurones (and nowhere else) by a corresponding, 180° out-of-phase velocity signal of PCs (Ito, 1982). Despite this seemingly simple scheme of the visually induced modulation of the VOR, it is still unclear if these control functions of floccular PCs are attributable to MF or CF input signals, or to a combination of both. Experiments in rabbits suggest that the visual signal of CFs mainly controls long-term, adaptive changes, and the signal of visual MFs short-term, immediate changes of the VOR (Ito, 1982; Miyashita and Nagao, 1984). Furthermore, as shown by anatomical studies, not only vestibular nerve but also vestibular nuclei neurones project to the flocculus. It is not known if these nuclei neurones (or at least some of them) are the target cells of floccular PCs (thus projecting information back to the flocculus), or if these neurones

carry vestibular signals not yet modulated by floccular output signals. We and others, based on neurophysiological experiments, have suggested that most or all of the vestibular MFs in the primate flocculus originate from "central" (secondary) and not from primary vestibular neurones (Waespe et al, 1981, 1985a; Langer et al., 1985a). These MFs are still activated by head velocity during visual suppression of the VOR. Similarly, "central" vestibular nuclei neurones highly sensitive to vestibular stimulation (threshold at or below 2.5 deg/s^2) are still modulated by head velocity despite visual suppression of the VOR even at very low accelerations of 5 or 10 deg/s^2 when vestibular information should be nullified by floccular output signals (Waespe and Henn, 1978; Buettner and Büttner, 1979). Thus, vestibular MFs in the flocculus and "central" vestibular neurones transmit head velocity signals during visual suppression of the VOR although there is no eye velocity at the output side, i.e. their vestibular in-

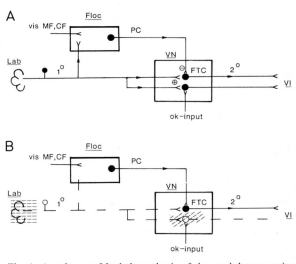

Fig. 1. A: scheme of Ito's hypothesis of the modulatory action of the flocculus upon secondary vestibular neurones. B: after bilateral labyrinthectomy or vestibular neurectomy the target cells of floccular PCs (FTC) in the vestibular nuclei should survive whereas "central" vestibular neurones involved in the "eye velocity storage" mechanism should be inactivated. 1°, 2°, primary and secondary vestibular neurones; VI, abducens motoneurones; VN, vestibular nuclei; Floc, flocculus.

formation is not yet nullified. It is rather unlikely, therefore, that these neurones are directly controlled by floccular PCs in such a way that their activity – as it should be according to Ito's hypothesis – always reflects the velocity of slow eye movements during visual-vestibular interaction. This seems also to be true for vertical vestibular nuclei neurones (Tomlinson and Robinson, 1984). It is presently unclear which of the secondary vestibular neurones are controlled by floccular output signals.

As noted above, signals of PCs may not always and necessarily be related to parameters of a motor act. This has been demonstrated for the "gaze-velocity" PCs of the primate flocculus. These PCs are modulated in relation to eye or gaze velocity

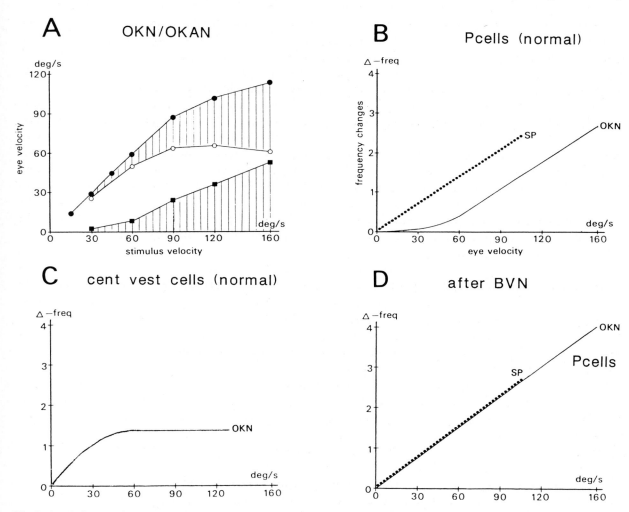

Fig. 2. A: relative contribution of the "eye velocity storage" component (open circles) and of the "short-time constant"-component ("direct" visual pathways, filled squares) to the slow phase velocity of steady-state OKN (filled circles) as a function of different constant stimulus velocities (abscissa). B,C: the curve characterizing the frequency changes (arbitrary values) of floccular PCs (B) or "central" vestibular neurones (C) as a function of slow phase velocity of steady-state OKN (abscissa) is of similar shape as that describing the relative contribution of the "storage" component or of the "short-time constant" component in A. D: after bilateral vestibular neurectomy (BVN) OKN is generated solely by that mechanism which is responsible for the "short-time constant" component. The strength of modulation of PCs as a function of eye velocity is similar during SP and OKN.

but only for specific stimulus conditions and not for others. Simple spike (SS) activity is more or less linearly related to eye velocity during smooth pursuit (SP) eye movements provided these are greater than 8 deg/s (Fig. 2B), and to head (or gaze) but not eye velocity during VOR-suppression (Lisberger and Fuchs, 1978; Miles et al., 1980). Furthermore, during steady-state optokinetic nystagmus (OKN), these same "gaze-velocity" PCs are modulated only over specific ranges of eye velocities. They are not modulated over those ranges of velocities which are mediated by the "eye velocity storage" element (Büttner and Waespe, 1984). Only when OKN slow phase velocities reach values above the saturation velocity of the "storage" element (about 40 – 60 deg/s) are they active (Fig. 2B; Waespe and Henn, 1981; Waespe et al., 1985a). Consequently, after bilateral vestibular neurectomy or labyrinthectomy, which abolishes the "velocity storage" mechanism but leaves the "short-time constant" component of OKN intact, the gaze-velocity PCs are also modulated over those ranges of eye velocities of OKN that do not cause a response in normal monkey (Waespe et al., 1985a). Thus, in labyrinthectomized or neurectomized monkeys with no eye velocity storage, the strength of modulation of floccular PCs is comparable during SP and OKN for any tracking eye velocity (Fig. 2D). This suggests that the short-time constant component (or "direct" visual pathway) utilizes neural mechanisms similar, if not identical, to those employed by the smooth-pursuit system. If in normal monkey the optokinetic stimulus is stopped abruptly with lighting left on, optokinetic afternystagmus (OKAN) and all activity of the velocity storage element built up during optokinetic stimulation are rapidly suppressed. During this period of active suppression of OKAN and of activity of the eye velocity storage, PCs are deeply modulated and this modulation cannot be related to gaze-, eye-, or head-velocity. Instead, it is rather related to the process of suppression of OKAN and of the activity within the storage element (Büttner and Waespe, 1984).

In summary, activity of floccular PCs can be related directly to the oculomotor output (eye or gaze velocity) for certain stimulus conditions (SP and VOR-suppression), but not for other conditions (OKN). Instead, modulation during OKN and conditions of visual-vestibular interaction is complementary to signals of central vestibular neurones (Fig. 2C) and the so-called eye velocity storage element than to those of vestibular nerve neurones, thereby extending the range of adequate slow eye velocity responses for gaze stabilization (Fig. 2). Floccular PCs indeed mediate signals for the efficient attainment of (oculo-)motor purposes. Modulation of "central" and second-order vestibular neurones is unlikely to be significantly controlled by floccular gaze-velocity PCs because the latter's strength of modulation can always be dissociated from slow eye velocities during OKN and conditions of visual-vestibular interaction. Without further processing their velocity signals cannot account for the oculomotor velocity responses. The question arises therefore where the target cells of floccular PCs involved in the regulation of horizontal eye movements are located and what their characteristics are. In a further attempt to address this problem we recorded the activity of vestibular nuclei neurones in monkeys after bilateral vestibular neurectomy (labyrinthectomy).

Theoretical background

The occurrence of reflex-like optokinetic nystagmus (OKN) and of optokinetic afternystagmus (OKAN) is a function of a so-called velocity storage mechanism within the vestibulooptokinetic system (Fig. 2A). The neural structure and location of this mechanism is unknown, it seems to be mediated by extracerebellar or at least extrafloccular structures as it is more or less unchanged after (para)flocculectomy (monkeys: Waespe et al., 1983; rat: Hess et al., 1988). Its dynamics are changed after nodul-/uvulectomy (Waespe et al., 1985b). The integrity of the storage mechanism, however, depends on that of the labyrinth and the primary vestibular neurones

(Cohen et al., 1973; Waespe and Wolfensberger, 1985). The permanent loss of reflex-like OKN and of OKAN after bilateral labyrinthectomy or vestibular neur(on)ectomy is assumed to be due to inactivation (= loss of spontaneous firing) of secondary vestibular neurones (Fig. 1B; Robinson, 1981; Collewijn, 1976). The operatively induced inactivation of primary vestibular neurones alone cannot account for these deficits because the primary neurones are not modulated by optokinetic whole-field stimulation (Büttner and Waespe, 1981). Central (second-order) vestibular neurones, as mentioned above, are activated by optokinetic stimulation (Fig. 2C). During OKAN the activity of these neurones changes with the slow phase velocity of nystagmus (Waespe and Henn, 1977a,b). Floccular PCs, on the other hand, are crucial for the mediation of velocity command signals for SP eye movements. These signals are not altered after bilateral labyrinthectomy or vestibular neurectomy (Waespe et al., 1985a). Therefore, their target cells in the vestibular nuclei (FTC in Fig. 1) must be intact after the operation and still be able to relay the PCs' eye velocity command signals. We expected after bilateral vestibular neurectomy (BVN): (i) to find a severe loss of neuronal activity within the vestibular nuclei for second-order vestibular neurones which are involved in the storage mechanism and which are not target cells of floccular PCs; and, due to this inactivation, (ii) to be able to identify more easily neurones which could be target cells of floccular PCs, because they mediate and/or integrate PCs' eye velocity command signals during SP and post-BVN OKN. As PCs exert an inhibitory control on their target cells and as they mostly (more than 90%) show increased activity for *ipsi*lateral SP eye movements and OKN slow phases, their target cells should increase activity for *contra*lateral smooth eye movements.

Methods

Experiments were performed on two monkeys (*Macaca mulatta*). Under general anaesthesia the following were chronically implanted: silver — silver chloride electrodes in the bony orbit to monitor horizontal and vertical eye position, bolts on top of the skull for immobilizing the head during experiments, and a well for a microelectrode carrier (for details see Waespe and Henn, 1977a). In the two monkeys the superior and inferior branches of the vestibular nerve on both sides were cut peripheral to Scarpa's ganglion using a translabyrinthine approach.

Single cell recordings were started 2 months postoperatively and extended over a period of approximately 9 months in each monkey. For details of single cell recordings, test protocol and data acquisition, see Waespe et al., 1985a. The monkeys were trained to fixate and to follow the movements of a single light-point. To locate the recording site, the nucleus abducens was identified before and repeatedly after the operation. Using a vertical approach with respect to the stereotaxic plane (*not* with respect to the brainstem), a field extending 2.5 mm laterally and 3.5 mm posteriorly to the nucleus abducens was systematically explored with eletrodes on one side of the brainstem. Cells were sampled to a depth of approximately $2-3$ mm below the floor of the 4th ventricle. Neural activity beneath the vestibular nuclei was irregular, and unrelated to eye movement parameters, and was characterized by large spike potentials. At the conclusion of cell recordings, small amounts of HRP were injected at the sites of the most successful recordings. Histological reconstruction showed that these marks were placed in the centre of the medial vestibular nucleus (MVN).

For computer-assisted data processing filtered unit recordings and other relevant signals as turntable, light point, and eye position were stored on a six channel analogue magnetic tape. For off-line analysis these signals were led through analogue-to-digital converters into digital storage on 20 Megabyte hard disc of an IBM/AT 2 computer.

Results

Postoperatively, horizontal and vertical vestibular

responses (to peak accelerations of 250 deg/s^2) as well as optokinetic afternystagmus (OKAN) were abolished. Postoperatively, OKN was quite irregular and a continuous, sustained response could not be elicited.

The activity of 829 neurones (4.8 cells per penetration; Table 1) located mainly within the medial vestibular nucleus (MVN) was recorded. We grouped neurones according to their eye position and eye velocity sensitivities during SP and OKN, and, qualitatively, according to their activity changes during saccades (no change, bursts, pauses). Despite the lack of vestibular responses in these neurones, which made classification more uncertain, we could allocate neurones to classes which have been defined in normal monkey (Fuchs

and Kimm, 1975; Waespe et al., 1977; Waespe and Henn, 1979a,b; Lisberger and Miles, 1980; Tomlinson and Robinson, 1984).

15% of all neurones ($n = 126$) could tentatively be classified as (vestibular)-pause [(V)P] and tonic-(vestibular-)pause [T(V)P] cells (Table 1); i.e. these cells behaved similarly to VP cells and TVP cells in normal monkey except for their lack of a vestibular response. Neurones were silenced for saccades in a specific or in each direction. The activity of a vertical T(V)P cell during vertical SP eye movements is shown in Fig. 3. Most of the horizontal T(V)P cells increased activity for eye positions to the contralateral side; i.e. in the normal monkey the cells could have been type I TVP cells. Mean resting discharge, mean eye position

TABLE 1

Summary of all classes and their characteristics after BVN

		Monkey 1	2	total	%	Resting discharge, mean (S.D.)		Eye position sensitivity, mean (S.D.)	Eye velocity sensitivity, mean (S.D.)	
									SP	OKN
Penetrations		74	99	173	100					
Cells		343	486	829	100					
Cells per penetration		4.6	4.9	4.8	–					
(V)P		10	23	33	4	99	(45)	0	0	0
T(V)P	horizontal	8	18	26	3.1	83	(30)	0.88 (0.46)	0.34 (0.19)	0.37 (0.24)
	vertical	36	27	63	7.6	104	(29.5)	1.95 (1.06)	0.47 (0.35)	–
	oblique	–	4	4	0.5	–		–	–	–
				126	15					
Tonic	contra (eII)	33	49	82	10	46	(29)	1.07 (0.82)	0.42 (0.32)	0.41 (0.35)
Tonic	ipsi (eI)	46	117	163	19.7	56	(45)	2.95 (1.57)	0.67 (0.64)	0.69 (0.69)
Tonic	vertical	24	22	46	5.6	42	(36)	–	–	–
Tonic	oblique (contra-down)	11	7	18 (15)	2.2	44	(34)	1.32 (0.44)*	0.89 (0.36)	0.96 (0.44)
				309	38					
Pure		86	129	215	26	40.5 (28)		0	0	0
Saccade-related		73	84	157	19	32	(31)	0	0	0
				372	45					
Complex		15	7	22	2.5	–		–	–	–

* Vertical: 2.06.

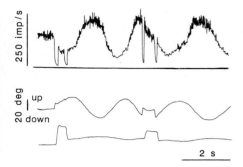

Fig. 3. Instantaneous activity (first trace) of a vertical T(V)P cell during vertical smooth pursuit. Second and third trace: vertical and horizontal eye position.

and slow eye velocity sensitivities are given in Table 1. Average eye position sensitivity of vertical T(V)P cells was twice that of horizontal T(V)P cells. The characteristics of presumably vertical T(V)P cells are comparable to those of vertical TVP cells in normal monkey (Tomlinson and Robinson, 1984). It is noteworthy that slow eye velocity sensitivities during SP and OKN were comparable and low. Horizontal TVP cells in normal monkey show a much stronger modulation during OKN (Waespe and Henn, 1979a,b) than T(V)P cells after BVN. Neuronal activity changes of T(V)P cells were strictly related to slow phase velocity of OKN and not to retinal slip velocity or to sustained activity within a velocity storage element as in normal monkey (Waespe and Henn, 1977a,b, 1979a,b).

Around 20% of all neurones increased their activity with eye positions to the recording side (tonic ipsilateral neurones, eI-cells; Table 1). Average eye position sensitivity was 2.95 impulses (imp)/s/deg. The spectrum of activity changes during saccades was large. Some neurones were not modulated at all (= pure tonic eye position neurones) and other neurones burst vigorously for ipsilateral saccades and paused for contralateral saccades (= burst-tonic cells). Slow eye velocity sensitivities during SP and OKN were comparable and averaged 0.69 imp/s/deg/s. Most of these eI-neurones were located in the most medial part of the MVN

posteriorly to the nucleus abducens, i.e. in a region believed to be important for the integration of eye velocity signals (Cannon and Robinson, 1986). Another 10% of the recorded neurones increased activity with contralateral eye positions (tonic contralateral neurones, eII-cells). Average eye position sensitivity was lower than that of tonic ipsilateral neurones and averaged 1.07 imp/s/deg. Usually neurones showed some weak burst activity for contralateral directed saccades and some inhibition for ipsilateral directed saccades. Slow eye velocity sensitivities during SP and OKN were also comparable and averaged 0.42 imp/s/deg/s. In about 2/3 of the eII-cells eye position and eye velocity sensitivities were weak and below 1.0 imp/s/deg and 0.5 imp/s/deg/s, respectively. There was no modulation due to retinal slip velocity in eII-neurones. Many of the eII-neurones could be type I-vestibular-eye movement related neurones (vI/eII-cells according to the nomenclature of Lisberger and Miles, 1980) in normal monkey. 26% of the recorded neurones were not modulated by any of the eye movement parameters. Judged from the regular firing rate these cells could constitute the class of pure-vestibular neurones in normal monkey. Another 20% of all neurones with or without a resting discharge rate exhibited activity changes during saccades only. The neurones of the latter two classes were not modulated during SP and OKN in relation to eye position or eye velocity. Two cells only showed a weak bidirectional and sustained modulation during optokinetic stimulation which was probably related to retinal slip velocity as the same neurones were not modulated during SP eye movements. Other classes of neurones with a more complex behaviour which were not analysed are listed in Table 1.

In summary, after BVN, activity is still present in the vestibular nuclei, in particular, MVN neurones display a rich variety of activity patterns. All classes of neurones defined in normal monkey could be recognized from their neurophysiological characteristics in the absence of vestibular responses. Our expectation of a severe decrease in neural activity was not fulfilled, although we cannot exclude the possibility that some central (second-order) vestibular neurones are silenced by BVN. We believe however that we can exclude absence of activity for an entire class of neurones. Neurones tentatively classified as (V)P, T(V)P and eII-neurones could represent in the normal monkey VP, TVP and type I-vestibular-eye movement related (vI/eII-) neurones (Waespe and Henn, 1979a,b; Lisberger and Miles, 1980; Tomlinson and Robinson, 1984). Characteristics such as average resting firing rate, eye position and eye velocity sensitivities during SP, and modulation with saccades are comparable. As an example, vertical TVP cells in normal monkey (Tomlinson and Robinson, 1984) have an average resting firing rate of 115 imp/s, after BVN it is 104 imp/s for T(V)Ps. Eye position and eye velocity sensitivities are 2.4 imp/s/deg and 0.4 imp/s/deg/s, respectively in normal monkeys, after BVN the respective values are 1.95 imp/s/deg and 0.47 imp/s/deg/s. Differences appear for the OKN response and are due to BVN or inactivation of the velocity storage. After BVN, the neurones are no longer continuously modulated during optokinetic stimulation and they are also not modulated during suppression of OKN. Ongoing modulation during OKN-suppression, and a strong modulation during optokinetic stimulation are typical characteristics of central vestibular neurones in normal monkey (Waespe and Henn, 1977b, 1979b; Buettner and Büttner, 1979). Sensitivity to optokinetic stimulus (and eye) velocity is on average 1.3 imp/s/deg/s for vestibularly driven neurones which also encode eye position (Waespe and Henn, 1979a,b). After BVN, eye velocity sensitivity during OKN and SP is between 0.3 and 0.4 imp/s/deg/s. Vestibular MFs recorded in the flocculus of normal monkeys have a similarly weak eye velocity sensitivity during SP of 0.22 imp/s/deg/s. The same MFs have, however, a much higher sensitivity during OKN of around 1.4 imp/s/deg/s (Waespe et al., 1985a).

Two findings are noteworthy after BVN: (i) neurones not encoding eye positions were also not modulated during SP and OKN with slow eye velocity; and (ii) in the neurones encoding eye posi-

tion the eye velocity sensitivity was comparable during SP and OKN. In normal monkeys, pure-vestibular neurones related to horizontal canal activation are always also modulated by optokinetic stimulation, pure (-vestibular) neurones after BVN were not.

With respect to our second assumption regarding the location of PC target cells, most of the horizontal T(V)P cells and the eII-neurones (i.e. about 10 − 15% of all neurones) could be target-cells of floccular "gaze-velocity" or "eye-movement-only" (see Miles et al., 1980) PCs. Their eye velocity sensitivities during SP and OKN are, however, quite low and on average between 0.3 and 0.4 imp/s/deg/s. Only 4 eII-neurones had an eye velocity sensitivity higher than 1.0 imp/s/deg/s (i.e. in the range of that of floccular PCs after BVN; Waespe et al., 1985a).

Discussion

This discussion is restricted to the question of the characteristics and the localization of target cells of floccular PCs in the vestibular nuclei. The strictly ipsilateral projection of the inhibitory PCs, and the expected polarity of modulation of possible target cells during horizontal SP and OKN after BVN, reduces consideration to horizontal T(V)P- and eII-cells. 10 − 15% of all neurones belong to these two classes. T(V)P cells are most likely TVP cells in normal monkey. In about 2/3 of the eII-neurones the eye position and eye velocity sensitivities were weak and below 1.0 imp/s/deg and 0.5 imp/s/deg/s, respectively. These low sensitivities, the regular firing rate and the weak modulation with saccades suggest that many of these eII-neurones could be vestibular type I-eye movement related neurones (vI/eII-cells) in normal monkey. Only 4 eII-cells (i.e. less than 1% of all neurones) had an eye velocity sensitivity above 1.0 imp/s/deg/s in the range of that of floccular PCs after BVN (Waespe et al., 1985a). The number and strength of modulation of horizontal T(V)P-and eII-cells during SP and OKN is so small that we have difficulty in imagining that these neurones are the main and sole relay neurones for the mediation and integration of horizontal smooth eye velocity command signals of floccular PCs after BVN, assuming that the flocculus has such a crucial role in the control of SP and OKN. The same discrepancies were encountered in normal monkey. TVP-cells are generally not regarded as the main target cells of gaze-velocity PCs because they are strongly modulated with head velocity during VOR-suppression (King et al., 1976; Waespe and Henn, 1978; Tomlinson and Robinson, 1984). Similarly, vestibularly driven nuclei neurones with a weak eye position sensitivity below 1.0 imp/s/deg (vI/eII-cells) are unlikely to be significantly modulated by gaze-velocity PCs. These vI/eII-neurones are also, like horizontal TVP cells, strongly modulated by vestibular signals during visual suppression of the VOR. Furthermore, during constant-velocity OKN these neurones usually saturate at low stimulus velocities (at lower velocities than the pure-vestibular neurones) so that the relative changes in firing rate and the relative increases in slow phase velocity of OKN strongly dissociate at higher stimulus velocities (Buettner and Büttner, 1979; Waespe et al., 1979a,b). The same holds true for sinusoidal stimulation at higher frequencies (Boyle et al., 1985). When "eye velocity storage" is intact, vI/eII-neurones and TVP-cells are highly sensitive to optokinetic stimulation for velocities below the saturation level (sensitivity of 1.3 imp/s/deg/s). In contrast, after BVN, eye velocity sensitivity is only between 0.3 and 0.4 imp/s/deg/s. Obviously, modulation in these eye position coding neurones is normally mainly related to slow phase velocities of reflex-like OKN for which the velocity storage mechanism is responsible. In summary, there is little indication in normal monkey that a large number of "central" (second-order) vestibular neurones are significantly controlled by "gaze-velocity" PCs. By "significantly" we mean that activity changes of these target cells are so closely related to eye velocity over the full range of stimulus velocities and frequencies that they can be regarded, according to Ito's hypothesis, as truly

premotor neurones for ocular motoneurones. That is, their relative frequency changes should no longer be dissociated from relative eye velocity changes during visual-vestibular stimulation. Lisberger recently suggested that simple spike (SS) activity of primate floccular PCs is "very sensitive to large, retinal slip" and that PCs send a "major" visual motion signal to their target cells in the brainstem (Lisberger, 1988). In our experimental paradigm using continuous rotation of a large-field visual surround either with or without suppression of OKN we failed to find a significant SS modulation of floccular PCs which could be attributed to retinal slip and/or target velocity in space (Büttner and Waespe, 1984; Waespe et al., 1985a). When the moving large-field stimulus was suddenly presented to the monkey, PCs were rapidly activated with latencies shorter than those of the accompanying slow eye movements. There was, however, no activation when the monkey suppressed the initiation of the slow eye movement by fixation. We interpreted these results to indicate that floccular PCs transmit rather a motor command signal (acceleration and velocity) than a visual motion signal (Waespe et al, 1985a). Similarly, after BVN we failed to find cells in the MVN which were responsive to retinal slip and carried a "major" visual motion signal. Neuronal activity was strictly related to parameters of the oculomotor response. It could be argued that visual motion information is encoded only by PCs and their target cells when it is behaviourally relevant to the monkey. But in fact, modulation of PCs and of cells in the MVN after BVN was related to eye velocity and not retinal slip when monkey performed SP and OKN, even when slow eye movements did not match stimulus velocity. It seems, therefore, that retinal slip drive is disabled upstream from floccular PCs (in contrast to vermal PCs, see Suzuki and Keller, 1988). Floccular PCs are rather situated within the "oculomotor driving circuit", i.e. whenever PCs are activated during SP and OKN, there will necessarily be a corresponding eye tracking movement. As mentioned in the Introduction, this is not true when the

234

optokinetic stimulus is stopped in the light and OKAN is rapidly suppressed.

In conclusion, we have difficulty in reconciling the seemingly low number of vestibular nuclei neurones on which floccular PCs could exert their main oculomotor control functions, either in normal monkey or after BVN, with the histologically demonstrated dense projection of the flocculus to the vestibular nuclei (Langer et al., 1985b). Many of the floccular PCs could naturally be involved in the regulation of functions other than oculomotor. However, bilateral (para)floccular lesions have minimal or no effect on postural control and the coordination of limb movements (Waespe, unpublished data). Presently, we can offer no simple solution to our dilemma, because, on experimental grounds, we assume that: (i) PCs exert an inhibitory control on their target cells; and (ii) the primate flocculus projects to the vestibular nuclei only (and the Y-group and a cell group called the basal interstitial nucleus of the cerebellum (Langer, 1985; Langer et al., 1985b)). To (i) the most densely labelled region after injections of anterograde tracer substances into the primate flocculus is the medial part of the MVN and the border zone between the MVN and the prepositus hypoglossi nucleus (see Fig. 2 in Langer et al., 1985b). Almost half of the neurones in this region (after BVN) are of the eI-type, i.e. they show increased activity for eye positions and velocities to the ipsilateral side like most of the horizontal gaze-velocity PCs. This region is believed to contain cells of the horizontal "eye position integrator" (Cannon and Robinson, 1987). If floccular PCs (or at least some) could also exert an excitatory action upon their target cells, our dilemma would be lessened. It would imply that floccular PCs directly contact cells of the "integrator" region. To (ii) the boundaries of the primate flocculus are rather uncertain. According to the atlas of Madigan and Carpenter (1971), which neurophysiologists usually use, the primate flocculus consists of 10 folia. Other authors, however, restrict the primate flocculus to 5 folia (folia 1 – 5; Larsell, 1970; Brodal and Brodal, 1985; Gerrits and Voogd, 1987). Un-

fortunately, in monkeys the sites of floccular recordings were not precisely located, so that one cannot exclude that "floccular" single cell studies also included a region containing folia 5 – 10. These belong, according to the latter authors, to the ventral paraflocculus. As anatomically it is not clear if the ventral paraflocculus receives a vestibular MF input or not (for discussion see Brodal, 1981), it is important to note that the flocculus-paraflocculus region where gaze-velocity PCs were recorded contained vestibular MF activity. The ventral paraflocculus, which corresponds to the tonsil in humans, projects to the dentate nucleus (Brodal, 1981). Thus, it could be that horizontal gaze velocity PCs project to structures other than the vestibular complex.

Acknowledgement

Supported by a grant from the Swiss National Foundation (3.510 – 0.86)

References

Boyle, R., Büttner, U. and Makert, G. (1985) Vestibular nuclei activity and eye movements in the alert monkey during sinusoidal optokinetic stimulation. *Exp. Brain Res.*, 57: 362 – 369.

Brodal, A. (1981) *Neurological Anatomy, 3rd Edn.* Oxford Press, New York, Oxford.

Brodal, A. and Brodal, P. (1985) Observations on the secondary vestibulocerebellar projections in the macaque monkey. *Exp. Brain Res.*, 58: 62 – 74.

Buettner, U. and Büttner, U. (1979) Vestibular nuclei activity in the alert monkey during suppression of vestibular and optokinetic nystagmus. *Exp. Brain Res.*, 37: 581 – 593.

Büttner, U. and Waespe, W. (1981) Vestibular nerve activity in the alert monkey during vestibular and optokinetic nystagmus. *Exp. Brain Res.*, 41: 310 – 315.

Büttner, U. and Waespe, W. (1984) Purkinje cell activity in the primate flocculus during optokinetic stimulation, smooth pursuit eye movements and VOR-suppression. *Exp. Brain Res.*, 55: 197 – 204.

Cannon, S.C. and Robinson, D.A. (1987) Loss of the neural integrator of the oculomotor system from brain stem lesions in monkey. *J. Neurophysiol.*, 57: 1383 – 1409.

Cohen, B., Uemura, T. and Takemori, S. (1973) Effects of labyrinthectomy on optokinetic nystagmus (OKN) and optokinetic after-nystagmus (OKAN). *Equilibrium Res.,* 3: 88 – 93.

Collewijn, H. (1976) Impairment of optokinetic (after-) nystagmus by labyrinthectomy in the rabbit. *Exp. Neurol.,* 52: 146 – 156.

Eccles, J.C., Ito, M. and Szentagothai, J. (1967) *The Cerebellum as a Neuronal Machine.* Springer, Berlin, Heidelberg, New York.

Fuchs, A.F. and Kimm, J. (1975) Unit activity in vestibular nucleus of the alert monkey during horizontal angular acceleration and eye movement. *J. Neurophysiol.,* 38: 1140 – 1161.

Gerrits, N.M. and Voogd, J. (1987) The topographical organization of climbing and mossy fiber afferents in the flocculus and the ventral paraflocculus in rabbit, cat and monkey. Abstr. presented at the *Symposium on Olivocerebellar system in motor control,* Turin.

Hess, B.J.M., Savio, T. and Strata, P. (1988) Dynamic characteristics of optokinetically controlled eye movements following inferior olive lesions in the brown rat. *J. Physiol. (London),* 397: 349 – 370.

Holmes, G. (1939) The cerebellum of man. *Brain,* 62: 1 – 30.

Ito, M. (1972) Neural design of the cerebellar motor control system. *Brain Res.,* 40: 81 – 84.

Ito, M. (1982) Cerebellar control of the vestibulo-ocular reflex- Around the flocculus hypothesis. *Ann. Rev. Neurosci.,* 5: 275 – 296.

Ito, M. (1984) *The Cerebellum and Neural Control.* Raven Press, New York.

King, W.M., Lisberger, S.G. and Fuchs, A.F. (1976) Responses of fibers in medial longitudinal fasciculus (MLF) of alert monkeys during horizontal and vertical conjugate eye movements evoked by vestibular or visual stimuli. *J. Neurophysiol.,* 39: 1135 – 1149.

Langer, T.P. (1985) Basal interstitial nucleus of the cerebellum: Cerebellar nucleus related to the flocculus. *J. Comp. Neurol.,* 235: 38 – 47.

Langer, T., Fuchs, A.F., Scudder, C.A. and Chubb, M.C. (1985a) Afferents to the flocculus of the cerebellum in the Rhesus macaque as revealed by retrograde transport of horseradish peroxidase. *J. Comp. Neurol.,* 235: 1 – 25.

Langer, T., Fuchs, A.F., Chubb, M.C., Scudder, C.A. and Lisberger, S.G. (1985b) Floccular efferents in the rhesus macaque as revealed by autoradiography and horseradish peroxidase. *J. Comp. Neurol.,* 235: 26 – 37.

Larsell, O. (1970) *The Comparative Anatomy and Histology of the Cerebellum from Monotremes Through Apes.* Univ. of Minnesota Press, Minneapolis.

Lisberger, S.G. (1988) The neural basis for motor learning in the vestibulooocular reflex in monkeys. *Trends Neurosci.,* 11: 147 – 152.

Lisberger, S.G. and Fuchs, A.F. (1978) Role of primate flocculus during rapid behavioral modification of vestibulo- ocular reflex. I. Purkinje cell activity during visually guided horizontal smooth-pursuit eye movement and passive head rotation. *J. Neurophsyiol.,* 41: 733 – 763.

Lisberger, S.G. and Miles, F.A. (1980) Role of primate medial vestibular nucleus in long-term adaptive plasticity of vestibuloocular reflex. *J. Neurophysiol.,* 43: 1725 – 1745.

Madigan, J.C. and Carpenter, M.B. (1971) *Cerebellum of the Rhesus Monkey.* University Park Press, Baltimore, London, Tokyo.

MacKay, W.A. and Murphy, J.T. (1979) Cerebellar modulation of reflex gain. *Prog. Neurobiol.,* 13: 361 – 417.

Miles, F.A., Fuller, J.H., Braitman, D.J. and Dow, B.M. (1980) Long-term adaptive changes in primate vestibulo- ocular reflex. III. Electrophysiological observations in flocculus of normal monkey. *J. Neurophysiol.,* 43: 1437 – 1476.

Miyashita, Y. and Nagao, S. (1984) Analysis of signal content of Purkinje cell responses to optokinetic stimuli in the rabbit cerebellar flocculus by selective lesions of brainstem pathways. *Neurosci. Res.,* 1: 223 – 241.

Robinson, D.A. (1981) Control of eye movements. In V.B. Brooks (Ed.), *Handbook of Physiology, The Nervous System., Vol II, Part 2.,* Williams and Wilkins, Baltimore, pp. 1275 – 1320.

Suzuki, D.A. and Keller, E.L. (1988) The role of the posterior vermis of monkey cerebellum in smooth-pursuit eye move- ment control. II. Target velocity-related Purkinje cell activi- ty. *J. Neurophysiol.,* 59: 19 – 40.

Tomlinson, R.D. and Robinson, D.A. (1984) Signals in vestibular nucleus mediating vertical eye movements in the monkey. *J. Neurophysiol.,* 51: 1121 – 1136.

Waespe, W. and Henn, V. (1977a) Neuronal activity in the vestibular nuclei of the alert monkey during vestibular and optokinetic stimulation. *Exp. Brain Res.,* 27: 523 – 538.

Waespe, W. and Henn, V. (1977b) Vestibular nuclei activity during optokinetic after-nystagmus (OKAN) in the alert monkey. *Exp. Brain Res.,* 30: 323 – 330.

Waespe, W. and Henn, V. (1978) Conflicting visual-vestibular stimulation and vestibular nucleus activity in alert monkey. *Exp. Brain Res.,* 33: 203 – 211.

Waespe, W. and Henn, V. (1979a) The velocity response of vestibular nucleus neurons during vestibular, visual, and combined angular acceleration. *Exp. Brain Res.,* 37: 337 – 347.

Waespe, W. and Henn, V. (1979b) Motion information in the vestibular nuclei of alert monkeys: Visual and vestibular in- put vs optomotor output. *Prog. Brain Res.,* 50: 683 – 693.

Waespe, W. and Henn, V. (1981) Visual-vestibular interaction in the flocculus of the alert monkey. II. Purkinje cell activity. *Exp. Brain Res.,* 43: 349 – 360.

Waespe, W. and Wolfensberger, W. (1985) Optokinetic nystagmus (OKN) and optokinetic after-responses after bilateral vestibular neurectomy in the monkey. *Exp. Brain Res.,* 60: 263 – 269.

Waespe, W. and Martin, P. (1987) Pursuit eye movements in a patient with a lesion involving the vestibular nuclear complex. *Neuro-Ophthalmology,* 7: 195 – 202.

Waespe, W., Henn, V. and Miles, T.S. (1977) Activity in the vestibular nuclei of the alert monkey during spontaneous eye movements and vestibular or optokinetic stimulation. In R. Baker and A. Berthoz (Eds.), *Control of Gaze by Brain Stem Neurons, Dev. Neurosci. Vol.* 1: 269 – 278.

Waespe, W., Büttner, U. and Henn, V. (1981) Visual-vestibular interaction in the flocculus of the alert monkey. I. Input activity. *Exp. Brain Res.,* 43: 337 – 348.

Waespe, W., Cohen, B. and Raphan, T. (1983) Role of the flocculus and paraflocculus in optokinetic nystagmus and visual-vestibular interactions: Effects of lesions. *Exp. Brain Res.,* 50: 9 – 33.

Waespe, W., Rudinger, D. and Wolfensberger, W. (1985a) Purkinje cell activity in the flocculus of vestibular neurectomized and normal monkeys during optokinetic nystagmus (OKN) and smooth pursuit movements. *Exp. Brain Res.,* 60: 243 – 262.

Waespe, W., Cohen, B. and Raphan, T. (1985b) Dynamic modification of the vestibulo-ocular reflex by the nodulus and uvula. *Science,* 228: 199 – 202.

SECTION III

Spinal Integration

J.H.J. Allum and M. Hulliger (Eds.)
Progress in Brain Research, Vol. 80
© 1989 Elsevier Science Publishers B.V. (Biomedical Division)

Overview and critique of Chapters 20 and 21

A. Taylor

London, England

Amjad et al.

Notwithstanding its title this paper is an outline presentation of some of the methods of statistical signal analysis applicable to the study of neural connections. Its main message is that though frequency domain manipulations are mostly mathematically interchangeable with the better known time domain ones, the former may nevertheless have some important practical advantages. It is intended to demonstrate that analysis of neural connections would benefit considerably from a combined frequency/time domain approach.

The authors constitute a group of workers well-respected for their ability to implement these methods and one presumes that the underlying purpose of the paper is to encourage the use of their skills amongst neurophysiologists. In the reviewer's opinion it is not likely to be entirely successful in this for two reasons. First, the theoretical explanations are too incomplete to instruct the novice, but through the use of unduly laborious and unmemorable symbolism act as a barrier to understanding the new and important material. Second, the examples chosen to illustrate the advantages of the methods do not seem to be worth so much sophisticated effort. These two criticisms will be expanded below, hopefully in constructive style and followed by the expression of some very positive views of the importance of the authors' work to modern neurophysiology.

A. Theoretical explanations

Within the space available one could not expect to have provided formal derivations of the mathematical theory required for neuronal signal analysis. The reader is indeed referred to some of the most appropriate sources, but then instead of simply listing the relations to be used in compact form for ease of reference, the authors make some attempts at basic definitions and derivations which take up much space, perhaps better devoted either to practical considerations or to quantitative demonstrations of the relative advantages of the different methods. The basic problem here seems to be that what is intended as an explanation often makes things more difficult for at least one reader. For example, it does not help to be told that cross-correlation, usually approximated by the cross-correlation histogram, when properly normalized, can be interpreted as the joint probability of occurrence of the times of spikes in one train separated by a time u from spikes in a second train. This is followed by the bald statement that " . . . in the frequency domain the correlation between the Fourier transforms of the individual spike trains provides an alternative measure of the strength of the association between them to that estimated by the cross-correlation histogram." No help is given in visualizing what is meant by the correlation between Fourier transforms of the individual spike trains. Most workers with some background in signal analysis understand the relationship between a regularly sampled function of time, its autocorrelation function and its Fourier transform and the extensions of these to two different functions. What is difficult to grasp is how one makes the transition, both theoretically and practically, from these to their equivalents for point processes. If this could be explained in straightforward practical terms, the need for much of the remaining formal introduction would disappear and more space could have been given to the important problems for example of deducing confidence levels of estimates.

The explanations tend to be couched in unnecessarily obscure mathematical jargon, which makes the work difficult to read. One can see that the authors feel compelled to be mathematically exact so as to avoid errors which have apparently arisen in some recent physiological interpretations of the methods, but for the rigorous explanations one would have to consult the original sources in any case. For example, in introducing stochastic point processes, after an unhelpful preliminary definition we are invited to "let $\{\tau \mathrm{j}\}$ $(j = 1, 2, \ldots)$ represent the set of the times of the occurrences of the spikes in a sample from the spike train N, the counting measure $N(t)$ gives the number of spikes between time 0 and time t and can be written as: $N(t) = \# \{\tau \mathrm{j}, 0 < \tau \mathrm{j} \leqslant t\}$ where $\# \{ \}$ denotes the number of events (spikes) in the interval $(0, t]$." The reader may struggle with the five new variable names and the significance of three types of brackets and four implied mathematical operators and still not know what has been achieved beyond agreeing to represent the number of spikes up to time t by $N(t)$. In any case, none of this explanation is necessary to what follows, so the struggle was pointless.

Another example of the redundant explanation is the third paragraph under "Stochastic point process parameters". There seems no reason why the assumption of stationarity in practice should depend on the arbitrariness of the choice of origin. In the lines which follow also, the laborious statement regarding the long range independence in a point process is unnecessarily burdened with algebra which is difficult to reconcile with the previous definitions, referring as it does to "the number of events in the *interval* (sic) $\mathrm{d}N(t + u)$."

As the theme develops, more and more defini-

tions and arbitrary symbols are introduced, which may be desirable for mathematical rigour, but seem to be unduly hostile to the non-expert. Where symbolism is necessary, could it not be made more acceptable by making choices with some phonetic relation to the variable, parameter or operation names represented. Why choose λ for frequency when its use for wavelength is so well established and f and ω are commonly used for cyclic and angular frequency? Is the Fourier transform not more generally and obviously represented by bold or italic upper case F?

B. The examples of applications

The reviewer must admit to a sympathy with the philosophy by which methods are devised to solve problems, rather than problems found to utilize methods. From this biased standpoint it is difficult to be impressed with the examples presented here. They are concerned with interactions between the firing of muscle spindle Ia afferents and α motoneurones. The effects of Ia afferents on α motoneurones are probably the most extensively studied of synaptic mechanisms. The need to know the distribution and detailed properties of individual Ia synapses led Mendell and Henneman to devise the since widely-used spike-triggered averaging method. This has probably been pressed to the limit of its useful sensitivity in detecting mono- and disynaptic connections with the summation of very large numbers of responses. It would be valuable to know if the frequency domain methods would be more efficient in this respect either from the point of view of obtaining greater significance with less data or of estimating properties such as latency with greater objectivity. The authors chose rather to look for interaction of pairs of Ia afferents on a motoneurone or of pairs of motor units on the firing of a Ia afferent. It has not yet been made apparent why details of this kind are likely to be important physiologically and are not merely epiphenomena. It is certainly very difficult to see how such data could ever be synthesized to predict the effect of these detailed interactions on the feedback functions of the muscle spindle.

It could be argued that these are merely illustrative examples to show the versatility of the methods. In this case a useful purpose in supporting the cause of frequency domain methods might have been served if there had been presented a specific comparison of frequency and time domain processing.

C. The way forward

Having been mainly negative in the views expressed above it is only fair to point out that the authors do in fact offer some very important prospects for advance in statistical data processing. Their virtuosity in applying such methods will make it possible for more workers to rapidly gain experience and to determine which processes are most useful for each type of problem. Specifically the possibilities of handling more than two spike trains using frequency domain methods could be very significant, though the interpretation of results will present formidable problems. Plotting the regression of phase upon frequency as a means of objectively estimating latency objectively also could be valuable, though no consideration was given to the problems of distinguishing a "transport delay" from a region of relatively linear phase/frequency plot often occurring in dynamic systems without such a delay. Probably the most interesting technique of all which sets frequency domain methods apart from time domain methods is the extraction of partial coherence. By this means it is possible to deduce whether covariation of two spike trains is due to a cause and effect relationship or rather to a common influence of a third process. A problem which could arise is that the theoretical basis for this separation appears to require conditions of linearity. It is not made clear in this paper whether there is a way around such difficulties.

In summary, through its subject matter this paper deserves to be influential. Its contribution may be considerable, but only if readers are already very mathematically expert, or are prepared to take the time to study the original literature in depth.

Eken et al.

The second paper deals with the possible functions of transmitter-controlled plateau potentials in α-motoneurones.

It has been convenient in the past to assume for the mammalian α motoneurone rather simple membrane properties by which excitatory and inhibitory postsynaptic currents can summate linearly to give a firing frequency reflecting the net inward synaptic current (see Granit et al., 1966). Such a simple assumption was undoubtedly valid in studies of the effects of intracellularly injected currents and of simple reflex inputs in anaesthetized or spinalized cats (for review see Granit, 1970) and this result was eagerly embraced by those hoping to apply linear systems analysis theory to motor control. In these terms (see e.g. Houk et al., 1970; Taylor, 1972) the motoneurone could be regarded as a "summing junction" for excitatory and inhibitory feedback pathways with descending command signals. One weakness of this approach was first indicated by the experiments of Hultborn and his collaborators commencing 14 years ago (Hultborn et al., 1975) and now reviewed and extended in the present paper. In the earlier work (reviewed by Hultborn and Wigström, 1980) it was discovered that a brief barrage of Ia input, which in the anaesthetized or spinal preparation caused the expected short lasting reflex response, in decerebrate cats caused the onset of a long-maintained firing of motoneurones which could be brought to an end by cutaneous nerve stimulation. The mechanism for the effect was evidently in the spinal cord, but supported by some facilitation from the brain stem, because it could also be demonstrated in spinal animals treated with precursors of 5-HT or noradrenaline. The most likely mechanism was argued at this time to be a prolonged excitatory synaptic bombardment of the motoneurones from a reverberating network of interneurones. In accordance with this, intracellular recordings showed prolonged depolarization and an appearance of greatly increased synaptic noise.

Subsequently the views expressed regarding the

242

origin of the prolonged motoneurone excitation have changed, with the emphasis now on an intrinsic motoneurone membrane property. A new look at the phenomenon was evidently stimulated by a series of papers by Schwindt and Crill (1980a,b,c), analysing persistent inward currents in cat motoneurones. Hultborn and his collaborators now find that a prolonged excitation, apparently the same as that previously produced by a Ia barrage, can also be induced at the single cell level by current injection, so effectively eliminating the original proposal for a reverberating network. This phenomenon also requires a background of serotonergic facilitation. Accordingly it is now referred to as "transmitter-controlled plateau potential" rather than the original "long latency autogenetic Ia excitation."

This is a most interesting development, with far-reaching implications. However, whatever this mechanism may prove to be, the prolonged excitatory effects have the same functional implications. Thus it is shown that in conscious animals tonic activity can be switched on by a brief excitatory afferent input and maintained without further effort till ended by an inhibitory input. Such a way of generating a motor output would be attractively economical, but it should be noted that it seems to be a bistable, non-graded effect whereas it was originally reported (Hultborn and Wigström, 1980) that it was "possible to maintain many levels of activity (its excited state is graded)". In this connection it is surprising that such bistable firing behaviour of motor units in chronic EMG recordings has not previously been reported.

An attractive feature of the original proposals which now seems to have been lost sight of is the integrating property of the mechanism. By this one could expect that the output could increase continuously as long as an excitatory input occurred but was then held at whatever level had been reached at the end of the input. This behaviour as an integrator with respect to time does not now seem to be available if only two stable firing rates exist. If, however, on further investigation, the originally described graded behaviour can be demonstrated,

then the possibility of the existence in other situations (such as the vestibulo-ocular reflex pathway) of such a mechanism should be carefully considered.

A surprising feature of the intracellular recordings in the present as in the earlier work, is the very large amplitude membrane noise. On the basis of the earlier theory of reverberating circuits, this could easily be explained as synaptic noise. Now, however, since it can be evoked by current injection it must represent current channel noise. The channels must be relatively very large to produce such gross irregularities. Detailed study of this aspect might be rewarding.

Finally, one is led to wonder whether the plateau potentials are restricted to S type motoneurones, because the resulting prolonged tonic discharges would not seem appropriate for FF or FR units.

References

Granit, R. (1970) *The Basis of Motor Control.* Academic Press, London, pp. 346.
Granit, R., Kernell, D. and Lamarre, Y. (1966) Algebraical summation in synaptic activation of motoneurones firing within the "primary range" to injected currents. *J. Physiol. (London),* 187: 379–399.
Houk, J.C., Singer, J.K. and Goldman, M.R. (1970) An evaluation of length and force feedback to soleus muscles of decerebrate cats. *J. Neurophysiol.,* 33: 784–811.
Hultborn, H. and Wigström, H. (1980) Motor response with long latency and maintained duration evoked by activity in Ia afferents. In J.E. Desmedt (Ed.), *Spinal and Supraspinal Mechanisms of Voluntary Motor Control and Locomotion,* Karger, Basel, pp. 99–116.
Hultborn, H., Wigström, H. and Wangberg, B. (1975) Prolonged activation of soleus motoneurones following a conditioning train in soleus Ia afferents — a case for reverberating loop? *Neurosci. Lett.,* 1: 147–152.
Schwindt, P. and Crill, W. (1980a) Role of persistent inward current in motoneuron bursting during spinal seizures. *J. Neurophysiol.,* 43: 1296–1318.
Schwindt, P. and Crill, W.E. (1980b) Effects of barium on cat spinal motoneurons studies by voltage clamp. *J. Neurophysiol.,* 44: 827–846.
Schwindt, P. and Crill, W.E. (1980c) Properties of a persistent inward current in normal and TEA-injected motoneurons. *J. Neurophysiol.,* 43: 1700–1724.
Taylor, A. (1972) Muscle receptors in the control of movement. *Paraplegia,* 9: 167–172.

J.H.J. Allum and M. Hulliger (Eds.)
Progress in Brain Research, Vol. 80
© 1989 Elsevier Science Publishers B.V. (Biomedical Division)

CHAPTER 20

A framework for the analysis of neuronal networks

A.M. Amjad, P. Breeze, B.A. Conway, D.M. Halliday and J.R. Rosenberg

Departments of Physiology and Statistics, University of Glasgow, Glasgow G12 8QQ, Scotland, U.K.

The object of this work is to consider the application of some methods of spike train analysis that are not widely known, and are concerned with the description of the interactions between spike trains and the determination of causal connections between them. The notation and terminology follow conventions established in the statistical literature. The examples given are based on in-continuity recordings of the spontaneous activity of single Ia afferents from the soleus muscle and single motor units from the same muscle. Cumulant densities are shown to be simple extensions of the traditional cross-correlation methods, and are useful in characterizing the pattern of activity in one spike train that influences that in another, and to reveal interactions between spike trains that would not be apparent from the correlation histogram alone. Parameters based on the Fourier transforms of the spike trains are shown to be useful in determining timing relations between them, and in inferring patterns of connectivity not possible by correlation methods alone.

Key words: Correlation; Coherence; Fourier analysis; Ia afferent; Motor unit; Neuronal network; Partial coherence; Partial spectrum; Point process; Spike train

Introduction

The most widely used approach to describe functional coupling or interactions between neuronal spike trains is that based on cross-correlation methods (some recent examples include Bryant et al., 1973; Ellaway and Murthy, 1985; Michalski et al., 1983; Toyama et al., 1981a,b). This method of analysis follows from a consideration of the correlation between the time of spikes in one train with those in a second displaced in time by a variable interval u. This correlation is usually approximated by the cross-correlation histogram, which, when properly normalized, can be interpreted as the joint probability of occurrence of the times of spikes in one train separated by a time u from spikes in a second train. In physiological terms the cross-correlation histogram counts the number of spikes that occur in a given neurone with some fixed delay (u) relative to those recorded from another neurone.

Alternatively, one may approach the problem of characterizing coupling between neurones by considering the correlation between a derived function of the times of occurrence of the spikes in the trains. For example, in the frequency domain the correlation between the Fourier transforms of the individual spike trains provides an alternative measure of the strength of association between them to that estimated by the cross-correlation histogram. In addition, the application of the Fourier transform to spike train data provides the basis for types of analyses involving three or more spike trains which are not possible by the traditional cross-correlation methods alone.

There are, therefore, two complementary methods for the analysis of neuronal interactions — one group of measures based on the correlation between the times of occurrence of events in different spike trains, and one based on the correlation between the frequency components in the different spike trains. The former are examples of time-domain methods, whereas the latter are known as Fourier or frequency domain-methods. It is often assumed that because these methods are, in some sense, mathematically equivalent, one need only use one of the methods, and, consequently, because of their widespread familiarity time-domain methods are used almost exclusively. However, since one is working with finite amounts of data the estimates of the time domain parameters may not represent or emphasize features of the data in exactly the same way as the corresponding estimates in the frequency-domain (for examples see Rosenberg et al., 1983; Rosenberg and Rigas, 1985).

The object of the present report, therefore, is to demonstrate that time- and frequency-domain methods taken together provide a powerful collection of analysis techniques, and that a detailed examination of neuronal interactions would benefit considerably from a combined time/frequency approach. Three questions associated with the analysis of neuronal networks will be discussed: (1) the assessment of the importance of pattern of neuronal activity in one cell in influencing the response of a second cell, (2) the characterization of the interaction between neuronal spike trains, and (3) the determination of the influence that one or several spike trains may have on the activity in another spike train or on a number of other spike trains. The presentation will emphasize methodological considerations and is based on some extensions of the familiar cross-correlation methods, and the introduction of some novel frequency-domain techniques. The presentation is formulated within the mathematical framework of the theory of stochastic point processes (Cox and Isham, 1980; Cox and Lewis, 1968, 1972). Our notation and terminology follows the conventions established in the statistical literature (e.g. Brillinger, 1972; Cox and Lewis, 1972). Derivations of some of the mathematical expressions which are listed and

discussed below will be found in Rosenberg et al. (1989). The examples are taken from both real and model generated data with the analysis procedures concentrating on extracting features of the data not necessarily available to the simple correlation methods commonly in use. However the detailed physiological implications of the experimental data presented cannot be discussed in the space available.

Stochastic point process parameters

The subsequent analytical work is based entirely on the relations between the sequences of the times of occurrence of the extracellularly recorded action potentials from several spike trains. From this point of view a spike train can be represented as the mathematical object known as a stochastic point process, which considers the properties of events occurring in some random but prescribed manner in time.

We therefore begin by setting down some definitions of the parameters that are used to characterize stochastic point processes. If we let $\{\tau_j\}$ $(j = 1, 2, \ldots)$ represent the set of the times of occurrence of the spikes in a sample from the spike train N, the counting measure $N(t)$ gives the number of spikes between time 0 and time t, and can be written as

$$N(t) = \# \{\tau j, 0 < \tau j \leqslant t\}$$

where $\# \{ \}$ denotes the number of events (spikes) in the interval $(0, t]$.

Differential increments of the process N, $dN(t)$, are useful in defining certain point process parameters, (e.g., Eqn. 5 below), and are defined as

$$dN(t) = N(t + dt) - N(t) = N(t, t + dt]$$

where $dN(t)$ gives the number of events in a small interval of time dt.

The mean intensity, P_N, of a point process is defined as

$$P_N = \lim_{h \to 0} \text{Prob} \{N \text{ point in } (t, t + h]\}/h \qquad (1)$$

where h is a small interval of time.

Since the choice of the origin for the measurement of spike times is arbitrary, the process N is assumed to be stationary. This assumption implies that the properties of the process are independent of the time at which the process is observed. It is also assumed that increments of the process N well separated in time are independent, i.e. for u large the number of events in the interval $dN(t + u)$ is independent of the number of events in the interval $dN(t)$, and finally it is also assumed that points of the process N do not occur simultaneously. A full discussion of these assumptions may be found in Cox and Isham (1980) and Cox and Lewis (1972).

Consider now two points processes (e.g., spike trains). The second-order cross-product density at lag u between processes N and M, $P_{NM}(u)$, is defined as

$$P_{NM}(u) = \lim_{h' \to 0} \text{Prob } \{N \text{ point in } (t+u, \ t+u+h] \\ \text{and } M \text{ point in } (t, \ t + h']\}/hh' \quad (2)$$

The cross-product density is usually estimated by a histogram referred to in the neurophysiological literature as the cross-correlation histogram or in the case of stimulus driven processes as the pre- and post-stimulus time histogram or the peristimulus time histogram. Estimation procedures for product densities have been discussed by Cox (1965) and Brillinger (1976), where methods for setting confidence intervals are given.

In addition, a conditional intensity may be defined as

$$m_{NM}(u) = \lim_{h \to 0} \text{Prob } \{N \text{ point in } (t+u, \ t+u+h] \\ \text{given an } M \text{ point at } t\}/h \quad (3)$$

and also written as

$$m_{NM}(u) = \frac{P_{NM}(u)}{P_M} \quad (4)$$

The cross-product density and conditional intensity provide useful measures of association between two processes.

If $\{\tau_j\}$ is the set of spike times for the sample of process N corresponding to the period of observation T, the empirical Fourier transform of this sample is defined as

$$d_N^T(\lambda) = \int_0^T e^{-i\lambda t} \, dN(t) = \sum_j e^{-i\gamma\tau_j} \quad (5)$$

where $i = \sqrt{-1}$ and λ is frequency.

The cross-spectrum between processes N and M may then be defined as

$$f_{NM}(\lambda) = \frac{1}{2\pi T} \lim_{T \to \infty} E \left\{ d_N^T(\lambda) \ \overline{d_M^T(\lambda)} \right\} \quad (6)$$

where E{ } denotes mathematical expectation and the overbar "——" complex conjugate (Bartlett, 1963; Brillinger, 1972). The auto-spectrum of process N may be obtained by replacing M by N in Expression 6. The cross-spectrum may be interpreted as the covariance between the components at frequency λ of the processes N and M. Various estimation procedures for point process spectra have been summarized in Halliday (1986), Rosenberg et al. (1983) and Rigas (1983).

Experimental methods

The experimental data, obtained from decerebrated cats, is derived from single motor unit recordings from soleus and lateral gastrocnemius muscles, and from single Ia afferents from the same muscles recorded in continuity with the spinal cord. The spike trains from the motor units and Ia afferents were digitized and stored in computer files as the ordered times of occurrences of the pulses. The duration of the recordings varied from one to three minutes.

Applications of cumulant densities

The cross-product density of order-2 defined by Expression 2 may be extended to examine the interaction between three processes. For example, given the three processes, N_1, N_2, N_3 with lags u,v as indicated in Fig. 1, the product density of order-3 may be defined as

$$P_{N_1 N_2 N_3}(u, v) = \lim_{h_1, h_2, h_3 \to 0} \text{Prob } \{N_1 \text{ point in}$$
$$(t+u,\ t+u+h_1] \text{ and } N_2 \text{ point in}$$
$$(t+v,\ t+v+h_2] \text{ and } N_3 \text{ point in}$$
$$(t,\ t+h_3]\}/h_1, h_2, h_3 \qquad (7)$$

The information contained in the third-order product density may be seen to be similar to that obtained by using the conditional-test pulse experimental paradigm. Estimation procedures and approximate confidence intervals for third-order product densities are discussed in Brillinger (1975a), Halliday (1986) and Rigas (1983), with further examples given by Abeles (1983), Gerstein and Perkel (1972), Rosenberg et al., (1983) and Windhorst and Schwestka (1982).

As we shall see in the following examples, when describing how the pattern of spike times in one train or the interaction between two spike trains may affect the activity in another process the third-order product density may be misleading. The second-order product density is based on counting the number of pairs of spikes separated by a time u. Third-order product densities, however, are based on counting the number of occurrences of various triplets of spike times, defined by the range of values of u,v (Fig. 1). When dealing with three spike trains, however, one must be careful in interpreting the third-order product density. Triplets with particular spacings may occur when two of the processes are associated but independent of the third. Yet such cases all contribute to the estimated third-order product density.

Therefore, when assessing the importance of patterns of neuronal activity or interactions it is often better to use cumulant densities as measures of the joint statistical dependence of the times of occurrence of the spikes in the different trains. Cumulants for stochastic point processes are defined in Brillinger (1972). The third-order cumulant density, for example, may be thought of as pro-

viding a measure of the statistical dependency between three processes not accounted for by lower-order interactions, and may be written as

$$q_{N_1 N_2 N_3}(u, v) = P_{N_1 N_2 N_3}(u,v) - P_{N_1 N_2}(u-v)$$
$$P_{N_3} - P_{N_1 N_3}(u)P_{N_2} - P_{N_2 N_3}(v)P_{N_1}$$
$$+ 2 P_{N_1} P_{N_2} P_{N_3}, \quad u \neq v \qquad (8)$$

Expression 8 will be zero if the three processes are independent or if any one process is independent of the other two. Expression 8 also indicates explicitly how the third-order cumulant differs from the third-order product density by taking into account the lower-order contributions to the third-order product density. Note also, that the cumulant may take on both positive and negative values suggesting, in the correct physiological context, timing sequences where facilitatory or inhibitory interactions may occur.

Several third-order cumulants may be examined depending on the choice of N_1, N_2, N_3. If N_2 and N_3 are taken to be the same spike train, then one is led to considering how the spacing in one process, the N_2 process for example, influences the times of occurrence of spikes in a third process, the N_1 process.

If N_1, N_2 and N_3 are taken to be separate processes, then, for example, one may examine how the timing of events in process N_2 relative to those of N_3 affects the times of occurrence of events in process N_1.

An example where N_2 and N_3 are taken to be the same process is shown in Fig. 2. The elevated

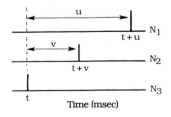

Fig. 1. Diagrammatic representation of the convention used to represent the relative times of occurrence of spikes from three processes N_1, N_2, and N_3.

region of Fig. 2a illustrates combinations of Ia interspike intervals that are effective in facilitating the discharge of the motor unit, i.e., leading to more motor unit spikes than would be expected on the basis of the summed independent effects of single Ia spikes. The region of significant facilitation is shown in more detail in the contour plot by the three cross-hatched peaks in Fig. 2b. The position of these peaks indicates that small changes in the spacing of the Ia afferent discharge relative to the motor unit discharge may be effective in facilitating this discharge.

A further example contrasting product density and cumulant density is illustrated in Fig. 3 which describes how the interaction between the activity from two motor units alters the response of a Ia afferent. Fig. 3a is an example of a third-order product density where the $u - v$ axis represents the time of the discharge of one of the motor units (α_1) prior to the Ia response, and the u axis gives the time of the discharge of the second motor unit (α_2) relative to the Ia response. This product density suggests regions where there may be an interaction between the discharge from the two motor units and the Ia response. One of these regions cor-

responds to the area around the main diagonal where $u - v$ does not differ greatly from u, and where the two motor units are firing nearly synchronously. The other two are represented by the elevated regions away from the main diagonal. Points to the left of the diagonal correspond to α_1 firing prior to α_2, whereas, for points to the right of the diagonal α_2 precedes α_1. The inserts in Fig. 3a, which show the product density plotted for $u = 6$ and $u - v = 6$, are similar to the kind of figures used by Windhorst and Schwestka (1982) to represent the combined effects of the discharge of two motor units on the response of a single Ia afferent to independent stimulation of the two motor units.

The elevated region to the left of the main diagonal in Fig. 3a for $u - v$ large and u small appears to be an area where the interaction between the discharge of the two motor units influences the Ia response. However, the insert in Fig. 3a for $u = 6$ shows that only a few of the points lie outside the 95% confidence interval for the product density under the assumption of independence, whereas the insert for $u - v = 6$ shows that for u large all of the points lie outside the 95% con-

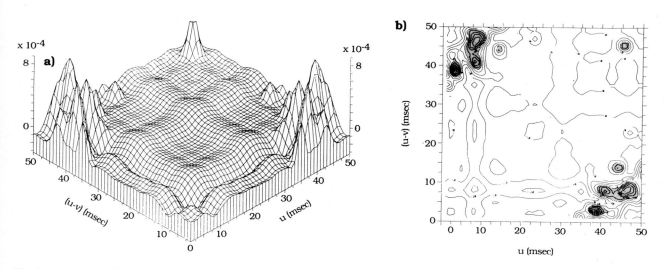

Fig. 2. a: estimated third-order cumulant, density where $u - v$ and u are the times of Ia spikes relative to the times of a motor unit spike. b: contour plot of the estimated third-order cumulant density in a illustrating the full pattern of interaction between Ia spike times and their effect on the motor unit discharge.

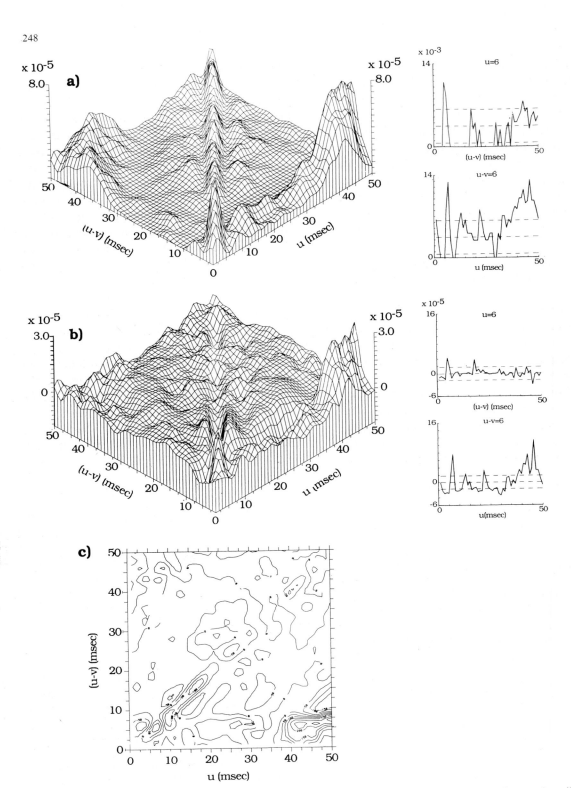

Fig. 3. Estimated third-order product density (a) and third-order cumulant density (b) where $u - v$ and u are the spike times from two different motor units relative to the time of occurrence of a Ia afferent spike. The inserts in (a) and (b) are for $u - v = 6$ and $u = 6$ and show the approximate 95% confidence interval (horizontal dashed lines) for the product density and cumulant density for these fixed values of $u - v$ and u, under the assumption that the two processes are independent. The inserts simply represent a single curve through the surface in a plane cutting the $(u - v)$, u plane at right angles at a fixed value of u or v. c: contour diagram corresponding to the cumulant density illustrated in b.

fidence interval, suggesting an interactive effect on the Ia discharge when α_2 precede α_1, but not in the reverse order. The cumulant (Fig. 3b), however, reveals more clearly the complexity of the pattern of interaction between the two motor units. First, the absence of symmetry with respect to the main diagonal confirms that the order of the discharge of the two motor units is an important feature of the interaction between their effects on the Ia response. Secondly, the insert for $u = 6$ indicates a significant decrease in the expected number of Ia spikes at $u - v = 46$, whereas the insert for $u - v = 6$ shows a significant increase in the number of Ia spikes at $u = 46$, therefore, a reversal in the order of the motor unit discharge, keeping their relative timing the same, reverses the effect of the interaction. Finally, points near the main diagonal trough in the cumulant suggest spindle unloading when the two motor units discharge nearly synchronously — a different conclusion might be drawn by examining the product density alone. The full details of the α_1/α_2 interaction are displayed in the contour plot of the cumulant (Fig. 3c). Note particularly for $u = 47$ ms, changing $u - v$ from 5 ms to 12 ms reverses the sign of the cumulant.

In the above two examples cumulants were used to extract significant patterns of activity from the spontaneously recorded discharge of single motor units and muscle spindle Ia afferents, but they may also be used to examine the interaction between the effects of stimulus driven activity on neuronal discharges. In addition, cumulants may be used to define the spectra of spike trains, giving an alternative definition to that of Expression 6. For example, the second-order cumulant between processes M and N is

$$q_{NM}(u) = P_{NM}(u) - P_N P_M \qquad (9)$$

and its Fourier transform defines the cross-spectrum between M and N as

$$f_{NM}(\lambda) = \frac{1}{2\pi} \int q_{NM}(u) \, e^{-i\lambda u} \, du \qquad M \neq N \quad (10)$$

The inverse relation

$$q_{NM}(u) = \int f_{NM}(\lambda) \, e^{i\lambda u} \, d\lambda \qquad M \neq N \quad (11)$$

along with Expression 10 shows explicitly the sense in which the time- and frequency-domain measures of association are mathematically equivalent. Spectra of higher-order are also defined as the Fourier transforms of the appropriate cumulants (Brillinger, 1972). We shall see however that mathematical equivalence does not imply an equivalent ability to display features of interest.

Applications of spectra

The time to the peak of the estimated cross-intensity is conventionally used to measure the latency between a stimulus and a response or the average delay between two processes. In systems whose behaviour is dominated by a delay the use of the cross-spectrum provides an alternative means of estimating latencies or delays. For example, suppose the process N is a delayed version of process M, then the set of spike times for N may be written as $\{\sigma_j + \tau\}$ where τ represents the time delay between the two processes, and $\{\sigma_j\}$ the set of spike times for process M. The cross-spectrum between N and M is

$$f_{NM}(\lambda) = e^{-i\lambda\tau} f_{NM}(\lambda) \qquad (12)$$

The phase, defined as the argument of the cross-spectrum, is then given as

$$\phi(\lambda) = -\lambda\tau \qquad (13)$$

If the relation between two processes is dominated by a delay, this delay may be estimated as the slope of the least squares line relating $\phi(\lambda)$ to λ, and elementary regression theory may then be used to estimate the standard error of the delay. Fig. 4 is an example of an application of the use of the cross-intensity and the phase to estimate the delay between two processes in a situation where the peak in the cross-intensity is particularly well defined. The time to the peak of the cross-intensity gives an estimated delay of approximately 7 ms. The delay estimated from the slope of the linear regression line is 6.68 ms with a 95% confidence interval of (6.56, 6.80). The method used to estimate the delay from the cross-intensity does not allow one to set a confidence interval for the estimate, and, therefore, limits the usefulness of this method. When the peak of the cross-intensity is broad and not well-defined it is better to estimate the delay between two processes as the slope of the fitted linear phase curve, which has the advantage of being based on more of the available data than the time of occurrence of a single point in the cross-intensity; particularly in cases where the peak of the cross-intensity is not well defined.

The frequency-domain measure of the strength of association between two spike trains is called the

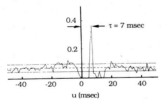

a) Sq-Rt. of cross intensity function

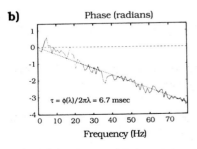

b)

Fig. 4. (a) The square-root of the estimated cross-intensity and (b) the estimated phase between a group I spike train from medial gastrocnemius and the response from a single motor unit in lateral gastrocnemius. The solid horizontal lines in a are the approximate 95% confidence intervals for the cross-intensity on the assumption that the two processes are independent. The dashed line in b is the least squares line fitted to the estimated phase curve.

coherence, denoted as $|R_{NM}(\lambda)|^2$, and defined as the magnitude squared of the correlation at frequency λ between the Fourier transforms of the two processes. The coherence may be expressed in terms of the finite Fourier transforms of the samples of spike trains N and M as

$$|R_{NM}(\lambda)|^2 = \lim_{T \to \infty} |\,\text{corr}\{\,d_N^T(\lambda), d_M^T(\lambda)\}\,|^2 \quad (14)$$

where "corr" denotes correlation. The coherence takes on values from 0 to 1, with 0 occurring when the two processes are independent. Development of Expression 14 indicates how the coherence may also be written in terms of the basic cross- and auto-spectra of the component processes as

$$|R_{NM}(\lambda)|^2 = \frac{|f_{NM}(\lambda)|^2}{f_{NN}(\lambda)f_{MM}(\lambda)} \quad (15)$$

The above method of defining the coherence may be extended to examine the question of how one or several processes may separately or together affect the strength of association and timing between two related processes. Suppose, for example, three processes, L, N_1, N_2, are pairwise correlated. Consider the question of deciding whether N_1 and N_2, for example, are directly connected, or if the observed correlation is simply the consequence of a common input L. This problem can be attacked by using an extension of the coherence called the partial coherence.

The partial coherence of order-1 may be defined as the coherence between processes N_1 and N_2 after removing the linear time invariant effects of process L from both N_1 and N_2 and, (suppressing the dependencies on λ), is written as

$$|R_{N_1 N_2 . L}|^2 = \lim_{T \to \infty} |\,\text{corr}$$
$$\left\{ d_{N_1}^T - \frac{f_{N_1 L}}{f_{LL}} d_L^T, d_{N_2}^T - \frac{f_{N_1 L}}{f_{LL}} d_L^T \right\}|^2 \quad (16)$$

The coefficients $f_{N_1 L}/f_{LL}$ and $f_{N_2 L}/f_{LL}$, where $f_{N_1 L}$, $f_{N_2 L}$, and f_{LL} are the basic cross- and auto-spectra of the component processes, give the best linear predictors of $d_{N_1}^T(\lambda)$ and $d_{N_2}^T(\lambda)$ in terms of $d_L^T(\lambda)$ for T large (Brillinger, 1983). The partial coherence takes on values between 0 and 1. If process L accounted entirely for the correlation between N_1 and N_2, one could expect the sample partial coherence to be close to zero. Partial coherences for point process data were introduced by Brillinger (1975b).

Expression 16 for the partial coherence of order-1 may be expanded in terms of ordinary coherences as

$$| R_{N_1 N_2 . L} (\lambda) |^2 =$$

$$\frac{| R_{N_1 N_2} (\lambda) - R_{N_1 L}(\lambda) R_{L N_2}(\lambda) |^2}{(1 - | R_{N_1 L} (\lambda) |^2) \, (1 - | R_{L N_2}(\lambda) |^2)} \qquad (17)$$

Expression 17 may, in turn, be further developed to give the partial coherences in terms of the cross-spectra and auto-spectra of the component processes. The partial coherence of order-1, suppressing the dependencies on λ, may then be written as

$$| R_{N_1 N_2 . L} |^2 = \frac{| f_{N_1 N_2 . L} |^2}{f_{N_1 N_1 . L} f_{N_2 N_2 . L}} \qquad (18)$$

where

$$f_{N_a N_b . L} = f_{N_a N_b} - \frac{f_{N_a L} f_{L N_b}}{f_{LL}} \qquad (19)$$

for a,b = 1,2.

Expression 19 defines partial cross-spectra and partial auto-spectra of order-1 for processes N_1 and N_2 taking into account the contribution of process L. Partial auto-spectra are useful in identifying the contribution that one process may make to another. The argument of the partial cross-spectrum, called the partial phase, may be used to examine how a third process affects the timing between two other processes.

Partial coherences and partial spectra of order-1 may be further generalized to provide descriptions of how several processes taken together may affect the strength of association and timing relation between two processes. For example, the partial coherence of order-2 between processes N_1 and N_2 taking into account the contribution from processes K and L may be written in terms of the partial coherences of order-1, after suppressing the dependencies on λ, as

$$| R_{N_1 N_2 . KL} |^2 =$$

$$\frac{| R_{N_1 N_2 . K} - R_{N_1 L . K} R_{L N_2 . K} |^2}{(1 - | R_{N_1 L . K} |^2) \quad (1 - | R_{L N_2 . K} |^2)} \qquad (20)$$

A simple extension of Expression 20 provides partial coherences of order-3 and higher, as well as the associated partial spectra. Once the basic cross-spectra and auto-spectra of the component processes have been estimated, the coherence, phase, partial coherences and partial phases of all orders may be estimated. Partial parameters for ordinary time series are discussed in Brillinger (1975c) and Jenkins and Watt (1968).

The following Figures illustrate applications of coherence, and partial spectra.

The computer generated data used in Fig. 5 was constructed so that in one case a periodic spike train at 20 Hz was delayed with respect to itself by approximately 10 ms. Both the reference and the delayed spike trains were superimposed on independent Poisson processes. A second pair of spike trains was generated with the same delay of 10 ms between them, but each at a frequency of 64 Hz and both superimposed on independent Poisson processes. The number of spikes from the pairs of periodic processes was small compared with the number of spikes used for the independent Poisson processes. As would be expected the estimated cross-intensities (Fig. 5a,b) for the two cases are the same, since the delay of 10 ms is common to both pairs of processes. The coherences, however, are different and provide the additional information that in one case the processes are coupled at 20 Hz (insert Fig. 5a) and in the other at 64 Hz (insert Fig. 5b). This example clearly illustrates how the coherence reveals the strength of association between two processes at a particular frequency. The application of partial coherence to real data is illustrated in Amjad et al. (1987) and in Brillinger et al. (1976).

The next two examples (Figs. 6 and 7) demonstrate how the partial auto-spectrum can be used to identify the contribution that one process may make to another process. In the first example (Fig. 6) the spontaneous activity of a single Ia afferent from the soleus muscle was recorded in continuity along with the spontaneous discharge of two motor units from the same muscle. The mean rate

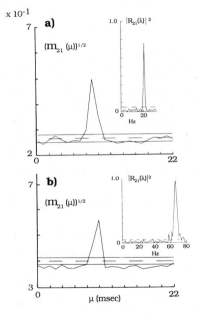

Fig. 5. Estimated cross-intensities and coherences (inserts) for computer generated spike trains consisting of a periodic process superimposed on a Poisson process, and a second periodic process of the same frequency as the first delayed by a fixed time and superimposed on a second independent Poisson process. In both a and b the periodic processes are delayed with respect to each other by approximately 10 ms, whereas in a the periodic process composed is at 20 Hz and in b at 64 Hz. The solid horizontal lines associated with the cross-intensities in a and b are the approximate 95% confidence intervals for the cross-intensities on the assumption that the two processes are independent. The horizontal dashed lines in the coherence plots are the approximate 95% confidence intervals for the coherence under the assumption that the two processes are independent.

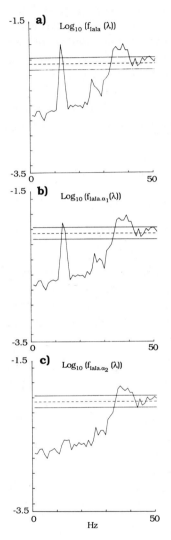

Fig. 6. a: the estimated auto-spectrum, $f_{\text{IaIa}}(\lambda)$, of a spontaneously discharging Ia afferent from lateral gastrocnemius recorded in continuity with the spinal cord in the presence of two spontaneously discharging motor units from the same muscle. b: first-order partial auto-spectrum of the Ia discharge taking into account the presence of the discharge of one of the motor units, $f_{\text{IaIa} \cdot \alpha_1}(\lambda)$. c: first-order partial auto-spectrum of the Ia discharge taking into account the presence of the discharge of the other motor unit, $f_{\text{IaIa} \cdot \alpha_2}(\lambda)$. Solid horizontal lines in a–c are approximate 95% confidence intervals for the auto-spectra.

of the Ia discharge was about 35 Hz, the two motor units were firing almost synchronously at about 12 Hz, and both appeared to be coupled to the Ia activity given the peak at the same frequency (12 Hz) in the Ia auto-spectrum (Fig. 6a). The partial auto-spectrum of the discharge of the Ia taking into account the activity of one of the motor units (Fig. 6b) remains largely unchanged, suggesting that the activity from this motor unit does not greatly affect the Ia response. The partial auto-spectrum of the Ia response taking into account the activity from the other motor unit (Fig. 6c) does not have a peak at 12 Hz, and strongly suggests that the peak at 12 Hz in the Ia auto-spectrum (Fig. 6a) can be attributed to the activity from this motor unit. The contribution that motor unit activity can make to the response of a Ia afferent has been demonstrated when stimulating electrically the axons of single motor units in cut ventral root filaments (Christakos et al., 1984). The above example shows that the partial auto-spectrum allows the same kind of information to be obtained from recordings of the spontaneous activity of intact muscle spindle afferents and motor units.

Fig. 7 is a second example of the application of partial auto-spectra based on the recordings from a Ia afferent and motor unit from a different experiment to that used for Fig. 6. Fig. 7a,b gives the auto-spectra of the motor unit and Ia afferent discharges, respectively. These auto-spectra exhibit strong peaks in the neighbourhood of 10 Hz. The partial auto-spectrum of the motor unit discharge taking into account the activity of the Ia afferent (Fig. 7c) shows a significant reduction in the peak at 10 Hz compared with that at 10 Hz in the motor unit auto-spectrum (Fig. 7a). The reduction in this peak may be attributed to the contribution that the Ia afferent makes to the motor unit discharge. Conversely, the reduction in the peak in the partial auto-spectrum of the Ia discharge taking into account the presence of the motor unit activity indicates a strong contribution from the motor unit to the Ia discharge. The partial auto-spectra in this example allow an assessment of the contribution that the Ia afferent makes to the motor unit

discharge as well as the contribution that the motor unit makes to the Ia afferent discharge — this information being extracted from the spontaneous activity of Ia afferent and motor unit. It is difficult to see how a similar analysis could be made by time-domain methods alone. A full discussion of partial parameters (coherence and phase) along with a number of examples from real data will be found in Rosenberg et al. (1989).

Concluding remarks

The examples presented above indicate how some direct extensions and alternatives to cross-correlation methods are useful for the analysis of

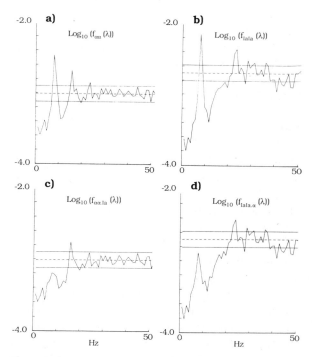

Fig. 7. Estimated auto-spectra of the spontaneous discharge of (a) single motor unit discharge and (b) Ia afferent discharge recorded in continuity with the spinal cord and the estimated partial auto-spectra of (c) the motor unit discharge taking into account the effect of the Ia discharge, and of (d) the Ia afferent discharge taking into account the effect of the motor unit discharge. Solid horizontal lines in a – d are approximate 95% confidence intervals under the assumption of independence.

neuronal interactions. One may still ask, however, why should the spectral methods proposed in this report be adopted, particularly when their very novelty may also carry with it a number of pitfalls not at all obvious to the uninitiated, and when in any case the cross-correlation methods give answers to all the questions under consideration. In our experience the spectral methods take no more time to learn than the time required to attain a proper understanding of the valid application and limitations of the traditional time-domain methods. Fourier based methods can be easily used to examine the relation between continuous signals such as changes in muscle length, joint angle, or membrane potential and single or multiple spike train activity. Further, the frequency-domain methods described above, particularly the partial parameters do not have, to our knowledge, useful time domain analogues, and therefore considerably extend the range of analyses that can be applied to the behaviour of neuronal circuits, particularly questions of causality that cannot be treated by correlation methods alone.

Note

If the analytical methods set out above are of interest to the reader, the authors are prepared to do a sample analysis on data sets sent to them. Details of the appropriate format for data transmission can be obtained from the authors.

Acknowledgements

This work was supported in part by a grant from the Medical Research Council of Great Britain. A.M.A. is supported by a grant from the Federal Government of Pakistan and the Provincial Government of Baluchistan, Pakistan. D.M.H is supported by the Wellcome Trust.

References

Abeles, M. (1983) The quantification and graphic display of correlations among three spike trains. *IEEE Trans. Biomed.*
Eng., BME-30: 235 – 239.

Amjad, A.M., Breeze, P., Gladden, M.H., Halliday, D.M. and Rosenberg, J.R. (1987) The application of partial coherence to the analysis of the association between spike trains. *J. Physiol. (London)*, 392: 9P.

Bartlett, M.S. (1963) The spectral analysis of point processes. *J. R. Statist. Soc.*, B25: 264 – 280.

Brillinger, D.R. (1972) The spectral analysis of stationary interval functions. In L.M. Lecamm, J. Neyman and E. Scott (Eds.), *Proc. 6th Berkeley Symp. Math. Statist. Probab., Vol. 1*, University of California Berkeley Press, Berkeley, pp. 483 – 513.

Brillinger, D.R. (1975a) Estimation of product densities. *Proc. Computer Science and Statistics 8th Annual Symp. on the Interface*. Health Science Computing Facility, U.C.L.A., pp. 431 – 438.

Brillinger, D.R. (1975b) The identification of point process systems. *Ann. Probab.*, 3: 909 – 929.

Brillinger, D.R. (1975c) *Time series – Data Analysis and Theory*. Holt, Rinehart and Winston, New York, 500 pp.

Brillinger, D.R. (1976) Estimation of second-order product densities. *J.R. Statist. Soc.*, B38: 60 – 66.

Brillinger, D.R., Bryant, H.L. Jr. and Segundo, J.P. (1976) Identification of synaptic interactions. *Biol. Cybernetics*, 22: 213 – 228.

Bryant, H.L. Jr., Ruiz Marcos, A. and Segundo, J.P. (1973) Correlations of neuronal spike discharges produced by monosynaptic connections and by common inputs. *J. Neurophysiol.*, 42: 1251 – 1263.

Christakos, C.N., Rost, I. and Windhorst, U. (1984) The use of frequency domain techniques in the study of signal transmission in skeletal muscle. *Pflügers Arch.*, 400: 100 – 105.

Cox, D.R. (1965) On the estimation of the intensity function of a stationary point process. *J.R. Statist. Soc.*, B27: 332 – 337.

Cox, D.R. and Isham, V. (1980) *Point Processes*. Chapman and Hall, London, 188 pp.

Cox, D.R. and Lewis, P.A.W. (1968) *Statistical Analysis of Series of Events*. Methuen, London, 285 pp.

Cox, D.R. and Lewis, P.A.W. (1972) Multivariate Point Processes. In L.M. LeCamm, J. Neyman and E. Scott (Eds.), *Proc. 6th Berkeley. Symp. Math. Statist. Probab., Vol. 3*, University of California Berkeley Press, pp. 401 – 448.

Ellaway, P.H. and Murthy, K.S.K. (1985) The origins of cross-correlated activity between γ-motoneurones in the cat. *Q. J. Exp. Physiol.*, 70: 219 – 232.

Gerstein, G.L. and Perkel, D.H. (1972) Mutual temporal relationships among spike trains. Statistical techniques for display and analysis. *Biophys. J.*, 12: 453 – 473.

Halliday, D.M. (1986) Application of point process system identification techniques to complex physiological systems. *Ph.D. Thesis*, University of Glasgow.

Jenkins, G. and Watt, D.G. (1968) *Spectrum Analysis and its Applications*. Holden-Day, San Francisco, 525 pp.

Michalski, A., Gerstein, G.L., Czarkowska, J. and Tarnecki,

R. (1983) Interactions between cat striate cortex neurones. *Exp. Brain Res.*, 51: 97 – 107.

Rosenberg, J.R. and Rigas, A. (1985) Spectral composition of muscle spindle Ia responses to combined length and fusimotor inputs. In I.A. Boyd and M.H. Gladden (Eds.), *The Muscle Spindle*, Macmillan, London, pp. 397 – 402.

Rosenberg, J.R., Murray-Smith, D.J. and Rigas, A. (1983) An introduction to the application of system identification techniques to elements of the neuromuscular system. *Trans. Inst. M.C.*, 4: 187 – 201.

Rosenberg, J.R., Amjad, A.M., Breeze, P., Brillinger, D.R. and Halliday, D.M. (1989) The Fourier approach to the identification of functional coupling between neuronal spike trains. *Prog. Biophysics. Mol. Biol.*, 51: 1 – 31.

Rigas, A.G. (1983) Point processes and time series analysis: Theory and applications to complex biological problems. *Ph.D. Thesis*, University of Glasgow.

Toyama, K., Kimura, M. and Tanaka, K. (1981a) Cross-correlation analysis of interneuronal connectivity in cat visual cortex. *J. Neurophysiol.*, 46: 191 – 201.

Toyama, K., Kimura, M. and Tanaka, K. (1981b) Organization of cat visual cortex as investigated by cross-correlation techniques. *J. Neurophysiol.*, 46: 202 – 214.

Windhorst, U. and Schwestka, R. (1982) Interactions between motor units in modulating discharge patterns of primary muscle spindle endings. *Exp. Brain Res.*, 45: 417 – 427.

J.H.J. Allum and M. Hulliger (Eds.)
Progress in Brain Research, Vol. 80
© 1989 Elsevier Science Publishers B.V. (Biomedical Division)

CHAPTER 21

Possible functions of transmitter-controlled plateau potentials in α motoneurones

T. Eken, H. Hultborn and O. Kiehn

Department of Neurophysiology, The Panum Institute, Blegdamsvej 3, DK-2200 Copenhagen N, Denmark

An increasing number of vertebrate central neurones has been shown to possess complex membrane properties. However, the functional significance of such properties is unclear. The aim of the present paper is to review some old and new findings in this field from this laboratory. First, a bistability in α motoneurones in reduced preparations is described. Thereafter we present some new data on a bistable behaviour in motor units in unrestrained intact animals during posture. Finally, the possible role of motoneuronal bistability in locomotion and in spasticity is discussed. Recently a bistable firing behaviour in motoneurones was described in the unanaesthetized decerebrate cat. This behaviour is generated by a plateau potential, which causes long-lasting excitability increase and can be initiated and terminated by short-lasting synaptic excitation and inhibition respectively, and is contingent upon activity in descending noradrenergic and serotonergic systems. In an in vitro preparation of the turtle spinal cord the plateau potential was shown to be serotonin dependent and generated by a voltage-dependent non-inactivating calcium conductance. In order to elucidate possible functional consequences of a bistable firing behaviour in the intact animal, the firing pattern of individual soleus motor units was studied by means of chronic EMG registration in awake unrestrained rats during quiet standing. Implanted electrodes allowed the delivery of excitatory and inhibitory stimulus trains to the motoneurones. It was found that short-lasting synaptic stimulation could induce maintained shifts between two stable levels of motoneurone firing frequencies, as in the decerebrate cat. Spontaneous shifts between the same two levels were also present. It seems most likely that plateau potentials are responsible for this bistable firing property in intact animals. The role of plateau potentials in locomotion is difficult to study. At present there are no clear indications of the utilization of plateau potentials in locomotion in intact animals. However, "clamped frequency" bursts which are observed in fictive locomotion in spinal cats might be explained by plateaus. The existence of plateau potentials in motoneurones may also be of importance in spasticity. Therefore, the development of spasticity in two spinalized cats was followed for 3 weeks. Acute experiments demonstrated plateau potentials in some motoneurones in this preparation.

Key words: Calcium conductance; Electrophysiology; 5-Hydroxytryptamine; Locomotion; Motoneurone; Motor unit; Noradrenaline; Posture; Spasticity; Spinal cord

Introduction

In the early 1950s Eccles and his collaborators used the intracellular recording technique in a pioneering analysis of the cat spinal α motoneurone, then regarded as a model neurone of the mammalian central nervous system. This work led to the notion that the membrane in the area of the synaptic contacts is essentially passive allowing a "linear" summation of the synaptic input at the spike generating region of the initial segment. Soon afterwards it was realized that most invertebrate neurones possess very complex membrane properties (e.g. bursting pacemaker properties). The apparent difference between vertebrates and invertebrates has led to the suggestion that the complex tasks of the nervous system could be solved either by a very large number of simple and similar neurones or by a much smaller number of neurones with more complex and specialized properties.

However, further investigations of vertebrate (including mammalian) central neurones in complex brain structures have now revealed equally intricate and specialized membrane properties as for invertebrate neurones (see Llinas, 1981; Jahnsen, 1986). Most of these studies were performed in very reduced preparations, often in vitro, and on types of neurones for which the function is still unclear. Therefore, we still do not understand the functional significance of the complex membrane properties.

Ironically, from a historical point of view, it has now been shown that vertebrate motoneurones also possess complex membrane properties. Schwindt and Crill (1980a,b,c, 1984) demonstrated that prolonged plateau potentials and self-sustained firing could be induced in motoneurones by reducing the K^+-conductance by inorganic channel blockers or by penicillin, and by increasing inward Ca^{2+}-currents. In a series of experiments in our laboratory it has been demonstrated that plateau potentials and self-sustained firing in motoneurones in the decerebrate unanaesthetized cat can be initiated and terminated by short-lasting excitation and inhibition (Hounsgaard et al., 1984, 1986, 1988; Crone et al., 1988). The plateau potentials cannot be expressed unless the motoneurones are influenced by an active innervation from the descending serotonergic system (Hounsgaard et al., 1984, 1988; Crone et al., 1988), or by injection of serotonergic or noradrenergic precursors (Hounsgaard et al., 1988; Conway et al., 1988). With this background, and the knowledge of motoneuronal control of muscular contraction, the "final common pathway" now seems to be an excellent starting point for evaluating the possible functional significance of complex neuronal properties.

In order to give a necessary background we shall first summarize our main findings on the transmitter-controlled plateau potentials in vertebrate motoneurones (Section 1). In the following part (Section 2) we provide new experimental evidence that plateau potentials contribute to motoneuronal activity during normal standing in the intact rat. In the last two sections we consider the participation of plateau potentials in locomotion (Section 3) and the role of plateau potentials in the pathophysiology of spasticity (Section 4).

Section 1. Plateau potentials in motoneurones of the cat and the turtle

Fig. 1 shows responses of a triceps surae motoneurone in a decerebrate unanaesthetized cat to brief trains of synaptic excitation (Ia EPSPs) and synaptic inhibition (skin afferents or muscle group II afferents). In B the brief train of Ia EPSPs triggered a maintained firing which was terminated by a short period of synaptic inhibition. In the following the nerve stimuli initiating or terminating the maintained firing are referred to as "on" and "off" stimuli, respectively.

When the excitability of the motoneurone was increased by current injection through the recording microelectrode, a slow tonic firing (14 Hz) was obtained before any nerve stimulation (Fig. 1C). The same "on" stimulus as in B now caused an abrupt and maintained increase in the firing frequency (from 14 to 24 Hz) which lasted until it was reset to the initial frequency by the "off" stimulus. When the spikes were inactivated by a period of excessive depolarization it was possible to visualize an all-or-none depolarizing potential, 10 – 15 mV in amplitude (Fig. 1D), triggered by the "on" stimulus. If the holding potential is appropriate this plateau potential is maintained until terminated by the "off" stimulus (Fig. 1D). With more negative holding potentials the plateau potential terminates spontaneously; with increasingly more negative holding potentials the duration of the plateau potential becomes successively shorter and finally the "on" stimulus fails to trigger the plateau.

The response to "on" and "off" stimuli could not be graded. This was shown both for the plateau potential (visualized following inactivation of the spike, Fig. 1D) and for the maintained fre-

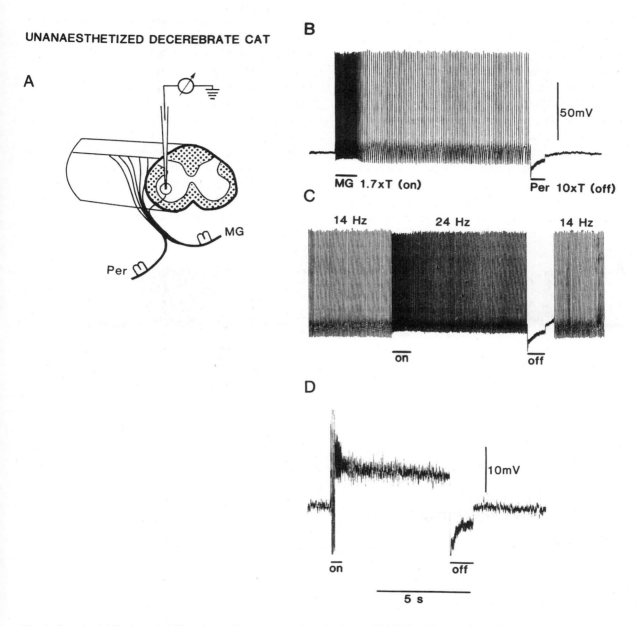

UNANAESTHETIZED DECEREBRATE CAT

Fig. 1. Sustained shifts in excitability triggered by postsynaptic excitation and inhibition. A: experimental arrangement. B: excitability increase in an LG-Sol motoneurone induced and terminated by short trains of stimuli to the medial gastrocnemius nerve and the peroneal nerve, respectively. C: same cell at a more depolarized level displaying a bistable firing pattern in response to "on" and "off" stimuli. D: after prior inactivation of the spike-generation mechanism by excessive depolarization a sustained shift in membrane potential was initiated by synaptic excitation and terminated by synaptic inhibition. The timing of the "on" stimulus (medial gastrocnemius $1.7 \times T$, 300/s) and the "off" stimulus (peroneal nerve $10 \times T$, 200/s) are marked below the intracellular recording. The time calibration in D applies for all records in B–D. Records in B and C from same cell (modified from Hounsgaard et al., 1984).

quency (from rest, Fig. 1B, or from low frequency steady firing, Fig. 1C). This alternation between two stable levels of firing frequencies is referred to as *bistable firing behaviour*.

That the self-sustained firing is due to intrinsic properties in the individual neurones is directly illustrated in Fig. 2, in which intracellular current pulses — and not synaptic excitation and inhibition — were used to stimulate the motoneurones. Fig. 2A shows self-sustained discharge following a short depolarizing pulse through the microelectrode; the firing was terminated by a short hyperpolarizing pulse. When the spike mechanism was

inactivated, brief intracellular current pulses generated maintained potential shifts (Fig. 2B) similar to those evoked synaptically (Fig. 1D).

In addition to the "on" and "off" responses described above we also observed a peculiar firing behaviour in response to long-lasting triangular current pulses. The firing frequency for any given current was much larger during the descending phase than during the initial ascending phase (Fig. 2C). When the instantaneous frequency was plotted against injected current the frequency/current relation showed an obvious counter-clockwise hysteresis (Fig. 2D), opposite to that expected

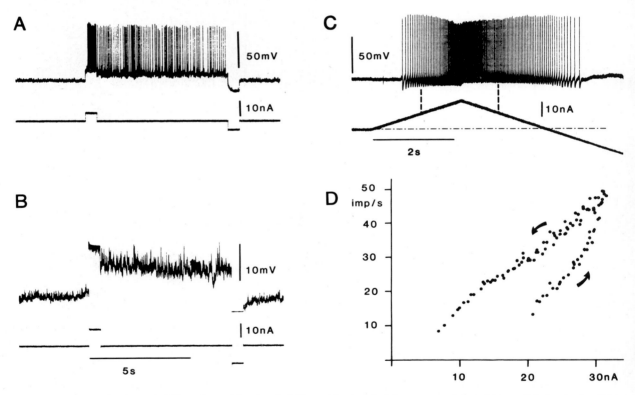

Fig. 2. Sustained shifts in excitability triggered by depolarizing and hyperpolarizing currents injected intracellularly. In A – C intracellular recordings from motoneurones are displayed in upper traces and injected current in lower traces. A: sustained firing initiated by a short depolarizing current pulse and terminated by a short hyperpolarizing current pulse. B: in the same cell this sequence of current pulses evoked and terminated a depolarizing shift after prior inactivation of the spike generating mechanism by excessive depolarization. C: hysteretic firing during a triangular current pulse. The intracellular signal was passed through a 5 Hz AC filter for reproduction. D: instantaneous frequency as a function of current during triangular current injection. Note the counter-clockwise hysteresis. Data taken from the records in C; arrows indicate the time sequence. Records in A and B are from the same cell; the cell in C and D is the same as illustrated in Fig. 1B – C (from Hounsgaard et al., 1984).

from the late adaptation described by Kernell and Monster (1982). It seemed likely that the sustained excitability increase due to short-lasting current pulses and the hysteresis during triangular pulses were caused by the same basic mechanism.

The bistable properties of the α motoneurones seen in the decerebrate cat are contingent upon an active serotonergic raphe-spinal innervation in this preparation. Thus, it has been shown that injection of methysergide prevents bistable firing behaviour (judged from recordings from the peripheral nerve; Crone et al., 1988), and the bistable firing behaviour also disappears after an acute spinal transection, but returns after injection of the serotonin precursor 5-HTP (Hounsgaard et al., 1984, 1988). Intravenous injection of a noradrenergic precursor (L-DOPA) and receptor agonist (clonidine) induces similar plateau potentials in α motoneurones as seen with 5-HTP (Conway et al., 1988). This indicates that both serotonergic and noradrenergic systems are active in regulating the membrane properties of motoneurones.

In an in vitro preparation of the turtle spinal cord the basic mechanisms underlying the plateau potentials and their dependence on monoaminergic innervation were analysed (Hounsgaard and Kiehn, 1985). In normal medium motoneurone firing appeared very similar to the classical description of the cat α motoneurone firing. When serotonin was added to the superfusion the motoneurones displayed bistable firing properties and plateau potentials (Hounsgaard and Kiehn, 1985). Subsequent analysis utilizing selective blockers of sodium and calcium channels led to the conclusion that the plateau potentials are caused by a voltage-dependent, non-inactivating Ca^{2+}-channel (Hounsgaard and Kiehn, 1985, 1989).

Section 2. Bistable firing pattern of soleus motor units during quiet standing

In order to evaluate whether a bistable firing pattern is present in the intact animal we have used a recently developed technique (Hennig and Lømo, 1985), which allows single motor unit recording in freely moving rats. Fine EMG-electrodes were implanted in the soleus muscle. A cuff-electrode around the tibial nerve and subcutaneously placed electrodes in the foot permitted stimulation of afferent fibres. All wires were led subcutaneously to

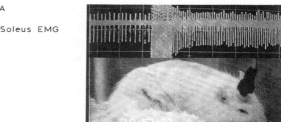

A

Soleus EMG

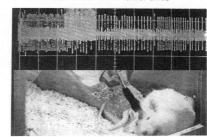

B

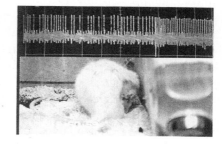

C

Fig. 3. Sustained shifts in soleus motor unit firing in intact rats. Hard copies of composite video picture with simultaneous display of raw EMG (upper part) and rat (lower part). A: maintained increase in firing frequency (from 10 to 20 Hz) in response to a short-lasting stimulation of the tibial nerve (150/s). B: maintained decrease in firing frequency (from 30 to 12 Hz) in response to a short-lasting activation of skin afferents in the foot. C: spontaneous frequency jump (from 10 to 22 Hz) during quiet standing. Records in A, B and C from different rats. Time scale for the EMG records is 0.5 s/div. (Previously unpublished results of Eken and Kiehn.)

the head and to a swivel, which allowed the animal to move freely. Using two video cameras and a signal mixer, the EMG-signal and rat movements were displayed synchronized on a monitor (see Fig. 3). So far we have only studied the firing behaviour during quiet standing (Eken et al., 1988; Eken and Kiehn, 1989).

The record in Fig. 3A shows a motor unit firing at a low steady rate (around 10 Hz). In the middle of the trace a brief train of weak stimuli was delivered to the tibial nerve (note artefacts). Off-line analysis showed that the firing frequency accelerated to about 20 Hz during the stimulus train due to the direct excitation from muscle spindle Ia afferents. Following termination of the stimulus train the motor unit continued firing with a frequency around 20 Hz – the record resembles closely the intracellular recording in Fig. 1C. It is important to note that the weak stimuli did not cause any gross movement of the limb either by direct activation of motor axons or by triggering a "voluntary" reaction in the rat.

When the tibial nerve "on" stimulus was repeated the frequency did not increase further. The response could not be graded, but appeared in an all-or-none fashion and typically consisted of a frequency jump of around 10 Hz.

Fig. 3B illustrates another soleus motor unit firing at around 30 Hz. A train of weak stimuli to the skin around the foot caused a maintained decrease of the firing frequency to around 12 Hz. If the same "off" stimulus trains were repeated there was no further decrease in frequency.

Based on the analysis of more than 40 soleus motor units we conclude that *maintained* shifts between two stable firing frequencies can be initiated by *short*-lasting synaptic excitation (Ia afferents in the tibial nerve) or inhibition (stimulation of skin afferents).

Most of the soleus motor units were tonically active for extended periods of time during postural activity. The distribution of interspike frequencies displayed as a frequency histogram often showed two peaks at 10 – 14 and 20 – 25 Hz respectively, corresponding to the two stable frequencies described above. It is important to note that a normal frequency modulation is also present, but it seems to be superimposed onto the two preferred frequencies. During quiet standing – and without any external stimuli – there were often sudden spontaneous frequency changes corresponding to the frequency shifts triggered by "on" and "off" stimulus trains. One example of a spontaneous frequency jump is illustrated in Fig. 3C where the frequency abruptly shifted from 10 Hz to 22 Hz.

These observations certainly demonstrate the occurrence of a bistable firing pattern in the intact animal during posture, and it seems most likely that the plateau potentials described in Section 1 are responsible for this pattern of activity. We propose that the large maintained depolarization provided by the plateau potentials substantially reduces the need for continuous synaptic excitation during quiet standing.

Section 3. Plateau potentials during fictive locomotion

Are plateau potentials in motoneurones also activated during phasic voluntary movement? This question is not easily answered – especially not by the indirect methods of analysing the firing pattern of individual motor units. Firstly, it is technically more difficult to obtain selective recordings from individual units during phasic motor activity; secondly, it is much more difficult to determine whether changes in firing frequency are due to changes in synaptic input or to intrinsic motoneuronal properties. Probably this question is most easily approached for "simple" alternating movements such as locomotion or respiration, which can be studied in intact as well as in reduced preparations.

There is already some relevant material available in the case of locomotion. By recording from individual motor axons innervating the "anterior thigh" Hoffer et al. (1987) have studied the activity patterns in the intact cat during treadmill walking. They found that the instantaneous firing rates of most motoneurones were lowest upon recruitment and increased progressively during a burst as long as the EMG was still increasing. Firing rates peaked midway through each burst and tended to decline toward the end of the burst. In other words, the modulation in firing rate of every motoneurone was found to be closely related to the smoothed electromyogram of its target muscle. Finally, when appropriately scaled depolarizing currents of similar shape as the smoothed electromyogram were applied intracellularly in motoneurones in acute spinal cats, these motoneurones generated bursts of action potentials resembling the bursts recorded during locomotion in the intact cat. Hoffer et al. (1987) therefore concluded that "fluctuations normally observed in EMG reflect ongoing changes in a central driving function that is common to the entire active motoneurone pool".

The situation is strikingly different in the high decerebrate cat made to walk on a moving belt by electrical stimulation of the mesencephalic locomotor region. In this preparation both Severin et al. (1967) and Zajac and Young (1980) reported that motor units attained a rather steady "preferred discharge rate" shortly after recruitment. Similar observations have also been reported during fictive locomotion in mesencephalic cats (Jordan, 1983) and spinal cats injected with L-DOPA (Edgerton et al., 1976). Since plateau potentials are easy to evoke in both the decerebrate preparation and the acute spinal DOPA-treated preparation (see Section 1) it seems likely that the more or less clamped firing frequency throughout the burst indeed reflects recruitment of plateau potentials by the synaptic depolarization from the rhythm generator. Many of the published intracellular recordings from such preparations show synaptic depolarizations nicely graded in parallel with the concomitant gross electromyogram (see Jordan, 1983 for references). However, some records display almost rectangular-shaped depolarizations reminiscent of plateau potentials (e.g. Fig. 1 in Schomburg et al., 1981).

Fig. 4 illustrates one such example from a knee flexor motoneurone during fictive locomotion in the low spinal cat treated with nialamide and DOPA. Following a few initial spikes in each cycle the spike mechanism is inactivated, revealing the underlying depolarization. Note that this depolarization is not modulated in parallel with the corresponding electroneurogram and that the onset and termination of the depolarization in relation to the nerve-burst varies much from one cycle to another. Most likely these large rectangular depolarizations are plateau potentials superimposed on underlying synaptic excitation.

To summarize, in reduced preparations in which plateau potentials can be easily evoked, circumstantial evidence suggests that plateau potentials indeed add to the active phase of locomotion. Similar signs have not been observed during treadmill locomotion in the intact cat. It seems premature, however, to conclude that plateau potentials

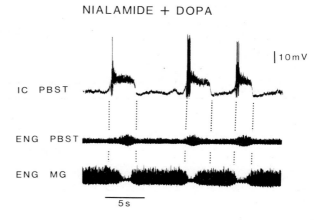

Fig. 4. Membrane fluctuations in an α-motoneurone correlated with alternating activity in flexor and extensor nerves during fictive locomotion in an acute spinal cat. The hindlimb was extensively denervated and the cat was paralysed and artificially ventilated. Rhythmic activity was induced by intravenous administration of the monoamine oxidase inhibitor nialamide (50 mg/kg) followed by L-DOPA (50 mg/kg). Upper trace shows intracellular recording from a posterior biceps – semitendinosus (IC PBST) motoneurone. Lower traces show simultaneous electroneurogram (ENG) recordings from ipsilateral flexor (middle trace; PBST) and extensor (lower trace; medial gastrocnemius) nerves. The intracellular recording demonstrates the plateau-like membrane potential during fictive locomotion. (Previously unpublished results of Conway, Hultborn and Kiehn.)

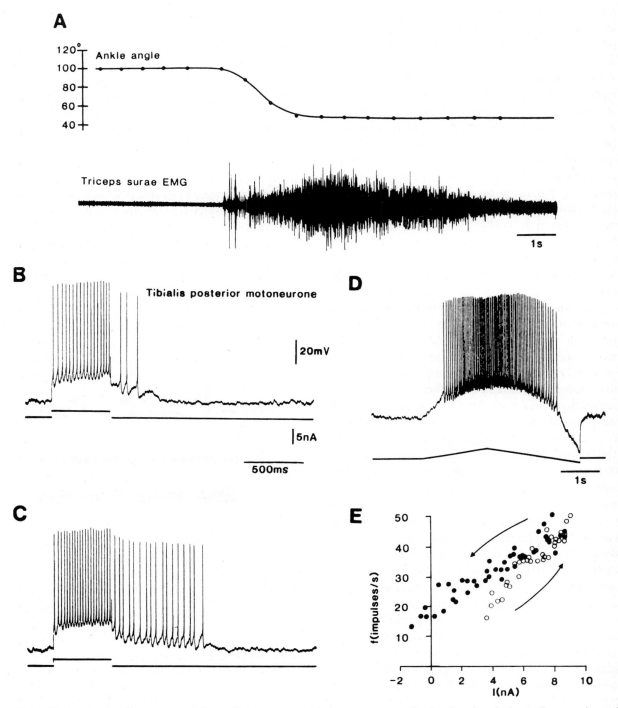

Fig. 5. Tonic stretch reflex motor activity and plateau potentials in motoneurones in the chronic spinal cat. For experimental preparation see text. A: tonic stretch reflex in the triceps surae muscle recorded in the "intact" cat 3 weeks following a complete spinal transection. Lower trace shows the raw EMG (recorded with surface electrodes) during a manual flexion of the ankle joint

are lacking during normal locomotion until additional experiments are carried out with the primary aim of studying this problem. If confirmed, the difference regarding the presence of plateau potentials during posture (Section 2) and locomotion may be functional (i.e. task related), but possibly it may also be attributed to differences in descending drive from the monoaminergic systems in different situations and in different motoneurone pools (e.g. soleus versus "anterior thigh").

Section 4. Plateau potentials in the chronic spinal cat

From clinical experience it is well known that large spinal lesions lead to an immediate depression of spinal reflex activity ("spinal shock"), but also that flexor reflexes and tonic stretch reflexes return and become exaggerated after weeks and months. A similar spastic syndrome can be reproduced following complete chronic (3 – 4 weeks) spinal transection in cats (Bailey et al., 1980). In such preparations short-lasting synaptic excitation by vibration or trains of group I stimuli can result in a long-lasting motor discharge (Crone et al., 1983 and unpublished) reminiscent of the response in the decerebrate preparation (Crone et al., 1988). This may suggest that the exaggerated reflexes seen in the chronic spinal state are related to the development of plateau potentials in motoneurones or interneurones.

Therefore we have recently followed the development of the clinical symptoms in 2 cats during 3 weeks after a complete spinal transection at low thoracic level. Shortly after the spinal transection only phasic stretch reflexes (tendon taps) could be evoked, but after about 2 weeks more tonic stretch

reflexes were regularly recorded. This is exemplified in Fig. 5A, which shows the triceps surae EMG during a manual flexion of the ankle joint. The lower part of the figure shows intracellular responses in a motoneurone of the same cat the following day. In B and C it is illustrated that the firing outlasts the stimulating current pulse. With slightly stronger depolarizing bias current the firing after the pulse was maintained. The frequency – current relation in response to a triangular current injection showed a counterclockwise hysteresis as in the decerebrate cat with intact spinal cord or in acute spinal cats treated with 5-HTP or L-DOPA (Hounsgaard et al., 1988; Conway et al., 1988). These findings in the chronic spinal state are in sharp contrast to the lack of any signs of bistability in the acute spinal cat (Hounsgaard et al., 1988). In the chronic spinal preparations monoaminergic innervation of the spinal cord is lacking (Andén et al., 1964) and the seeming reappearance of plateau potentials under such circumstances may then be attributable to slow changes at the level of intracellular messenger systems.

Concluding remarks

With an appropriate serotonergic and/or noradrenergic innervation the voltage-dependent noninactivating Ca^{2+}-conductance underlying the plateau potential (Hounsgaard and Kiehn, 1989; Hounsgaard et al., 1989) can be expected to provide a large amplification of synaptic excitation. With an amplitude ranging from 5 – 15 mV plateau potentials are likely to be of major importance in providing an increase in the gain of motoneuronal activity. Further experiments on reduced prepara-

---

as indicated in upper trace. B – E: responses of an extensor α motoneurone to injection of rectangular and triangular current pulses in the same cat as illustrated in A. Upper traces in B – D illustrate intracellular recordings and lower traces the injected current. The amplitude of bias current was increased from + 4 nA in B to + 6 nA in C. Note the accelerated firing during the rectangular current injection and the afterdischarge after termination of the current pulse. In E the instantaneous frequency measured in the record in D is plotted against current. The direction of the arrows indicate the ascending (○) and descending (●) phase of the triangular waveform. The frequency – current relation shows a counter-clockwise hysteresis. The current and voltage calibrations in B applies for all records in B – D. (Previously unpublished results of Eken, Hultborn, Kiehn and Tóth.)

tions investigating the control of plateau potential threshold and amplitude by monoaminergic innervation are now critical. In this context it is interesting that motor nuclei which innervate muscles with pronounced tonic activity have a very dense serotonergic innervation (Kojima et al., 1983). Also, from this point of view it seems probable that plateau potentials may be significant in postural control by maintaining tonic activity with a minimum of ongoing synaptic excitation.

A "gain-setting" role has previously been attributed to the descending monoaminergic innervation of motoneurones by several authors (McCall and Aghajanian, 1979; VanderMaelen and Aghajanian, 1982; Kuypers and Huismann, 1982). This notion rests on the observation that iontophoretic application of serotonin or noradrenaline does not excite motoneurones but that it dramatically potentiates the action of excitatory amino acids (McCall and Aghajanian, 1979; VanderMaelen and Aghajanian, 1982; White and Neuman, 1980, 1983). Individual raphe-spinal neurones seem to have widespread projections to cervical, thoracic and lumbosacral segments (Huismann et al., 1981), and they receive afferent inputs from several brain regions, as do nuclei coeruleus and subcoeruleus (for refs. see Kuypers and Huismann, 1982; see however Aston-Jones et al., 1986 for results indicating a restricted afferent control of nucleus coeruleus). Based on the physiological experiments of Aghajanian and colleagues, as well as on the connections to and from the relevant brain stem nuclei Kuypers and Huismann (1982) proposed that the monaminergic systems could serve as a special "gain-setting" component to the motor system "instrumental in providing motivational drive in the execution of movements".

In this context it would be of great interest to record the activity of the descending monoaminergic neurones innervating the ventral horn during various types of motor performance in the intact animal. The technique for doing this is available and has been used to study the normal activity of neurones in other parts of the raphe nuclei (Jacobs, 1982).

Acknowledgements

This work was supported by the Danish Medical Research Council, the Danish Multiple Sclerosis Society, Købmand Sven Hansen og hustru Ina Hansens Foundation, Familien Hede Nielsens Foundation and the Warwara Larsen Foundation. T.E. was supported by the Norwegian Research Council for Science and the Humanities and Nordiska Forskarkurser.

References

Andén, N.-E., Häggendal, J., Magnusson, T. and Rosengren, E. (1964) The time course of the disappearance of noradrenaline and 5-hydroxytryptamine in the spinal cord after transection. *Acta Physiol. Scand.*, 62: 115 – 118.

Aston-Jones, G., Ennis, M., Pieribone, V.A., Nickell, W.T. and Shipley, M.T. (1986) The brain nucleus locus coeruleus: restricted afferent control of a broad efferent network. *Science*, 234: 734 – 737.

Bailey, C.S., Lieberman, J.S. and Kitchell, R.L. (1980) Response of muscle spindle primary endings to static stretch in acute and chronic spinal cats. *Am. J. Vet. Res.*, 41: 2030 – 2034.

Conway, B.A., Hultborn, H., Kiehn, O. and Mintz, I. (1988) Plateau potentials in α-motoneurones induced by intravenous injection of L-DOPA and clonidine in the spinal cat. *J. Physiol. (London)*, 405: 369 – 384.

Crone, C., Hultborn, H., Malmsten, J. and Mazieres, L. (1983) Tonic stretch reflexes and their dependence of polysynaptic excitation from muscle spindle Ia afferents. In E. Pedersen, J. Clausen and L. Oades (Eds.), *Actual Problems in Multiple Sclerosis Research*, FADL, Copenhagen, pp. 99 – 102.

Crone, C., Hultborn, H., Kiehn, O., Mazieres, L. and Wigström, H. (1988) Maintained changes in motoneuronal excitability by short-lasting synaptic inputs in the decerebrate cat. *J. Physiol. (London)*, 405: 321 – 343.

Edgerton, V.R., Griller, S., Sjöström, A. and Zangger, P. (1976) Central generation of locomotion in vertebrates. In R.M. Herman, S. Grillner, P.S.G. Stein and D.G. Stuart (Eds.), *Neural Control of Locomotion*, Plenum, New York, pp. 439 – 464.

Eken, T. and Kiehn, O. (1989) Bistable firing properties of soleus motor units in freely moving rats. *Acta Physiol. Scand.*, 136: 383 – 394.

Eken, T., Hultborn, H. and Kiehn, O. (1988) Bi-stable firing pattern of soleus motor units in rats during quiet standing. *J. Physiol. (London)*, 406: 29P.

Hennig, R. and Lømo, T. (1985) Firing patterns of motor units in normal rats. *Nature (London)*, 314: 164 – 166.

Hoffer, J.A., Sugano, N., Loeb, G.E., Marks, W.B., O'Donovan, M.J. and Pratt, C.A. (1987) Cat hindlimb motoneurones during locomotion. II. Normal activity patterns. *J. Neurophysiol.*, 57: 530–553.

Hounsgaard, J. and Kiehn, O. (1985) Ca^{2+} dependent bistability induced by serotonin in spinal motoneurones. *Exp. Brain Res.*, 57: 422–425.

Hounsgaard, J. and Kiehn, O. (1989) Serotonin-induced bistability of turtle motoneurones caused by a nifedipine-sensitive calcium plateau potential. *J. Physiol. (London)*, 414: 265–282.

Hounsgaard, J., Hultborn, H., Jespersen, B. and Kiehn, O. (1984) Intrinsic membrane properties causing a bistable behaviour of α-motoneurones. *Exp. Brain Res.*, 55: 391–394.

Hounsgaard, J., Hultborn, H. and Kiehn, O. (1986) Transmitter-controlled properties of α-motoneurones causing long-lasting motor discharge to brief excitatory inputs. In H.J. Freund, U. Büttner, B. Cohen and J. Noth (Eds.), *The Oculomotor and Skeletal-Motor Systems: Differences and Similarities, Prog. Brain Res., Vol. 64*, Elsevier, Amsterdam, pp. 39–49.

Hounsgaard, J., Hultborn, H., Jespersen, B. and Kiehn, O. (1988) Bistability of α-motoneurones in the decerebrate cat and in the acute spinal cat after intravenous 5-hydroxytryptophan. *J. Physiol. (London)*, 405: 345–367.

Huismann, A.M., Kuypers, H.G.J.M. and Verburgh, C.A. (1981) Quantitative differences in collateralization of the descending spinal pathways from red nucleus and other brain stem cell groups in rats as demonstrated with multiple fluorescent retrograde tracing technique. *Brain Res.*, 209: 271–286.

Jacobs, B.L. (1982) Recording serotonergic unit activity in the brains of freely moving cats. *J. Histochem. Cytochem.*, 30: 815–816.

Jahnsen, H. (1986) Responses of neurons in isolated preparations of the mammalian central nervous system. *Prog. Neurobiol.*, 27: 351–372.

Jordan, L.M. (1983) Factors determining motoneuron rhythmicity during fictive locomotion. In A. Roberts and B.L. Roberts (Eds.), *Neural Origin of Rhythmic Movements, Symposia of the Society for Experimental Biology 37*, Cambridge University Press, pp. 423–444.

Kernell, D. and Monster, A.W. (1982) Time course and properties of late adaptation in spinal motoneurones of the cat. *Exp. Brain Res.*, 46: 191–196.

Kojima, M., Takeuchi, Y., Kawat, M. and Sano, Y. (1983) Motoneurones innervating the cremaster muscle of the rat are characteristically densely innervated by serotonergic fibers as revealed by combined immunohistochemistry and retrograde fluorescence DAPI-labelling. *Anat. Embryol.*,

168: 41–49.

Kuypers, H.J.G.M. and Huismann, A.M. (1982) The new anatomy of the descending brain pathways. In B. Sjölund and A. Björklund (Eds.), *Brain Stem Control of Spinal Mechanisms 2*, Elsevier Biomedical Press, Amsterdam, pp. 29–54.

Llinas, R.R. (1981) Electrophysiology of the cerebellar networks. In J.M. Brookhart, V.B. Mountcastle and V.B. Brooks (Eds.), *Handbook of Physiology, The Nervous System, Vol. II, Motor Control, Part 2*, American Physiological Society, Bethesda, MD., U.S.A., pp. 831–876.

McCall, R.B. and Aghajanian, G.K. (1979) Serotonergic facilitation of facial motoneuron excitation. *Brain Res.*, 169: 11–27.

Schomburg, E.D., Behrends, H.-B. and Steffens, H. (1981) Changes in segmental and propriospinal reflex pathways during spinal locomotion. In A. Taylor and A. Prochazka (Eds.), *Muscle Receptors and Movement*, Macmillan, London, pp. 413–425.

Schwindt, P. and Crill, W. (1980a) Role of persistent inward current in motoneuron bursting during spinal seizures. *J. Neurophysiol.*, 43: 1296–1318.

Schwindt, P.C. and Crill, W.E. (1980b) Effects of barium on cat spinal motoneurons studied by voltage clamp. *J. Neurophysiol.*, 44: 827–846.

Schwindt, P.C. and Crill, W.E. (1980c) Properties of a persistent inward current in normal and TEA-injected motoneurons. *J. Neurophysiol.*, 43: 1700–1724.

Schwindt, P.C. and Crill, W.E. (1984) Membrane properties of cat spinal motoneurons. In R.A. Davidoff (Ed.), *Handbook of the Spinal Cord, Vols. 2 and 3, Anatomy and Physiology*, Marcel Dekker, New York, pp. 199–242.

Severin, F.V., Shik, M.L. and Orlovskii, G.N. (1967) Work of the muscles and single motor neurones during controlled locomotion. *Biophysics*, 12: 762–772.

Vandermaelen, C.P. and Aghajanian, G.K. (1982) Serotonin-induced depolarization of rat facial motoneurons in vivo: Comparison with amino acid transmitters. *Brain Res.*, 239: 139–152.

White, S.R. and Neuman, R.S. (1980) Facilitation of spinal motoneurone excitability by 5-hydroxytryptamine and noradrenaline. *Brain Res.*, 188: 119–127.

White, S.R. and Neuman, R.S. (1983) Pharmacological antagonism of facilitatory but not inhibitory effects of serotonin and norepinephrine on excitability of spinal motoneurones. *Neuropharmacology*, 22: 489–494.

Zajac, F.E. and Young, J.L. (1980) Discharge properties of hindlimb motoneurons in decerebrate cats during locomotion induced by mesencephalic stimulation. *J. Neurophysiol.*, 43: 1221–1235.

J.H.J. Allum and M. Hulliger (Eds.)
Progress in Brain Research, Vol. 80
© 1989 Elsevier Science Publishers B.V. (Biomedical Division)

Overview and critique of Chapters 22 and 23

Recurrent inhibition – in search of a function

H. Hultborn

Copenhagen, Denmark

The pioneering studies by Renshaw (1941) and Eccles et al. (1954) on recurrent inhibition of motoneurones were motivated by the possibilities to perform conclusive experiments on a neuronal circuit, rather than by any hypothesis on its role in motor control. During the following three decades a detailed description of the pathway has been achieved covering morphological, physiological and pharmacological aspects. Basic aspects of synaptic transmission, transmitter function and properties of interneurones were unravelled. In the '50s and '60s most of these results on Renshaw cells were unique in the sense that comparable studies on identified interneurones in other parts of the mammalian CNS were simply lacking. Progress in understanding the *role* of recurrent inhibition in motor control has been far less conspicuous. Although the general feature of a negative feedback is obvious, the implications of such a feedback are not. Several elaborate hypotheses on possible functions have centred around four themes (cf. reviews by Baldissera et al., 1981; Pompeiano, 1984; Windhorst, 1988): (1) control of the spatial pattern of motoneuronal activity (stretching from theories of a "sharpening of motor contrast" to the hypothesis that the particular distribution of recurrent inhibition may support specific "synergic" motor patterns); (2) control of the temporal pattern (e.g. synchronization of motoneuronal activity, suppression of oscillations; change of dynamic properties of motoneurones); (3) control of the relative activity of slow and fast motor units within a motoneurone pool; and (4) a proposal that the Renshaw system would serve as a variable gain regulator at the output level. Each of these many hypotheses rely on some (or several) aspects of our present knowledge (conflicting results often being disregarded) as well as on unproven assumptions.

Studies on the distribution of recurrent inhibition among motor nuclei innervating the cat's hindlimb (for review see Baldissera et al., 1981) certainly emphasize that the largest recurrent IPSPs are evoked in motoneurones of the same motor nucleus (homonymous recurrent IPSP). However, many motoneurones innervating other muscles (also acting at neighbouring joints) do receive strong inhibition. It is therefore an oversimplification to regard recurrent inhibition in terms of a simple feed-back system. It has been proposed that the more extended pattern would relate to more complex muscle synergies in various movements. This has motivated *Illert and Wietelmann* to investigate the distribution of recurrent inhibition among motor nuclei innervating the cat's forelimb, which is used in a much more versatile manner than the hindlimb. Their results add to, and partly change, the picture obtained from previous hindlimb studies. As for the hindlimb, close synergists (mutually linked by Ia connections) as well as synergists at different joints are often linked directionally by recurrent inhibition. The new findings concern the recurrent inhibition of supinators and pronators from both flexors *and* extensors of the elbow, and the lack of recurrent inhibition for radial motoneurones innervating muscles that act on the digits – also when these muscles were located in the distal forelimb. Since the long toe muscles of the hindlimb have quite sparse recurrent connections (both on the producing and receiving side) as compared to ankle and knee muscles this difference between fore- and hindlimb may be more quantitative than qualitative.

The present material on the forelimb certainly stresses the independence between the distributions of Ia connections and recurrent inhibition; the parallelism between these two systems has probably been overemphasized earlier. The results (re)emphasize that the distribution of recurrent inhibition relates to – and supports – specific motor patterns ("task groups"; Loeb, 1984). The fact that the distribution of recurrent inhibition and Ia excitation only partly overlaps may reflect that they indeed support (partly) different "task groups". The recent observation by Hamm (1988) on the recurrent connections to (and from) the two hindlimb motor nuclei to flexor digitorum longus (FDL) and flexor hallucis longus (FHL) are very important in this context. Despite being both mechanical synergists and linked in Ia synergism, they exhibit different activity patterns during locomotion; FHL behaves as an extensor, while FDL is active during the flexor phase (O'Donovan et al., 1982). Hamm's results show that the pattern of recurrent inhibition for these motor nuclei reflects their function during locomotion rather than their anatomical and Ia synergism. It is thus obvious that if studies on the distribution of recurrent inhibition between different motor nuclei shall help to achieve an understanding of this control circuit, they have to be combined with investigations of other reflex pathways and of the patterns of muscular activity during natural movements.

Windhorst (1989) has put forward the hypothesis that recurrent inhibition is of importance for "decoding" the information received (by motoneurones) from proprioceptors; especially the muscle spindle.

This hypothesis is discussed both at a general level and as a special case at the "microlevel" for small groups of motor units (or even single motor units). The following comments focus on the special case, which is sufficiently concrete to be tested experimentally.

This hypothesis sets out with the assumption that a similar distribution of Ia excitation and recurrent inhibition is the normal situation. As discussed above this parallelism may indeed have been overestimated earlier, although the patterns of distribution for the two systems certainly do overlap strongly. However, it may be dangerous to build a hypothesis on the combined function of "spinal subsystems" on such points of convergence. Lack of recurrent inhibition to motor nuclei with strong Ia excitation (e.g. the distal limb muscles, see Illert and Wietelmann, 1989, this volume) as well as the presence of recurrent inhibition without Ia excitation (phrenicus motoneurones; Lipski et al., 1985; see also Feldman, 1986) may not be exceptional, but rather emphasize that the "rules" underlying the distribution of Ia excitation and recurrent inhibition are basically independent, although often convergent.

Would Windhorst's hypothesis work in the common case with large homonymous Ia excitation and recurrent inhibition? This needs to be addressed experimentally, but I must confess to some pessimism. Recordings from Renshaw cells disclose an enormous convergence, not only from one, but several muscles (and not only the closest synergists) and therefore it seems unlikely that it could "sharpen" and "interpret" the localized muscle spindle feedback to "their own" motoneurones. Furthermore, even the *maximal* recurrent inhibition following a maximal antidromic motor volley (IPSP of about 3 mV, corresponding to 3 nA if the input resistance is 1 MΩ; Hultborn et al., 1988) is small in relation to the net excitation of motoneurones during movement (when considering that the firing frequency/current-relation is about 1 impulse/s/nA). How much effect would the minute fraction of the recurrent inhibition have, which is related to the output of topographically related motor units?

Sensorimotor partitioning within muscles often relates to obvious anatomical subunits, which are likely to have different mechanical effects. But how relevant is partitioning within homogeneous (parts of) muscles? In contrast, it seems that "task grouping" of muscles − and motor units within a muscle − is an important problem which is now receiving growing attention.

Which are the most urgent questions to address, in order to achieve a better understanding of recurrent inhibition in motor control? It may be impossible to give an answer to that question, but my bid would be that a further basic knowledge on the signal transmission from motor axon collaterals to Renshaw cells is crucial. Windhorst and colleagues and Cleveland and Ross (refs. in Windhorst, 1988) have contributed a series of papers covering static input-output relations as well as the dynamics of signal transmission. However, more information would be needed to predict how e.g. supraspinal facilitation/inhibition would influence the segmental circuit. In fact, further evaluation of most of the hypotheses, as summarized in four groups at the beginning of this commentary, would require further knowledge in this field.

References

Baldissera, F., Hultborn, H. and Illert, M. (1981) Integration in spinal neuronal systems. In J.M. Brookhart, V.B. Mountcastle and V.B. Brooks (Eds.), *Handbook of Physiology, The Nervous System, Vol. II, Motor Control, Part 1*, American Physiological Society, Bethesda, pp. 509 – 595.

Eccles, J.C., Fatt, P. and Koketsu, K. (1954) Cholinergic and inhibitory synapses in a pathway from motor-axon collaterals to motoneurones. *J. Physiol. (London)*, 126: 524 – 562.

Feldman, J.L. (1986) Neurophysiology of breathing in mammals. In V.B. Mountcastle and F.E. Bloom (Eds.), *Handbook of Physiology, The Nervous System, Vol. IV*, American Physiological Society, Bethesda, pp. 463 – 524.

Hamm, T.M. (1988) Recurrent inhibition to and from motoneurons innervating the flexor digitorum longus and flexor hallucis longus in the cat. *Soc. Neurosci. Abstr.*, 14: 794.

Hultborn, H., Katz, R. and Mackel, R. (1988) Distribution of recurrent inhibition within a motor nucleus. II Amount of recurrent inhibition in motoneurones to fast and slow units. *Acta Physiol. Scand.*, 134: 363 – 374.

Illert, M. and Wietelmann, D. (1989) Distribution of recurrent inhibition in the cat forelimb. In J.H.J. Allum and M. Hulliger (Eds.), *Afferent Control of Posture and Locomotion, Prog. Brain Res., Vol. 80*, Elsevier, Amsterdam, pp. 273 – 281.

Lipski, J., Fyffe, R.E.W. and Jodokowski, J. (1985) Recurrent inhibition of cat phrenic motoneurons. *J. Neurosci.*, 5: 1545 – 1555.

Loeb, G.E. (1984) The control and responses of mammalian muscle spindles during normally executed movements. *Exercise Sport Sci. Rev.*, 12: 157 – 204.

O'Donovan, M.J., Pinter, M.J., Dum, R.P. and Burke, R.E. (1982) Actions of FDL and FHL muscles in intact cats: functional dissociation between anatomical synergists. *J. Neurophysiol.*, 47: 1126 – 1143.

Pompeiano, O. (1984) Recurrent inhibition. In R.A. Davidoff (Ed.), *Handbook of the Spinal Cord, Vols. 2 and 3, Anatomy and Physiology*, Marcel Dekker, New York, pp. 461 – 557.

Renshaw, B. (1941) Influence of discharge of motoneurons upon excitation of neighboring motoneurons. *J. Neurophysiol.*, 4: 167 – 183.

Windhorst, U. (1988) *How Brain-like is the Spinal Cord? Interacting Cell Assemblies in the Nervous System*. Springer, Berlin, 334 pp.

Windhorst, U. (1989) Do Renshaw cells tell spinal neurones how to interpret muscle spindle signals? In J.H.J. Allum and M. Hulliger (Eds.), *Afferent Control of Posture and Locomotion, Prog. Brain Res., Vol. 80*, Elsevier, Amsterdam, pp. 283 – 294.

J.H.J. Allum and M. Hulliger (Eds.)
Progress in Brain Research, Vol. 80
© 1989 Elsevier Science Publishers B.V. (Biomedical Division)

CHAPTER 22

Distribution of recurrent inhibition in the cat forelimb

M. Illert and D. Wietelmann

Department of Physiology, University of Kiel, Olshausenstr. 40, D-2300 Kiel, F.R.G.

This chapter reviews experiments on the distribution of recurrent pathways from motor axon collaterals to α motoneurones in the brachial enlargement of the cat. In anaesthetized cats intracellular recording from identified forelimb motorneurones was used to reveal the pattern of recurrent inhibition or excitation following stimulation of muscle nerves. The recurrent connections of the motor nuclei acting on the elbow follow the tight mechanical agonism of the muscles involved. Extensive bidirectional recurrent inhibitory connections were found between motor nuclei innervating elbow and wrist muscles. It is suggested that one group of these connections supports the organization of limb extension, the other group organization of limb flexion. The supinator and the pronator teres motornuclei have identical recurrent connections. Co-convergence from elbow flexor and extensor motornuclei in one and the same motoneurone is frequent. It is suggested that this pattern may serve the stabilization of the radio-ulnar plane. Neither homonymous nor heteronymous recurrent actions were observed in the radial motornuclei acting on the digits, which suggests a lack of recurrent axon collaterals in these nuclei. These results draw attention to the fact that recurrent inhibition is not evenly distributed between all limb motor nuclei.

Key words: Recurrent inhibition; Recurrent facilitation; Renshaw cell; Forelimb; Cervical spinal cord; Intracellular recording; Ia pathway

Introduction

The inhibitory system activated by motor axon collaterals (Renshaw, 1941) is a basic neuronal circuit in the spinal cord. Via the Renshaw cells it can control spinal α and γ motoneurones, Ia inhibitory interneurones, ascending tract neurones and other Renshaw cells (for review see Baldissera et al., 1981). In the hindlimb, where the Renshaw system has been investigated most comprehensively, recurrent actions are present in the great majority of the motor nuclei to muscles acting on the hip, knee and ankle joints. However, anatomical and electrophysiological evidence shows that axon collaterals are missing in the short plantar flexor muscles (Cullheim and Kellerth, 1978), but it is an open question whether this indicates a general lack of recurrent pathways in intrinsic foot muscles. In addition to homonymous effects (actions from the

axons to the parent motor nucleus), most motor nuclei receive recurrent inhibition from a large number of other nuclei (heteronymous projection; Eccles et al., 1961), which are in many cases mechanical synergists. The function of the homonymous projection is mainly discussed in terms of limiting feedback control that stabilizes the motor output and can change the spatial and temporal pattern of the activity within a motoneuronal pool (Haase et al., 1975; Gelfand et al., 1963). The discussion of the heteronymous projection is dominated by the striking feature of the Renshaw system that recurrent effects evoked from the axons to one muscle are distributed in parallel to the effects evoked from the primary muscle spindle afferents (Ia) of the same muscle (Hultborn et al., 1971a). This suggested that the recurrent inhibitory system may control the expression of the full pattern of Ia actions (including heteronymous Ia excitation and reciprocal Ia inhibition).

The general validity of these different hypotheses is difficult to judge, since most of the relevant experiments have been performed in motor nuclei acting on hinge joints, which have a limited mechanical repertoire and display fixed and stereotyped synergistic or antagonistic relations between the different muscles. In contrast, the mechanical repertoire of the distal forelimb, with the ball-like construction of the wrist joint and the possibilities for pronation and supination, is much more versatile. It is an important question for the general function of the Renshaw system whether and how this mechanical mobility is reflected in the organization of the recurrent pathways. The experiments by Thomas and Wilson (1967) demonstrated the presence of Renshaw inhibition also in the upper extremity of the cat, but the study has concentrated on the motor nuclei acting on the elbow. Recent electrophysiological experiments on the recurrent connections between the motor nuclei to the distal forelimb muscles have now shown results which differ from the organization present in the hindlimb (Hahne et al., 1988; Illert and Wietelmann, 1988, and to be published).

The data were obtained in chloralose anaesthetized or decerebrate unanaesthetized cats with the dorsal roots cut between C6 and Th1. Forelimb muscle nerves were stimulated (abbreviations in Table 1) and recurrent inhibitory or excitatory potentials (RIPSPs or REPSPs) were recorded intracellularly from antidromically identified forelimb motoneurones. Fig. 1 summarizes the findings (for more detailed quantitative information refer to Table 1 in Hahne et al., 1988). The different connectivity patterns will be reviewed and discussed with respect to functional principles which could explain the organization of the Renshaw system in the cat forelimb.

Presence of the recurrent system in some motor-nuclei to the distal forelimb

It is generally assumed that the recurrent feedback is a mechanism which is of principle necessary for the control of the activity within a motoneuronal pool and for the integration in the reflex apparatus of the corresponding limb segments. This assumption is based on the findings from the cat hindlimb that the Renshaw system is present in the motor-nuclei to all major muscles (see Baldissera et al.,

TABLE 1

Abbreviations

Muscle nerves or nerve stems dissected	Abbreviation
M. biceps brachii	Bi
M. brachialis	Br
M. triceps brachii	Tri
long head	TLo
medial head	TM
lateral head	TLa
M. anconeus	An
N. radialis profundus	DR
M. brachioradialis	BRD
M. extensor carpi radialis	ECR
M. supinator	Sup
M. extensor digitorum communis	EDC
M. extensor digitorum lateralis	EDL
M. extensor carpi ulnaris	ECU
M. abductor pollicis longus	APL
M. extensor indicis proprius	EIP
EDC, EDL, EIP + APL	DEx
N. medianus	M
M. pronator teres	PrT
M. flexor carpi radialis	FCR
M. flexor digitorum profundus	FP
2nd head (median nerve)	FP2m
3rd – 5th head	FP3,4,5
M. palmaris longus	Pl
M. pronator quadratus	PQ
FP2m, Pl, FP3, FP4	MF1
N. ulnaris	Ul
M. flexor carpi ulnaris (humeral head)	FCUh
M. flexor carpi ulnaris (ulnar head)	FCUu
M. flexor digitorum profundus	FP
1st head	FP1
2nd head (ulnar nerve)	FP2u
intrinsic paw muscles supplied	
(ulnar nerve)	Ulp
FP1, FP2u	UF1

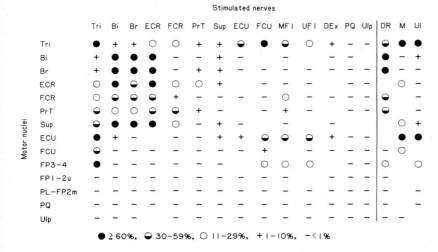

Fig. 1. Distribution of the recurrent inhibitory pathways between the different forelimb motor nuclei. The motor nuclei are listed from top to bottom, the stimulated nerves from left to right (for abbreviations see Table 1). The symbols indicate the relation of the cells receiving RIPSPs to the number of cells recorded from each motor nucleus. Combinations without symbols have not been tested. Effects with stimulation of the main nerve stems are illustrated in the three columns on the far right, separated by a vertical line.

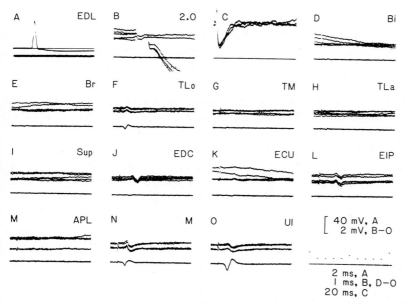

Fig. 2. Lack of recurrent effects in an EDL motoneurone. The upper traces are intracellular records (oscilloscope traces, five sweeps superimposed), the lower traces records from the dorsal root entry zone at the level of the motoneurones (the dorsal roots C6 – T1 were cut). In D – O the stimulated nerves (10 times threshold) are indicated above the specimen records. The voltage calibrations refer to the intracellular signals. Chloralose anaesthetized cat. Records A and B show, at two different magnifications, the antidromic spike upon stimulation of the EDL nerve at 2-times threshold. C illustrates the duration of the after-hyperpolarization of the antidromic spike.

1981; note, however, the absence of the recurrent system in the short plantar flexor muscles). There are now strong indications that in the cat forelimb the recurrent system might be absent in the radial motor nuclei to the extrinsic extensor muscles of the digits (EDC, EDL, APL, EIP). This is illustrated in the EDL motoneurone of Fig. 2. None of the antidromically stimulated nerves evoked any heteronymous RIPSPs. The same negative finding was obtained when averaging techniques were used or when a depolarizing current was intracellularly applied to reveal concealed RIPSPs. Also, there was no homonymous recurrent effect in the motoneurone of Fig. 2. Fig. 1 further shows that the respective motor nerves (combined under the label DEx = digit extensors) did not supply RIPSPs to any other motor nucleus of the limb (there was just one ECU motoneurone which received a very small RIPSP from EDL and EIP). Comparable findings were made in unanaesthetized, decerebrate cats where neither RIPSPs nor REPSPs were found. The most likely explanation for the absence of RIPSPs and REPSPs would be a complete lack of motor axon collaterals in the respective motor nuclei. However, additional results seem necessary to support this hypothesis. It cannot be excluded that Renshaw cells, although activated from motor axon collaterals, did not transmit since they were inhibited by some central control mechanism which was active in the functional state, which prevailed under the experimental conditions (note, however, that the full pattern of heteronymous RIPSPs was always present when the transmittability of the Renshaw system was tested in nearby located TLo motoneurones). In any case, whatever the explanation, the result is very interesting per se, since it shows that the organization of the recurrent feedback may be different between the major motor nuclei to the distal limb. RIPSPs were also absent in the PQ, FP1-2u, Pl-FP2m and Ulp motor nuclei (Fig. 1), but since the sample of recorded neurones is smaller in these combinations than in the radial motor nuclei described above, it would be premature to suggest a similar lack of axon collaterals also for these palmar motornuclei.

Pattern of recurrent inhibition

Recurrent inhibition is regular and prominent between the motor nuclei to muscles acting on the elbow (different Tri heads, Bi, Br, BRD), on the wrist (ECR, ECU, FCR, FCU) and on the radio-ulnar plane (PrT, Sup). It is sparse in the motor nuclei to the more distal muscles (FP3 – 4). The connectivity patterns and the quantitative relations are again summarized in Fig. 1. In the case of homonymous connections the evidence of quantitative relations is equivocal, since detection of RIPSPs depends on the threshold of the neurone for antidromic activation. In addition to the homonymous, the motor nuclei received heteronymous RIPSPs, sometimes from very wide fields. These recurrent connections were mostly bidirectional. The Sup motor nucleus is a remarkable exception from this rule, since it received strong and regular RIPSPs from a variety of different motornuclei, but supplied recurrent inhibition in only a few cases (Tri: 4/105 cells; Bi: 2/38; Br: 2/33; ECR: 1/43; ECU: 1/16).

It has been suggested that one of the functions of recurrent inhibition is to coordinate the activity between mechanical agonists (Renshaw, 1941). In fact, several heteronymous relations in the forelimb can be explained by a mechanical synergism between the muscles (identical action onto a common joint). This is obvious in the case of the strong and regular bidirectional recurrent connections between the different Tri motor nuclei (Fig. 1; refer to Table 1 of Hahne et al., 1988) and between the elbow flexors Bi and Br. However, many of the connections now described do not follow such simple mechanical principles. There are tight mechanical agonists, e.g. PrT and PQ, which have no recurrent interconnections. It seems therefore that the pattern of recurrent inhibitory actions reflects a functional synergism of the interconnected motor nuclei in extension and flexion of the forelimb. Yet, more differentiated movement patterns related to the manipulatory capacity of the paw are not evident in the distribution of the recurrent system.

Limb extension

The heteronymous inhibitory convergence on the elbow extensors, which are the prime movers in limb extension, is mainly supplied by motor nuclei to muscles located at the palmar side of the limb (MF1, UF1, FCU, FCR) and to the ECU (Fig. 1; incidence of effects below 10% being regarded as aberrant). The effects were regular and large (see also Fig. 3). Most of these relations are bi-directional. To a certain extent the FCR, ECU, FCU and FP3 – 4 motor nuclei are, in addition, connected with each other (Fig. 1). The muscles interconnected by these bi-directional recurrent pathways are all active during the stance phase of the locomotor step cycle (English, 1978; Hoffmann et al., 1985) and are therefore regarded as physiological extensors. We suggest therefore, that this recurrent neuronal network supports the coordination of the described motor nuclei in antigravity reactions of the limb. It is an important question to what extent palmar flexion of the wrist and digits is included in this network. The present, but still preliminary results, would indicate that the recurrent connections between the wrist and digit flexors are weak, if at all present. If this finding were substantiated it would suggest that the recurrent pathways between the physiological extensors mainly serve the organization of elbow extension, and are not concerned with organization of wrist and digit movements.

Elbow flexion

The bi-directional recurrent connections between the Bi and Br motor nuclei (Fig. 1) reflect the mechanical agonism of the respective muscles in elbow flexion. The heteronymous bi-directional relations of both nuclei with the ECR are more difficult to interpret. They could be discussed in the frame of a mechanical synergism, because the ECR muscle has a moderate elbow flexing action. On the other hand, extension of the wrist seems to be an invariable component of elbow flexion. This is concluded from the regular coactivation of the Bi, Br and ECR muscles during elbow flexion as it is observed in paw lifting movements (Hoffmann et

al., 1986) and during the flexion phase of locomotion (Hoffmann et al., 1985). Thus, these recurrent connections could be discussed in the broader context of limb flexion in a purposeful motor behaviour.

PrT and Sup motor nuclei

The incorporation of the Sup and PrT motor nuclei into the network of the recurrent inhibitory connections deserves separate consideration. In both nuclei heteronymous RIPSPs were evoked from the same muscle nerves, although there were quantitative differences in the projection patterns (Fig. 1). These actions are not distributed to different motoneurones of one motor nucleus, resulting in several subpopulations of neurones with different recurrent convergence patterns. The results rather indicate that the full patterns of RIPSPs is present in one and the same motoneurone. This organization requires a very differentiated control of the transmittability in the respective recurrent pathways.

PrT and Sup motor nuclei both receive recurrent inhibition from the antagonists at the elbow (Fig. 1). This surprising convergence is seen in relation with the stability of the radioulnar plane during limb movements. Since the forelimb rotates around the ulna, external or internal forces applied to the paw (e.g. during the stance phase) will change the radioulnar angle. The described pathways from the elbow motor nuclei may support a coordination of the elbow muscles with the Sup and PrT motor nuclei, and thus serve the stabilization of the radioulnar plane. A recurrent neuronal network supporting this function should include the PQ motor nucleus since this muscle is a strict agonist of the PrT and an important pronator of the forelimb. Future experiments will have to investigate these relations in more detail.

Pattern of recurrent facilitation

It is generally accepted that recurrent facilitation (Renshaw, 1941; Wilson and Burgess, 1962) mainly reflects a disinhibition of motoneurones, via an-

'tidromically activated Renshaw cells, from the inhibitory drive of tonically active Ia inhibitory interneurones (Hultborn et al., 1971b). In the forelimb REPSPs were observed so far only in motor nuclei acting on elbow muscles. The recordings of Fig. 3 from a TLo motoneurone in a chloralose anaesthetized cat illustrate REPSPs from the Ia antagonists Bi, Br and ECR (slightly larger REPSPs were present in the decerebrate unanaesthetized state). Comparable findings were obtained in Bi, Br and ECR motoneurones (REPSPs from the different Tri heads). Following stimulation of the M and Ul nerve stem minute REPSPs were sometimes present in ECR motoneurones, but there was no indication from which muscle nerve these effects originated. REPSPs were not found in motor nuclei to muscles acting on forelimb joints other than the elbow.

Comparison of the recurrent connections with the distribution of the Ia pathways

It is an interesting feature of the Renshaw system in the cat hindlimb that the recurrent inhibitory effects evoked from the axons to one muscle are in most cases distributed in parallel to the monosynaptic excitation evoked from the Ia afferents of the same muscle (Hultborn et al., 1971a). Minor discrepancies exist, with the Renshaw actions being more widely distributed than the Ia actions (see Fig. 3 in Baldissera et al., 1981). In the cat forelimb the situation is different (Fig. 4). The radial motor nuclei (EDC, EDL, EIP, APL) acting on the carpophalangeal and interphalangeal joints neither receive nor emit recurrent inhibitory actions. They have, however, very differentiated and complex monosynaptic Ia connections with each other (Fritz et al., 1989), which support the manipulatory capacity of the cat distal forelimb. The observed lack of recurrent connections in these radial motor nuclei strongly indicates that this Ia synergism does not depend on any recurrent inhibitory control.

The muscles located at the palmar side of the limb are organized by their Ia connections in three groups (Fritz et al., 1989). One group comprises

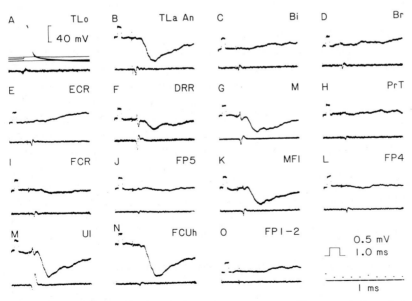

Fig. 3. Recurrent IPSPs and EPSPs in a TLo motoneurone. The nerves indicated above the specimen records were stimulated at 10-times threshold. Record A shows the antidromic spike with oscilloscope recordings, records B – O are averaged records (*n* = 16). Construction of the figure as in Fig. 2.

the flexors of the wrist (FCR, FCU, Pl), the second the extrinsic flexors of the paw (Pl, different FP heads), the third the intrinsic paw muscles. Within each group the muscles have bi-directional Ia connections with each other. It was argued that this organization would optimally serve a general extension synergism of the limb and support the animal against gravity. The pattern of the recurrent connections between these motor nuclei is less clear, since recurrent inhibition was found in some motor nuclei (FCR, FCU, FP3 − 4) but not in others (FP1, 2u, Pl − FP2m). It nevertheless seems to indicate that the distribution of the Ia pathways and of the recurrent inhibitory connections between the motor nuclei of wrist and digits is dif-

ferentially organized. Whereas the organization of the Ia system would serve an optimal exchange of the length information *between* the different palmar motor nuclei, this aspect seems to be of minor importance in the distribution of the recurrent system. The latter pathways rather serve the recurrent control of some palmar muscles (FCR, FCU, FP3 − 4) from the extensors of the elbow and vice versa (note in Fig. 4 that the relation between the Tri and FCR is the only connection in the Ia system which crosses the elbow joint to palmar located physiological extensors). In line with the observations on the lateral side of the limb, the coordination between the distal muscles is represented in the distribution of the Ia pathways, but it is not

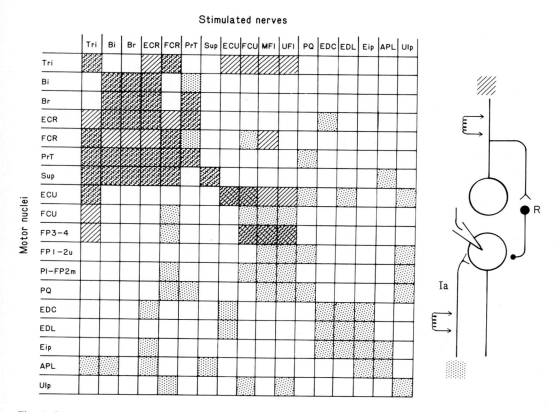

Fig. 4. Comparison of the patterns of monosynaptic excitation from muscle spindle Ia afferents and recurrent inhibition via motor axon collaterals in motor nuclei supplying various forelimb muscles in the cat. Experimental arrangement and neuronal circuits as illustrated in the scheme on the right. Motor nuclei recorded from are listed from top to bottom, the stimulated nerves from left to right. Heteronymous Ia excitation and recurrent inhibition are indicated by the stippled and hatched areas, respectively. For abbreviations refer to Table 1. The material on recurrent inhibition is taken from Fig. 1, but relations with RIPSP incidence below 10% have been omitted, since they are regarded as aberrant.

reflected in the pattern of the recurrent system, which appears to be lacking.

The bi-directional Ia relations between the different Tri heads are paralleled by corresponding bi-directional recurrent inhibitory pathways. In the Tri motor nuclei heteronymous recurrent inhibition is supplied from a more extended field than heteronymous Ia excitation. This resembles the situation in the hindlimb, where recurrent inhibition is more widely distributed than monosynaptic Ia excitation (Hultborn et al., 1971a). A parallel organization of monosynaptic Ia excitation and recurrent inhibition is also found between the Bi, Br and ECR motor nuclei. The bi-directional Ia relation between ECR and EDC and the unidirectional Ia excitation from ECR in EIP and APL motoneurones, which are not paralleled by recurrent inhibitory pathways, reflect the participation of the ECR in the Ia synergism supporting the manipulatory capacity of the distal forelimb. The distribution of recurrent facilitation between the different elbow muscles corresponds to the pattern of reciprocal Ia inhibition. Illert and Tanaka (1978) have shown that the elbow flexors Bi, Br, BRD and ECR evoke disynaptic inhibition in the different Tri motor nuclei via inhibitory Ia pathways and vice versa. Antidromic stimulation of the elbow flexor or extensor muscle nerves accordingly evoked REPSPs in the antagonistic motor nuclei.

A complete match between Ia excitation and recurrent inhibition is present in the connections of the PrT and Sup motor nuclei with the proximal limb muscles, but differences are found in the relations of the PrT and Sup with the more distally located muscles. Thus the bi-directional Ia connections of the Sup with the APL (which is a distal supinator of the limb) and of the PrT with the PQ have no correlates in respective recurrent inhibitory pathways.

Functional considerations

Reviewing earlier data, several new aspects on the function of the Renshaw system have been revealed in the present analysis. The proposed lack of ax-on collaterals in some distal forelimb muscles suggests that the recurrent feedback is no prerequisite for the coordination of activity within a motor nucleus and for the integration of motor activity within the spinal reflex apparatus. Although in some cases limitation of the discharge frequency of motoneurones and stabilization of the output from a motor nucleus may be functions of the recurrent system, it seems unlikely that these features are decisive organizing factors for the distribution of the Renshaw system.

Proximity of motor nuclei within the spinal cord has been discussed for a long time as being responsible for the distribution of the recurrent inhibitory pathways (Eccles et al., 1961; Thomas and Wilson, 1967). This hypothesis became unlikely when it was demonstrated, in the cat hindlimb, that the pattern of the recurrent inhibitory pathways closely correlates with the distribution of monosynaptic Ia excitation and of disynaptic Ia inhibition (Hultborn et al., 1971a; Baldissera et al., 1981). This has now been confirmed in the forelimb for the situation at the elbow. The parallel organization strongly suggests the participation of both systems in a common function. The presence of the recurrent pathways at the elbow, as well as the hip, knee and ankle joints suggests that organization of reciprocal alternating movements may be the function which is common to both systems. The movement repertoire of these joints is limited (restricted to one degree of freedom in case of the hinge joints) and the synergistic – antagonistic relations between the muscles are stereotyped and fixed. The similarities in the distribution of the Ia pathways and of the recurrent inhibitory connections strongly support the hypothesis that it may be the main function of the recurrent inhibition to control in parallel the activation of motoneurones and corresponding Ia inhibitory interneurones, as it was proposed in the concept of the motoneuronal output stage (Hultborn et al., 1979; Baldissera et al., 1981). If it is the balance between Ia supplied excitation of the synergists and inhibition of the antagonists which necessitates control by a recurrent feedback system, then the interesting question arises, why the differentiated and complex movements of the distal forelimb seem not to be represented in recurrent inhibitory pathways. One possible explanation could be that the reciprocal relations between the muscles acting on the wrist and digits are not organized in the rather rigid Ia inhibitory pathways but in other circuits, which are better adapted to the changing synergistic and antagonistic relations between the forelimb muscles. We have no real information about the reflex connections in the cat distal forelimb, but it is noteworthy that there is no direct evidence up to now for the presence of disynaptic Ia inhibitory pathways between the motor nuclei to distal forelimb muscles.

Acknowledgements

This research was supported by the Deutsche Forschungsgemeinschaft. Technical assistance was provided by Mrs. M. Wendisch. We thank Dr. P. Heepe for participation in some experiments.

References

Baldissera, F. Hultborn, H. and Illert, M. (1981) Integration in spinal neuronal systems. In J.M. Brookhart, V.B. Mountcastle and V.B. Brooks (Eds.), *Handbook of Physiology, Section I, The Nervous System, Vol. II, Motor Control, Part 1,* American Physiological Society, Bethesda, pp. 509 – 595.

Cullheim, S. and Kellerth, J.-O. (1978) A morphological study of the axons and recurrent axon collaterals of cat α-motoneurones supplying different hindlimb muscles. *J. Physiol. (London),* 281: 285 – 299.

Eccles, J.C., Eccles, R.M., Iggo, A. and Ito, M. (1961) Distribution of recurrent inhibition among motoneurones. *J. Physiol. (London),* 159: 479 – 499.

English, A.W.M. (1978) An electromyographic analysis of forelimb muscles during overground stepping in the cat. *J. Exp. Biol.,* 76: 105 – 122.

Fritz, N., Illert, M., de la Motte, S., Reeh, P. and Saggau, P. (1989) Pattern of monosynaptic Ia connections in the cat forelimb. *J. Physiol. (London),* in press.

Gelfand, I.M., Gurfinkel, V.S., Kots, Y.M., Tsetlin, M.L. and Shik, M.L. (1963) Synchronization of motor units and associated model concepts. *Biofizika,* 8: 475 – 486.

Haase, J., Cleveland, S. and Ross, H.-G. (1975) Problems of postsynaptic autogenous and recurrent inhibition in the mammalian spinal cord. *Rev. Physiol. Biochem. Pharmacol.,* 73: 74 – 129.

Hahne, M., Illert, M. and Wietelmann, D. (1988) Recurrent inhibition in the cat distal forelimb. *Brain Res.,* 456: 188 – 192.

Hoffmann, P., Illert, M. and Wiedemann, E. (1985) EMG recordings from the cat forelimb during unrestrained locomotion. *Neurosci. Lett., Suppl.* 22: S126.

Hoffmann, P., Illert, M. and Wiedemann, E. (1986) EMG pattern of cat forelimb muscles during target reaching and food taking movements. *Neurosci. Lett., Suppl.* 26: S215.

Hultborn, H., Jankowska, E. and Lindström, S. (1971a) Relative contribution from different nerves to recurrent depression of Ia IPSPs in motoneurones. *J. Physiol. (London),* 215: 637 – 664.

Hultborn, H., Jankowska, E., Lindström, S. and Roberts, W. (1971b) Neuronal pathway of the recurrent facilitation of motoneurones. *J. Physiol. (London),* 218: 495 – 514.

Hultborn, H., Lindström, S. and Wigström, H. (1979) On the function of recurrent inhibition in the spinal cord. *Exp. Brain Res.,* 37: 399 – 403.

Illert, M. and Tanaka, R. (1978) Integration in descending motor pathways controlling the forelimb in the cat. 4. Corticospinal inhibition of forelimb motoneurones mediated by short propriospinal neurones. *Exp. Brain Res.,* 31: 131 – 141.

Illert, M. and Wietelmann, D. (1988) Recurrent inhibition in the cat forelimb. *Pflügers Arch.,* 411: Suppl. 1, R136.

Renshaw, B. (1941) Influence of discharge of motoneurones upon excitation of neighboring motoneurones. *J. Neurophysiol.,* 4: 167 – 183.

Thomas, R.C. and Wilson, V.J. (1967) Recurrent interactions between motoneurons of known location in the cervical cord of the cat. *J. Neurophysiol.,* 30: 661 – 674.

Wilson, F.J. and Burgess, P.R. (1962) Effects of antidromic conditioning on some motoneurons and interneurons. *J. Neurophysiol.,* 25: 630 – 650.

J.H.J. Allum and M. Hulliger (Eds.)
Progress in Brain Research, Vol. 80
© 1989 Elsevier Science Publishers B.V. (Biomedical Division)

CHAPTER 23

Do Renshaw cells tell spinal neurones how to interpret muscle spindle signals?

U. Windhorst

Zentrum Physiologie und Pathophysiologie der Universität, Abteilung Neuro- und Sinnesphysiologie, 3400 Göttingen, F.R.G.

In vertebrates many α motoneurone pools are subjected both to recurrent inhibition via Renshaw cells and to proprioceptive feedback via muscle fibres and proprioceptors, particularly spindles. In these cases, the two feedback loops have a common input (α motoneurone output) and a common target (α motoneurones). This implies that the target α motoneurones receive a compound information despatched by the source α motoneurones, but processed in different ways via the two feedback paths. Since the Renshaw cells monitor the input to skeletal muscle, and the spindles (and Golgi tendon organs) monitor certain aspects of muscle output, both feedback paths in conjunction contain information about the mechanical state of skeletal muscle. Based on these interrelationships the following hypothesis is discussed. At a micro-level, muscle spindles might provide information about motor unit contractions to the homonymous α motoneurones. This information is filtered and enhanced by recurrent inhibition via Renshaw cells. This is effected by correlation of the signals which are propagated through the two feedback loops after having been initiated by firing of the same α motoneurone(s). The effects of the correlation can be strengthened by (a) topographical order in the feedback connections, (b) heterosynaptic modulation, and (c) tendencies towards synchronous discharge between motoneurones. The information about the unfused contractions of a muscle unit (or a small group of them), thus retrieved from the barrage of signals delivered by proprioceptive afferents, could then play a role in shaping the precise discharge pattern of the innervating motoneurone. This in turn may be of importance for mechanisms of optimal force production during muscle fatigue.

Key words: Motor control; Spinal cord; Recurrent inhibition; Renshaw cell; Proprioception; Muscle spindle; Tendon organ; Motoneurone: Motor unit; Muscle fatigue

Introduction

Motor control in mammals requires the solution of very complex problems. These problems are not only posed by the constraints originating from external forces and mechanical interactions between limb segments, but also by those implicated by the very means (e.g. muscles, tendons, joints etc.) which were developed by the organism to solve them. It is probable that, with increasing motor capabilities, the nervous system has developed particular solutions to cope with the properties of its own instruments.

State feedback

The mammalian motor control system is a multi-variable, nonlinear and time-varying system, of which Fig. 1A presents a very general scheme. The double-line arrows represent multi-path signal vectors, i.e., arrays of signal lines, among which topological relations represent spatial order. These vectors connect multi-input, multi-output subsystems, in which one input may influence several outputs, and vice versa. For example, many macroscopically defined limb muscles act on more than one joint angle and, conversely, one joint

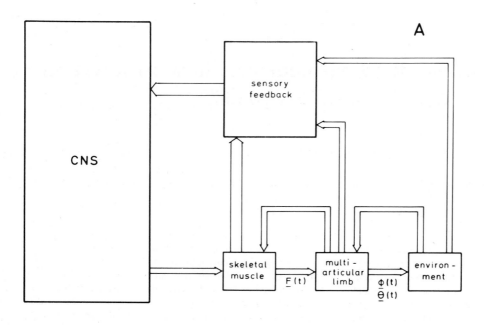

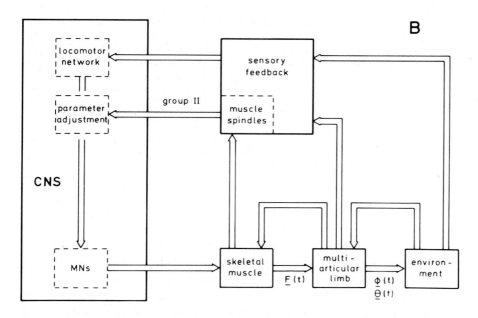

Fig. 1. General block diagrams of the motor control system. These schemes are so general as to incorporate lumped groups of muscles including antagonists. Part A emphasizes the multi-channel structure of signal transmission and processing by double lines. Also indicated are peripheral feedbacks from the environment on joint angles ($\Phi(t)$) and torques ($\Theta(t)$) and from the latter on muscle force production ($F(t)$). Vectors are indicated as underlined symbols. CNS, central nervous system. Part B emphasizes the idea that afferent state feedback serves to modulate (adjust) parameters (gains, thresholds etc.) of central neuronal networks (parameter adjustment), here exemplified by group II spindle afferents which, together with joint and skin afferents, might be involved in opening or closing central neural pathways during locomotion depending on hip joint angle. MN, motoneurones.

angle is often co-determined by the actions of more than one muscle. In general, then, all the signal transformations (e.g., from motor efferents to sensory afferents or from the latter back to the former) occur in higher-dimensional vector spaces. Also indicated is the fact that various (nonlinear) feedbacks occur at the peripheral level. For instance, joint angles ($\Phi(t)$, and their time derivatives) co-determine the properties of skeletal muscles as expressed in the well-known length-tension and force-velocity relations. Environmental factors in turn influence joint angles and torques ($\Theta(t)$), etc. Finally, muscles (and their nervous control) possess a number of plastic properties (see, e.g., Gottlieb and Agarwal, 1988).

For the solution of the control problems which arise from such complexity, the nervous system needs information about (a) the state of the position of the body and its parts relative to each other and to external space and possible obstacles, and (b) the internal state of its mechanical instruments (muscles in particular).

Various components of the feedback state vector arising from the variety of peripheral receptors are used in multiple and specialized ways, even at the same, but especially also at different levels of the central nervous system. An example of such a specialized use is illustrated in Fig. 1B. It has recently been hypothesized that during locomotion in cats the signals carried by group II afferents from muscle spindles (in conjuction with information from joint and skin receptors) are used by mid-lumbar interneurones to alter the gain of spinal reflex pathways as a function of hip angle (Edgley and Jankowska, 1987; also Jankowska, 1989, this volume). This is certainly only one of several functions of this particular component of the proprioceptive vector. More generally, this example illustrates how certain kinds of afferent signals may serve to adjust parameters of central neural networks.

In fact, much of the afferent state feedback can be thought of as adjusting parameters of central neural networks, such as thresholds, gains, dynamics, oscillation periods, and so on.

Integrative action of proprioceptive feedback and recurrent inhibition: general outline

If the state of skeletal muscles is an important determinant in the adjustment of central networks, how can it be determined? One possibility is to measure muscle input and output simultaneously and use this compound information for parameter adjustment. I here propose that spinal recurrent inhibition via Renshaw cells in conjunction with proprioceptive feedback from muscle spindles (and perhaps, in certain cases, from Golgi tendon organs) provides an integrated system suitable for such a task. An essential first step is to recognize that proprioceptive feedback provides information about the self-generated motor actions of the nervous system (Sherrington, 1906; Evarts, 1981). A second, more speculative step is to see that recurrent inhibition can help "interpret" the signals arising from proprioceptive feedback, particularly from spindle Ia afferents. These signals are not only determined by the efferent commands to the muscles, but also by complicated peripheral processes converting them into mechanical actions (see preceding section). The central nervous system, or certain parts of it, might read them more easily by "knowing" what efferent signals have been despatched to the muscles, which it indeed does know, given the information available from spinal recurrent feedback. This general idea is supported by the fact that Renshaw cells and, in particular, Ia fibres from primary muscle spindle endings converge on common spinal systems such as α motoneurones, reciprocal Ia inhibitory interneurones (see Hultborn, 1976) and on cells of origin of the ventral spinocerebellar tract (Lindström and Schomburg, 1973). In these cells, the two feedback signals interact whenever the related pathways are active concurrently. These facts call for a concept in which both feedback systems are seen as cooperating subsystems with partially matched properties.

Fig. 2 depicts a scheme comprising the two feedback systems. The controlled system of interest here is an array (vector) of skeletal (e.g., limb) muscles. Its input is measured by Renshaw cells as the signal vector $d_{MN}(t)$, which represents the spatial distribution of the activity operating on skeleto-motor fibres. Part of its output is measured by muscle spindles as the signal $d_{MF}(t)$, which represents the spatial distribution of muscle fibre lengths (see Hoffer et al., 1989, this volume). Note that the combination of the two signals, $d_{MF}(t)$ and $d_{MN}(t)$ (encircled), contains information on the properties of muscle that is not contained in either of them alone.

The combined outputs from the two feedback systems, denoted by $e_{RC}(t)$ and $e_{MS}(t)$ (encircled in Fig. 2, RC, Renshaw cells; MS, muscle spindle),

adapt the parameters (spatio-temporal excitability distributions, parameters of input – output relations, i.e., thresholds and gains, etc.) in some spinal neuronal networks, including skeleto- and fusi-motoneurones, reciprocal Ia inhibitory interneurones and Renshaw cells (Fig. 2).

Both measuring devices (Renshaw cells and muscle spindles) receive, via interneurones and fusi-motor neurones, additional inputs from descending and spinal afferent sources, designated $u_3(t)$ and $u_1(t)$, respectively. These additional inputs provide the context for the task to be executed.

The parameter adjustment is performed in accordance with the varying functional requirements

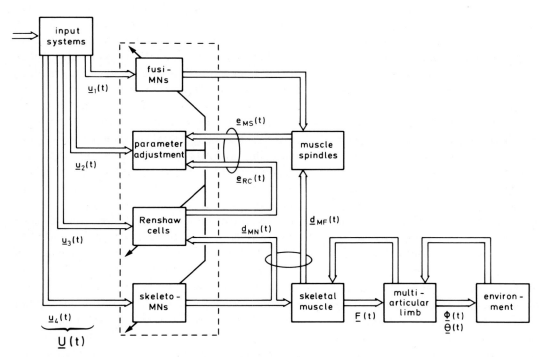

Fig. 2. General scheme of an adaptive motor control system incorporating recurrent inhibition. As in Fig. 1, all pathways are represented by double lines in order to indicate signal vectors. Skeleto-motoneurone (MN) output or muscle input is designated $d_{MN}(t)$ and sensed by Renshaw cells. The muscle output of interest here is designated $d_{MF}(t)$ and is sensed by muscle spindles. Renshaw cells and muscle spindles receive two components of the command input, $u_3(t)$ and $u_1(t)$, respectively. Their outputs, $e_{RC}(t)$ and $e_{MS}(t)$, are fed back to spinal networks, including skeleto- and fusi-motoneurones, Renshaw cells (and reciprocal Ia inhibitory interneurones, not represented for simplicity), for parameter adjustment, which is symbolized by the oblique arrows originating from the parameter-adjustment subsystem and drawn across the other subsystems. Anatomically, the parameter-adjustment subsystem is not sharply delineated from the other subsystems, as symbolized by the dashed box, but may contain further interneurones. It may thus also receive a separate input signal component $u_2(t)$, different from those to Renshaw cells, fusi-motoneurones and skeleto-motoneurones. The entire set of input vectors is designated $U(t)$.

of the tasks to be executed. This task-dependence is partially co-determined by the state of the peripheral system.

Integrative action of proprioceptive feedback and recurrent inhibition: special case

A specific "micro-level" example of a motor task in which recurrent inhibition may serve to "interpret" proprioceptive feedback is maintained voluntary muscle contraction. In this case, it could be desirable for homonymous α motoneurones to be able to detect the characteristics of their muscle unit contractions, for example, in order to adapt their firing patterns to changes of these characteristics during fatigue (see below).

The signalling of such changes to motoneurones via muscle spindle afferents is complicated by the convergence – divergence structure in the proprioceptive system (see Fig. 3B). Virtually the same structure is found in the recurrent inhibitory system (Fig. 3A). This means that the signal despatched by the firing of a particular motoneurone is dispersed − via motor axon collaterals and muscle fibres − to many muscle spindles in the first case, and − via motor axon collaterals − to many Renshaw cells in the second case. These in turn distribute their output to many homonymous α motoneurones. (These feedback connections of virtually all motoneurones with themselves are represented by the matrices labelled R and M in Fig. 3C. At first glance, it appears unlikely that a single motoneurone might filter out the self-generated feedback signals from the interfering signals generated by other motoneurones.

There are at least two solutions to this problem, which are not mutually exclusive. One is based on signal focusing resulting from inhomogeneous distributions of signal transmission gains through the above networks (Windhorst, 1978, 1979, 1988). The other employs signal correlation as a mechanism to enhance transmission reliability (Windhorst, 1978, 1988).

Signal focusing is a means of restricting the influence of interfering signals (see above). Topographical order in the recurrent inhibitory system of a single motor nucleus has been postulated (Windhorst, 1979) and confirmed recently (Hamm

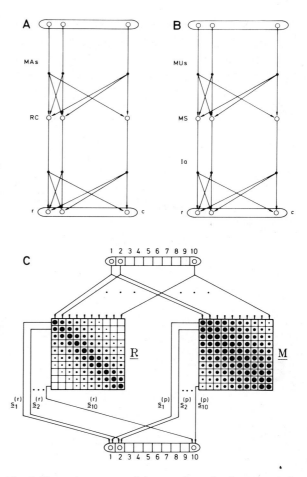

Fig. 3. Network structure of the proprioceptive (monosynaptic Ia) and recurrent inhibitory feedback systems. Part A schematically depicts the convergence-divergence structure within the recurrent inhibitory feedback system, part B that within the proprioceptive system. In each case, the motoneurone column ("cigar") is represented twice, at the top and at the bottom, for graphical reasons (r, rostral, c, caudal). Arrows indicate signal flow. Part C represents the subsystems in parts A and B as two parallel matrices, denoted R and M. Underlined symbols indicate matrices or vectors. For graphical simplicity, the motoneurone column has been divided into only 10 components. Hence, the matrices are of dimension 10×10. The dots of different size in the matrices symbolize the different gains within each motoneurone – motoneurone connection, which is formed by the two feedback networks. The concentration of high gains around the main diagonal in the recurrent network R indicates the focal localization of recurrent inhibition as experimentally demonstrated in the next figure. Each motoneurone in the lower array, say the second, receives two vector inputs. For instance, $\underline{s}^{(r)}_2$ is the array of recurrent signals $(s^{(r)}_{21}, s^{(r)}_{22}, \ldots, s^{(r)}_{210})$ originating from the 10 despatching motoneurones, and equivalently for the proprioceptive signal vector $\underline{s}^{(p)}_2$ (where all these signals are functions of time which, for brevity, is sometimes not made explicit in the formulation).

et al., 1987b). Fig. 4 presents a particularly marked example of the localized recurrent inhibitory effects that activation of a single skeleto-motor axon to the cat medial gastrocnemius muscle exerts on homonymous α motoneurones at various rostro-caudal distances. This topographically weighted distribution of recurrent inhibition may be due to two factors. (1) The response of the Renshaw cells

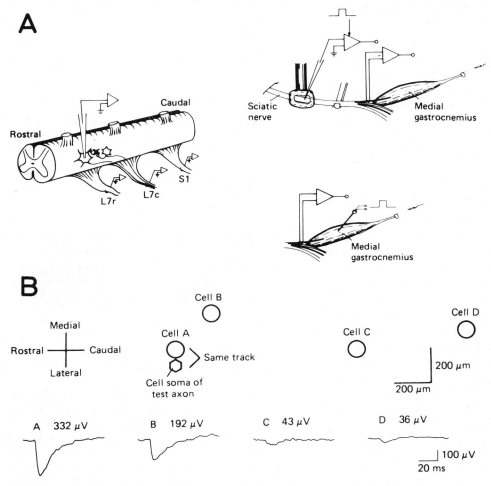

Fig. 4. Effects of topography within the recurrent Renshaw cell circuit of a single spinal motor nucleus. Part A shows the experimental arrangement for measurement of single-axon inhibitory postsynaptic potentials (IPSPs) in deeply anaesthetized or decapitate cats. The left side shows spinal arrangements for intracellular recording from a medial gastrocnemius (MG) motoneurone and three separate extracellular recordings from the L7 rostral (r), L7 caudal (c) and S1 ventral roots. The top right shows intra-axonal stimulation of single motor axons (or their myelin sheaths) innervating the medial gastrocnemius muscle, using a microelectrode. Alternatively, single motor axons were activated intramuscularly using a fine bipolar electrode as shown at the bottom right. For both techniques, the unitary nature of the stimulation was judged by observation of an extracellularly recorded action potential in one segment of the ventral roots. The upper sketch in part B shows medial-lateral and rostral-caudal distances between four medial gastrocnemius motoneurones (cells) from which single-axon IPSPs were recorded in the same experiment. The cell soma of the stimulated (test) axon was immediately dorsal to cell A (i.e., these two recordings were made along the same microelectrode track). The location of cells, B, C and D was progressively more caudal from the cell soma of the test axon (250, 1000 and 1600 μm from cell A). The corresponding recurrent IPSP measurements are shown below. Peak amplitude of each recurrent IPSP is in μV, the value progressively decreasing from cell A to cell D. In this example, the stimulated axon and the axons of all four cells were in the same portion of the ventral roots (S1). (With permission from Hamm et al., 1987a (A); their Fig. 1; and from Hamm et al., 1987b (B); their Fig. 2.)

interposed in each inhibitory intermotoneuronal cross-connection decreases with increasing distance between the motoneurones (decrease in gain of excitatory motor axon-Renshaw cell synaptic transmission). (2) The number of inhibitory synapses per cross-connection declines with increasing distance (decrease in gain of inhibitory Renshaw cell-motoneurone synaptic transmission). Such an inhomogeneous distribution of gains within the recurrent convergence-divergence network is symbolized in Fig. 3C by dots of different diameter in the recurrent connectivity matrix (labelled R). In the proprioceptive system (established by motor unit-muscle spindle and monosynaptic Ia-motoneurone connections), localization of this sort, if existent at all, is more diversified (depending on muscle structure and other factors) and usually not as strong (the matrix labelled M in Fig. 3C symbolizes a moderate degree of "muscle, sensory and reflex partitioning"; see Stuart et al., 1988; Windhorst, 1988). Signal focusing in either system alone is of little help in retrieving self-generated proprioceptive signals. But if the topographical structure within the recurrent system is matched to that within the proprioceptive system, then the recurrent feedback may – by cross-correlation – filter the proprioceptive signals so as to tell a motoneurone which of the signals are self-generated.

Cross-correlation of the proprioceptive signal to be detected with a (recurrent) "searchlight" signal will render detection easier. This idea is made particularly clear by the following mathematical formulation (after Bendat and Piersol, 1971).

Assume that an α motoneurone behaves like a linear constant-parameter (time-invariant) system, i.e., it sums up the synaptic inputs impinging on it. As schematically shown in Fig. 3C, the kth (e.g., the second) motoneurone in the lower array receives, via two matrices R and M, recurrent and proprioceptive signals despatched by the array of homonymous motoneurones (upper array). These two kinds of feedback signals are combined into two vectors, $s^{(r)}_k(t)$ and $s^{(p)}_k(t)$.

Each component of each vector is then transformed into a contribution to the kth motoneurone's membrane potential by the synaptic filtering process. Call such a contribution $m^{(r)}_{ki}$ for a recurrent signal component and $m^{(p)}_{kj}$ for a proprioceptive one. These contributions are then given by the convolution integrals

$$m^{(r)}_{ki}(t) = \int_0^\infty h^{(r)}_{ki}(\tau)s^{(r)}_{ki}(t-\tau)d\tau, \quad m^{(p)}_{kj}(t) = \int_0^\infty h^{(p)}_{kj}(\tau)s^{(p)}_{kj}(t-\tau)d\tau,$$

where $h^{(r)}_{ki}(\tau)$ and $h^{(p)}_{kj}(\tau)$ are weighting functions (or impulse responses).

Now all these contributions sum up to $m_k(t)$:

$$m_k(t) = \sum_{i,j=1}^{10} (m^{(r)}_{ki}(t) + m^{(p)}_{kj}(t))$$

$$= \sum_{l=1}^{10} m^{(\cdot)}_{kl}(t),$$

where, for simplicity, a dot has been put in the upper index of the right expression to substitute for r and p. Summation is to be carried out over both r and p.

The cross-correlation function, $R^{(\cdot)}_{kl}(\sigma)$, between the lth input $s^{(\cdot)}_{kl}(t)$ and the output $m_k(t)$ is defined as follows (with E denoting the expectation operation):

$$R^{(\cdot)}_{kl}(\sigma) = E(s^{(\cdot)}_{kl}(t) \cdot m_k(t+\sigma))$$

$$= E(s)^{(\cdot)}_{kl}(t) \sum_{n=1}^{10} \int_0^\infty h^{(\cdot)}_{kn}(\tau)s^{(\cdot)}_{kn}(t+\sigma-\tau)d\tau)$$

$$= \sum_{n=1}^{10} \int_0^\infty h^{(\cdot)}_{kn}(\tau)E(s^{(\cdot)}_{kl}(t) \cdot s^{(\cdot)}_{kn}(t+\sigma-\tau))d\tau$$

$$= \sum_{n=1}^{10} \int_0^\infty h^{(\cdot)}_{kn}(\tau)R^{(\cdot\ \cdot)}_{ln}(\sigma-\tau)d\tau \tag{1}$$

where $R^{(\cdot \ \cdot)}_{ln}(\sigma - \tau)$ is the cross-correlation function between two inputs with any combination of lower indices l and n and upper indices r and p (represented by two dots in the brackets).

Eqn. 1 is important because it shows that the lth (r or p) input, by being present in the other inputs through correlation, is also transmitted to the output via the corresponding weighting functions, $h^{(\cdot)}_{kn}(\tau)$.

Now consider the correlation between the kth motoneurone potential and the lth proprioceptive input, $R^{(p)}_{kl}(\sigma)$. Even under the condition that all the proprioceptive inputs (with upper index p) are uncorrelated and that the same also applies to all the recurrent inputs (with upper index r, which is the case for uncorrelated motoneurone discharge), the proprioceptive and recurrent inputs with equal lower index l will still be correlated since they are generated by the same source, i.e., the lth motoneurone. Thus:

$$R^{(p)}_{kl}(\sigma) = \int_0^\infty h^{(p)}_{kl}(\tau)R^{(pp)}_{ll}(\sigma - \tau)d\tau \ +$$

$$+ \int_0^\infty h^{(r)}_{kl}(\tau)R^{(rp)}_{ll}(\sigma - \tau)d\tau \qquad (2)$$

where $R^{(pp)}_{ll}(\sigma - \tau)$ is the auto-correlation function for the lth proprioceptive input, and $R^{(rp)}_{ll}(\sigma - \tau)$ is the cross-correlation function between the lth recurrent and proprioceptive signals. This then implies that the correlation $R^{(p)}_{kl}(\sigma)$ is augmented by a term (the second right-hand term in Eqn. 2) expressing the degree of correlation between the proprioceptive and recurrent signals of common origin.

It is important to note that the effect of this correlation is in turn weighted by the recurrent weighting functions, $h^{(r)}_{kl}(\tau)$, whose amplitudes are higher the closer the motoneurones with indices k and l (factor 2 responsible for the inhomogeneous distribution of gains in the recurrent connectivity matrix R; see above). If the despatching (l) and receiving (k) motoneurones are identical, the effect of the recurrent-proprioceptive

correlation is maximal. That is, the topography of the recurrent network interacts with, and thereby shapes, the significance of this correlation.

Whether Golgi tendon organ afferents contribute to the proprioceptive feedback in the above task is difficult to predict because of their more diffuse projection patterns mediated via group I non-reciprocal inhibitory interneurones (see Harrison and Jankowska, 1985, and references therein). But principally it is conceivable that correlations between Ia and Ib afferents arising from common inputs (motor units modulating the discharge of both types of afferents) serve to route the Ib signals through those interneurones to the appropriate motoneurones.

Nonlinear interactions between recurrent inhibitory and proprioceptive inputs

The above formulation is based on linear superposition. Indeed, nonlinearities might act so as to actually approximate the multiplicative functions required in cross-correlation. One such nonlinearity is the spike generating mechanism.

The average membrane potential changes evoked in an α motoneurone, via recurrent collaterals and Renshaw cells, by action potentials in a homonymous motor axon usually consist of inhibitory hyperpolarizations of surprisingly long time course, occasionally followed by a smaller depolarization (see Fig. 4B; also Hamm et al., 1987a). Corresponding membrane potential changes elicited via the proprioceptive loop, i.e., by activating homonymous motor units (under isometric conditions) and thereby modulating muscle afferent discharge, are occasionally more complicated in time course; but they are usually also dominated by a hyperpolarization component (Koehler et al., 1984). The time-related interaction of the two kinds of potential change elicited in the kth motoneurone by discharges of the lth motoneurone may well be nonlinear. To date, there is little data on the relation between the shape of hyperpolarizing potential changes and the firing probability of the postsynaptic cell, apart from the fact that this relation shows some nonlinearity (Gustafsson and McCrea, 1984). This is probably of significance for the effects of hyperpolarizations which nearly coincide from (at least) two sources.

Another nonlinearity could arise from heterosynaptic interactions between the recurrent inhibitory and proprioceptive feedbacks in central neurones. But, for lack of space, this cannot be further pursued here.

Correlations between motoneurone discharges

So far, only one form of correlation between inputs to a motoneurone has been considered: that between any two recurrent and proprioceptive signals originating from the discharge of an individual motoneurone. Another form may originate from correlation between the discharges of different motoneurones. Alpha motoneurones may show various forms and degrees of synchronized firing (reviewed in Windhorst, 1988). A prominent form is the short-term synchronization in which one motoneurone tends to show an increased firing probability within a few milliseconds of the firing of another. Synchronous discharges of two or more motoneurones will, probably nonlinearly, enhance the effects on spinal neurones exerted via their recurrent and proprioceptive pathways.

To support focused signal transmission, synchronization should favourably show a topographical pattern as well, i.e. it should be strongest between adjacent motoneurones and decline with rostrocaudal distance between motoneurones increasingly apart. A mechanism contributing to such a topographic pattern of synchronization is the monosynaptic cross-coupling between neighbouring motoneurones via recurrent axon collaterals (Cullheim et al., 1977). Khatib et al. (1986) suggested such cross-connections to be responsible for synchronizing cat phrenic motoneurones. Topographically ordered synchronization was also demonstrated between intercostal motoneurone pools (Kirkwood et al., 1982). This

pattern here resulted from the (synchronizing) presynaptic inputs being spatially restricted to part of the motoneurone pool. This may happen whenever a muscle contains subpools of motor units which are preferentially recruited in certain tasks and, furthermore, when they are spatially separated from each other (e.g., ter Haar Romeny et al., 1984). Note that intermotoneuronal synchronization reinstates the conditions for the more general Eqn. 1 (instead of Eqn. 2 discussed above).

Force optimization during motor unit fatigue

The filtering property of the recurrent inhibitory system discussed above may be put to use in a particular situation in which the contractile responses of motor units are particularly important, i.e., during developing muscle fatigue.

During fatigue of maximal voluntary muscle contractions in man, motor units show an adaptation of their firing rate (for reviews see Marsden et al., 1983; Bigland-Ritchie and Woods, 1984; see also Bigland-Ritchie et al., 1983a,b), although the neural command input to the motoneurones appears to remain constant and maximal (Bigland-Ritchie et al., 1983a,b). Since fatigue entails not only a reduction of the twitch force of the fatiguing motor units, but also a decrease in their contractile speed and especially in their relaxation velocity (Bigland-Ritchie et al., 1983b), it has been hypothesized that the firing rate reduction is a physiologically favourable adaptive mechanism which, by taking account of the reduced fusion frequency of the slowed motor units, optimizes force output ("muscular wisdom"; Marsden et al., 1983; Bigland-Ritchie and Woods, 1984).

At least three different mechanisms could contribute to the rate reduction and the ensuing force optimization. (1) Intrinsic motoneurone properties provide the required firing rate adaptation (Kernell and Monster, 1982). (2) Group II−IV afferents from ergo- and nociceptors reflexly inhibit the motoneurones (Bigland-Ritchie et al., 1986; Garland et al., 1988). (3) Since the discharge of muscle spindles and Golgi tendon organs is modulated by the unfused contractions of even a single motor unit (reviewed in Windhorst, 1988), these receptors are suited in principle to monitor some relevant parameters of motor unit contractions and their change during fatigue. The signals from these receptors could therefore be utilized by each homonymous motoneurone to reduce its firing rate in a manner that is optimally adapted to the changing contractility of its muscle fibres. As argued above, correlation with a matched recurrent inhibitory feedback should be of benefit and even necessary to extract, by filtering, the relevant information from proprioceptive feedback. Interestingly, the tendency towards motoneuronal firing synchrony increases in the course of longer-lasting muscle contractions (Mori, 1973; Milner-Brown et al., 1974; Jessop and Lippold, 1977; Bigland-Ritchie et al., 1983b). Clearly, these ideas are still hypothetical and need to be tested experimentally.

In summary, in certain motor tasks, spinal recurrent inhibition may filter proprioceptive signals, particularly those arising from muscle spindles, in such a way that α motoneurones can "see" self-generated motor effects. Hence, in these cases, Renshaw cells would tell spinal neurones how to interpret muscle spindle signals.

Discussion

This paper advances a general, and a specific, proposal on the integrative action of two spinal subsystems, i.e., recurrent inhibition and proprioceptive feedback, particularly from muscle spindles. Therefore, both proposals apply only for muscles which are subject to both feedback actions. There are muscles (in the cat) which lack either of them (see Windhorst, 1988; also Illert and Wietelmann, 1989, this volume). Certainly, these special cases will have to be explained as such within the framework of a general theory (see Windhorst, 1988). But, in the first place, a theory is required to account for the most frequent situation. It appears to be the rule that many α motoneurone pools generate as well as receive recurrent inhibition and proprioceptive feedback whose integrated

action needs functional explanation.

There are spinal neuronal systems (e.g., DSCT cells, nonreciprocal group I inhibitory interneurones and midlumbar cells with spindle and other sensory inputs; see Jankowska, 1989, this volume; also Windhorst, 1988; and Fig. 1B), which receive proprioceptive but no recurrent inhibitory feedback. This is not at variance with the present proposal. Firstly, proprioceptive feedback has multifarious roles, this paper dealing with only part (a vector component) of them. Secondly, proprioceptive feedback is distributed over several types of afferent and processed by various interneuronal systems because the mechanical periphery to be monitored is more diversified than α motoneurone output (Windhorst, 1988).

Concerning the specific proposal, it may not appear likely that contractions of single motor units have, via spindle and possibly tendon organ afferents, a significant feedback action on the discharge of their motoneurones. However, if such action indeed occurs, it is probably established by interaction with recurrent inhibition. More likely is that small groups of motor units associated by their tendency towards synchronous firing exert significant feedback action. Finally, even if the specific proposal in its strictest form does not hold true, the general interaction of recurrent inhibition and proprioceptive feedback as outlined in Fig. 3 is still of importance for mechanisms of physiological tremor. This needs to be further studied by computer simulations.

Acknowledgements

I am grateful to Prof. D.G. Stuart for encouragement, to Dr. C.N. Christakos for valuable suggestions on the manuscript, to Mrs. U. deBuhr for the preparation of the figures and to Mr. H. Schultens for scrutinizing the English.

References

Bendat, J.S. and Piersol, A.G. (1971) *Random Data: Analysis and Measurement Procedures*, Wiley, New York, pp. 147–153.
Bigland-Ritchie, B. and Woods, J.J. (1984) Changes in muscle contractile properties and neural control during human

muscular fatigue. *Muscle Nerve*, 7: 691–699.

Bigland-Ritchie, B., Johansson, R.S., Lippold, O.C.J. and Woods, J.J. (1983a) Changes in motoneurone firing rates during sustained maximal voluntary contractions. *J. Physiol. (London)*, 340: 335–346.

Bigland-Ritchie, B., Johansson, R.S., Lippold, O.C.J. and Woods, J.J. (1983b) Contractile speed and EMG changes during fatigue of sustained maximal voluntary contractions. *J. Neurophysiol.*, 50: 313–324.

Bigland-Ritchie, B., Dawson, N.J., Johansson, R.S. and Lippold, O.C.J. (1986) Reflex origin for the slowing of motoneurone firing rates in fatigue of human voluntary contractions. *J. Physiol. (London)*, 379: 451–459.

Cullheim, S., Kellerth J.-O. and Conradi, S. (1977) Evidence for direct synaptic interconnections between cat spinal alpha motoneurons via recurrent axon collaterals: a morphological study using intracellular injection of horseradish peroxidase. *Brain Res.*, 132: 1–10.

Edgley, S.A. and Jankowska, E. (1987) An interneuronal relay for group I and II muscle afferents in the midlumbar segments of the cat spinal cord. *J. Physiol. (London)*, 389: 647–674.

Evarts, E.V. (1981) Sherrington's concept of proprioception. *Trends Neurosci.*, 4: 44–46.

Garland, S.J., Garner, S.H. and McComas, A.J. (1988) Reduced voluntary electromyographic activity after fatiguing stimulation of human muscle. *J. Physiol. (London)*, 401: 547–556.

Gottlieb, G.L. and Agarwal, G.C. (1988) Compliance of single joints: elastic and plastic characteristics. *J. Neurophysiol.*, 59: 937–951.

Gustafsson, B.G. and McCrea, D. (1984) Influence of stretch-evoked synaptic potentials on firing probability of cat spinal motoneurones. *J. Physiol. (London)*, 347: 431–451.

Hamm, T.M., Sasaki, S., Stuart, D.G., Windhorst, U. and Yuan, C.-S. (1987a) The measurement of single motor-axon recurrent inhibitory post-synaptic potentials in the cat. *J. Physiol. (London)*, 388: 631–651.

Hamm, T.M., Sasaki, S., Stuart, D.G., Windhorst, U. and Yuan, C.-S. (1987b) Distribution of single-axon recurrent inhibitory post-synaptic potentials in a single motor nucleus in the cat. *J. Physiol. (London)*, 388: 653–664.

Harrison, P.J. and Jankowska, E. (1985) Sources of input to interneurones mediating group I non-reciprocal inhibition of motoneurones in the cat. *J. Physiol. (London)*, 361: 379–401.

Hoffer, J.A., Caputi, A.A., Pose, I.E. and Griffiths, R.I. (1989) Roles of muscle activity and load on the relationship between muscle spindle length and whole muscle length in the freely walking cat. In J.H.J. Allum and M. Hulliger (Eds.), *Afferent Control of Posture and Locomotion, Prog. Brain Res., Vol. 80,* Elsevier, Amsterdam, pp. 75–85.

Hultborn, H. (1976) Transmission in the pathway of reciprocal Ia inhibition to motoneurones and its control during tonic stretch reflex. In S. Homma (Ed.), *Understanding the Stretch Reflex, Prog. Brain Res., Vol. 44*, Elsevier, Amsterdam, pp. 235–254.

Illert, M. and Wietelmann, D. (1989) Distribution of recurrent inhibition in the cat forelimb. In J.H.J. Allum and M. Hulliger (Eds.), *Afferent Control of Posture and Locomotion, Prog. Brain Res., Vol. 80,* Elsevier, Amsterdam, pp. 273–281.

Jankowska, E. (1989) A neuronal system of movement control via muscle spindle secondaries. A brief review. In J.H.J. Allum and M. Hulliger (Eds.), *Afferent Control of Posture and Locomotion, Prog. Brain Res., Vol. 80,* Elsevier, Amsterdam, pp. 299–303.

Jessop, J. and Lippold, O.C.J. (1977) Altered synchronization of motor unit firing as a mechanism for long-lasting increases in the tremor of human hand muscles following brief, strong efforts. *J. Physiol. (London)*, 269: 20P.

Kernell, D. and Monster, A.W. (1982) Time course and properties of late adaptation in spinal motoneurones of the cat. *Exp. Brain Res.*, 46: 191–196.

Khatib, M., Hilaire, G. and Monteau, R. (1986) Excitatory interactions between phrenic motoneurons in the cat. *Exp. Brain Res.*, 62: 273–280.

Kirkwood, P.A., Sears, T.A., Stagg, D. and Westgaard, R.H. (1982) The spatial distribution of synchronization of intercostal motoneurones in the cat. *J. Physiol. (London)*, 327: 137–155.

Koehler, W., Hamm, T.M., Enoka, R.M., Stuart, D.G., Windhorst, U. (1984) Contractions of single motor units are reflected in membrane potential changes of homonymous α motoneurons. *Brain Res.*, 296: 379–384.

Lindström, S. and Schomburg, E.D. (1973) Recurrent inhibition from motor axon collaterals of ventral spinocerebellar tract neurons. *Acta Physiol. Scand.*, 88: 505–515.

Marsden, C.D., Meadows, J.C. and Merton, P.A. (1983) "Muscular wisdom" that minimizes fatigue during prolonged effort in man: peak rates of motoneuron discharge and slowing of discharge during fatigue. In J.E. Desmedt (Ed.), *Motor Control Mechanisms in Health and Disease*, Raven Press, New York, pp. 169–211.

Milner-Brown, H.S., Stein, R.B. and Lee, R.G. (1974) Synchronization of human motor units: possible roles of exercise and supraspinal reflexes. *Electroenceph. Clin. Neurophysiol.*, 38: 245–254.

Mori, S. (1973) Discharge patterns of soleus motor units with associated changes in force exerted by foot during quiet stance in man. *J. Neurophysiol.*, 36: 458–471.

Sherrington, C.S. (1906) On the proprio-ceptive system, especially in its reflex aspects. *Brain*, 29: 467–482.

Stuart, D.G., Hamm, T.M. and Vanden Noven, S. (1988) Partitioning of monosynaptic Ia excitation to motoneurons according to neuromuscular topography: generality and functional implications. *Prog. Neurobiol.*, 30: 437–447.

ter Haar Romeny, B.M., Denier van der Gon, J.J. and Gielen,

294

C.C.A.M. (1984) Relation between location of a motor unit in the human biceps brachii and its critical firing level for different tasks. *Exp. Neurol.*, 85: 631 – 650.

Windhorst, U. (1978) Considerations on mechanisms of focussed signal transmission in the multi-channel muscle stretch reflex system. *Biol. Cybern.*, 31: 81 – 90.

Windhorst, U. (1979) Auxiliary spinal networks for signal focussing in the segmental stretch reflex system. *Biol. Cybern.*, 34: 125 – 135.

Windhorst, U. (1988) *How Brain-like is the Spinal Cord? Interacting Cell Assemblies in the Nervous System*, Springer, Berlin, 334 pp.

J.H.J. Allum and M. Hulliger (Eds.)
Progress in Brain Research, Vol. 80

295

Overview and critique of Chapters 24 and 25

E.E. Fetz

Seattle, U.S.A.

The papers of Elzbieta Jankowska and Emmanuel Pierrot-Deseilligny both examine the organization of spinal reflex circuitry, but from quite different perspectives. Dr. Jankowska presents a comprehensive analysis of the synaptic organization of a new class of spinal interneurones, using intracellular recording and other acute techniques. Dr. Pierrot-Deseilligny describes the functional consequences of reflex circuitry on motor unit activity, tested in awake humans by cross-correlation methods. These two approaches provide complementary information on segmental circuitry, and suggest additional experimental strategies that could help to further clarify the underlying mechanisms.

Jankowska's paper summarizes the latest in her systematic series of studies to characterize different classes of spinal interneurones. We are certainly indebted to her for her prodigious and painstaking efforts to elucidate the synaptic organization of segmental circuitry. She has applied an awesome arsenal of state-of-the-art techniques to clarify the synaptic inputs and outputs of various spinal interneurones. These approaches are well represented in her present review of the experimental evidence on the so-called mid-lumbar or L4 group II interneurones. Intracellular recording of postsynaptic potentials reveal particularly strong inputs from group II muscle afferents on the L4 interneurones, although they also receive convergent input from virtually all other types of afferents, as well as most of the major descending pathways. An elegant confirmation of the effectiveness of input from spindle afferents involves selective activa-

tion of intrafusal fibres by ventral root stimulation. Of course the cells' function depends as much on their postsynaptic targets as their synaptic input. The output of the L4 interneurones to motoneurones has been documented by spike-triggered averaging of ventral root potentials. These post-spike potentials suggest that the L4 interneurones produce monosynaptic EPSPs or IPSPs in lower lumbar motoneurones. (An important assumption here is that the ventral root potentials reflect only the post-synaptic potentials of motoneurones, uncontaminated by wick recording of field potentials.) To further elucidate the input – output relations of these cells it would be of interest to know how the input to excitatory interneurones differs from that of the inhibitory interneurones. This information is difficult to obtain, but evidence so far indicates that both appear to receive similar inputs. If the same input does activate excitatory and inhibitory interneurones, they may still act synergistically if they affect different groups of motoneurones. The potential role of these interneurones in locomotion has been supported by evidence that they respond to supraspinal stimulation in the mesencephalic locomotor region, and that ionophoretic injection of monoamines (like L-DOPA, known for its ability to initiate locomotion) can preferentially modulate the synaptic effects of particular afferents.

One can hardly fault this impressive range of experimental results, so instead we might consider what additional methods could be brought to bear on the functional issues. The possible function of these interneurones is inferred largely from data obtained in acute experiments with intracellular recordings. These hypothetical functions could potentially be tested in behaving animals. A significant step in this direction has been taken with the mesencephalic cat preparation, which can be made to exhibit fictive locomotion, and which even provides sufficient stability for intracellular recording (Shefchyk et al., 1988). The candidate mid-lumbar interneurones can be identified by antidromic stimulation from motoneurone pools and by activation of group II inputs; curiously, many of these interneurones were not modulated during fictive locomotion (Shefchyk et al., 1987). However, this paralysed preparation eliminates the afferent input from peripheral receptors, so it seems worth investigating the activity of these cells in the intact, moving animal. Techniques are available for extracellular recording in spinal cord of awake behaving animals, using implanted recording chambers and stimulating electrodes (e.g., Bromberg and Fetz, 1977). The technical challenge would be to identify the same interneurones that have been studied in previous acute experiments. One can potentially characterize the output effects of interneurones on motoneurones by spike-triggered averaging of EMG. Their peripheral input can also be documented by innocuous stimulation of afferent nerves. Electrical stimulation of high-threshold afferents is precluded in awake animals, but may still be possible by anaesthetizing the animal (assuming the interneurones can be held through the transition from awake to anaesthetized). The descending inputs to these interneurones could also be confirmed by electrical stimulation of supraspinal centres or descending pathways. A major advantage of such a preparation is that the stimulating electrodes and recording chamber need be implanted only once and can be utilized repeatedly in successive recording sessions, maximizing the yield of data per preparation time. The response patterns of these cells in the intact animal during natural movements such as locomotion would provide crucial information concerning their active roles. Such a study would represent a welcome bridge between the detailed information on synaptic circuitry obtained in acute intracellular studies and the behavioural data obtainable in the unanaesthetized behaving preparation.

The paper by *Pierrot-Deseilligny* illustrates his elegant approach to reflex testing in conscious humans, a subject whose synaptic circuitry can only be examined by non-invasive means. The basic observables are the cross-correlation features produced by underlying postsynaptic potentials in motoneurones. The conditioning-testing paradigm can be used to probe the facilitation and suppression of the mediating interneurones. His experiments indicate the existence of non-monosynaptic excitation to motoneurones, possibly mediated by interneurones analogous to the C3 – C4 propriospinal neurones documented in the cat. Certainly his experimental evidence would suggest the existence of some excitatory interneurones receiving convergent input from descending and peripheral afferents in man. However, it seems remarkable that there is so little evidence for the existence of C3 – C4 propriospinal neurones in the subhuman primate. The intracellular recordings of Michael Illert and colleagues do not provide strong evidence of any propriospinal neurones contributing a disynaptic corticomotoneuronal EPSP (Fritz et al., 1985) in the macaque. The existence of these interneurones should manifest itself in the appearance of polysynaptic CM-EPSPs, which have not been reported to be a prominent feature in the primate studies of Preston and Whitlock (1961), Phillips and Porter (1977), or Shapovalov (personal communication). It remains possible that these interneurones were suppressed by anaesthesia, or that their effects were masked by disynaptic inhibition. In any case, the reflex testing experiments do suggest that later polysynaptic excitation can be evoked by nerve stimulation in waking humans.

Some properties of this polysynaptic excitation remain puzzling. It seems curious that the threshold for evoking this *di*synaptic excitation is less than the threshold for the *mono*synaptic EPSP. This is attributed to the activation of heteronymous non-monosynaptic low-threshold Ia afferents, but one would expect that the stimulus would also evoke monosynaptic effects via homonymous Ia afferents, which are recruited at slightly higher stimulus intensities. Their contribution would appear as a facilitation of the control firing probability, even for sub-threshold stimuli (as for example in Fig. 1b), so it seems remarkable that one can get a lower threshold for polysynaptic than monosynaptic activation. Some of these issues can perhaps be resolved by investigating the phenomenon in nonhuman primates, in which the mediating circuitry can be analysed by intraspinal recording. Certainly, the studies of Pierrot-Deseilligny provide much new information on these polysynaptic reflex pathways as they manifest themselves in humans, and confirm the importance of cat and monkey experiments for understanding human physiology.

An issue relevant to both papers is the effectiveness of transmission through polysynaptic pathways via interneurones. Intracellular recording of EPSPs and IPSPs have provided much quantitative evidence on the relative magnitude of synaptic input from various sources, but the quantitative effects of these synaptic potentials on the firing of interneurones remains unknown. The relation between postsynaptic potentials and the firing probability has been quantified in motoneurones (Fetz and Gustafsson, 1983; Cope et al., 1987). However, motoneurones and interneurones exhibit significant differences in their firing properties: in motoneurones the afterhyperpolarization following an action potential precludes threshold crossing by many EPSPs, and those that do cross threshold can trigger at most only one action potential. In contrast, interneurones may be triggered more frequently and may even fire repetitively during a single EPSP. This would indicate that similar-sized PSPs may have more potent effects in interneurones than in motoneurones. Knowing the effectiveness of synaptic inputs in spinal interneurones would also help interpret some of the evidence from reflex testing in humans.

References

Bromberg, M.A. and Fetz, E.E. (1977) Responses of single units in cervical spinal cord of alert monkeys. *Exp. Neurol.*, 55: 469–482.

Cope, T.C., Fetz, E.E. and Matsumura, M. (1987) Cross-correlation assessment of the synaptic strength of single Ia fibre connections with lumbar motoneurones in the cat. *J. Physiol. (London)*, 390: 161–188.

Fetz, E.E. and Gustafsson, B. (1983) Relation between shapes of postsynaptic potentials and changes in firing probability of cat motoneurones. *J. Physiol. (London)*, 341: 387–410.

Fritz, N., Illert, M., Kolb, F.P., Lemon, R.N., Muir, R.B., van der Burg, J., Wiedemann, E. and Yamaguchi, T. (1985) The corticomotoneuronal input to hand and forearm motoneurones in the anaesthetized monkey. *J. Physiol. (London)*, 366: 20P.

Phillips, C.G. and Porter, R. (1977) *Corticospinal Neurones*, Academic Press, London, 450 pp.

Preston, J.B. and Whitlock, D.G. (1961) Intracellular potentials recorded from motoneurones following precentral gyrus stimulation in primate. *J. Neurophysiol.*, 24: 91–100.

Shefchyk, S.J., McCrea, D.A., Kriellaars, D.J., Noge, B.R. and Jordan, L.M. (1987) Activity of L4 interneurones with group II input during fictive locomotion in the mesencephalic cat. *Soc. Neurosci. Abstr.*, 13: 826.

Shefchyk, S.J., McCrea, D.A., Kriellaars, D.J., Jordan, L.M. and Fortier, P. (1988) Activity of midlumbar group II interneurones during brainstem evoked fictive locomotion in the mesencephalic cat. *Soc. Neurosci. Abstr.*, 14: 265.

J.H.J. Allum and M. Hulliger (Eds.)
Progress in Brain Research, Vol. 80
© 1989 Elsevier Science Publishers B.V. (Biomedical Division)

CHAPTER 24

A neuronal system of movement control via muscle spindle secondaries

E. Jankowska

Department of Physiology, University of Göteborg, Göteborg, Sweden

A recently discovered spinal interneuronal system of movement control is briefly described. It includes a population of midlumbar interneurones with a predominant monosynaptic input from secondary muscle spindle afferents but supplied with information via several other afferent and descending neuronal systems as well. The neurones are in direct contact with both motoneurones and other interneurones. The evidence in favour for their involvement in locomotion is briefly summarized.

Key words: Spinal cord; Spinal reflex; Interneurone muscle spindle; Synaptic transmission; Locomotion; Noradrenaline; Serotonin; Locus coeruleus; Raphe nucleus

Introduction

Various populations of spinal interneurones receive different kinds of afferent information and affect different sets of other neurones, and are thus specialized to contribute to different aspects of movement control. The role played by several spinal interneuronal populations has already been discussed and is a subject of further attention in this volume. In cat, rats and primates this is particularly the case for interneurones mediating Ia reciprocal inhibition and Renshaw cells (see e.g. Pratt and Jordan, 1987; Noga et al., 1987), interneurones interposed in pathways from tendon organs (see e.g. Harrison and Jankowska, 1985), neurones with input from the flexion reflex afferents (see e.g. Lundberg et al., 1987) and cervical propriospinal neurones (see e.g. Alstermark et al., 1981). To these we may now add a population of interneurones with a predominant monosynaptic input from group II muscle afferents, interneurones which are located primarily in the 4th lumbar (L4) segment (Edgley and Jankowska, 1987b). The contribution of these interneurones to movement control has been investigated from several points of view, and using different experimental approaches; these will be briefly summarized.

Projections and actions

We have now evidence that many of L4 interneurones have direct excitatory or inhibitory actions upon lower lumbar motoneurones and are thus interposed in disynaptic reflex pathways from group II muscle afferents (Cavallari et al., 1987). This has been established by using records from motoneuronal populations (from ventral roots, with a sucrose gap technique) and spike triggered averaging. However, the study of axonal projections of these interneurones, after they have been injected with horseradish peroxidase, has revealed their terminal branching both within and outside motor nuclei and the additional possibility of their actions via other interneurones (Bras, Cavallari, Jankowska and Kubin, in preparation).

Afferent input

The input to L4 interneurones was investigated by using intracellular records from individual interneurones which were antidromically activated from motor nuclei in lower lumbar segments and excited by group II muscle afferents, while stimulating various groups of afferents. The interneurones were found to be most effectively excited by electrical stimulation of group II afferents of the following muscle nerves: quadriceps, sartorius, deep peroneal and flexor digitorum longus; these afferents made direct synaptic contacts with them (Edgley and Jankowska, 1987b). The receptor origin could only be defined for group II afferents of anterior tibial and extensor digitorum longus, and, partly, for those of the quadriceps. The afferents were found to be from receptors activated by small muscle stretches (Edgley and Jankowska, 1987a) or by stimulation of γ fusimotor axons within one of the ventral roots (Harrison et al., 1988). Although the two procedures activate both group Ia and II muscle spindle afferents, their effects could be limited to the latter when tested on neurones which lacked any input from group I afferents, or on field potentials evoked exclusively from group II afferents. The group II input in all the tested cases has been concluded to be primarily from the secondary muscle spindle afferents. We have generalized this conclusion for group II input to L4 interneurones from both the pretibial flexors and other muscles, and accordingly consider these interneurones as primarily monitoring muscle length.

Other sources of afferent input to the same interneurones have been found to include: primary muscle spindle (Ia) afferents of a variety of muscles and afferents in cutaneous, joint and interosseous nerves (Edgley and Jankowska, 1987b). This means that responses of these interneurones to muscle stretches will be modulated by signals concerning the rate of these changes and the resulting position of the limb. The modulation will involve both facilitation and depression of the responses to muscle stretches since either EPSPs or IPSPs are evoked from any of the tested afferents in individual interneurones. The most direct coupling with group I afferents is monosynaptic while with other afferents either disynaptic or monosynaptic.

Descending input

L4 interneurones with group II input were often found to be excited by nerve impulses in cortico-, rubro-, reticulo- and vestibulo-spinal tract fibres, mono- or polysynaptically (Brink et al., 1985 and personal communication; Edgley et al., 1988). Depending on the intensity of the descending actions these were discharging the interneurones either by themselves, or only on the background of their depolarization by afferent impulses. The monosynaptic input from the vestibulo-spinal system is of particular interest for the contribution of these L4 interneurones to postural reflexes, because it is very tightly linked to other labyrinthine and neck reflexes (Brink et al., 1985 and personal communication). Another source of the strong descending excitatory input to L4 interneurones with group II input is from the region of the cuneiform nucleus (within the mesencephalic locomotor region), favouring their activation during locomotion (Edgley et al., 1988).

Modulation of synaptic input to L4 interneurones by monoamines

The synaptic transmission from group II afferents to L4 interneurones is effectively modulated by monoamines. In one series of experiments this has been established while using recording of extracellular field potentials and extra- and intracellular recording of responses of individual interneurones to various stimuli, both before and after ionophoretic application of serotonin and noradrenaline and after either ionophoretic or intravenous application of the noradrenaline precursor L-DOPA (Edgley et al., 1988; Bras et al., 1988 and in preparation). All these drugs appeared to have very similar affects. They produced a marked depression of synaptic actions evoked from group II afferents, but practically no change in transmission from other (Ia) afferents with a similar monosynaptic coupling. In another series of experiments similar tests were used to assess effects of electrical stimulation in the areas of the locus coeruleus and of the raphe nuclei, the sources of the descending noradrenergic and serotonergic bulbo-spinal pathways (Bras, Jankowska and Noga, in preparation). Stimuli applied in these areas closely mimicked effects of the ionophoretically applied monoamines in that they depressed responses to group II but not to group I input (tested on extracellular field potentials). In addition these experiments have shown that the depression evoked by a short train of such stimuli (e.g. 6 stimuli at 400 Hz) may last less than 200 ms, in contrast to the much longer-lasting effects of ionophoretically applied drugs. Thus, following a brief synaptic activation of descending noradrenergic or serotonergic neurones the L4 interneurones might show lower responsiveness to muscle stretch during selected phases of movements.

Concluding comments

Taking into account both the input, and the sensitivity of L4 interneurones to the monoaminergic modulatory control, we have put forward the hypothesis that they play an essential role in locomotion (Edgley and Jankowska, 1987b; Edgley et al., 1988), although they would undoubtedly be involved in any feedback control of muscle activity based on information on muscle length, and in movements induced by those descending systems which activate them.

The peripheral input to these neurones closely corresponds to the input to interneurones required to mediate transition from the extension (stance) to the flexion (swing) phase of the step cycle and the phase dependent reflex reversal, i.e. opposite reflex actions of cutaneous stimuli applied during

various phases of the step cycle (for references see Grillner, 1981; Edgley and Jankowska, 1987b), for which information on hip position is apparently the main type of excitatory input. Such information ought to be provided in parallel by the various muscle, joint and cutaneous receptors, because only a small proportion of these afferents is sufficient for the adequate responses to appear. This requirement is fulfilled by a predominant group II input from hip muscles (quadriceps and sartorius) to L4 interneurones and by the extensive convergence of various types of afferents upon them. A further requirement of an additional excitatory input from pretibial flexors is likewise fulfilled. The inhibitory input from group Ib afferents of triceps surae (and of other antigravity muscles, which bear the body weight during the stance phase, and which prevent premature termination of this phase) and from cutaneous afferents has also been seen.

The strong excitatory input from within the mesencephalic locomotor region and their susceptibility to modulatory monoaminergic actions similarly point to the intimate relationship between L4 interneurones and the neuronal networks of locomotion, since stimulation of the same brain region and intravenous injection of L-DOPA very effectively initiate locomotion (see Lundberg, 1969; Grillner, 1981).

The depressive, rather than facilitatory actions of monoamines and similar effects of stimulation within the areas of origin of the descending monoaminergic pathways on L4 interneurones appeared first to be rather puzzling. However, since the effects of electrical stimuli in the nuclei of origin of the descending monoaminergic pathways are quite short-lasting, the depression of transmission from group II afferents to L4 interneurones may be limited to only some phases of the step cycle, either alternating or overlapping with the periods of excitation of these neurones by phasically active neurones of the mesencephalic locomotor region (see e.g. Armstrong, 1986). Functional consequences of the selective monoaminergic depression of transmission from group II muscle spindle afferents and its mechanisms remain to be investigated, but it will clearly allow the relative potency of the input from different sources to L4 interneurones to be graded during different phases of movement; it will, for example, make them relatively more dependent on dynamic aspects of muscle stretches (via Ia muscle spindle afferents or tendon organs), and on descending commands during periods of depressed transmission from group II muscle afferents.

The hypothesis of the essential role of L4 interneurones with group II input in locomotion is further supported by two groups of observations made during fictive locomotion. One group of these observations concerns the rhythmic, phase-locked activity of a high proportion of L4 neurones (see e.g. Deliagina et al., 1983). In these early studies the neurones were unidentified functionally but might well have included interneurones with group II input. The second group of observations have been made on L4 interneurones identified in the same way as the above described neurones with group II input. Several of them were found to be rhythmically active, in particular during the transition between the two phases of the locomotor cycle (Shefchyk et al., 1988, and personal communication). The activity of these interneurones, and their contribution to locomotion will, of course, be greatly influenced by the γ and β fusimotor systems and their actions on spindle group II input, and it may be a highly challenging problem to determine the interplay between the descending monoaminergic systems and the neuronal systems of control of fusimotor neurones to ensure the proper functioning of the locomotor networks.

Acknowledgement

This study was supported by the Swedish Medical Research Council (project 5648).

References

Alstermark, B., Lundberg, A., Norrsell, U. and Sybirska, E. (1981) Integration in descending motor pathways controlling the forelimb in the cat. 9. Differential behavioural defects after spinal cord lesions interrupting defined pathways from higher centres to motoneurones. *Exp. Brain Res.*, 42: 299 – 318.

Armstrong, D.M. (1986) Supraspinal contributions to the initiation and control of locomotion in the cat. *Prog. Neurobiol.*, 26: 273 – 361.

Bras, H., Cavallari, P. and Jankowska, E. (1988) An investigation of local actions of ionophoretically applied DOPA in the spinal cord. *Exp. Brain Res.*, 71: 447 – 449.

Brink, E.E., Suzuki, I., Timerick, S.J.B. and Wilson, V.J. (1985) Tonic neck reflex of the decerebrate cat: a role for propriospinal neurons. *J. Neurophysiol.*, 54: 978 – 987.

Cavallari, P., Edgley, S.A. and Jankowska, E. (1987) Postsynaptic actions of midlumbar interneurones on motoneurones of hind-limb muscles in the cat. *J. Physiol. (London)*, 389: 675 – 690.

Deliagina, T.G., Orlovsky, G.N. and Pavlova, G.A. (1983) The capacity for generation of rhythmic oscillations is distributed in the lumbosacral spinal cord of the cat. *Exp. Brain Res.*, 53: 81 – 90.

Edgley, S.A. and Jankowska, E. (1987a) Field potentials generated by group I and II muscle afferents in the middle lumbar segments of the cat spinal cord. *J. Physiol. (London)*, 385: 393 – 413.

Edgley, S.A. and Jankowska, E. (1987b) An interneuronal relay for group I and II muscle afferents in the midlumbar segments of the cat spinal cord. *J. Physiol. (London)*, 389: 675 – 690.

Edgley, S.A., Jankowska, E. and Shefchyk, S. (1988) Evidence that interneurones in reflex pathways from group II afferents are involved in locomotion in the cat. *J. Physiol. (London)*, 403: 57 – 73.

Grillner, S. (1981) Control of locomotion in bipeds, tetrapods and fish. In J.M. Brookhart, V.B. Mountcastle and V.B. Brooks (Eds), *Handbook of Physiology – the Nervous System, Vol. II, Motor Control, Part 1*, William and Wilkins, Baltimore, pp. 1179 – 1236.

Harrison, P.J. and Jankowska, E. (1985) Organization of input to the interneurones mediating group I non-reciprocal inhibition of motoneurones in the cat. *J. Physiol. (London)*, 361: 403 – 418.

Harrison, P.J., Jami, L. and Jankowska, E. (1988) Further evidence for synaptic actions of muscle spindle secondaries in middle lumbar segments of the cat spinal cord. *J. Physiol. (London)*, 402: 671 – 686.

Lundberg, A. (1969) Reflex control of stepping. *The Nansen Memorial Lecture V*, Universitetsforlaget, Oslo, pp. 1 – 42.

Lundberg, A., Malmgren, K. and Schomburg, E.D. (1987) Reflex pathways from group II muscle afferents. 3. Secondary spindle afferents and the FRA; a new hypothesis. *Exp. Brain Res.*, 65: 294 – 306.

Noga, B.R., Shefchyk, S.J., Jamal, J. and Jordan, L.M. (1987) The role of Renshaw cells in locomotion: antagonism of their excitation from motor axon collaterals with intravenous mecamylamine. *Exp. Brain Res.,* 66: 99 – 105.

Pratt, C.A. and Jordan, L.M. (1987) Ia inhibitory interneurons and Renshaw cells as contributors to the spinal mechanisms of fictive locomotion. *J. Neurophysiol.,* 57: 56 – 71.

Shefchyk, S.J., McCrea, D.A., Kriellaars, D.J., Jordan, L.M. and Fortier, P. (1987) Activity of midlumbar group II interneurons during brainstem evoked fictive locomotion in the mesencephalic cat. *Soc. Neurosci. Abstr.,* 14: 265.

J.H.J. Allum and M. Hulliger (Eds.)
Progress in Brain Research, Vol. 80
© 1989 Elsevier Science Publishers B.V. (Biomedical Division)

CHAPTER 25

Peripheral and descending control of neurones mediating non-monosynaptic Ia excitation to motoneurones: a presumed propriospinal system in man

E. Pierrot-Deseilligny

Clinical Neurophysiology, Department of Rééducation, Hôpital de la Salpêtrière, Paris Cedex 13, France

Evidence for a non-monosynaptic Ia excitation of wrist flexor and quadriceps motoneurones (MNs) in man has been provided while using two independent methods: construction of post-stimulus time histograms (PSTHs) of voluntarily activated motor units and the spatial facilitation of the H-reflex. This non-monosynaptic Ia excitation has a long central latency (3 – 6 ms) and a very low threshold. Neurones mediating this effect seem to receive a strong descending excitation at the onset of voluntary movement and it is argued that they might mediate part of the descending command to MNs. In contrast, increasing the afferent input produces an inhibition of the transmission in this pathway. Several characteristics of the non-monosynaptic excitation and its depression bear resemblance to those of the C3 – C4 propriospinal system in the cat, which is used as a model for the discussion of the present results.

Key words: Propriospinal neurone; Spinal interneurone; Reflex pathway; Muscle spindle Ia afferent; Cutaneous afferent; Descending pathway; Voluntary movement; Motor control; Post-stimulus time histogram; Human upper limb

Introduction

The traditional view is that certain spinal interneurones are part of reflex pathways. However, the main function of other interneurones is to transmit the descending motor command from the brain. Since these neurones also receive projections from primary afferents, the descending command to the motoneurones (MNs) can be modified en route by the afferent activity at a pre-moto-neuronal level (Jankowska and Lundberg, 1981). A good example of such a system is furnished by the C3 – C4 propriospinal neurones which have been shown to mediate target-reaching movements in the cat and to receive both excitation and inhibition from forelimb afferents (see Lundberg, 1979). Evidence for a similar system has been sought in man.

Non-monosynaptic Ia excitation of MNs

Responses of individual motoneurones

Single motor unit recordings in man
The PSTH method. The effect of a given stimulus on a voluntarily activated MN can be determined by constructing a histogram of occurrence of MN spikes following repeated presentation of the stimulus. The resulting post-stimulus time histogram (PSTH) extracts from the naturally occurring spike train only those changes in firing probability which are time-locked to the stimulus (Stephens et al., 1976; Fetz and Gustafsson, 1983).

Monosynaptic EPSPs. Stimulation of the homonymous nerve at motor threshold ($1 \times MT$) evokes in most motor units (MUs) a large increase in firing probability (Fig. 1A, open columns) with a latency exactly corresponding to that of the H-reflex. It has been shown that this early peak can be attributed to the monosynaptic Ia excitatory post-synaptic potential (EPSP) (Mao et al., 1984).

Experimental design to study non-monosynaptic EPSPs. For the purposes of this study it was necessary to hinder the

monosynaptic discharge since the following refractoriness would prevent any subsequent non-monosynaptic EPSP from discharging the MN. This was achieved both by reducing the intensity of stimulation and by delivering it at a fixed delay after the previous spike (Fournier et al., 1986). This delay was adjusted so that the afterhyperpolarization (AHP) following the previous MN discharge would reduce the firing probability due to the monosynaptic EPSP evoked by the stimulation, but that it would have less effect on any non-monosynaptic EPSPs since

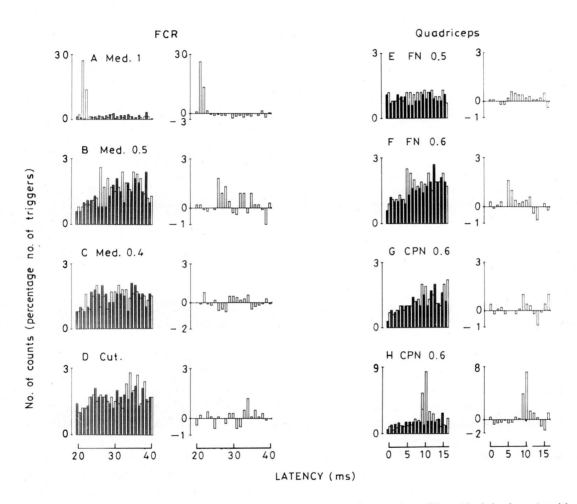

Fig. 1. Time histograms of the discharge of voluntarily activated MUs in control conditions (shaded columns) and in response to stimulation (open columns), and difference between these two histograms (open columns on the right in each pair). The number of counts, expressed as a percentage of the number of triggers (A 300, B – D 1000, E 1500, F – G 800, H 600), is plotted against the latency from the stimulation (A – D) or from the monosynaptic latency (E – H). A – D, responses of the same FCR MU to various stimuli applied either to the median nerve (Med.) (A 1 × MT, B 0.5 × MT, C 0.4 × MT) or to the skin (Cut.) (D). Note that the scale of the ordinate is smaller in B – D than in A. E – H, responses of 3 different Q MUs (E, F – G, H) to stimuli applied either to the femoral nerve (FN) (E 0.5 × MT, F 0.6 × MT) or to the common peroneal nerve (CPN) (G – H 0.6 × MT). (A – D adapted from Malmgren and Pierrot-Deseilligny, 1987; E adapted from Fournier et al., 1986; F – H adapted from Forget et al., 1989.)

they would occur later when the AHP had decayed further. The latency of these late EPSPs is expressed as the time in excess of the monosynaptic latency in the histograms shown in Fig. 1 E–H, and Figs. 4 and 5.

Histograms were also constructed in a control situation (without stimulation), and conditioned and control situations were randomly alternated within a sequence. In the control situation (shaded columns in Figs. 1 and 5), the "spontaneous" firing progressively increased with increasing time intervals, reflecting the post-spike trajectory of the MN membrane potential. Histograms following stimulations (open columns) were compared to this background firing probability. To clarify the differences between the two situations the value obtained in the control situation was subtracted from that obtained after stimulation in each 1 ms bin, and the results of these subtractions are shown on the right of the corresponding histograms (Figs. 1 and 5). In Fig. 4 only the results of these subtractions are shown.

Non-monosynaptic Ia EPSPs in wrist flexor MNs
Late EPSPs.   Fig. 1 A–C shows the changes in firing probability of a flexor carpi radialis (FCR) MU following median nerve stimulations at various intensities. At $1 \times$ MT (Fig. 1A) there was an early (21 ms) peak attributed to the monosynaptic Ia EPSP (see above). At $0.5 \times$ MT (Fig. 1B) the monosynaptic response had disappeared whereas a second peak appeared with a sharp onset at a latency (26 ms) which was 5 ms longer than the monosynaptic one. This second peak was much smaller than the monosynaptic peak (note the different scale of the ordinates in A and B) but highly significant ($P < 0.001$). At $0.4 \times$ MT (Fig. 1C) median nerve stimulation was ineffective. Such late excitation was found in 60% of the 70 MUs recorded from, with latencies ranging between 3 and 6 ms. FCR MUs received late excitation mainly from the median nerve whereas flexor carpi ulnaris (FCU) MUs received late excitation about as often from the ulnar nerve (Malmgren and Pierrot-Deseilligny, 1988a).

The late excitation was not cutaneous in origin since pure cutaneous stimulation, mimicking the sensation evoked by median nerve stimulation, produced an increase in firing probability which was much smaller and which occurred later (Fig. 1-D). The onset of the late excitation may therefore be ascribed to low threshold muscle (group I) afferents. The threshold of the late excitation was usually lower than that of the monosynaptic Ia peak which indicates a contribution from the lowest threshold afferents.

Non-monosynaptic group I excitation.   A decrease in the size of the monosynaptic Ia EPSP, due to the low intensities used, cannot be responsible for a shift of several ms in latency, since it has been shown in the cat that decreasing the size of the EPSP does not delay the corresponding increase in firing probability by more than 0.35 ms (Fetz and Gustaffson, 1983). Similarly in man, reducing the stimulus intensity to $0.6 \times$ MT has been shown to delay the monosynaptic peak by less than 1 ms (see Malmgren and Pierrot-Deseilligny, 1988b, their Fig. 2). Thus the long latency reflects, with all likelihood, an activation of interneurones.

Non-monosynaptic Ia EPSPs in quadriceps MNs
Homonymous EPSPs.   Stimulation of the femoral nerve (FN) may evoke in quadriceps (Q) MUs a non-monosynaptic excitation occurring with a central latency of 4–5 ms (Fournier et al., 1986), but this excitation is both smaller (Fig. 1E) and less frequent (only 20% of the MUs) than in wrist flexor MUs. In this case too, this non-monosynaptic excitation was caused by the lowest threshold group I afferents.

Heteronymous EPSPs from the common peroneal
nerve (CPN).   The effects of a weak stimulation to the FN and CPN on the firing probability of the same Q MU are compared in Fig. 1F,G; here the excitation evoked by CPN stimulation was weak, but it was often much larger in other units (Fig. 1H). This CPN stimulation-induced excitation occurred at a latency 9 ms longer than that of the FN stimulation-induced monosynaptic Ia EPSP, i.e. 4–5 ms later than the non-monosynaptic excitations evoked by FN stimulation. This delay corresponds to the extra afferent conduction time of the CPN volley, from the more distal stimulation site to the spinal cord. Hence, non-monosynaptic excitation evoked by CPN and FN stimulations

have a similar central latency, which suggests that they could be mediated through similar neuronal systems (Forget et al., 1989).

Responses of a MN population

Spatial and temporal facilitation technique

In animal experiments, the spatial facilitation technique has been used to demonstrate convergence from two different fibre systems onto common interneurones while recording EPSPs in MNs (see Lundberg, 1975): the EPSPs evoked by two conditioning stimuli applied separately or together are compared and summation at a pre-motoneuronal level is inferred when the EPSP on combined stimulation is larger than the algebraic sum of the EPSPs evoked by separate stimuli. The same principle can be used in man when the synaptic effects are assessed with the H-reflex technique. However, if the facilitation of the reflex on combined stimulation is larger than the algebraic sum of the effects evoked by the two separate stimuli, the problem is to determine whether the extra facilitation (i.e. the part of the facilitation exceeding the algebraic sum) represents a summation at a pre-motoneuronal level or a non-linear summation at the MN level (see Fournier et al., 1986).

Extra facilitation of the H-reflex

Fig. 2A – E shows the spatial facilitation of the FCR H-reflex when conditioned by two stimuli: one conditioning stimulus (C1) was applied to the median nerve (0.5 × MT, 5 ms conditioning-test interval) and the other (C2) to the ulnar nerve (0.6 × MT, 4 ms conditioning-test interval). The amount of reflex facilitation, i.e. the difference between conditioned reflex and unconditioned reflex (expressed as a percentage of the control reflex value), was compared when conditioning stimuli were applied separately and together. When applied alone, neither C1 (Fig. 2B) nor C2 (Fig. 2C) evoked any significant facilitation of the test reflex. By contrast, a large reflex facilitation appeared on combined stimulation (C1 + C2) (Fig. 2E). The difference between this facilitation

and the algebraic sum by separate stimuli is indicated by the double-headed arrow in Fig. 2E and represents the extra facilitation of the reflex on combined stimulation. Cutaneous afferents were shown not to contribute to this effect. Moreover, similar results were obtained while using weak tendon taps, which indicates that Ia afferents contribute to the extra facilitation of the reflex (Malmgren and Pierrot-Deseilligny, 1988a).

Results from another experiment are used to illustrate the time course of the extra facilitation of

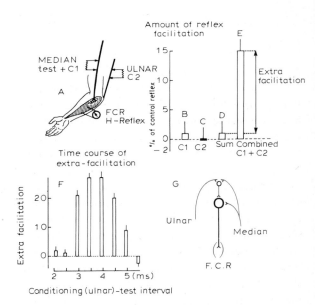

Fig. 2. Spatial facilitation of the FCR H-reflex. A, general experimental arrangement: two conditioning stimuli, to the median (C1) and ulnar (C2) nerves, are used. B – E, the amount of reflex facilitation (conditioned reflex -unconditioned reflex) is expressed as a percentage of the size of the control reflex. B – C, effect of C1 (0.5 × MT) and C2 (0.5 × MT) when applied alone. D, algebraic sum of effects by separate stimuli. E, facilitation of the reflex on combined stimulation; the double-headed arrow represents the difference between E and D, i.e. the extra facilitation of the reflex on combined stimulation. F, extra facilitation on combined stimulation (C1 0.6 × MT, C2 1 × MT) is plotted against the time interval between C2 and the test volley (C1-test interval is constant at 5 ms). B – F, each column represents the mean of 40 measurements. Vertical bars one standard error (S.E.) of the mean (adapted from Malmgren and Pierrot-Deseilligny, 1988a). G, sketch of the presumed connections.

the reflex (Fig. 2F). When applied alone C1 (0.6 × MT) evoked a large homonymous reflex facilitation whereas C2 (1 × MT) was ineffective (not illustrated). The amount of extra facilitation of the reflex on combined stimulation is plotted against the time interval (at spinal level) between C2 and the test volley (the interval between C1 and the test volley being constant at 5 ms). Extra facilitation had a long central latency (3 ms) and a sharp onset. A similar extra facilitation of the Q H reflex, with a central latency of 3 – 5 ms, was observed when combining a volley to the FN either with a weak tap to the Q tendon (Fournier et al., 1986) or with CPN stimulation (Forget et al., 1989).

The long central latency observed here rules out the possibility that the extra facilitation of the reflex is caused by non-linear summation of monosynaptic Ia EPSPs at the MN level since, in such a case, extrafacilitation should occur at monosynaptic latency. A summation at a premotoneuronal level is therefore suggested. In the case of the upper limb this would indicate that group I fibres from the median and ulnar nerve converge onto common excitatory interneurones projecting on FCR MNs (Fig. 2G).

Conclusion

Two independent methods have been used to provide evidence for non-monosynaptic Ia excitation of human MNs. On the basis of the similarities between the results obtained with the two methods (same central latency, same very low threshold) it is argued that the late EPSP in PSTH experiments and the extra facilitation of the reflex are mediated through the same pre-motoneuronal pathway.

In both PSTH (Fig. 1B) and reflex (Fig. 2B – E) experiments the threshold of the late Ia excitation was below that of the monosynaptic excitation. An explanation for this finding might be that the Ia fibres activated by the weak stimuli which were used, could be heteronymous and lack monosynaptic projections onto the MNs recorded from, whilst projecting to the interneurones mediating the late excitation; given the large number of muscles sup-

plied by the median and the ulnar nerves, this appears plausible.

Possibly, the non-monosynaptic Ia excitation could be mediated through a system similar to the C3 – C4 propriospinal neurones. In the cat, however, propriospinal neurones receive their main excitatory input from descending tracts and the main effect from primary afferents is inhibition (cf. Fig. 6). Therefore evidence for descending excitation and peripheral inhibition of the neurones mediating the effect described above was sought in further experiments.

Descending facilitation of the transmission in the pathway of non-monosynaptic Ia excitation during movement

The time course of the variations in the FCR H-reflex when preceded by a conditioning stimulation to the ulnar nerve (0.6 × MT) was compared at rest and at the onset of a voluntary wrist flexion of moderate force (20% of the maximal force) (Baldissera and Pierrot-Deseilligny, 1989). At rest (Fig. 3, ○) the ulnar nerve volley was almost inef-

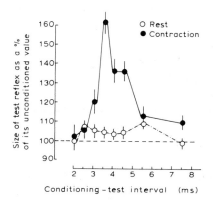

Fig. 3. The time course of the variations in the FCR H-reflex when preceded by a conditioning stimulus to the ulnar nerve (0.6 × MT) is compared at rest (○) and at the onset of a voluntary wrist flexion (●). The size of the test reflex expressed as a percentage of its control value is plotted against the conditioning-test interval at the spinal level. Each symbol represents the mean of 20 measurements. Vertical bars 1 S.E. of the mean (adapted from Baldissera and Pierrot-Deseilligny, 1989).

310

fective, whereas at the onset of contraction it evoked a large reflex facilitation (Fig. 3, ●), which occurred at a latency of 3 ms (conditioning-test interval at the spinal level) and had a short duration (2 ms). As it was shown that cutaneous afferents did not contribute to this reflex facilitation, it can be attributed to group I muscle afferents. The 3 ms central latency speaks against the possibility that the reflex facilitation might be due to a decrease in either Ib inhibition or presynaptic inhibition of Ia terminals since these mechanisms have been shown to first manifest themselves at intervals below 1 ms (Fournier et al., 1983; Hultborn et al., 1987). In fact the reflex facilitation has a time course which corresponds to that of the non-monosynaptic Ia excitation described above. This suggests that there might be a facilitation of the transmission in the pathway of non-monosynaptic Ia excitation to FCR MNs at the onset of voluntary wrist flexion. Non-monosynaptic Ia excitation to Q MNs was similarly facilitated at the onset of very weak Q contractions (Hultborn et al., 1986).

In these experiments the conditioning volley was triggered by the first voluntary EMG potential. i.e. probably before any group I discharge evoked by the contraction (Vallbo, 1971). It can therefore be assumed that the reflex facilitation seen at the onset of movement is due to a descending excitation of the interneurones mediating the Ia excitation to MNs.

Inhibition of non-monosynaptic Ia excitation

Evidence for inhibition

In PSTH experiments, increasing the afferent input regularly depressed the non-monosynaptic Ia excitation (Malmgren and Pierrot-Deseilligny, 1988b). The inhibitory effect of increasing the intensity of stimulation is illustrated in Fig. 4 (note that in Figs. 4 and 5, zero on the abscissa corresponds to the monosynaptic latency): the significant non-monosynaptic excitation observed in one FCU MU when stimulating the median nerve at 0.4 × MT (Fig. 4A) disappeared when the stimulus in-

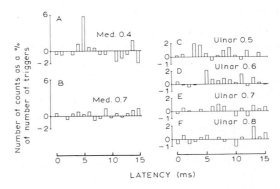

Fig. 4. Time histograms of the discharge of two different FCU MUs (A – B and C – F) when the intensity of the stimulation to the median (A – B) or the ulnar (C – F) nerve is increased. Ordinate and abscissa, same legend as in Fig. 1 E – H. Note that only the difference between the values obtained after stimulation and those obtained in control conditions is represented. Number of triggers: A 180, B 580, C – F 500 (adapted from Malmgren and Pierrot-Deseilligny, 1988b).

tensity was increased to 0.7 × MT (Fig. 4B). Also the early part (first two bins) of the excitation evoked by the ulnar nerve stimulation at 0.5 × MT in another MU disappeared when the intensity was increased to 0.6 × MT (Fig. 4 C,D). With further increases in the intensity there was no trough in the firing probability at the latency of the early excitation, although the depression became more and more manifest at longer latencies (Fig. 4 E,F).

A strong depressive effect was also observed on combined stimulation of two nerves. So, in the case of the FCU MU illustrated in Fig. 5, the non-monosynaptic excitation evoked by separate stimulation of the median nerve at 0.5 × MT (Fig. 5A) disappeared on combined stimulation of the median and ulnar nerves (Fig. 5C) (note that separate stimulation of the ulnar nerve did not evoke any early effect, Fig. 5B). A similar depression was observed in 80% of the MUs in which separate stimulation of one or both nerve(s) evoked a non-monosynaptic excitation. Occlusion in the excitatory pathway cannot explain this depression since the effect on combined stimulation was smaller than the largest of the two separate effects (cf. C with A in Fig. 5). Hence an inhibitory

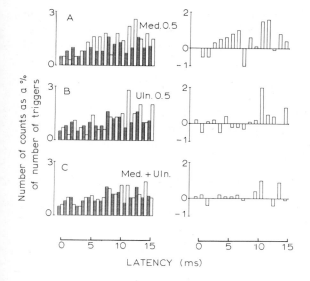

Fig. 5. Time histograms of the discharge of an FCU MU. The effects evoked by two stimuli evoked separately (A: median 0.5 × MT; B ulnar 0.5 × MT) and together (C) are compared. Left and right, ordinate and abscissa, same legend as in Fig. 1 E – H. Number of triggers: 700 (adapted from Malmgren and Pierrot-Deseilligny, 1988b).

mechanism is implied. Presynaptic inhibition of one volley by the other is excluded by the extremely brief latency of the effect (the two volleys were timed to reach the MNs simultaneously). A post-synaptic inhibition is therefore implied.

This inhibition had the same low threshold as the excitation. Both cutaneous and group I afferents were able to evoke it, but the inhibitory action of cutaneous afferents was clearer. The onset of the inhibition was found to vary systematically with the latency of the excitation: whatever the latency of the excitation (range 3 – 6 ms) the first bin of excitation was always depressed, but the inhibition on combined stimulation was never preceded by a trough in the PSTH (Malmgren and Pierrot-Deseilligny, 1988b, Fig. 4).

Non-monosynaptic excitation of Q MNs evoked by stimulation of one nerve (FN and/or CPN) was also depressed on combined stimulation of the two nerves (Forget et al., 1989).

Inhibition is exerted at the pre-motoneuronal level

An inhibitory post-synaptic potential (IPSP) at the MN level is expected to manifest itself as a trough in which the firing rate falls below baseline rate (Fetz and Gustafsson, 1983). An early trough was sometimes seen (latency 1 ms in Fig. 5A). Because of its short latency and duration and of the low stimulus intensity required this inhibition was probably of Ib origin.

However, there was never any trough in the PSTH at the latency of the non-monosynaptic excitation: whatever the amount of the afferent input the inhibition could at the very most suppress the excitation (Fig. 4 C – F). This is taken to support the idea that the inhibition is exerted at a pre-motoneuronal level. Another argument in favour of this interpretation is the finding that the onset of the inhibition varied systematically with that of the excitation. Also, there was never any inhibition (appearing as a trough in the PSTH) on combined stimulation in those recordings where there was no excitation.

All these findings are best explained by an inhibition exerted at a pre-motoneuronal level. Such a disfacilitation can be revealed at the MN level only if the interneurones mediating the excitation are fired: accordingly it would only appear against a background of non-monosynaptic excitation and then only as a depression of it. Also, if the inhibition affects the earliest interneuronal excitation, its onset would be expected to vary with the latency of the excitation, as was indeed demonstrated.

If the neurones interposed in the excitatory pathways had mediated part of the descending command to the MN studied in the PSTH, their inhibition — if strong enough — could have reduced (below the control level) the excitatory input to the MN, with the consequent disclosure of a trough in the PSTH. To explain the finding that the inhibition never manifests itself as a trough it was postulated that these neurones were not fired during the very weak (one MU) contraction studied. This seemingly contradicts the results reported above (Fig. 3). However, these results concerned stronger contractions (20% of the maximal force) and the neurones in question might be more or less easily recruited in contractions of different strength.

In conclusion, the characteristics of the depression of the non-monosynaptic Ia excitation are well explained by postulating an inhibition of the transmission in the neuronal pathway mediating this excitation to MNs.

Depression of the homonymous Ia facilitation of the FCR H-reflex by an ulnar nerve volley

As seen above (Fig. 2) an extra facilitation of the FCR H-reflex can be observed when two conditioning stimuli applied to the median (C1) and the ulnar (C2) nerves are applied together. However, this occurred only when C1 preceded C2 at the spinal level (intervals below 5 ms in Fig. 2F where the C1-test interval was kept constant at 5 ms). By contrast, an opposite result was obtained when an ulnar nerve volley, ineffective by itself, preceded a median nerve volley evoking, when applied alone, a large homonymous facilitation of the reflex: on combined stimulation this facilitation was significantly reduced. It has been argued that this result is compatible with the above interpretation (disfacilitation): the non-monosynaptic part of the homonymous Ia facilitation would be inhibited by the ulnar nerve volley (Malmgren and Pierrot-Deseilligny, 1988b).

Possible pathway

The long central latency of the non-monosynaptic Ia excitation described here (3 – 6 ms) might be taken to entail polysynaptic transmission. However, the very low threshold and sharp onset of the effect suggest that the excitation is not mediated through a long chain of interneurones. The long latency could instead be explained by a long conduction distance between MNs and interneurones located at different spinal segments.

In this context propriospinal neurones may be good candidates. Rostral hindlimb neurones have been recently described in the lumbar cat spinal cord: they project to hindlimb MNs and receive excitation from both hindlimb afferents and descending tracts (see Cavallari et al., 1987). However, the best known of the propriospinal systems is the system of C3 – C4 neurones, which project monosynaptically onto forelimb MNs and receive extensive excitatory convergence from descending tracts. They also receive both monosynaptic excitation (Illert et al., 1978) and disynaptic inhibition

(Alstermark et al., 1984) from low threshold forelimb afferents, but inhibition is very prominent. A reason for choosing the C3 – C4 system as a model is that, since it is so well defined, it provides a framework for the discussion of the present results. The organization of the C3 – C4 propriospinal system in the cat is schematically represented in Fig. 6 and parallels can be drawn between our results and this system.

(1) Like C3 – C4 propriospinal neurones, neurones mediating Ia excitation to MNs seem to receive strong descending excitation.

(2) Also the present results fit with a system similar

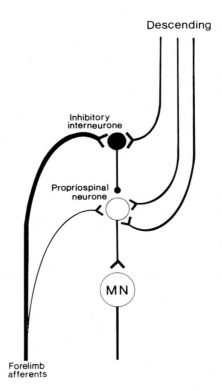

Fig. 6. Schematic diagram of some excitatory (bars) and inhibitory (small filled circles) connections to C3 – C4 propriospinal neurones in the cat. Monosynaptic projection of propriospinal neurone to a forelimb motoneurone (MN) is represented. Large filled circle, inhibitory interneurone. Primary afferents evoke both excitation and inhibition of propriospinal neurones, but inhibitory effects are very prominent (thick line). (Modified from Lundberg, 1979, and adapted from Malmgren and Pierrot-Deseilligny, 1988b.)

to that providing feedback inhibition from peripheral afferents to C3 – C4 propriospinal neurones in the cat. Supposing that the excitation to the propriospinal neurones had a somewhat lower threshold than the inhibition, which involves one more synapse, excitation will dominate at low stimulus intensity (Figs. 4A,C). The finding that disfacilitation appears when the afferent input is increased (Figs. 4B,E,F, 5C) might indicate that the interneurones mediating inhibition are more strongly activated by an increasing afferent input than are the excitatory (propriospinal) neurones. This would lead to an increased size and a reduced latency of the IPSP, which could then arrive early enough to prevent propriospinal neurones from firing in response to the afferent volley.

Functional significance

The system of C3 – C4 propriospinal neurones has been shown to function as a relay station transmitting target-reaching movements of the cat (Alstermark et al., 1981). The strong descending excitation of the neurones mediating non-monosynaptic Ia excitation to human MNs at the onset of voluntary contraction suggests that these neurones might mediate part of the descending command to MNs. Convergence from upper limb afferents onto these neurones could then be viewed as a peripheral sensory feedback aiming at regulating the descending command en route to the MNs.

For example, the inhibition by cutaneous afferents of the neurones in question could play an important role in the termination of a movement: the exteroceptive activity resulting from the contact with the target (or with an unexpected obstacle) could inhibit the descending command at the propriospinal neurone level, thus contributing to curtail the movement. As emphasized by Alstermark et al. (1984), delegating part of the task of termination of the movement, which the brain does not easily and reliably plan ahead of movement execution, to spinal cord mechanisms would be an elegant solution.

References

Alstermark, B., Lundberg, A., Norrsell, U. and Sybirska, E. (1981) Integration in descending motor pathways controlling the forelimb in the cat. 9. Differential behavioural defects after spinal cord lesions interrupting defined pathways from higher centres to motoneurones. *Exp. Brain Res.*, 42: 299 – 318.

Alstermark, B., Lundberg, A. and Sasaki, S. (1984) Integration in descending motor pathways controlling the forelimb in the cat. 12. Interneurones which may mediate descending feed-forward inhibition and feed-back inhibition from the forelimb to C3-C4 propriospinal neurones. *Exp. Brain Res.*, 56: 308 – 322.

Baldissera, F. and Pierrot-Deseilligny, E. (1989) Facilitation of transmission in the pathway of non-monosynaptic Ia excitation to wrist flexor motoneurones at the onset of voluntary movement in man. *Exp. Brain Res.*, 74: 437 – 439.

Cavallari, P., Edgley, S.A. and Jankowska, E. (1987) Post-synaptic actions of midlumbar interneurones on motoneurones of hind-limb muscles in the cat. *J. Physiol. (London)*, 309: 675 – 689.

Fetz, E.E. and Gustafsson, B. (1983) Relation between shapes of post-synaptic potentials and changes in firing probability of cat motoneurones. *J. Physiol. (London)*, 341: 387 – 410.

Forget, R., Pantiou, R., Pierrot-Deseilligny, E., Shindo, M. and Tanaka, R. (1989) Facilitation of quadriceps motoneurones by group I afferents from pretibial flexors in man. 1. Possible interneuronal pathway. *Exp. Brain Res.*, 78: 10 – 20.

Fournier, E., Katz, R. and Pierrot-Deseilligny, E. (1983) Descending control of reflex pathways in the production of voluntary isolated movement in man. *Brain Res.*, 288: 375 – 377.

Fournier, E., Meunier, S., Pierrot-Deseilligny, E. and Shindo, M. (1986) Evidence for interneuronally mediated Ia excitatory effects to human quadriceps motoneurones. *J. Physiol. (London)*, 377: 143 – 169.

Hultborn, H., Meunier, S., Pierrot-Deseilligny, E. and Shindo, M. (1986) Changes in polysynaptic Ia excitation to quadriceps motoneurones during voluntary contraction in man. *Exp. Brain Res.*, 63: 436 – 438.

Hultborn, H., Meunier, S., Morin, C. and Pierrot-Deseilligny, E. (1987) Assessing changes in presynaptic inhibition of Ia fibres: a study in man and the cat. *J. Physiol. (London)*, 389: 729 – 756.

Illert, M., Lundberg, A., Padel, Y. and Tanaka, R. (1978) Integration in descending motor pathways controlling the forelimb in the cat. 5. Properties of and monosynaptic excitatory convergence on C3-C4 propriospinal neurones. *Exp. Brain Res.*, 33: 101 – 130.

Jankowska, E. and Lundberg, A. (1981) Interneurones in the spinal cord. *Trends Neurosci.*, 4: 230 – 233.

Lundberg, A. (1975) Control of spinal mechanisms from the brain. In D.B. Tower (Ed.), *The Nervous System, The Basic Neurosciences,* Vol. 1, Raven Press, New York, pp. 253 – 265.

Lundberg, A. (1979) Integration in a propriospinal motor centre controlling the forelimb in the cat. In H. Asanuma and V.J. Wilson (Eds.), *Integration in the Nervous System,* Igaku Shoin, Tokyo, pp. 47 – 64.

Malmgren, K. and Pierrot-Deseilligny, E. (1987) Evidence that low threshold afferents both evoke and depress polysynaptic excitation of wrist flexor motoneurones in man. *Exp. Brain Res.,* 67: 429 – 432.

Malmgren, K. and Pierrot-Deseilligny, E. (1988a) Evidence for non-monosynaptic Ia excitation of wrist flexor motoneurones, possibly via propriospinal neurones. *J. Physiol. (London),* 405: 747 – 764.

Malmgren, K. and Pierrot-Deseilligny, E. (1988b) Inhibition of neurones transmitting non-monosynaptic Ia excitation to human wrist flexor motoneurones. *J. Physiol. (London),* 405: 765 – 783.

Mao, C.C., Ashby, P., Wang, M. and McCrea, D. (1984) Synaptic connections from large muscle afferents to the motoneurones of various leg muscles in man. *Exp. Brain Res.,* 56: 341 – 350.

Stephens, J.A., Usherwood, T.P. and Garnett, R. (1976) Technique for studying synaptic connections of single motoneurones in man. *Nature (London),* 263: 343 – 344.

Vallbo, Å.B. (1971) Muscle spindle response at the onset of voluntary isometric contractions in man. Time difference between fusimotor and skeletomotor effects. *J. Physiol. (London),* 218: 405 – 431.

J.H.J. Allum and M. Hulliger (Eds.)
Progress in Brain Research, Vol. 80
© 1989 Elsevier Science Publishers B.V. (Biomedical Division)

Overview and critique of Chapters 26 and 27

Parameter adaptation in the spinal cord?

U. Windhorst

Göttingen, F.R.G.

After the establishment of the basic principles of synaptic transmission, a period of research has started which is still in full rush and is concerned with "modulatory" actions (in a wide sense) of classical neurotransmitters. A prominent trias among these are acetylcholine, noradrenaline and serotonin. They are found ubiquitously at different levels of the nervous system throughout the phylum, and are involved in a variety of functions, from gating functions in the establishment of topographic and other maps during a sensitive "imprinting" period in early ontogeny (e.g. Bear and Singer, 1986) to modulation of signal transmission at various levels, e.g. in the cerebellum (Ito, 1984) or the spinal cord (Wallén et al., 1989, this volume; Pompeiano, 1989, this volume).

The work of *Wallén and his coworkers* on the locomotor rhythm generation in the lamprey paradigmatically illustrates the rapid advance that has been made over the past decades in elucidating the basic mechanisms of rhythmic motor behaviours. From invertebrates to mammals there are examples, in which this research has succeeded in identifying and classifying specialized types of neurones, in characterizing their anatomy and firing patterns, the underlying specific membrane properties, and in describing, at least in part, their synaptic interconnections including the electrical or transmitter interactions involved.

An important aspect of the present authors' work is the computer simulation in which they try to reverse the analytical direction of their experimental work by reassembling the bits and pieces into a coherent model. Indeed, this synthetic approach is a necessary complement of the analysis and serves to validate, in quantitative terms, intuitive ideas about the functioning of a network. As yet, this model is rather simple and certainly needs improvement (see Grillner et al., 1988). However, models need to be simplified representations of reality since otherwise they would be useless (see Agarwal and Gottlieb, 1982).

The present computer model supported the idea that the modulatory actions of serotonin on the network's rhythm originated from its effects at the membrane level. The suppression of the late afterhyperpolarization at the single-cell level then elicits, via synaptic interactions, the oscillatory behaviour of the network. This beautifully exemplifies the "emergent" properties of a network and supports the notion that the generation of a particular rhythm results not only from intrinsic properties of specialized "pacemaker" cells, but from a complicated interplay of cellular (intrinsic), synaptic and network properties (Getting, 1988). This result is also in keeping with Davis' (1985) recent considerations who concluded, from work on the network generating feeding behaviour in the sea mollusc *Pleurobranchaea,* that emergent network properties predominate over intrinsic neurone properties.

Davis (1985) also emphasized that certain functions are distributed across a number of neurones, so that each of these exerts multiple functions.

These notions, if generally valid (see Getting, 1988), imply that a degree of redundancy and ambiguity is introduced into the network design. This in turn imposes difficulties of system identification in more complicated cases. Specifically, multiple function is a property of neurones that, at least in higher vertebrates, is carried over to the entire network. For, the central pattern generator is not isolated, but connected with other systems, even if, in the simplest case, it is merely modulated by afferent or other influences. For example, the modulatory serotonergic system whose effects were studied by Wallén et al. is split into a reticulospinal and a proprioceptive subsystem. Quite apart from the present ignorance about the functional meaning of this division, it is not yet known whether and how these two subsystems receive different central and sensory inputs and are thus integrated in different task- and context-dependent control systems. An example in mammals is the respiratory rhythm generator (e.g. Richter, 1986), which is intimately related with the cardiovascular control system and, in man, with voluntary control of posture and speech. Thus, the network may be used in different contexts (see also Getting, 1988).

For problems, such as the generation of a rhythm, there are usually a number of different solutions in terms of neural network implementation (Getting, 1988). It is therefore very difficult to decide whether a particular implementation is a necessary and specific adaptation to specific demands of a particular organism, or rather a chance variation of some unknown prototype. Indeed chance should not be underestimated as a source of phylogenetic variation in network design (e.g. Ebbesson, 1984). Chance variations indeed might prevent a complete understanding of locomotor and other networks.

Pompeiano summarizes in his paper a number of studies in the cat on the effects exerted from the locus coeruleus region on spinal (hindlimb) motoneurones and recurrent inhibition during slow excitation of the labyrinths. These studies supplement former investigations on a modulatory cholinergic system (Boyle and Pompeiano, 1984; Pompeiano et al., 1985a,b), which are first briefly reviewed.

The studies were all conducted using the same paradigm, i.e., sinusoidal head rotation in decerebrate cats with neck afferents cut. Responses of gastrocnemius motoneurones, Renshaw cells linked to them, and of spindle afferents from the gastrocnemius muscles were recorded. Based on these results Pompeiano et al. (1985b) proposed the following hypothetical system organization. Two supraspinal nuclei are mainly involved: the lateral vestibular (Deiters) nucleus, and the medullary inhibitory area of Magoun and Rhines. Vestibulospinal neurones, which are excited by ipsilateral macular (utricular) labyrinth receptors, increase their firing rates on ipsilateral head-down movements and decrease it on upwards movement (α-response). They in turn excite the ipsilateral extensor (e.g., gastrocnemius) α and γ motoneurones mono- and polysynaptically (for references see Grillner, 1969, and Boyle and Pompeiano 1984), where the motor response also is of the α type. In contrast, the ipsilateral medullary reticulospinal system shows a β-response (approximately 180° out of phase with the α-response) to head-down movement, the stronger, the more it is facilitated by a pontine cholinergic system. This β-response results from excitatory input to the reticulospinal neurones from the contralateral labyrinth. The reticulospinal system is postulated to excite the Renshaw cells coupled to the ipsilateral extensor (gastrocnemius) α motoneurones. Therefore, during ipsilateral head-down movement, extensor α and γ motoneurones are excited from the vestibulospinal tract, and the α motoneurones are, in addition, disinhibited by reduced Renshaw firing. Pompeiano's present results now add another pathway from the labyrinths down to the spinal ''motor output stage'' (Hultborn et al., 1979), that from the locus coeruleus region.

It should first be noted that the response classification into α- or β-types (an unfortunate choice of terms) is meaningful only if defined as a population average: the phase relations of the individual unit responses (of vestibulospinal, locus coeruleus, and Renshaw cells or spindle afferents) to sinusoidal head or body rotation vary over a wide range and — at least in part — depend on rotation frequency (Boyle and Pompeiano, 1984; Pompeiano, 1989, this volume). Provided the units within each population commonly converge on postsynaptic units, an algebraical vector sum of their output could be of the defined type. Indeed, representation of signals in multi-dimensional vector spaces almost certainly is a common principle up to cortical motor levels (e.g., in the neural representation of voluntary goal-directed movements; see Georgopoulos, 1986). However, weighted or even selective convergence, effected by topographical or other factors ("partitioning": see Windhorst, 1989, this volume; Windhorst, 1988; Windhorst et al., 1989), would defy the simple definition of average α- and β-types, but, on the other hand, it could account for the variance of response patterns in each postsynaptic population.

Both the work of Wallén et al. and Pompeiano appear to provide clear evidence for what may be called parameter adaptation, a term borrowed from systems theory (see, e.g., Inbar, 1972). Across species there are "modulatory systems" (serotonergic, cholinergic and noradrenergic in the present studies), which change and adjust parameters of neural subsystems. In the lamprey, serotonin changes the input–output characteristics at the single-neurone level which — through the network's emergent properties — leads to changes in the parameters of the locomotor rhythm. In the cat, supraspinal cholinergic and noradrenergic systems seem to alter the input–output characteristics (e.g., gain) of the Renshaw cells and, consequently, of the motoneurone pool subject to this adjustable negative feedback (see also Inbar, 1972; Hultborn et al., 1979). In interpreting his findings, Pompeiano adopts the view of Hultborn et al. (1979) who envisage recurrent inhibition as a variable gain regulator acting at the motor output stage. However, his results do not, in the strict sense, allow the conclusion that the gain of recur-rent inhibition and thereby of the motoneurone pool is altered. For instance, by elevating the output of the pontine cholinergic system, Pompeiano et al. (1985b) could change the Renshaw cell firing type during sinusoidal head rotation from α to β. Such a drastic phase shift (of 180°) cannot be due to a change in gain. Instead, it may result from a — not necessarily linear — vector summation of two sinusoidally modulated inputs (from the labyrinths) to Renshaw cells: that mediated via vestibulospinal tract and α motoneurones, and that mediated via reticulospinal tracts. If any gain is varied, it is that of the reticulospinal pathway. A parallel argument holds for the effects mediated via the locus coeruleus region. Switching the perspective, one may view the effects from the reticulo- and coeruleospinal tracts as additional inputs to α motoneurones via Renshaw cells. Together with the excitatory effects of the vestibulospinal tract on ipsilateral extensor α and γ motoneurones, and via spindles back to α motoneurones, the pattern of macular influence on α motoneurones might be envisaged as a "triple-input system" (Windhorst, 1988). In this context, the vestibulospinal and reticulospinal systems have been adduced as an example, where supraspinal systems (here the macular afferents) exert matched actions on fusimotor and Renshaw cells coupled to the same motoneurone pool. Such an organization would support the notion of a close cooperation between proprioceptive and recurrent inhibitory feedback (Windhorst, 1988; see also Windhorst, 1989, this volume). The supplementation of the reticulospinal system by a coeruleospinal system with opposite action on (extensor-related) Renshaw cells would endow the triple input-system with a high degree of flexibility (by alterable balance between the descending signals), including a partial independence of the inputs to Renshaw cells and to α and γ motoneurones (for independence of inputs to α and γ motoneurones see Hulliger et al., 1989, this volume; Taylor and Donga, 1989, this volume).

However, all this does by no means exclude the possibility of a true gain adjustment of Renshaw cells and, hence, of the motoneurone pools by reticulo- and coeruleospinal systems. Yet it has to be investigated with the appropriate quantitative methods, i.e., by measuring the parameters of the input – output relations of Renshaw cells and motoneurones with and without the action of a modulating system. In this respect, it is important to measure not only static characteristics (as considered in the hypothesis of Hultborn et al., 1979), but also the dynamic ones. Renshaw cells exhibit particular dynamics (Cleveland and Ross, 1977; Christakos et al., 1987), whose adaptability by modulating input systems have not yet been assessed. Since these dynamics will codetermine the dynamics of the closed-loop motoneurone-Renshaw cell system (Windhorst and Koehler, 1983), the relevant effects of the modulating inputs will have to be measured. Mutatis mutandis, this also applies to lamprey spinal neurones whose dynamic response characteristics and their modulation by serotonin (and other modulatory substances) need to be described in quantitative terms.

It appears that the cholinergic and noradrenergic modulatory systems in the cat are fairly unspecific. For the latter, this is supported by the fact that the locus coeruleus region exerts its effects on both extensors and flexors, ipsi- and contralaterally, as noted by Pompeiano. In this respect, they are much less specific than the vestibulospinal tract (from Deiters nucleus) itself. This does not prevent the discharge of locus coeruleus neurones (and via these that of the cholinergic dorsal pontine neurones) from also being modulated by macular afferent input. It fits in with this picture of unspecific modulatory effects from the labyrinth that, in addition to this intricate system, ipsilateral semicircular canal afferents also have an inhibitory action on Renshaw cells, both those related to extensor and to flexor α-motoneurones (Ross and Thewissen, 1987).

References

Agarwal, G.C. and Gottlieb, G.L. (1982) Mathematical modeling and simulation of the postural control loop: Part I. *CRC Crit. Rev. Biomed. Engin.,* 8: 93 – 134.

Bear, M.F. and Singer, W. (1986) Modulation of visual cortical plasticity by acetylcholine and noradrenaline. *Nature (London),* 320: 172 – 176.

Boyle, R. and Pompeiano, O. (1984) Discharge activity of spindle afferents from the gastrocnemius-soleus muscle during head rotation in the decerebrate cat. *Pflügers Arch., European J. Physiol.,* 400: 140 – 150.

Christakos, C.N., Windhorst, U., Rissing, R. and Meyer-Lohmann, J. (1987) Frequency response of spinal Renshaw cells activated by stochastic motor axon stimulation. *Neuroscience,* 23: 613 – 623.

Cleveland, S. and Ross, H.G. (1977) Dynamic properties of Renshaw cells: frequency response characteristics. *Biol. Cybern.,* 27: 175 – 184.

Davis, W.J. (1985) Central feedback loops and some implications for motor control. In W.J.P. Barnes and M.H. Gladden (Eds.), *Feedback and Motor Control in Invertebrates and Vertebrates,* Croom Helm, London, pp. 13 – 33.

Ebbesson, S.O.E. (1984) Evolution and ontogeny of neural circuits. *Behav. Brain Sci.,* 7: 321 – 331.

Georgopoulos, A.P. (1986) On reaching. *Ann. Rev. Neurosci.,* 9: 147 – 170.

Getting, P.A. (1988) Comparative analysis of invertebrate central pattern generators. In A.V. Cohen, S. Rossignol and S. Grillner (Eds.), *Neural Control of Rhythmic Movements in Vertebrates,* Wiley, New York, pp. 101 – 127.

Grillner, S. (1969) Supraspinal and segmental control of static and dynamic γ-motoneurones in the cat. *Acta Physiol. Scand.,* Suppl., 327: 1 – 34.

Grillner, S., Buchanan, J.T., Wallén, P. and Brodin, L. (1988) Neural control of locomotion in lower vertebrates. From behavior to ionic mechanisms. In A.V. Cohen, S. Rossignol and S. Grillner (Eds.), *Neural Control of Rhythmic Movements in Vertebrates,* Wiley, New York, pp. 1 – 40.

Hulliger, M., Dürmüller, N., Prochazka, A. and Trend, P. (1989) Flexible fusimotor control of muscle spindle feedback during a variety of natural movements. In J.H.J. Allum and M. Hulliger (Eds.), *Afferent Control of Posture and Locomotion, Prog. Brain Res., Vol. 80,* Elsevier, Amsterdam, pp. 87 – 101.

Hultborn, H., Lindström, S. and Wigström, H. (1979) On the function of recurrent inhibition in the spinal cord of the cat. *Exp. Brain Res.,* 37: 399 – 403.

Inbar, G.F. (1972) Muscle spindles in muscle control. 3. Analysis of adaptive system model. *Kybernetik,* 11: 130 – 141.

Ito, M. (1984) *The Cerebellum and Neural Control.* Raven Press, New York, 580 pp.

Pompeiano, O. (1989) Relationship of noradrenergic locus coeruleus neurones to vestibulospinal reflexes. In J.H.J. Allum and M. Hulliger (Eds.), *Afferent Control of Posture and Locomotion, Prog. Brain Res., Vol. 80,* Elsevier, Amsterdam, pp. 329 – 343.

Pompeiano, O., Wand, P. and Srivastava, U.C. (1985a)

Responses of Renshaw cells coupled with hindlimb extensor motoneurons to sinusoidal stimulation of labyrinth receptors in the decerebrate cat. *Pflügers Arch., Eur. J. Physiol.,* 403: 245 – 257.

Pompeiano, O., Wand, P. and Srivastava, U.C. (1985b) Influence of Renshaw cells on the response gain of hindlimb extensor muscles to sinusoidal labyrinth stimulation. *Pflügers Arch., Eur. J. Physiol.,* 404: 107 – 118.

Richter, D.W. (1986) Zur Frage der Rhythmogenese der Atmung. *Physiologie aktuell,* 2: 201 – 218.

Ross, H.-G. and Thewissen, M. (1987) Inhibitory connections of ipsilateral semicircular canal afferents onto Renshaw cells in the lumbar spinal cord of the cat. *J. Physiol. (London),* 388: 83 – 99.

Taylor, A. and Donga, R. (1989) Central mechanisms of selective fusimotor control. In J.H.J. Allum and M. Hulliger (Eds.), *Afferent Control of Posture and Locomotion, Prog. Brain Res., Vol. 80,* Elsevier, Amsterdam, pp. 27 – 35.

Wallén, P., Christenson, J., Brodin, L., Hill, R., Lansner, A. and Grillner, S. (1989) Mechanisms underlying the serotonergic modulation of the spinal circuitry for locomotion in lamprey. In J.H.J. Allum and M. Hulliger (Eds.), *Afferent Control of Posture and Locomotion, Prog. Brain Res., Vol. 80,* Elsevier, Amsterdam, pp. 321 – 327.

Windhorst, U. (1988) *How brain-like is the Spinal Cord? Interacting Cell Assemblies in the Nervous System.* Springer-Verlag, Berlin, 334 pp.

Windhorst, U. (1989) Do Renshaw cells tell spinal neurones how to interpret muscle spindle signals? In J.H.J. Allum and M. Hulliger (Eds.), *Afferent Control of Posture and Locomotion, Prog. Brain Res., Vol. 80,* Elsevier, Amsterdam, pp. 283 – 294.

Windhorst, U. and Koehler, W. (1983) Dynamic behaviour of α-motoneurone sub-pools subjected to inhomogenous Renshaw cell inhibition. *Biol. Cybern.,* 46: 217 – 228.

Windhorst, U., Hamm, T.M. and Stuart, D.G. (1989) On the function of muscle and reflex partitioning. *Behav. Brain Sci.* (in press).

J.H.J. Allum and M. Hulliger (Eds.)
Progress in Brain Research, Vol. 80
© 1989 Elsevier Science Publishers B.V. (Biomedical Division)

CHAPTER 26

Mechanisms underlying the serotonergic modulation of the spinal circuitry for locomotion in lamprey

P. Wallén, J. Christenson, L. Brodin, R. Hill, A. Lansner[1] and S. Grillner

Nobel Institute for Neurophysiology, Karolinska Institute, and [1]Department of Numerical Analysis and Computer Technology, Royal Institute of Technology, Stockholm, Sweden

The central nervous system of the lamprey contains serotonergic (5-hydroxytryptamine, 5-HT) neurones both in the spinal cord and in the brainstem. Endogenously released 5-HT from these systems modulates the pattern of fictive locomotion induced in the in vitro preparation; the burst rate is lowered and burst discharges become longer and of higher intensity. Local application of 5-HT, mimicking activation of the 5-HT systems, has a specific effect on the late phase of the afterhyperpolarization (AHP) in motoneurones and interneurones. 5-HT markedly reduces the amplitude of the late AHP without affecting passive membrane properties or the shape or threshold of the action potential. This 5-HT effect appears to result from a direct action on the calcium-dependent potassium channels underlying the late phase of the AHP. A reduction of the amplitude of the AHP will result in altered spike discharge characteristics, with potentiation of the response (discharge rate) to a given excitatory input in all neurones influenced by 5-HT. It is suggested that the modulatory effect of 5-HT on fictive locomotion can be attributed to its action on the late AHP and thereby to the potentiation of excitability in excitatory and inhibitory interneurones in the generator circuitry. This has been further corroborated in computer simulation studies of a network model, where the action of 5-HT was simulated by decreasing AHP amplitude, resulting in a slowing of the rhythm analogous to the effect demonstrated experimentally.

Key words: Spike frequency regulation; After-hyperpolarization; Neuronal membrane property; Modulation of rhythmic activity; Locomotion; Interneuronal network; 5-Hydroxytryptamine; Spinal cord; Lamprey; Computer simulation

Introduction

The in vitro preparation of the lamprey CNS can produce the rhythmic motor pattern corresponding to the alternating swimming movements of the intact animal (Wallén and Williams, 1984; Grillner et al., 1988b). Even though such fictive locomotion is generated by the spinal generator circuitry in the absence of any feedback signals, the rhythmic pattern can be powerfully influenced from different kinds of modulatory inputs. One such input is the movement-related feedback arising from stretch receptive elements, notably the edge cells located along the lateral margin of the spinal cord (Grillner et al., 1984). Another modulatory input to the spinal generator circuitry comes from the reticulo-spinal, descending neurones of the brainstem (see Grillner et al., 1988b). This chapter will deal with yet another type of input which appears capable of strongly modulating the efferent motor pattern of the spinal cord, and which originates from central serotonergic nerve terminals. The anatomical relations as well as the cellular mechanisms underlying this modulatory input to the spinal circuitry will be briefly described.

5-HT systems in the lamprey CNS

In the ventromedial portion of the lamprey spinal cord, close to the central canal, a large number of

322

small 5-HT positive neurones have been found in immunohistochemical studies (Van Dongen et al., 1985a). These neurones form a dense, ventromedial fibre plexus along the length of the spinal cord. Fig. 1A shows the 5-HT fibre plexus on either side of the central canal as a stereo pair computer reconstruction, after immunofluorescence labelling and scanning in a confocal laser

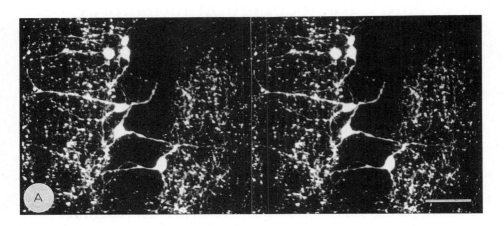

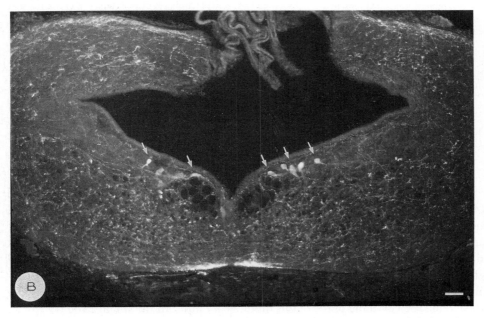

Fig. 1. 5-Hydroxytryptamine immunoreactive neurones in lamprey brainstem and spinal cord. A: stereopair showing a three-dimensional reconstruction of intraspinal 5-HT neurones. The spinal cord was incubated as a wholemount in 5-HT antiserum followed by FITC-coupled secondary antibodies. The reconstruction was obtained by scanning the preparation in sequential focal planes using a confocal laser microscope system. The projection is from a dorsal view, and processes extending from the cell bodies can be followed down towards the 5-HT-immunoreactive fibre plexus near the ventral spinal cord surface. B: micrograph showing a section from the caudal rhombencephalon incubated with 5-HT antiserum. Immunoreactive cell bodies (arrows) which project to the lateral and ventromedial columns of the spinal cord are present in the posterior rhombencephalic reticular nucleus. Scale bars, 50 μm.

scanning microscope (Wallén et al., 1988a). There is also a descending projection of 5-HT neurones in the brainstem contributing to the serotonergic innervation of the lateral and ventral spinal cord, as well as an afferent system with cell bodies in spinal ganglia supplying the dorsal horn − dorsal column (Brodin et al., 1986; and unpublished). Descending 5-HT neurones have been found in two different brainstem areas − one in the posterior reticular nucleus of the rhombencephalon (Fig. 1B) and another rostral to the trigeminal motor nucleus (Brodin et al., 1986).

As evidenced from studies combining 5-HT immunohistochemistry and intracellular labelling, many neurones of the grey matter send dendrites into close proximity with the 5-HT fibres (Van Dongen et al., 1985b). The question whether the 5-HT fibres form point-to-point synapses with these neurones was investigated in a study using peroxidase immunohistochemistry and electron microscopy (Christenson et al., 1988). No synaptic specializations were observed on the 5-HT varicosities, suggesting that the serotonergic fibres exert their effect by a diffuse release rather than via traditional synaptic contacts.

Endogenous release of 5-HT modulates the fictive locomotor pattern

It has been demonstrated previously that bath application of 5-HT during fictive locomotion in the in vitro preparation of the lamprey spinal cord will markedly influence the burst pattern (Grillner and Wilén, as cited in Grillner et al., 1988b; Harris-Warrick and Cohen, 1985). The rate of bursting is slowed down, and both intensity and duration of the burst discharges will increase.

By blocking the 5-HT uptake system, similar effects on the fictive burst pattern have recently been demonstrated (Fig. 2; Wallén et al., 1988b; Christenson et al., unpublished). This finding suggests that an endogenous release of 5-HT from the spinal cord fibres, and hence any natural activation of them, may modulate the locomotor activity.

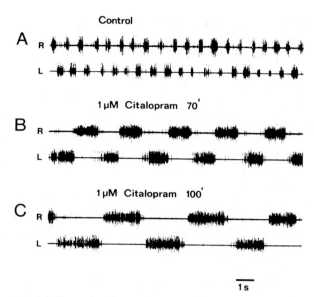

Fig. 2. Effects of 5-HT uptake blockade on fictive locomotion. A: ventral root control recordings from the left and right side of the same spinal segment during fictive locomotion induced by bath application of NMDA (100 μM). B,C: burst pattern after reperfusion with the 5-HT uptake blocker Citalopram (1 μM) for 70 and 100 min, respectively.

Cellular mechanisms underlying the effects of 5-HT on fictive locomotion

It is thus clear that 5-HT will in some way influence the activity of the neurones responsible for generating the locomotor rhythm. To investigate how individual neurones will be affected, intracellular studies have been performed where a release of 5-HT was mimicked by local droplet application near the ventral surface of the spinal cord, while recording from individual neurones (Van Dongen et al., 1986; Wallén et al., 1986, 1989).

The membrane input resistance was found to remain unaffected following 5-HT application, and no effect was observed with regard to the shape or the threshold of the action potential. Thus, the resting membrane properties as well as the mechanisms underlying the action potential appear not to be influenced by 5-HT. In contrast, when investigating the afterhyperpolarization (AHP) following the action potential, a marked effect was revealed. Within seconds after the 5-HT application, the amplitude of the AHP was substantially reduced (Fig. 3). Whenever the early and late phases of the AHP in these cells could be distinguished, it was seen that only the late phase was reduced by 5-HT (Fig. 3A,B).

The detailed neuronal mechanisms underlying this specific effect of 5-HT on the AHP have recently been investigated (Wallén et al., 1986, 1989). Like in several other types of CNS neurones, the AHP in these lamprey neurones is associated with an increase in membrane conductance (cf. Gustafsson, 1974). Local application of 5-HT markedly reduces this conductance increase, which indicates that the ionic currents underlying the AHP are being blocked by 5-HT. The late phase of the AHP is in general attributed to the activation of calcium-dependent potassium channels (Meech, 1978; for lamprey, see Hill et al., 1985), and it was found that this holds true also for the lamprey neurones studied here (Wallén et al., 1989).

A possible mechanism by which 5-HT could reduce the amplitude of the AHP could be a blockade of the entry of calcium during the action potential. The other alternative is that 5-HT would act later in the chain of events and prevent, directly or indirectly, the activation of the calcium-dependent potassium channels. When 5-HT was droplet-applied in the presence of tetraethylam-

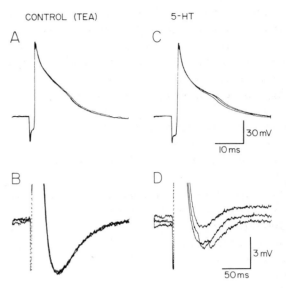

Fig. 4. The reduction of the AHP by 5-HT appears not to be due to a blockage of Ca^{2+} entry. A: the action potential of a motoneurone was prolonged by TEA and exhibited a large Ca^{2+}-component during the falling phase. B: the AHP of the TEA action potential. C: after local application of 5-HT, the duration of the action potential was little affected, but the AHP was markedly reduced (D). In A – D, three sweeps were superimposed. Calibrations in C,D also apply to A,B, respectively. Modified from Wallén et al., 1989.

monium (TEA), which blocks the "early" potassium channels and leads to increased calcium entry during a much prolonged action potential, the spike remained prolonged (Fig. 4A,C) and thus the entry of calcium does not appear to be blocked by 5-HT. Still, the AHP was depressed after 5-HT application (Fig. 4B,D). From these experiments one may thus conclude that 5-HT appears to exert its action after calcium has entered the cell.

The possibility that 5-HT might act via a second messenger system, as is the case for the corresponding effect of noradrenaline and acetylcholine on hippocampal neurones (Madison and Nicoll, 1982, 1986a,b; Malenka et al., 1986), was tested with regard both to cyclic AMP, cyclic GMP, diacylglycerol, and arachidonic acid (Wallén et al., 1986, 1989). No evidence was obtained for an involvement of any of these second messenger

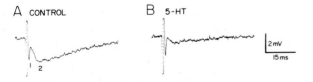

Fig. 3. Local application of 5-HT affects the late phase of the AHP. A: control record from a motoneurone before 5-HT, illustrating the early (1) and late (2) phases of the AHP following an action potential elicited by a brief depolarizing current pulse. B: after application of 5-HT to the ventral surface of the spinal cord near the medial dendrites of the motoneurone, the late phase of the AHP was markedly reduced, while the early phase remained unaffected. Modified from Wallén et al., 1989.

systems, nor for a mediation via a pertussis toxin sensitive G-protein (cf. Dunlap et al., 1987). It thus appears likely that the 5-HT effect on the late phase of the AHP results from a direct action on the calcium-dependent potassium channels.

It is not known which type of 5-HT receptor is involved in mediating the effect on the AHP. The 5-HT$_2$ receptor blocker cinanserin did not influence the 5-HT action and methysergide, a blocker of 5-HT$_1$ and 5-HT$_2$ receptors had a slight agonist effect (Wallén et al., 1989), which makes 5-HT$_3$ receptors a plausible candidate. This receptor type appears to mediate similar direct effects in other systems (Fozard, 1987). However, the receptor identity remains to be investigated in direct experiments with specific blockers.

The firing properties of the individual neurone are influenced by 5-HT

The size of the afterhyperpolarization is a major factor determining the spike frequency characteristics of the neurone (Kernell, 1965; Baldissera and Gustafsson, 1974; Madison and Nicoll, 1982). 5-HT would therefore be expected to influence the spike response to a given excitatory input. Fig. 5 shows that the response to a long, depolarizing stimulus pulse is markedly altered after 5-HT application: the number of spikes is more than doubled. Note also the reduction in size of the late AHP (arrows). The same excitatory input thus results in a more powerful spike response when the neurone

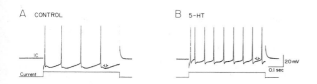

Fig. 5. 5-HT potentiates the spike response characteristics. A: before 5-HT, a 7 nA, 500 ms-long depolarizing current pulse elicited 4 to 5 spikes in a motoneurone. The late AHP was prominent (arrow). B: after 5-HT application the late AHP decreased (arrow), and the frequency of firing increased to 8 or 9 spikes in response to an identical pulse. Note also the greater reduction of the first interval. Modified from Wallén et al., 1989.

is under the influence of 5-HT. The input–output relation, or the "gain" of the neurone is altered by 5-HT, in other words, the response to excitatory inputs in each neurone that is affected by 5-HT is potentiated.

Effects on the spinal generator circuitry – simulation studies

A release of 5-HT will potentiate the spike response of both motoneurones and interneurones with dendrites in the region of the 5-HT fibres. In addition to motoneurones, lateral interneurones and CC-interneurones, both of which are inhibitory premotor interneurones, are influenced by 5-HT as described above, i.e. the late phase of the AHP is markedly reduced and the response characteristics (gains) are potentiated. Both these interneurone types are part of the circuitry proposed as a model neuronal network for the generation of the locomotor rhythm in the lamprey (Grillner et al., 1987, 1988a). CC-interneurones (having a crossed, caudally projecting axon; Buchanan, 1982) inhibit the network neurones on the contralateral side of the spinal cord, thereby assuring alternating activity. Lateral interneurones inhibit CC-interneurones on the same side, terminating their burst activity and thereby allowing the contralateral side to become active. Both types of inhibitory interneurones are excited by local excitatory interneurones, which are also an integral part of the model network (Buchanan and Grillner, 1987).

5-HT will increase the excitability in both excitatory and inhibitory neurones. Furthermore, the AHP is likely to play an important role in the circuitry as a burst-terminating factor (Grillner et al., 1988a). To investigate the possible influence of these factors, experiments were carried out, with a computer program model which simulates the rhythm-generating network of the lamprey spinal cord and which is based on experimentally established neuronal properties and connectivity (Grillner et al., 1988a). When a release of 5-HT was simulated by reducing the size of the AHP in the neurones of the network model, the burst rate decreased, and bursts were prolonged and more spikes were fired at a higher frequency (Grillner et al., 1988a). These effects are analogous to those found experimentally with 5-HT uptake blockade or bath application of 5-HT (cf. above). It thus appears that the modulatory effects of 5-HT on the locomotor burst pattern can be ascribed to the reduction of the AHP in the neurones of the generator circuitry. Also the motoneurones will be influenced by a release of 5-HT (Van Dongen et al., 1986; Wallén et al., 1989), which will further increase spike frequency and burst intensity. The effects on the motoneurones will, however, not contribute to the alteration in burst rate, since the motoneurones themselves are not part of the generator circuitry (Wallén and Lansner, 1984).

Concluding remarks

5-HT may thus influence neurones of the lamprey spinal cord in a very specific manner: the amplitude of the late phase of the AHP is markedly attenuated, without any influence on passive membrane properties or on the action potential per se. The size of the late AHP appears to be modulated through a direct action on the underlying calcium-dependent potassium channels.

As suggested by computer simulation experiments, the reduction in size of the AHP will lead to a slowing down of the rhythmic activity, with an increased intensity and duration of the burst discharges. This is in good agreement with experimental findings with either externally applied 5-HT or after blocking 5-HT uptake to increase endogenous levels. Taken together, these results thus suggest that the 5-HT systems of the lamprey CNS may modulate the efferent rhythmic activity underlying locomotion by simply regulating the amplitude of the AHP in the different neurone types involved in motor activity. It may here be noted that 5-HT does not affect the AHP in dorsal cells and edge cells, both of which are primary sensory neurones (Wallén et al., 1989).

Regulation of the AHP-amplitude appears to be a simple and straightforward strategy by which a modulatory control of the motor activity can be accomplished. Whenever the external demands require that the locomotor movements be altered, perhaps when the resistance to the movements increases as during burrowing, activation of the 5-HT fibres will change the firing characteristics of the involved neurones by influencing one particular ionic conductance, the calcium-dependent potassium channels responsible for the late phase of the AHP. Further experimentation is needed to clarify how and under what circumstances the 5-HT fibres are naturally activated, and it also remains to be investigated what are the specific roles of the different 5-HT systems.

References

Baldissera, F. and Gustafsson, B. (1974) Firing behaviour of a neurone model based on the afterhyperpolarization conductance time course and summation. Adaptation and steady state firing. *Acta Physiol. Scand.*, 92: 27–47.

Brodin, L., Buchanan, J.T., Hökfelt, T., Grillner, S. and Verhofstad, A.A. (1986) A spinal projection of 5-hydroxytryptamine neurons in the lamprey brainstem; evidence from combined retrograde tracing and immunohistochemistry. *Neurosci. Lett.*, 67: 53–57.

Buchanan, J.T. (1982) Identification of interneurons with contralateral caudal avons in the lamprey spinal cord: synaptic interactions and morphology. *J. Neurophysiol.*, 47: 961–975.

Buchanan, J.T. and Grillner, S. (1987) Newly identified "glutamate interneurons" and their role in locomotion in the lamprey spinal cord. *Science*, 236: 312–4.

Christenson, J., Cullheim, S., Grillner, S. and Hökfelt, T. (1988) 5-HT varicosities in the lamprey spinal cord have no synaptic specializations. *Eur. J. Neurosci.*, Suppl.: 137.

Dunlap, K., Holz, G.G. and Rane, S.G. (1987) G proteins as regulators of ion channel function. *Trends Neurosci.*, 10: 241–244.

Fozard, J.R. (1987) 5-HT: The enigma variations. *Trends Pharmacol. Sci.*, 8: 501–506.

Grillner, S., Williams, T. and Lagerbäck, P.-Å. (1984) The edge cell, a possible intraspinal mechanoreceptors. *Science*, 223: 500–503.

Grillner, S., Wallén, S., Dale, N., Brodin, L., Buchanan, J. and Hill, R. (1987) Transmitters, membrane properties and network circuitry in the control of locomotion in lamprey. *Trends Neurosci.*, 10: 34–41.

Grillner, S., Buchanan, J.T. and Lansner, A. (1988a) Simulation of the segmental burst generating network for locomotion in lamprey. *Neurosci. Lett.*, 89: 31 – 35.

Grillner, S., Buchanan, J.T., Wallén, P. and Brodin, L. (1988b) Neural control of locomotion in lower vertebrates – from behavior to ionic mechanisms. In A.H. Cohen, S., Rossignol. and S. Grillner (Eds.), *Neural Control of Rhythmic Movements in Vertebrates,* John Wiley & Sons, NY, pp. 1 – 40.

Gustafsson, B. (1974) Afterhyperpolarization and the control of repetitive firing in spinal neurons of the cat. *Acta Physiol. Scand.,* Suppl. 416.

Harris-Warrick, R.M. and Cohen, A.H. (1985) Serotonin modulates the central pattern generator for locomotion in the isolated lamprey spinal cord. *J. Exp. Biol.,* 116: 27 – 46.

Hill, R.H., Århem, P. and Grillner, S. (1985) Ionic mechanisms of 3 types of functionally different neurons in the lamprey spinal cord. *Brain Res.,* 358: 40 – 52.

Kernell, D. (1965) The limits of firing frequency in cat lumbosacral motoneurones possessing different time course of afterhyperpolarization. *Acta Physiol. Scand.,* 65: 87 – 100.

Madison, D.V. and Nicoll, R.A. (1982) Noradrenaline blocks accommodation of pyramidal cell discharge in the hippocampus. *Nature (London),* 299: 636 – 638.

Madison, D.V. and Nicoll, R.A. (1986a) Actions of noradrenaline recorded intracellularly in rat hippocampal CA1 pyramidal neurones, in vitro. *J. Physiol. (London),* 372: 221 – 244.

Madison, D.V. and Nicoll, R.A. (1986b) Cyclic adenosine 3′,5′-monophosphate mediates beta-receptor actions of noradrenaline in rat hippocampal pyramidal cells. *J. Physiol. (London),* 372: 245 – 260.

Malenka, R.C., Madison, D.V., Andrade, R. and Nicoll, R.A. (1986) Phorbol esters mimic some cholinergic actions in hippocampal pyramidal neurons. *J. Neurosci.,* 6: 457 – 480.

Meech, R.W. (1978) Calcium-dependent potassium activation in nervous tissues. *Ann. Rev. Biophys. Bioeng.,* 7: 1 – 18.

Van Dongen, P.A., Grillner, S. and Hökfelt, T. (1986) 5-Hydroxytryptamine (serotonin) causes a reduction in the afterhyperpolarization following the action potential in lamprey motoneurons and premotor interneurons. *Brain Res.,* 366: 320 – 5.

Van Dongen, P.A., Hökfelt, T., Grillner, S., Verhofstad, A.A., Steinbusch, H.W., Cuello, A.C. and Terenius, L. (1985a) Immunohistochemical demonstration of some putative neurotransmitters in the lamprey spinal cord and spinal ganglia: 5-hydroxytryptamine-, tachykinin-, and neuropeptide-Y-immunoreactive neurons and fibers. *J. Comp. Neurol.,* 234: 501 – 22.

Van Dongen, P.A., Hökfelt, T., Grillner, S., Verhofstad, A.A. and Steinbusch, H.W. (1985b) Possible target neurons of 5-hydroxytryptamine fibers in the lamprey spinal cord: immunohistochemistry combined with intracellular staining with Lucifer yellow. *J. Comp. Neurol.,* 234: 523 – 35.

Wallén, P. and Lansner, A. (1984) Do the motoneurones constitute a part of the spinal network generating the swimming rhythm in the lamprey? *J. Exp. Biol.,* 113: 493 – 497.

Wallén, P. and Williams, T.L. (1984) Fictive locomotion in the lamprey spinal cord in vitro compared with swimming in the intact and spinal animal. *J. Physiol. (London),* 347: 225 – 239.

Wallén, P., Buchanan, J.T., Grillner, S. and Hökfelt, T. (1986) 5-HT modifies frequency regulation and inherent membrane potential oscillations in lamprey neurons. *Proc. 1st Internat. Congr. Neuroethology,* Tokyo.

Wallén, P., Carlsson, K., Liljeborg, A. and Grillner, S. (1988a) Three-dimensional reconstruction of neurons in the lamprey spinal cord in whole-mount, using a confocal laser scanning microscope. *J. Neurosci. Methods,* 24: 91 – 100.

Wallén, P., Christenson, J., Cullheim, S. and Grillner, S. (1988b) Endogenous release of 5-HT modulates fictive locomotion in lamprey spinal cord by altering the input-output relation of individual neurons. *Soc. Neurosci. Abstr.,* 14: 264.

Wallén, P., Buchanan, J.T., Grillner, S., Hill, R.H., Christenson, J. and Hökfelt, T. (1989) Effects of 5-hydroxytryptamine on the afterhyperpolarization, spike frequency regulation, and oscillatory membrane properties in lamprey spinal cord neurons. *J. Neurophysiol.,* 61: 759 – 768.

J.H.J. Allum and M. Hulliger (Eds.)
Progress in Brain Research, Vol. 80
© 1989 Elsevier Science Publishers B.V. (Biomedical Division)

CHAPTER 27

Relationship of noradrenergic locus coeruleus neurones to vestibulospinal reflexes

O. Pompeiano

Dipartimento di Fisiologia e Biochimica, Universita' di Pisa, 56100 Pisa, Italy

The electrical activity of presumably noradrenergic locus coeruleus (LC) neurones was recorded in decerebrate cats during roll tilt of the animal at 0.15 Hz, $\pm$ 10°, leading to sinusoidal labyrinth stimulation. Among the tested units, some of which projected to the lumbosacral spinal cord, 56.7% responded to animal tilt. Most of these neurones were activated during side-up and depressed during side-down tilt of the animal, while a smaller proportion of units showed the opposite response pattern. This predominant response pattern of LC neurones and coeruleospinal (CS) neurones to animal tilt was opposite in activation polarity to that of vestibulospinal (VS) neurones projecting to the same segments of the spinal cord. Both the VS and the CS neurones exert a direct excitatory influence on ipsilateral limb extensor motoneurones. However, VS neurones excite corresponding Renshaw (R) cells, though due to activation of limb extensor motoneurones and their recurrent collaterals, the CS neurones may inhibit them. It appears, therefore, that during side-down animal tilt, the motoneurones innervating the ipsilateral limb extensors are excited by the increased discharge of VS neurones, while the corresponding R-cells are disinhibited due to the reduced discharge of CS neurones. The functional coupling between ipsilateral limb extensor motoneurones and the corresponding R-cells would then increase, just at the time in which these motoneurones are driven by the excitatory VS volleys, thus limiting the response gain of limb extensors to labyrinth stimulation. This hypothesis is supported by two facts: (1) R-cells linked with limb extensor motoneurones discharge during side-down tilt, thus firing in phase with the excitatory VS volleys, and (2) functional inactivation of the noradrenergic LC neurones increases the gain of the vestibulospinal reflexes acting on limb extensors.

Key words: Central noradrenergic system; Locus coeruleus; Lateral vestibular nucleus; Descending control; Recurrent inhibition; Renshaw cell; Labyrinth input; Vestibulospinal reflex

Introduction

Experiments performed in precollicular decerebrate cats have shown that slow rotation about the longitudinal axis of the animal (roll) or rotation of the head after neck deafferentation produces contraction of ipsilateral forelimb extensors during side-down tilt and relaxation during side-up tilt (cf. Schor and Miller, 1981; Manzoni et al., 1983a). The peak of response was closely related to the extreme animal or head displacement, thus being attributed to stimulation of position-sensitive macular (utricular) receptors. As to the hindlimb extensors, myographic (Boyle and Pompeiano, 1984) and electromyographic experiments (Manzoni et al., 1984; D'Ascanio et al., 1985; Pompeiano et al., 1985a,b) have shown that these muscles either did not respond or displayed only a small amplitude modulation of their activity during slow roll tilt of the animal or head rotation after neck deafferentation. In these instances, the response pattern of the hindlimb extensors to a given labyrinth signal was similar to that of the forelimb extensors, although the gain was smaller in size.

The main structure which transmits the

vestibular afferent volleys to limb extensor moto-neurones is the lateral vestibular nucleus (LVN), whose excitatory vestibulospinal (VS) projection acts mono- and polysynaptically on ipsilateral limb extensor motoneurones (Lund and Pompeiano, 1968; cf. Pompeiano, 1975).

In addition to the LVN, there are structures located in the dorsolateral pontine tegmentum, such as the locus coeruleus (LC) and the locus sub-coeruleus (SC), which also exert a prominent facilitatory influence on posture. These structures contain, in the cat, catecholaminergic neurones (cf. Jones and Friedman, 1983), which are not only noradrenergic (Miachon et al., 1984) but also norepinephrine (NE)-sensitive, due to the existence of self-inhibitory synapses which act on α_2-adrenoceptors by utilizing mechanisms of recur-rent and/or lateral inhibition (cf. Foote et al., 1983; Ennis and Aston-Jones, 1986a).

After the demonstration that the LC complex contributes to a direct coeruleospinal (CS) projec-tion (cf. Holstege and Kuypers, 1987), whose aminergic terminals are in close contact with ven-tral horn neurones (Mizukawa, 1980). Evidence has been presented indicating that the correspon-ding neurones exert a facilitatory influence on posture. In particular, anatomical or functional in-activation of the LC complex produced either by electrolytic lesion of this structure (D'Ascanio et al., 1985) or by local injection of clonidine (Pom-peiano et al., 1987), which acts as an α_2-adrenergic agonist thus inhibiting the activity of the corresponding noradrenergic neurones, decreased the decerebrate rigidity in the ipsilateral limbs. On the other hand, stimulation of the LC complex exerted a facilitatory influence on ip-silateral limb extensor (and flexor) motoneurones (Fung and Barnes, 1981, 1984, 1987; Chan et al., 1986), an effect which has been attributed, at least in part, to a direct excitatory influence of noradrenergic CS neurones on spinal motoneurones (White and Neumann, 1980, 1983), in part to suppression of the tonic discharge of in-hibitory interneurones acting on motoneurones (Jordan et al., 1977). Some of these interneurones

could be involved in the transmission of flexion reflex afferent volleys to motoneurones (cf. Lund-berg, 1982). An additional possibility, however, is that the CS pathway acts on Renshaw (R)-cells anatomically linked with extensor motoneurones. Finally, experiments of unit recording have shown that an increased or a decreased discharge of LC-complex neurones is associated with parallel changes of postural activity in the decerebrate cat (Pompeiano and Hoshino, 1976; cf. Pompeiano, 1980).

The experiments summarized in the present report were performed to find out: (1) whether the CS neurones, as well as the VS neurones, respond to sinusoidal stimulation of macular labyrinth receptors; (2) whether the CS influences on posture are at least in part mediated through R-cells coupl-ed with extensor motoneurones; and finally (3) whether the noradrenergic LC system intervenes in the gain regulation of the vestibulospinal reflexes.

Responses of vestibulospinal and coeruleospinal neurones to sinusoidal stimulation of labyrinth receptors

The activity of single units located either in the LVN or in the LC complex was recorded in precollicular decerebrate cats paralysed with gallamine triethiodide and ventilated artificially. Stimulating electrodes were implanted into the lateral funiculi of both sides at $T_{12} - L_1$ for an-tidromic activation of VS and CS neurones. Each unit was tested during roll tilt of the animal. The unit activity was averaged over several cycles and processed on-line with a computer system equip-ped with a Fourier analyser. A spectral analysis of the angular input (table rotation) and of the output (unit activity) was performed and the gain (ab-solute change of the mean discharge rate per degree of tilt in impulses per second (i.p.s.)/degree) and of the phase angle of the first harmonic responses (expressed in degrees with respect to the peak of the side-down position of the animal) were evaluated.

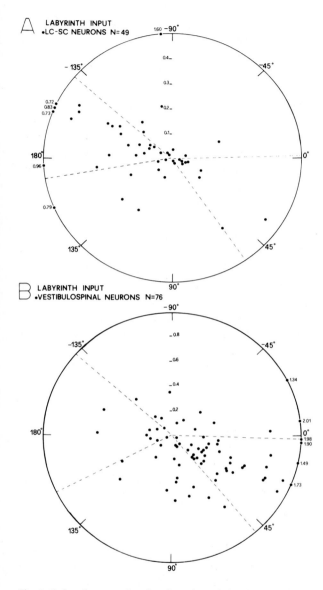

Responses of lateral vestibular nucleus neurones

The responses of VS neurones originating from the LVN to animal tilt were recorded by several investigators (cf. Pompeiano, 1984a). However, in order to relate the response pattern of LVN neurones with the postural adjustments, we shall refer here only to the results of experiments in which the recorded units were found to project to the lumbosacral segments of the spinal cord (Marchand et al., 1987). It was shown that among the 129 VS neurones antidromically activated by stimulation of the spinal cord at $T_{12} - L_1$, 76 units (58.9%) underwent a periodic modulation of their firing rate during animal tilt at the frequency of 0.026 Hz, $\pm$ 10°. The average gain of these unit responses was 0.47 $\pm$ 0.44 (S.D.) i.p.s./degree.

Most of the units responded to the extreme animal displacements (Fig. 1B). In particular, 51 units (67.1%) were excited during side-down tilt of the animal (α-responses), while 15 units (19.7%) by side-up tilt (β-responses); both populations of neurones fired with an average phase lead of the first harmonic of responses of $+21.0 \pm 27.2$ degrees with respect to the extreme animal displacements. The remaining 10 units (13.2%) showed intermediate phase angle of the responses. The gain of the VS units showing α-responses (0.57 $\pm$ 49 i.p.s./degree) was on the average higher than that of the units displaying β-responses (0.26 $\pm$ 0.19 i.p.s./degree).

The phase angle of the VS neurones to animal tilt either remained unmodified or showed a

Fig. 1. Polar diagrams showing the gain and the phase angle of responses of LC_d-SC neurones (A) and LVN neurones (B) to slow sinusoidal tilt of the animal at 0.026 – 0.15 Hz, $\pm$ 10 degree amplitude in precollicular decerebrate cats. Among the recorded units, 10 LC_d-SC neurones and all the LVN neurones were antidromically identified as projecting to the lumbosacral segments of the spinal cord. The response gain of each unit is indicated by the distance of the corresponding symbol to the centre of the diagram (see the scale along the vertical meridian); 6 units in A had a gain higher than 0.5 and 6 units in B had a gain higher than 1.0. The relative position of the symbol with respect to 0° meridian indicates in degrees the phase lead (positive values) or the phase lag (negative values) of responses with respect to the extreme side-down position of the animal. The dashed lines outline the standard deviation of the phase angle of response of the main populations of units responsive to animal tilt in A and B. In particular, the mean phase angle of the LC_d-SC units excited during side-down and side-up animal tilt in A corresponded to $+ 27.0 \pm 27.6$, S.D., degrees ($n = 13$) and $- 163.9 \pm 25.2$ degrees ($n = 31$), respectively, while that of the LVN units displaying the same response patterns in B corresponded to $+ 25.0 \pm 23.8$ degrees ($n = 51$) and $- 172.6 \pm 33.9$ degrees ($n = 15$), respectively. From Marchand et al. (1987) and Pompeiano et al. (1988b).

decrease in phase lead for increasing frequency of tilt from 0.008 to 0.32 Hz, thus indicating that the responses were due to stimulation of macular, utricular receptors. In some instances, however, the phase lead of the responses increased, as if the units received a convergent input from the canal receptors (cf. Manzoni et al., 1987).

Responses of locus coeruleus-complex neurones

Pompeiano et al. (1988a,b) have recently studied the effects of animal tilt on the activity of 141 LC-complex neurones, 41 of which were histologically located in the LC dorsalis (LCd), 67 in the LC_α and 33 in the SC. This is the region in which spinally projecting neurones are located (Holstege and Kuypers, 1987). The LC-complex neurones recorded these experiments satisfied one or more of the criteria attributed to noradrenergic neurones (cf. Foote et al., 1983), namely: (1) they showed a prolonged extracellular spike wave duration ($\geq$ 2 ms); (2) they had a slow and regular resting discharge; and (3) they responded to a nociceptive input elicited by compression of the paws with a transient excitatory response followed by a cessation of firing. A proportion of these neurones (16/141) were activated antidromically by electrical stimulation of the spinal cord between T_{12} and L_1, thus projecting to the lumbosacral segments of the spinal cord.

A large number of LC-complex neurones (80/141, i.e. 56.7%) responded to roll tilt of the animal at the frequency of 0.15 Hz, $\pm$ 10°. In particular, the gain of the first harmonic of responses corresponded on the average to 0.19 $\pm$ 0.26 i.p.s./degree. However, the proportion of units responsive to standard parameters of tilt as well as the response gain were on the average higher in the SC (24/33, i.e. 72.7% and 0.32 $\pm$ 0.36 i.p.s./degree) and the LCd (25/41, i.e. 61.0% and 0.19 $\pm$ 0.23 i.p.s./degree) than in the LC_α (31/67, i.e. 46.3% and 0.09 $\pm$ 0.13 i.p.s./degree). While the LC_α units did not respond with any predominant phase angle, a large proportion of SC and LCd neurones responded to the extreme animal displacements (Fig. 1A). In particular, 31 units

(63.3%) were excited during side-up tilt of the animal (β-responses), while 13 units (26.5%) by side-down tilt (α-responses); both populations of neurones fired with an average phase lead of the first harmonic of responses of +19.3 $\pm$ 26.1 degrees with respect to the extreme animal displacements. The remaining 5 units (10.2%) showed intermediate phase angle of the responses. Among the positional-sensitive SC and LCd units, those excited by side-up tilt of the animal showed more than a twofold larger gain (n = 31; 0.28 $\pm$ 0.26 i.p.s./degree) with respect to the units excited by side-down tilt (n = 13; 0.12 $\pm$ 0.17 i.p.s./degree). Over increasing frequency of sinusoidal tilt from 0.008 to 0.32 Hz at the fixed amplitude of $\pm$ 10°, the LC-complex neurones either showed no change or only a slight increase in the response gain.

Similar response properties were also found for 11 out of the 16 antidromically identified CS neurones which responded to animal tilt. In fact, the majority of these neurones were located in the SC and the LCd (n = 10 units) and showed large amplitude β-responses (n = 8 units).

In conclusion, it appears that the majority of the LC-complex units, including those projecting to the lumbosacral segments of the spinal cord, responded with a pattern (β-responses) which was just opposite to that of the VS neurones projecting to the same segments of the spinal cord (α-responses). Since even the primary afferents originating from the utricular macula showed mainly α-responses to tilt, in apparent agreement with the morphological polarization of the majority of the corresponding receptors (cf. Goldberg and Fernández, 1984), it appears that the macular input of one side is transmitted not only to the ipsilateral LVN, but also via a crossed pathway (cf. Pompeiano, 1979) to the contralateral LC complex. This effect could be mediated through the ventral aspect of the contralateral medullary reticular formation (Manzoni et al., 1983b), whose neurones may at least in part project to the LC complex (Aston-Jones et al., 1986), where they exert a prominent excitatory influence on NE-containing neurones (Ennis and Aston-Jones, 1986b, 1987). We cannot exclude, however, that the responses of the LC-complex neurones to tilt are due to direct afferent projections from the vestibular nuclei to the LC-complex (Cedarbaum and Aghajanian, 1978; Clavier, 1979; Morgane and Jacobs, 1979; Fung et al., 1987b; cf. however, Sakai et al., 1977; Aston-Jones et al., 1986).

Vestibulospinal and coeruleospinal influences on recurrent inhibition and Renshaw cells

In order to understand the functional significance of the reciprocal pattern of response of the LVN neurones as well as of the LC-complex neurones during the vestibulospinal reflexes, we should consider that both the lateral VS neurones (cf. Pompeiano, 1975) as well as the CS neurones (cf. Fung and Barnes, 1984) exert a direct excitatory in-

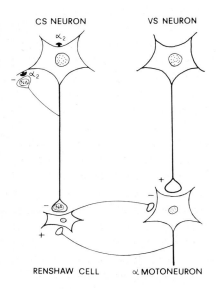

Fig. 2. Schematic representation of vestibulospinal (VS) and coeruleospinal (CS) neurones exerting an antagonistic influence on the same Renshaw (R)-cell. While the VS neurone excites the α motoneurone innervating an ipsilateral limb extensor muscle and then, through its recurrent collateral, the related R-cell, the CS neurone exerts a direct inhibitory influence on this inhibitory interneurone. Note that the CS neurone is provided by a self-inhibitory mechanism, which utilizes noradrenaline (NA) acting on α_2-adrenoceptors.

fluence on ipsilateral limb extensor motoneurones and, for the CS projection, also on flexor motoneurones. The same pathways, however, exert an antagonistic influence on R-cells linked with limb extensor motoneurones (Fig. 2). In fact, while the lateral VS neurones act indirectly on the recurrent inhibitory circuit by exciting first the limb extensor motoneurones and then, through their recurrent collaterals, the related R-cells, the CS neurones exert a direct inhibitory influence on these inhibitory interneurones, as shown in the following section.

Locus coeruleus influences on recurrent inhibitory pathways in the lumbar spinal cord

Fung et al. (1987a, 1988) have studied the effects of LC stimulation on recurrent inhibition in the lumbar spinal cord. In precollicular decerebrate cats, both hindlimbs were denervated, except for the left gastrocnemius-soleus (GS) and common peroneal (CP) nerves, which were dissected free for stimulation, while the ventral roots (VR) L6 – S1 were sectioned intradurally. Stable control monosynaptic reflexes (MRs), which were adjusted to half-maximal amplitudes, were recorded from the proximal end of the split VR bundle of L7 of the left side by stimulating the central cut end of either the GS or the CP nerve with single or double shocks (0.1 – 0.2 ms pulses), while recurrent inhibition was achieved by conditioning the test MR with a single volley delivered to the remaining bundle of the L7 VR or the adjacent VR (for additional methodological details see Fung et al. 1987a, 1988).

With a given set of VR and GS (or CP) stimulus strengths, the most conspicuous effect of recurrent inhibition occurred at a conditioning-test interval of 6.1 – 18.3 ms; beyond that point the inhibitory effect declined progressively. The time course of the recurrent inhibition curves resembled that reported originally by Renshaw (1941) in his monosynaptic reflex studies and by Eccles et al. (1954) for the inhibitory postsynaptic potentials recorded in cat motoneurones.

Typically, the VR-induced recurrent inhibition

was regularly counteracted by LC preconditioning stimuli. Such a decrease in recurrent inhibition, involving both extensor (GS) and flexor (CP) motor nuclei, was generally observed to exceed the LC-evoked reflex facilitation. Thus the observed reduction of the recurrent inhibition may be attributed to an LC suppressive effect on R-cell activity, which, in some cases, may be admixed with concurrent LC facilitation of test MRs. Support for the former hypothesis is provided by the fact that distinct weakening in recurrent inhibition was evident despite the lack of any measurable facilitation. Furthermore, the magnitude of LC-induced disinhibition was significantly correlated with that of this VR-induced recurrent inhibition (coefficient of correlation, $r = 0.70$; $P < 0.005$; $n = 145$), suggesting a strong interactive link between the LC and the R cell-motoneurone system. This proposed interaction was evident from direct recordings of R-cells with intracellular electrodes filled with 3 M potassium chloride. Upon LC conditioning, the characteristic high-frequency discharges of the R-cell in response to single VR

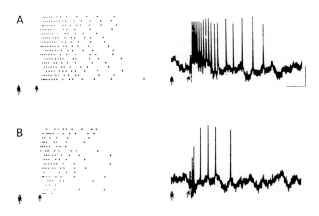

Fig. 3. Inhibitory LC influence on Renshaw (R)-cell firing in a precollicular decerebrate cat. A and B (left records): raster-dot displays of 16 consecutive sweeps (from top downwards) of control and conditioned R-cell discharges evoked by single ventral root volleys, respectively. Corresponding intracellular records were shown in A and B (right records). Single arrows, ventral root shocks; double arrows, LC stimuli (100 μA $\times$ 4 pulses at 770/s). Calibrations: 10 ms, 5 mV. From Fung et al. (1987a).

volleys (Fig. 3A) were significantly inhibited. This inhibition was clearly demonstrated by decrements in both the number of spikes and the duration of evoked R-cell responses (Fig. 3B).

The LC-induced removal of recurrent inhibition was, at least in part, attributed to an inhibitory LC control on the R-cell activity, uncoupling it from corresponding input motoneurones. This is in accord with early findings showing that R-cell activities were inhibited by iontophoretically applied norepinephrine (Biscoe and Curtis, 1966; Engberg and Ryall, 1966; Weight and Salmoiraghi, 1966), a putative transmitter of CS synapses (cf. Fung and Barnes, 1984). The same finding may also contribute to the CS activation of motoneurones (Chan et al., 1986; Fung and Barnes, 1981, 1984, 1987).

Responses of Renshaw cells to sinusoidal stimulation of labyrinth receptors

Since during the vestibulospinal reflexes there is a contraction of ipsilateral limb extensors during side-down tilt of the animal and extensor relaxation during side-up tilt (Schor and Miller, 1981; Manzoni et al., 1983a), one may postulate that the motoneurones innervating the ipsilateral limb extensors are excited by an increased discharge of VS neurones during side-down tilt. However, the R-cells anatomically linked with these extensor motoneurones would be disinhibited by a reduced discharge of CS neurones for the same direction of animal orientation, thus becoming more prominently linked with the ipsilateral limb extensor motoneurones. This hypothesis is supported by the results of unit recording experiments. In particular, Pompeiano et al. (1985a) have recorded the electrical activity of R-cells anatomically linked with GS motoneurones in precollicular decerebrate cats submitted to bilateral neck deafferentation, immobilized with pancuronium bromide and artificially ventilated. Both hindlimbs were denervated except for the nerves supplying the left GS muscle, which was deefferented by section of the ventral roots L6 – S2.

In these experiments, the discharge of 47 R-cells

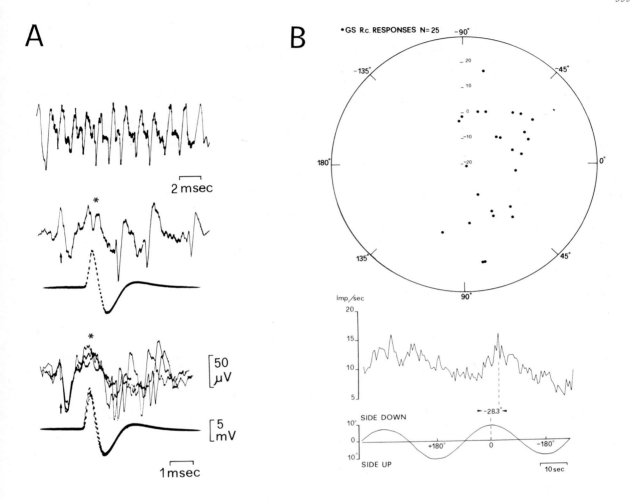

Fig. 4. Response pattern to slow head rotation (at 0.026–0.15 Hz, ± 10°) of Renshaw (R)-cells anatomically coupled with GS motoneurones (GS R-cells). Precollicular decerebrate cats with bilateral neck deafferentation, paralysed with pancuronium bromide. A: antidromic response of a single R-cell following single-shock stimulation of the central end of L7 ventral root with 0.2 ms pulse duration, 1.6-times the α threshold (upper trace) and single or superimposed orthodromic responses of the same R-cell to stimulation of the ipsilateral GS nerve with 0.2 ms pulses, 2-times the threshold (T) for the group I afferents (middle and lower traces). The arrows indicate the field potential due to the orthodromic group I volley and the asterisks indicate the field potential due to monosynaptic activation of the GS motoneurones, which coincides with the segmental monosynaptic reflex recorded simultaneously from the ipsilateral ventral root L7. The response of the R-cell appears with a latency of 0.88 ms with respect to the peak of the segmental monosynaptic reflex, indicating that the reflex discharge of the GS motoneurones monosynaptically excited the R-cell. B: polar diagram showing the dynamic characteristics of 25 groups of averaged responses (ARs) recorded from 15 GS R-cells. The sensitivity of each response, defined as the percentage change of the mean firing rate per degree of displacement, is represented by the distance of the corresponding symbol from the centre of the diagram (see the scale along the vertical meridian in decibels). The relative position of the symbols with respect to the 0° meridian indicates in degrees the phase lead (positive values) or the phase lag (negative values) of responses with respect to the extreme side-down head displacement. Below the diagram, the upper record represents a sequential pulse density histograms (SPDH) (average of 8 sweeps, using 128 bins with 0.6 s bin width) showing the response of a single GS R-cell to head rotation at 0.026 Hz, ± 10°, while the lower trace indicates the head position. In this instance the mean discharge rate or base frequency (BF) was 11.0 i.p.s., the response gain 0.24 i.p.s./degree and the phase angle corresponded to a lag of −28.3° with respect to the extreme side-down head displacement. From Pompeiano et al. (1985a,b).

was recorded from L7 and upper S1 spinal cord segments, both in the animal at rest as well as during bidirectional rotation of the head on the coronal plane (at 0.026 – 0.15 Hz, ± 10°), while the body remained fixed horizontally; due to neck deafferentation, the head displacement led to selective stimulation of labyrinth receptors. Averaged responses (AR) of single units were recorded during successive cycles of rotation. Among those R-cells which responded monosynaptically to antidromic ventral root stimulation, 22 units were disynaptically excited by the orthodromic group I volleys induced by single shock stimulation of the ipsilateral GS nerve, thus indicating that they were under the direct control of the recurrent collaterals of GS motoneurones monosynaptically driven by the orthodromic group Ia volleys (Fig. 4A) (Ross et al., 1972; Pompeiano et al., 1975).

Of the 47 R-cells tested, 9 units (2 of which coupled with GS motoneurones) were silent at rest and did not respond to head rotation, while the remaining 38 units (20 of which coupled with GS motoneurones) showed a spontaneous discharge at rest. Among these spontaneously firing R-cells, 31 units (16 of which coupled with GS motoneurones) responded to head rotation at either one or both the parameters indicated above. In resting animals with the ankle joint fixed at 90° dorsiflexion, all spontaneously active R-cells fired at a low rate, and their discharge rate closely corresponded to the mean firing rate evaluated during head rotation at 0.026 Hz, ± 10°. In particular, the mean firing rate evaluated for 24 spontaneously active units responsive to this stimulus (15 of which coupled with the GS motoneurones) corresponded on the average to 5.90 ± 5.35 (S.D.) i.p.s., while the gain of the first harmonic responses to head rotation at 0.026 Hz, ± 10° corresponded on the average to 0.075 ± 0.059 i.p.s./degree (35 groups of AR). The mean firing rate as well as the gain were on the average slightly higher for the 15 R-cells coupled with the GS motoneurones (25 groups of AR) than for the 9 unidentified R-cells (10 groups of AR).

As to the phase angle of the first harmonic of responses of R-cells to head rotation, most of the averaged responses (27 out of 35 groups of AR, i.e. 77.1%) recorded from 17 out of the 24 R-cells were characterized by an increased discharge during side-down head rotation and a decreased discharge during side-up rotation and showed a phase angle which ranged from ± 90° to 0° with an average lead of +3.1 ± 54.3 degrees with respect to the extreme side-down head displacement (α-responses) (Fig. 4B, lower traces). On the other hand, the responses recorded from the remaining 7 R-cells (8 AR, i.e. 22.9%) showed a phase angle which varied from ± 90° to 180°, with an average lag of −157.7 ±69.6 degrees (β-responses). Similar results were also obtained from the averaged responses of R-cells coupled with GS motoneurones, the majority of which (22 out of 25 groups of AR, i.e. 88.0%) recorded from 13 out of 15 R-cells showed α-responses (Fig. 4B, polar diagram).

The low firing rate of the R-cells linked with limb extensor motoneurones as recorded in decerebrate animals at rest can be partly attributed to the tonic inhibitory influence exerted on them by the spontaneously firing LC and SC neurones, leading to disinhibition of the corresponding extensor motoneurones. As to the labyrinthine influences, the observation that most of the R-cells coupled with GS motoneurones increased their discharge rate during side-down head rotation can only in part be attributed to the discharge of lateral VS neurones acting on ipsilateral limb extensor motoneurones and then, through their recurrent collaterals, on the related R-cells, since this modulation of R-cells activity occurred even in preparations in which the GS muscle did not show any EMG modulation prior to the ventral radicotomy. Therefore, the increased discharge of R-cells during side-down head rotation (α-response) can be attributed, at least in part, to the reduced firing rate of the CS neurones (β-response) leading to disinhibition of these interneurones.

In conclusion, it appears that in normal decerebrate cats the motoneurones innervating the ipsilateral limb extensors are excited by an increased discharge of VS neurones during side-down tilt, but this effect is, at least in part, attenuated by the reduced discharge of the CS neurones leading to disinhibition of the related R-cells. In this instance the R-cells would be more prominently coupled with the ipsilateral limb extensor motoneurones, a finding which should reduce the response gain of the corresponding limb extensors to labyrinth stimulation. Indeed in precollicular decerebrate cats, in which there is a tonic discharge of the CS neurones, the gain of the vestibulospinal reflexes is quite small in forelimb extensors (Manzoni et al., 1983a) and almost negligible or absent in hindlimbs (Boyle and Pompeiano, 1984; Manzoni et al., 1984; D'Ascanio et al., 1985; Pompeiano et al., 1985a,b).

Increase in gain of vestibulospinal reflexes after inactivation of NE-sensitive locus coeruleus-complex neurones

If one of the main roles of the CS neurones is to modify the functional coupling between R-cells and the related extensor motoneurones, one might expect that for a given amount of labyrinth signal, the amplitude of the EMG modulation of limb extensors depends on the background discharge of the CS neurones. In particular, the higher the firing rate of these units in the animal at rest, the greater the disinhibition which would affect the R-cells related to limb extensor motoneurones during side-down animal tilt. In this instance the resulting increase in firing rate of the R-cells would reduce the response of limb extensor motoneurones to the excitatory VS volleys, thus leading to a reduced gain of the vestibulospinal reflexes. Just the opposite result would occur following inactivation of the LC neurones.

It is known that α_2-adrenergic receptors are present within the LC, on the basis of histoimmunochemical observations (Young and Kuhar, 1980). Iontophoretic application of the α_2-adrenergic agonist clonidine into the LC inhibits the activity of the corresponding NE-containing neurones (Svensson et al., 1975; Guyenet, 1980).

These and other findings have led to postulate that the LC neurones are self-inhibitory, due to the fact that NE, which is released by the LC neurones as a consequence of impulse activity, acts on α_2-adrenoceptors of the same or neighbouring neurones, thus leading to recurrent and/or lateral suppression of their activity (cf. Foote et al., 1983). Recently, Pompeiano et al. (1987) investigated the effects of functional inactivation of the noradrenergic and NE-sensitive LC-complex neurones, produced by local injection of the α_2-adrenergic agonist clonidine, on posture as well as on the vestibulospinal reflexes.

In precollicular decerebrate cats, injection of 0.25 μl of the clonidine solution at the concentration of $0.012 - 0.15$ μg/μl of saline (marked with 5% pontamine) into the LC-complex of one side decreased the postural activity in the ipsilateral limbs, but greatly increased the amplitude of modulation and thus the gain of the multiunit EMG response of the ipsilateral triceps brachii to labyrinth stimulation (at 0.15 Hz, $\pm$ 10°). In particular, in four experiments, the gain of the averaged multiunit responses (AR) of the triceps brachii to animal tilt increased from the mean value of 0.66 ± 0.26 i.p.s./degree (42 groups of AR) to 1.73 ± 1.07 i.p.s./degree (60 groups of AR) (t-test, $P < 0.001$). Moreover, a slight decrease in phase lead of the responses was observed, which changed on the average from $+ 3.5 \pm 14.8$ degrees before injection to $+ 1.4 \pm 9.8$ degrees after injection of clonidine (Fig. 5, left traces).

The increased gain of the VS reflexes did not depend on the decrease in postural activity of the extensor muscle following injection of the α_2-adrenergic agonist, since it was still observed when the reflex contraction produced by an increased static stretch of that muscle compensated for the reduced EMG activity. The effects described above were first observed $10 - 15$ min after injection of clonidine in the ipsilateral LC; the highest value was reached in about $30 - 60$ min and persisted for more than 2 h after the injection.

The increase in the response gain produced by clonidine affected not only the ipsilateral but also

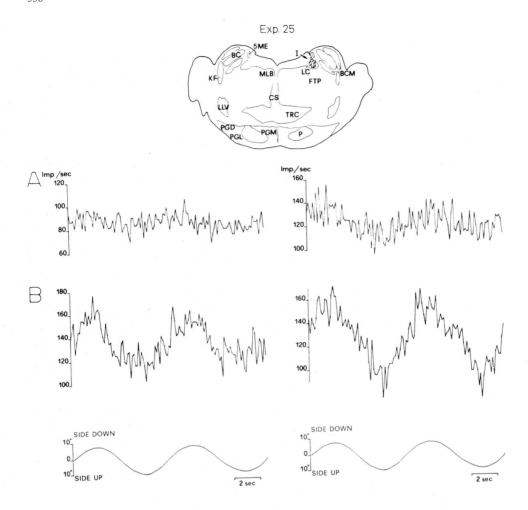

Fig. 5. Effects of local injection of clonidine into the LC of one side on the response gain of the ipsilateral and the contralateral triceps brachii to roll tilt of a precollicular decerebrate cat. Schematic representation of a transverse section of the pons, in which the tip of the cannula (arrow) was surrounded by a shaded area, indicating the spread of 0.25 µl of clonidine solution at the concentration of 0.012 µg/µl of saline stained with 5% pontamine. The site of the injection (I) was located within the LC of the left side (corresponding to the right side of the figure). Below this scheme there are SPDHs showing the averaged multiunit responses of the left triceps brachii (left side traces) and of the right triceps brachii (right side traces) to roll tilt of the animal at 0.15 Hz, ± 10°. Each record is the average of 6 sweeps, using 128 bins with 0.1 s bin width, while the lower trace in each column indicates the animal displacement. A: SPDHs recorded in the control situation. The mean base frequency (BF) evaluated from the left triceps brachii was 85.8 i.p.s., the response gain 0.41 i.p.s./degree, while the phase angle of the response corresponded to a lead of +45.2° with respect to the extreme side-down tilt of the animal. In the same experiment, the mean BF from the right triceps brachii was 122.7 i.p.s., the gain 0.87 i.p.s./degree, while the phase angle corresponded to a lead of +14.9°. B: SPDHs recorded 6 and 10 min, respectively, after local injection of clonidine into the LC of the left side (as shown above). In this instance the mean BF evaluated from the left triceps brachii was 136.1 i.p.s., the response gain 1.71 i.p.s./degree, while the phase angle of the response corresponded to a lead of +22.7° with respect to the extreme side-down tilt of the animal. The mean BF from the right triceps brachii was 127.6 i.p.s., the gain 2.80 i.p.s./degree, while the phase angle corresponded to a lead of +8.7°. In this experiment, the decrease in EMG activity of the ipsilateral triceps brachii after injection of clonidine was compensated for by the reflex discharge induced by an increased static stretch of the muscle. From Pompeiano et al. (1987).

the contralateral triceps brachii (Fig. 5, right traces). There was, however, a slight increase in phase lead of the responses with respect to the control values, which contrasted with the slight decrease in phase lead of the responses recorded ipsilaterally to the side of the injection. These reflex changes usually followed the same time course as that obtained from the ipsilateral triceps brachii.

The effects of clonidine were not due to irritative phenomena, since no postural and reflex changes were observed following local injection of 0.25 μl of saline into the LC complex. On the other hand, the described effects were dose-dependent and side-specific. The effective area included both the LC and the SC, as well as the dorsal pontine reticular formation located immediately ventral to the LC complex. This finding can easily be explained, since in the cat noradrenergic and NE-sensitive neurons are not exclusively located within the LC and the SC; moreover, clonidine may act on α_2-receptors located not only on the cell body but also on terminals of NE-containing neurones.

The conclusion that the effects produced by local injection of the α_2-adrenergic agonist clonidine into the LC complex were due to reduction or suppression of the spontaneous discharge of the corresponding neurones is supported by the results of previous experiments showing that postural and reflex changes similar to those induced by clonidine were obtained following electrolytic lesion of the LC of one side (D'Ascanio et al., 1985).

We postulate, therefore, that functional inactivation of the LC and the SC neurons produced by local injection of clonidine, releases the R-cells from the suppressive influence exerted by the noradrenergic terminals. The resulting increase in firing rate of these inhibitory interneurones would reduce the postural activity in the ipsilateral (and the contralateral) limbs in the animal at rest. Moreover, the lack of vestibular modulation of the CS neurones would prevent the increase in functional coupling between these inhibitory interneurones and the corresponding limb extensor motoneurones during side-down animal tilt. These

extensor motoneurones would then respond more efficiently to the same excitatory VS volleys elicited by this direction of animal orientation, thus increasing the response gain of limb extensors to labyrinth stimulation.

Discussion

The experiments summarized in the present report have shown that both the VS neurones originating from the LVN as well as the CS neurones originating from the LC complex contribute to the postural adjustments during the vestibulospinal reflexes.

It is known that the VS neurones exert a direct excitatory influence on ipsilateral limb extensor motoneurones (Lund and Pompeiano, 1968; cf. Pompeiano, 1975) and then though their recurrent collaterals on the related Renshaw (R)-cells. CS neurones, whose noradrenergic terminals are in close contact with ventral horn neurones (cf. Holstege and Kuypers, 1987), also exert an excitatory influence on ipsilateral limb extensor (and flexor) motoneurones (Fung and Barnes, 1981, 1984, 1987; Chan et al., 1986). This effect, however, through probably directly mediated (While and Neuman, 1980, 1983), can be attributed at least in part to an inhibitory control of the noradrenergic CS neurones on R-cell activity, thus leading to disinhibition of spinal cord motoneurones (Fung et al., 1987a, 1988). Indeed, selective stimulation of the LC, in which NE-containing neurons are located, produced a consistent reduction of ventral root-induced recurrent inhibition of monosynaptic reflexes in both extensor (GS) and flexor (CP) motor nuclei. The magnitudes of the LC-induced decrease in recurrent inhibition, functional disinhibition, and recurrent inhibition were significantly correlated. Moreover, direct recordings from R-cells indicated that LC stimulation decreased the number of spikes and the duration of firing in response to single antidromic (ventral root) volleys. These results suggested that the LC depression of the recurrent inhibitory pathway depended, at least in part, upon coeruleospinal inhibitory influences on R-cell activity. This is in accord with early findings showing that R-cell activity was inhibited by iontophoretically applied NE (Biscoe and Curtis, 1966; Engberg and Ryall, 1966; Weight and Salmoiraghi, 1966).

The demonstration that the LC exerts an inhibitory action on R-cells coupled to both extensor (and flexor) motoneurones, thus releasing these motoneurones from their related recurrent inhibition, suggested that this structure could play a role in regulating the gain setting of the output stage of the motor system during the vestibulospinal reflexes (Pompeiano, 1984b; cf. also Hultborn et al., 1979).

In order to test this hypothesis, the activity of LC and SC neurones, particularly projecting to the spinal cord, was recorded in decerebrate cats to find out whether, in addition to the lateral VS neurones, the CS neurones also responded to natural stimulation of macular labyrinthine receptors, thus being involved in the postural adjustments induced by labyrinth stimulation. In particular, the activity of a large number of LVN neurones, as well as of LC-complex neurones, was recorded during roll tilt of the animal leading to sinusoidal stimulation of labyrinth receptors. A large proportion of both LVN and LC-complex neurones responded to animal tilt, the responses being attributed to stimulation of macular utricular receptors. However, while the majority of VS neurones projecting to the lumbosacral segments of the spinal cord showed α-responses (excitation during side-down tilt), the majority of the LC-complex neurones, some of which were identified antidromically as CS neurones by stimulation of the spinal cord at $T_{12} - L_1$, showed β-responses (excitation during side-up tilt). Since during the vestibulospinal reflexes there is a contraction of ipsilateral limb extensors during side-down tilt of the animal, it appears that the increased discharge of VS neurones would increase the activity of the ipsilateral limb extensor motoneurones and the related R-cells. However, the reduced discharge of CS neurones for the same direction of

animal orientation would lead to disinhibition of the R-cells linked with these extensor motoneurones, thus enhancing the functional coupling of these inhibitory interneurones with the corresponding extensor motoneurones; just the opposite results would occur during side-up animal tilt.

It is of interest that in precollicular decerebrate cats the continuous and regular discharge of the LC-complex neurones (cf. also Pompeiano and Hoshino, 1976) led to a low firing rate of the R-cells linked with limb extensor motoneurones (Pompeiano et al., 1985a). Moreover, in the same preparation, these R-cells were excited during side-down tilt, which explains why the amplitude of the EMG modulation and thus the response gain of limb extensors to animal tilt was quite small in amplitude in the forelimbs (Manzoni et al., 1983a) and almost negligible or absent in the hindlimbs (Boyle and Pompeiano, 1984; Manzoni et al., 1984; D'Ascanio et al., 1985; Pompeiano et al., 1985a,b).

This interpretation of the experimental findings is supported by the results of experiments performed in decerebrate cats, showing that functional inactivation of the corresponding noradrenergic neurones produced by local injection into the LC-complex of minute doses of the α_2-adrenergic agonist clonidine (Pompeiano et al., 1987), which acts on the somatodendritic α_2-adrenoceptors by enhancing recurrent and/or lateral inhibition of the corresponding NE-containing neurones (cf. Foote et al., 1983; Ennis and Aston-Jones, 1986a), decreased the postural activity, but greatly increased the gain of the vestibulospinal reflexes.

In order to explain these findings we postulated that inactivation of the LC-complex neurones would release the R-cells from the suppressive influence exerted by the CS terminals, thus reducing the postural activity of the extensor limb musculature in the animal at rest. Moreover, due to lack of vestibular modulation of LC activity, the functional coupling between R-cells and limb extensor motoneurones would not undergo periodic fluctuations during animal tilt; in particular, this coupling would not increase during side-down animal tilt. The extensor motoneurones would then respond more efficiently to the same excitatory VS volleys elicited by this direction of animal tilt, thus increasing the response gain of limb extensors to labyrinth stimulation.

In summary, while in normal decerebrate cats the reduced discharge of LC and SC neurones during side-down animal tilt would lead to disinhibition of R-cells, thus enhancing the recruitment of these inhibitory interneurones during the motoneuronal discharge elicited by the VS volleys, after functional inactivation of the LC complex produced by clonidine injection a derecruitment of the R-cells would occur for the same direction of animal tilt. Obviously, in the first instance, the increased coupling of R-cells with the extensor motoneurones during side-down tilt would *limit the response gain* of the GS muscle to labyrinth stimulation, while in the second instance the reduced coupling of R-cells with the extensor motoneurones for the same direction of animal orientation would *enhance the response gain* of the GS muscle to labyrinth stimulation. The CS system may thus operate as a variable gain regulator, modulating motoneuronal activation during the vestibular reflexes. Since the LC and SC neurones undergo spontaneous fluctuations in their firing rate (cf. Hobson and Steriade, 1986) leading to changes in postural activity (cf. Pompeiano, 1967) during the sleep – waking cycle, they may well intervene in order to adapt the gain of the vestibulospinal reflexes to the animal state.

It is worth mentioning that the LC could act in more than one way to modify the response gain of extensor muscles to labyrinth stimulation. In addition to the reported LC-induced inhibition of R-cell activity (Fung et al., 1987a, 1988), another means involves the LC enhancement of firing efficacy of extensor motoneurones (Fung and Barnes, 1981, 1984, 1987; Chan et al., 1986), modifying the excitatory vestibulospinal drive to extensors. Another means depends on the LC inhibition of dorsal pontine reticular neurones and the related medullary inhibitory reticulospinal (RS)

neurones (D'Ascanio et al., 1985; Pompeiano et al., 1987; cf. D'Ascanio et al., 1988). The latter neurones may actually inhibit the extensor motoneurones by exciting the corresponding R-cells (cf. Pompeiano et al., 1985b). Through this interplay among VS, CS and RS systems, it becomes possible for the animals to execute balanced postural adjustments in response to labyrinthine signals.

Acknowledgements

This study was supported by the NIH grant NS 07685-21 and a grant from the Ministero della Pubblica Istruzione, Roma, Italy.

References

Aston-Jones, G., Ennis, M., Pieribone, V.A., Nickell, W.T. and Shipley, M.T. (1986) The brain nucleus locus coeruleus: restricted afferent control of a broad efferent network. *Science,* 234: 734 – 737.

Biscoe, T.J. and Curtis, D.R. (1966) Noradrenaline and inhibition of Renshaw cells. *Science,* 151: 1230 – 1231.

Boyle, R. and Pompeiano, O. (1984) Discharge activity of spindle afferents from the gastrocnemius-soleus muscle during head rotation in the decerebrate cat. *Pflügers Arch.,* 400: 140 – 150.

Cedarbaum, J.M. and Aghajanian, G.K. (1978) Afferent projections to the rat locus coeruleus as determined by a retrograde tracing technique. *J. Comp. Neurol.,* 178: 1 – 16.

Chan, J.Y.H., Fung, S.J., Chan, S.H.H. and Barnes, C.D. (1986) Facilitation of lumbar monosynaptic reflexes by locus coeruleus in the rat. *Brain Res.,* 369: 103 – 109.

Clavier, R.M. (1979) Afferent projections to the self-stimulation regions of the dorsal pons, including the locus coeruleus, in the rat as demonstrated by the horseradish peroxidase technique. *Brain Res. Bull.,* 4: 497 – 504.

D'Ascanio, P., Bettini, E. and Pompeiano, O. (1985) Tonic inhibitory influences of locus coeruleus on the response gain of limb extensors to sinusoidal labyrinth and neck stimulations. *Arch. Ital. Biol.,* 123: 69 – 100.

D'Ascanio, P., Pompeiano, O. and Stampacchia, G. (1988) Noradrenergic and cholinergic mechanisms responsible for the gain regulation of vestibulospinal reflexes. In O. Pompeiano and J.H.J. Allum (Eds.), *Vestibulospinal Control of Posture and Locomotion. Prog. Brain Res., Vol. 76,* Elsevier, Amsterdam, pp. 361 – 374.

Eccles, J.C., Fatt, P. and Koketsu, K. (1954) Cholinergic and inhibitory synapses in a pathway from motor-axon collaterals to motoneurones. *J. Physiol. (London),* 126: 524 – 562.

Engberg, I. and Ryall, R.W. (1966) The inhibitory action of noradrenaline and other monoamines on spinal neurones. *J. Physiol. (London),* 185: 298 – 322.

Ennis, M. and Aston-Jones, G. (1986a) Evidence for self- and neighbor-mediated postactivation inhibition of locus coeruleus neurones. *Brain Res.,* 374: 299 – 305.

Ennis, M. and Aston-Jones, G. (1986b) A potent excitatory input to nucleus locus coeruleus from the ventrolateral medulla. *Neurosci. Lett.,* 71: 299 – 305.

Ennis, M. and Aston-Jones, G. (1987) Two physiologically distinct populations of neurones in the ventrolateral medulla innervate the locus coeruleus. *Brain Res.,* 425: 275 – 282.

Foote, S.L., Bloom, F.E. and Aston-Jones, G. (1983) Nucleus locus coeruleus: New evidence of anatomical and physiological specificity. *Physiol. Rev.,* 93: 844 – 914.

Fung, S.J. and Barnes, C.D. (1981) Evidence of facilitatory coerulospinal action in lumbar motoneurons of cats. *Brain Res.,* 216: 299 – 311.

Fung, S.J. and Barnes, C.D. (1984) Locus coeruleus control of spinal cord activity. In C.D. Barnes (Ed.), *Brainstem Control of Spinal Cord Function. Research Topics in Physiology, Vol. 6,* Academic Press, Orlando, pp. 215 – 255.

Fung, S.J. and Barnes, C.D. (1987) Membrane excitability changes in hindlimb motoneurons induced by stimulation of the locus coeruleus in cats. *Brain Res.,* 402: 230 – 242.

Fung, S.J., Pompeiano, O. and Barnes, C.D. (1987a) Suppression of the recurrent inhibitory pathway in lumbar cord segments during locus coeruleus stimulation in cats. *Brain Res.,* 402: 351 – 354.

Fung, S.J., Reddy, V.K., Bowker, R.M. and Barnes, C.D. (1987b) Differential labeling of the vestibular complex following unilateral injections of horseradish peroxidase into the cat and rat locus coeruleus. *Brain Res.,* 401: 347 – 352.

Fung, S.J., Pompeiano, O. and Barnes, C.D. (1988) Coeruleospinal influence on recurrent inhibition of spinal motonuclei innervating antagonistic hindleg muscles. *Pflügers Arch.,* 412: 346 – 353.

Goldberg, J.M. and Fernández, C. (1984) The vestibular system. In *Handbook of Physiology, Section 1. The Nervous System, Vol. III,* American Physiological Society, Bethesda, MD, pp. 977 – 1022.

Guyenet, P.G. (1980) The coeruleospinal noradrenergic neurones: anatomical and electrophysiological studies in the rat. *Brain Res.,* 189: 121 – 133.

Hobson, J.A. and Steriade, M. (1986) Neuronal basis of behavioral state control. In F.E. Bloom (Ed.), *Intrinsic Regulatory System of the Brain. Handbook of Physiology, Section 1, The Nervous System, Vol. IV,* American Physiological Society, Bethesda, MD, pp. 701 – 823.

Holstege, J.C. and Kuypers, H.G.J.M. (1987) Brainstem projections to spinal motoneurons: an update. *Neuroscience,* 23: 809 – 821.

Hultborn, H., Lindström, S. and Wigström, H. (1979) On the function of recurrent inhibition in the spinal cord. *Exp. Brain Res.,* 37: 399 – 403.

Jones, B.E. and Friedman, L. (1983) Atlas of catecholamine perikarya varicosities and pathways in the brainstem of the cat. *J. Comp. Neurol.,* 215: 382 – 396.

Jordan, L.M., McCrea, D.A., Steeves, J.D. and Menzies, J.E. (1977) Noradrenergic synapses and effects of noradrenaline on interneurones in the ventral horn of the cat spinal cord. *Can. J. Physiol. Pharmacol.,* 55: 399 – 412.

Lund, S. and Pompeiano, O. (1968) Monosynaptic excitation of alpha motoneurons from supraspinal structures in the cat. *Acta Physiol. Scand.,* 73: 1 – 21.

Lundberg, A. (1982) Inhibitory control from the brain stem of transmission from primary afferents to motoneurons, primary afferent terminals and ascending pathways. In B. Sjölund and A. Björklund (Eds.), *Brain Stem Control of Spinal Mechanisms,* Elsevier, Amsterdam, pp, 179 – 224.

Manzoni, D., Pompeiano, O., Srivastava, U.C. and Stampacchia, G. (1983a) Responses of forelimb extensors to sinusoidal stimulation of macular labyrinth and neck receptors. *Arch. Ital. Biol.* 121: 205 – 214.

Manzoni, D., Pompeiano, O., Stampacchia, G. and Srivastava, U.C. (1983b) Response of medullary reticulospinal neurons to sinusoidal stimulation of labyrinth receptors in decerebrate cat. *J. Neurophysiol.,* 50: 1059 – 1079.

Manzoni, D., Pompeiano, O. Srivastava, U.C. and Stampacchia, G. (1984) Gain regulation of vestibular reflexes in fore- and hindlimb muscles evoked by roll tilt. *Boll. Soc. Ital. Biol. Sper.,* 60: Suppl. 3, 9 – 10.

Manzoni, D., Marchand, A.R., Pompeiano, O. and Stampacchia, G. (1987) Coding of the velocity signal by lumbar projecting vestibulospinal neurons in the decerebrate cats. *Neuroscience,* 22: Suppl., S739.

Marchand, A.R., Manzoni, D., Pompeiano, O. and Stampacchia, G. (1987) Effects of stimulation of vestibular and neck receptors on Deiters neurons projecting to the lumbosacral cord. *Pflügers Arch.,* 409: 13 – 23.

Miachon, S., Berod, A., Leger, L., Chat, M., Hartman, B. and Pujol, J.F. (1984) Identification of cetecholamine cell bodies in the pons and pons-mesencephalon junction of the cat brain, using tyrosine hydroxylase and dopamine-β-hydroxylase immunohistochemistry. *Brain Res.,* 305: 369 – 374.

Mizukawa, K. (1980) The segmental detailed topographical distribution of monoaminergic terminals and their pathways in the spinal cord of the cat. *Anat Anz.,* 147: 125 – 144.

Morgane, P.J. and Jacobs, M.S. (1979) Raphe projections to the locus coeruleus in the rat. *Brain Res. Bull.,* 4: 519 – 534.

Pompeiano, O. (1967) The neurophysiological mechanisms of the postural and motor events during desynchronized sleep. *Res. Publ. Ass. Nerv. Ment. Dis.,* 45: 351 – 423.

Pompeiano, O. (1975) Vestibulospinal relationships. In R.F. Naunton (Ed.), *The Vestibular System,* Academic Press,

New York, San Francisco, London, pp. 147–180.

Pompeiano, O. (1979) Neck and macular labyrinthine influences on the cervical spino-reticulocerebellar pathway. In R. Granit and O. Pompeiano (Eds.), *Reflex Control of Posture and Movement, Prog. Brain Res., Vol. 50,* Elsevier, Amsterdam, pp. 501–514.

Pompeiano, O. (1980) Cholinergic activation of reticular and vestibular mechanisms controlling posture and eye movements. In J.A. Hobson and M.A.B. Brazier (Eds.), *Reticular Formation Revisited, IBRO Monograph Series, Vol. 6,* Raven Press, New York, pp. 473–512.

Pompeiano, O. (1984a) A comparison of the response characteristics of vestibulospinal and reticulospinal neurones to labyrinth and neck inputs. In C.D. Barnes (Ed.), *Brainstem Control of Spinal Cord Function, Research Topics in Physiology, Vol. 6,* Academic Press, Orlando, pp. 87–140.

Pompeiano, O. (1984b) Recurrent inhibition. In R.A. Davidoff (Ed.), *Handbook of the Spinal Cord, Vols. 2 and 3,* Marcel Decker, New York, pp. 461–557.

Pompeiano, O. and Hoshino, K (1976) Tonic inhibition of dorsal pontine neurons during the postural atonia produced by an anticholinesterase in the decerebrate cat. *Arch. Ital. Biol.,* 114: 310–340.

Pompeiano, O., Wand, P. and Sontag, K.-H. (1975) Response of Renshaw cells to sinusoidal stretch of hindlimb extensor muscles. *Arch. Ital. Biol.,* 113: 205–237.

Pompeiano, O., Wand, P. and Srivastava, U.C. (1985a) Responses of Renshaw cells coupled with hindlimb extensor motoneurons to sinusoidal stimulation of labyrinth receptors in the decerebrate cat. *Pflügers Arch.,* 403: 245–257.

Pompeiano, O., Wand, P. and Srivastava, U.C. (1985b) Influence of Renshaw cells on the gain of hindlimb extensor muscles to sinusoidal labyrinth stimulation. *Pflügers Arch.,* 404: 107–118.

Pompeiano, O., D'Ascanio, P., Horn, E. and Stampacchia, G. (1987) Effects of local injection of the α_2-adrenergic agonist clonidine in the locus coeruleus complex on the gain of vestibulospinal and cervicospinal reflexes in decerebrate cats. *Arch. Ital. Biol.,* 125: 225–269.

Pompeiano, O., Manzoni, D., Barnes, C.D., Stampacchia, G. and D'Ascanio, P. (1988a) Labyrinthine influences on locus coeruleus neurons. *Acta Otolaryngol. (Stockholm),* 105: 576–581.

Pompeiano, O., Manzoni, D., Barnes, C.D., Stampacchia, G. and D'Ascanio, P. (1988b) Responses of locus coeruleus and subcoeruleus neurons on sinusoidal stimulation of labyrinth receptors in decerebrate cat. *Neuroscience,* in press.

Renshaw, B. (1941) Influence of discharge of motoneurons upon excitation of neighboring motoneurons. *J. Neurophysiol.,* 4: 167–183.

Ross, H.-G., Cleveland, S. and Haase, J. (1972) Quantitative relation of Renshaw cell discharges to monosynaptic reflex height. *Pflügers Arch.,* 332: 73–79.

Sakai, K., Touret, M., Salvert, D., Leger, L. and Jouvet, M. (1977) Afferent projections to the cat locus coeruleus as visualized by the horseradish peroxidase technique. *Brain Res.,* 119: 21–41.

Schor, R.H. and Miller, A.D. (1981) Vestibular reflexes in neck and forelimb muscles evoked by roll tilt. *J. Neurophysiol.,* 46: 167–178.

Svensson, T.H., Bunney, B.S. and Aghajanian, G.K. (1975) Inhibition of both noradrenergic and serotonergic neurons in brain by the α-adrenergic agonist clonidine. *Brain Res.,* 92: 291–306.

Weight, F.F. and Salmoiraghi, G.C. (1966) Adrenergic responses of Renshaw cells. *J. Pharmacol. Exp. Ther.,* 154: 391–397.

White, S.R. and Neuman, R.S. (1980) Facilitation of spinal motoneurone excitability by 5-hydroxytryptamine and noradrenaline. *Brain Res.,* 188: 119–127.

White, S.R. and Neuman, R.S. (1983) Pharmacological antagonism of facilitatory but not inhibitory effects of serotonin and norepinephrine on excitability of spinal motoneuron. *Neuropharmacology,* 22: 489–494.

Young, W.S. III and Kuhar, M.J. (1980) Noradrenergic α_1 and α_2 receptors: light microscopic autoradiographic localization. *Proc. Natl. Acad. Sci. U.S.A.,* 77: 1696–1700.

Interaction of Visual, Vestibular and Proprioceptive Inputs

J.H.J. Allum and M. Hulliger (Eds.)
Progress in Brain Research, Vol. 80
© 1989 Elsevier Science Publishers B.V. (Biomedical Division)

Overview and critique of Chapters 28 and 29

F.J.R. Richmond

Kingston, Canada

"How are neck muscles used to produce normal head movements?" This question has been addressed in the two following studies by examining EMG patterns in alert, chronically-instrumented cats. Such studies yield large quantities of data that tell us much about the activity of neck muscles that could not be predicted from studies on reduced, anaesthetized or immobilized preparations. For example, *Roucoux and his colleagues* demonstrate that EMG patterns in neck muscles are quite different when the cat's head is free to follow a visual target than when the head is held fixed. *Peterson and his co-workers* show that patterns of neck-muscle recruitment are more variable and difficult to predict from one cat to the next when the cat moves its head voluntarily than when it makes corrective movements driven by vestibulocollic reflexes. However, many questions still remain concerning the control of neck muscles. The strengths and limitations of the EMG studies conducted so far can perhaps be appreciated more easily if we parse the central question into its components, and then consider how thoroughly each of the experiments presented here addresses those components.

How are *neck muscles* used to produce normal head movements?

First, what are the relevant muscles? Most attention has been paid so far to the dorsal muscles attaching to the lambdoidal crest of the skull. Such a focus may be justifiable when studies are confined to small nodding or turning movements made primarily across the atlantoaxial and atlantooccipital joints. However, in more complex but more typical movements, it is important to know the recruitment patterns of all relevant muscles, if the contribution of any single muscle is to be evaluated in an appropriate context. For example, attention is seldom paid to muscles attaching to lower cervical vertebrae, even though cats commonly elevate their heads by bending the neck across the cervicothoracic flexure located caudal to C3. Without knowing the contribution of more caudally located muscles, it may be difficult to evaluate the relative role played by muscles inserting onto the skull.

Second, is it enough to record from a neck muscle using a single pair of electrodes implanted indiscriminately? Many neck muscles are known to contain several compartments of motor units. Roucoux and coworkers point out quite correctly that in-series compartments have shown similar patterns of recruitment in the few studies where compartments have been examined concurrently in alert cats (Wilson et al., 1983; Loeb et al., 1987). However, some neck muscles are compartmentalized in parallel, by specializations in fibre-type distribution or mechanical action. For example, in obliquus capitis caudalis, superficial layers are composed almost exclusively by fast fibres, whereas deep layers have a predominance of slow fibres. In our experiments (Loeb et al., 1987), EMG records taken from these two regions differ substantially. Superficial regions have phasic bursts of discharge, whereas deep regions can show a maintained activity. Thus, the intramuscular location of electrodes will influence the comparability of results from one animal to another. In the experiments of Roucoux and colleagues, intramuscular electrodes might be expected to sample from deep fibre fascicles, whereas in the experiments of Peterson and coworkers, patch electrodes would record preferentially from fast, superficial regions.

How are neck muscles *used to produce* normal head movements?

In the studies reported here, the use of a muscle has been assessed by EMG recordings. In other motor systems, such EMG signals are commonly cross-referenced to biomechanical measures of muscle performance, by appropriate placement of tension transducers on tendons, length gauges alongside muscles or force-plates to be engaged by the moving skeletal part. In the neck, such monitoring devices are much more difficult to use and inferences about muscle behaviour become much more dependent on EMG records alone. Therefore, it is particularly important to bear in mind the strengths and problems associated with EMG recording when such results are interpreted. Almost any two leads implanted randomly in muscle will generate EMG records. The challenge is to ensure that the records are representative and accurate. Thus, the onus must be on the investigator to prove that each original record is (1) free of cross-talk from other muscles, (2) free of artifact, (3) taken from site(s) that represent adequately the different histochemical or functional compartments of a muscle, (4) calibrated in a way that permits comparisons between behaviours, preparations and investigators. This can be difficult to ensure when highly processed summary figures must be constructed in order to reduce the length of published work.

EMG activation is only one of the variables that govern force development in a muscle. The strength of contraction will also depend on other factors such as (1) the activation history of the muscle, (2) the lengths of muscle fibres and (3) the velocity of shortening or lengthening motion. Consequently, a similar level of EMG activity can produce quite different levels of performance depending on the conditions under which the muscle is working. This problem is often not considered when comparing patterns of recruitment during different motor tasks. Without information about the biomechanics of the system, studies of muscle function based on recruitment cannot advance beyond a certain level of descriptive generality.

How are neck muscles used to produce *normal head movements?*

In the cat, head movements are required for many behavioural tasks, such as fighting, grooming, and carrying prey. However, in the laboratory it is often only practical to study simple, controlled head movements such as those made to track a visual target or follow a drinking tube. These gentle behaviours require little force and much less orchestration than the more complex behaviours that lie at the root of the cat's survival. The comparative anatomist would probably remind us that the architecture of a muscle is often shaped not by the requirements of the simplest tasks, but rather the needs of the most difficult ones. Studies of unobstructed head turns and lifts give much information about the activity of a small population of motoneurones that presumably operate at the base of the recruitment ladder, but they may give little insight into the performance of the rest of the motor-unit population. This problem becomes most clear when studying muscles such as trapezius or sternomastoideus that contain few type SO fibres (Richmond and Vidal, 1988) and are seldom found to be active during small, controlled head movements.

When cats make more complex head movements, motion is seldom confined to a single joint. Instead, the movements can involve combined or even antiphasic motions across a complex column of bones interspaced by eight cervical joints. It may be true to say that "the head can move in, at most, 6 degrees of freedom". However, the muscles producing that movement are also acting on the cervical vertebral column, and each cervical joint may have at least three degrees of freedom in addition. Thus, the movement that can be generated between the head and the trunk can become biomechanically much more complicated than might be guessed simply by plotting the position of the head. Further, a single "head" movement may require a different pattern of muscle synergy according to the initial posture of the head with respect to the body because the underlying movements of the neck will be quite different. A thorny question of methodology concerns the manner in which the relative movements across cervical joints can be monitored and evaluated together with information about neck-muscle recruitment, because the patterning of muscle activity is presumably related to the neck movement, as well as the head movement that must be made. To use the hindlimb system as an analogy, it would be difficult to understand the biomechanical and neural events underlying locomotion if the investigator only monitored the trajectory of the paw.

Studies of head and neck movements in the alert cat are still in their infancy. The studies outlined her underline the feasibility of such methods, but emphasize that recruitment patterns are not always simple to understand. They also point to the problems of modelling a complex biomechanical system using analytical approaches and simplifying assumptions that remove biological realism, and at the same time, perhaps ignore the kinesiological variables that the neuromuscular system must control during voluntary head movements.

References

Loeb, G.E., Yee, W.J., Pratt, C.A., Chanaud, C.M. and Richmond, F.J.R. (1987) Cross-correlation of EMG reveals widespread synchronization of motor units during some slow movements in intact cats. *J. Neurosci. Methods,* 21: 239 – 249.

Richmond, F.J.R. and Vidal, P.R. (1988) The motor system: joints and muscles of the neck. In B.W. Peterson and F.J.R. Richmond (Eds.), *Control of Head Movement,* Oxford University Press, New York, pp. 1 – 21.

Wilson, V.J., Precht, W. and Dieringer, N. (1983) Responses of different compartments of cat's splenius muscle to optokinetic stimulation. *Exp. Brain Res.,* 50: 153 – 156.

J.H.J. Allum and M. Hulliger (Eds.)
Progress in Brain Research, Vol. 80
© 1989 Elsevier Science Publishers B.V. (Biomedical Division)

CHAPTER 28

Neck muscle activity in eye – head coordinated movements

A. Roucoux, M. Crommelinck and M.-F. Decostre

Laboratoire de Neurophysiologie, University of Louvain, Brussels, Belgium

The electromyographic (EMG) activity of different neck muscles in relation to gaze orientation has been studied in alert trained cats. When the head is kept fixed, the activity of these muscles is proportional to eye eccentricity in the horizontal as well as in the vertical planes. On basis of this tonic activity, a preferential orientation can be attributed to each muscle: upward and lateral for biventer, rectus and complexus, and downward and lateral for longissimus, splenius and obliquus capitis cranialis. Fluctuations in this modulation of the EMG activity by eye position can be observed. When the head is free to move, the muscles show phasic discharges having similar preferential orientations. For a given muscle, this orientation covers a quite large angle: many muscles contribute to a given movement. The timing of the discharge of the different muscles as a function of the direction of the head movement was examined. It was found that the latency, i.e. the delay between the discharge and movement onset, progressively increases as the movement direction diverges from the preferential orientation of the muscle. It has been noted that the muscles having an upward preferential orientation may show, in relation to downward movements, inhibition occurring prior to the onset of the head movement. The same muscles may also increase their activity around the midcourse of downward movements. Thus, the head motor system controls the direction and amplitude parameters not only by selectively activating the appropriate muscles but also by sequencing their activity in a subtle way to start, control the trajectory and stop the movement, reminiscent of what has been described for limb movements.

Key words: Electromyographic activity; Eye-head coordination; Eye movement; Gaze control; Head movement; Neck muscle; Orientation; Visuo-motor response

Introduction

Neck muscles are implicated in the control of gaze. Indeed, most eye orienting movements are accompanied by synchronized and coordinated head movements: this combination of movements enlarges the angle through which gaze can move and, with the help of the vestibulo-ocular reflex, enables the eye to come back in the vicinity of its primary position. In this behaviour, the head plays an ancillary role: indeed, the controlled parameter is gaze position in space, i.e. the position of the visual axis with respect to the body. Achieving this control requires precise coordination mechanisms between eye and head and a motor programme adapted to the characteristics of the head musculature.

The properties of this particular motor activity of the neck are still largely unknown in natural conditions. There are only a few studies on the subject. Bizzi et al. (1972) recorded the activity of splenius muscles during horizontal head orientation in monkeys. They described two modes of eye-head coupling: a "triggered" mode, in response to an unexpected visual target, where the agonist splenius showed a phasic discharge, followed, after a short pause, by a tonic activity, where the antagonist splenius activity was suppressed. The other mode was called "predictive": it was observed when the monkey, after a long training period, oriented his head towards an expected target. In this case, there was a gradual increase in activity of the agonist muscle and a progressive decrease of activity in the antagonist. No mention of active braking by the antagonist is made (Bizzi et al., 1976). Crommelinck et al. (1982) described the activity of obliquus capitis muscles, in the cat, during spontaneous exploratory behaviour. These authors observed that tonic activities were associated with eccentric head positions, that phasic bursts occurred during fast head rotations, and that mean discharge was related to head velocity during visual scanning. As these head movements are very complex, no consistent quatification could be made. Roucoux et al. (1985) and Roucoux and Crommelinck (1988) studied in alert, head free, trained cats, the activity of 7 pairs of neck muscles during gaze orientation. They observed that phasic discharges were predominant when the head moved: the intensity of this discharge depended on direction, amplitude and initial position of the head. Richmond et al. (1985) showed, in unrestrained alert cats, that tonic activity related to stationary posture of the head was only present in a few muscles. When the head moved, the muscles were recruited in a complex way, depending on several factors such as direction, amplitude, starting position, speed, etc. of the movements. Loeb and Richmond (1986), in the same preparation, described during slow head movements (grooming) rhythmic bursts having a frequency of 25 to 30 Hz, that were synchronized between different muscles. In man, Hannaford et al. (1984) analysed the EMG activity of several neck muscles under various conditions, in a task where the controlled variable was not gaze but head rotation amplitude, velocity and load (stereotyped head movements). They showed that, for fast horizontal head movements, splenius muscles displayed a triphasic pattern of activity, analogous to what has been described for arm movements. They also studied some of the relationships between EMG and movement dynamics.

In the head-fixed cat, Roucoux et al. (1981), Roucoux et al. (1982) and Vidal et al. (1982) reported that neck EMG activity was strongly correlated with horizontal eye position during spontaneous, vestibular or optokinetic oculomotor activity. Wilson et al. (1983) showed that, in these conditions, all the compartments of the splenius muscle behaved similarly. Lestienne et al. (1984), in the head-fixed monkey, found very similar results.

The results that are presented in this current study concern the "spatial" distribution and temporal sequencing of EMG activity in a series of neck muscles of alert, head free cats, during visual orientation in various directions. In order to "control" as much as possible the reproducibility of head movements, the animals have been trained, in an operant paradigm, to foveate visual targets.

Methods

These data were collected from 3 cats. The animals were first implanted, under anaesthesia, with eye coils, a head fixation device and EMG electrodes in neck muscles. After recovery, they were trained to acquire and fixate visual targets. When a satisfactory level of performance was attained, recording sessions took place.

Eye and head movement recording

Eye movements were recorded by the magnetic search-coil technique. Head movements were measured by the same technique, a coil being affixed to the head implant, as close as possible to the recorded eye. By subtracting head position signal from eye or gaze signal, eye position in orbit was measured. Head position records were easily calibrated, as the head coil could be stereotactically positioned. The head was in its "zero" position when its sagittal plane corresponded to the sagittal plane of the cat's body, and its horizontal Horsley-Clarke plane parallel to the earth's horizontal. Eye position was calibrated by an optical method in such a way that the eye was said to be at "zero", or primary position, when its optical axis (the axis passing through the centre of the area centralis and the optical centre) was horizontal and parallel to the sagittal body plane. The signals originating from the two coils were digitized at a rate of 500 Hz. The total bandwidth of the recording system was 0 to 100 Hz (-3 dB).

Neck muscle EMG recording

Pairs of braided stainless steel wires, insulated with teflon, were inserted, under control of vision, into 6 pairs of muscles: biventer cervicis, complexus, longissimus capitis, obliquus capitis superior, rectus capitis anterior major and splenius. The exposed part of the wires was about 2 mm long and each wire of a pair was placed about 6 to 10 mm apart, according to the muscle size. Each pair of wires was sutured to the muscle, to avoid any displacement during contraction. The wires were led subcutaneously to connectors embedded in the head implant. The signals were amplified (bandwidth 10 Hz to 3 kHz), rectified and integrated. The output of the integrators was digitized at a rate of 500 Hz. After each sample, the computer reset the integrators; no data was thus lost and the temporal resolution of the EMG was identical to that of eye and head position signals. EMG amplitude is either expressed in mV, or in percentage of the maximum discharge measured, for a given muscle, in isometric conditions (head fixed).

Experimental paradigm

After having recovered from surgery, the cats were trained daily to foveate and fixate small spots of light. Animals sat crouched in a box, which restrained most of their body or limb movements. The anterior part of the box constituted a sort of loose "carcan" restraining movements of the scapular girdle while leaving the neck free. With the help of the head implant, the head could be fixed in its "zero" position. The cat, in the dark, faced a translucent tangent screen located 1 m away. Spots of light having a size of 0.5 degree were retroprojected upon this screen. The spots were generated, under computer control, by a high resolution XY analogue monitor (Tektronix 606A). A typical trial consisted of the presentation

of the spot somewhere within the central 40 degrees of the visual field for a duration of 3 s, followed by a sudden jump of the spot to another position where it remained on for another 3 s, and then disappeared. If the cat fixated the two successive spots within a given time and with the precision required, a small amount of food (beef baby food) was delivered through a tubing attached to the head, in the head fixed condition, or poured onto a small plate located slightly under the chin, at the midline, when the head was free. If not, the trial was aborted and no reward given. A "window" around the target, increasing with target eccentricity, allowed a certain error of fixation. A recording session consisted in 30 successive trials. This procedure had the advantage of keeping the animals fully alert and motivated and also helped to control gaze movements rather precisely.

Data analysis

Horizontal and vertical eye, head and target positions, as well as four pairs of muscle signals could be sampled and stored (on disk) simultaneously. These signals were later displayed for analysis on a colour monitor. With the help of cursors, different parameters could be measured and their values stored, manipulated and plotted.

Results

Modulation of neck EMG activity with eye position when the head is fixed

All the neck muscles recorded to date in head fixed condition show a striking modulation of their activity related to eye position. In the cat engaged in a visual task, the coupling of neck and eye is always observed. Fig. 1 shows an example of this phenomenon for four pairs of muscles. The first position of the target is 10 degrees down and left; it jumps to 10 degrees to the right, in the same horizontal plane. The eye makes a 15 degree horizontal saccade, undershooting the target by 5 degrees. Given the "window" around the target, the cat is however rewarded after a fixation of 3 s. Longissimus, obliquus and splenius muscles all show a shift of their tonic activity from the left side to the right. Biventers are almost completely silent: this is due to the fact that the eye remains around 15 degrees down. When the eye is directed upward, Biventers strongly discharge.

Each of these muscles discharge preferentially for certain positions of the eye in the orbit. This is illustrated by Fig. 2. The mean discharge corresponding to different eye positions is represented for the 6 left muscles (the right muscles behave symmetrically). It is clear that the biventer, for instance, only discharges for upward and leftward eye positions, whereas the obliquus is active for left and downward eye fixations. One may consider that each muscle has a preferential direction, in relation with eye eccentricity.

It appears that the change in the EMG (increase or decrease) occurs around the onset of saccade. Fig. 3 illustrates the latency of the discharge for 2 muscles, for various directions of the saccades, and shows that the latency is quite variable: the range spans from − 100 ms (early discharge) to 100 ms (late discharge). For a number of saccades, the modulation of EMG occurs during the movement, even in the preferential direction of the muscle. This is quite noticeable for the rectus. The splenius shows many ''early'' latencies, except for downward saccades, for which ''late'' discharges predominate.

We tried to determine if a relation between muscle discharge and saccade velocity existed. Comparing the maximal level of discharge during saccades and during the fixation that followed, we were unable to ascertain a ''phasic'' activity in relation with eye velocity. However, in some cases, a very small burst preceded the saccade by about 30 ms, but was immediately followed by a large increase of discharge. In Fig. 1, a transient increase of activity in the right longissimus and obliquus appears to be correlated with a small corrective saccade.

The mean level of activity of all the muscles, in the head fixed condition, was very high, compared to the activity observed in the more natural head free condition. Possible explanations for this will be discussed later.

At the end of a successful trial, as soon as the target was turned off, the cat received a food reward: the discharge in many muscles then progressively decreased to zero, as if the coupling between neck and eye, no longer necessary in absence of foveal vision of the target, was abandoned.

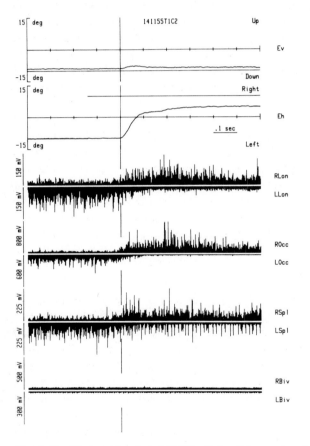

Fig. 1. Rectified and integrated EMG activity of four pairs of neck muscles (Lon, longissimus; Occ, obliquus capitis superior; Spl, splenius; Biv, biventer cervicis) recorded in head fixed trained cat, along with vertical (Ev) and horizontal (Eh) eye position. The occurrence and position of the two successive visual targets (10° left and down and 10° right and down) are indicated by horizontal lines. Vertical lines mark saccade onset.

Neck EMG activity when the head is free

Once the head was released, the configuration of neck muscle activity changed dramatically. The large tonic activity observed with head fixed was

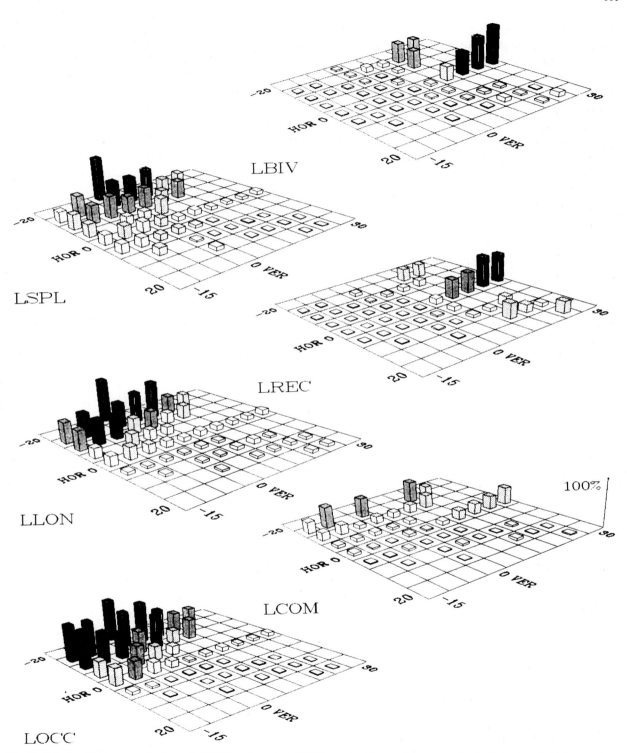

Fig. 2. Relationship between horizontal (HOR) and vertical (VER) eye position and mean maximal discharge of 6 left muscles measured during fixations lasting at least 250 ms. Muscle discharge is calibrated in percentage, as described in Methods. Negative eye positions correspond to left or down deviations.

356

absent and instead, phasic discharges correlated with shifts of gaze predominated. Fig. 4 illustrates two examples. In the right example, the gaze movement is horizontal and has an amplitude of 40 degrees. The head movement, however, though having a roughly horizontal direction, has a rather complex trajectory. The bursts in the right obliquus and splenius start about 30 to 50 ms before the head movement onset. They are terminated just before the head attains its maximal velocity. In this example, there is no antagonist or braking activity visible. The right splenius pulse is clearly biphasic.

In the left example, the gaze movement is horizontal, has an amplitude of 35 degrees and stops around the centre. It is made in the preferential direction of the right splenius. A clear biphasic activity can be observed on the pair of splenius muscles: a first agonist burst on the right side is followed by a burst on the left side. The agonist burst shows a tendency to split into two com-

ponents, but not as clearly as on the right example. This doubling of the burst is related to the amplitude and velocity of the head movement. In this example, note the presence of an antagonist "braking" pulse appearing in the left splenius, slightly before the end of the gaze shift and the maximal velocity of the head. The left complexus also shows a long latency burst, synchronized with the left splenius one. The right complexus does not seem to be involved in the control of this movement.

The intensity of the agonist burst depends on the direction, amplitude and initial position of the head. This is illustrated for three left muscles in Fig. 5. Head movements have been divided into two categories. Centrifugal movements originate from an area of 3 degrees around the zero position of the head and terminate at different eccentric locations. Centripetal movements start from various positions in the visual field and stop close to the centre (within a window of 2.5 degrees). All

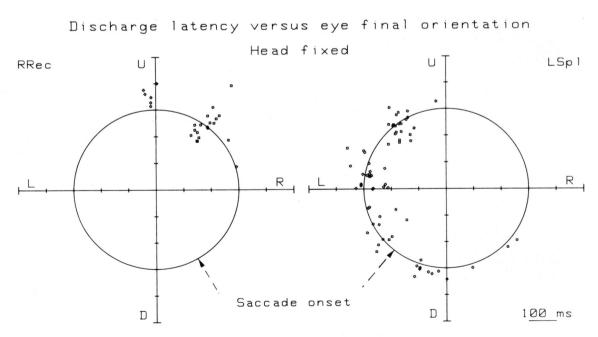

Fig. 3. Polar diagram illustrating the relation between the latency of the EMG discharge with respect to saccade onset and eye final orientation, for 2 muscles (right rectus and left splenius) in head fixed cat. The circle corresponds to saccade onset; symbols drawn inside the circle represent negative latencies. U, up; L, left; D, down; R, right.

357

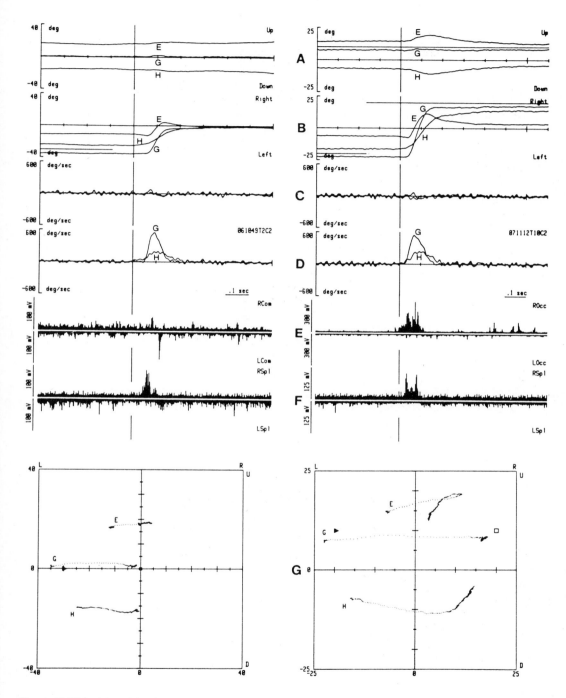

Fig. 4. EMG activity of 3 pairs of muscles (E and F: complexus, splenius and obliquus capitis) recorded in head free trained cat. A and B: vertical and horizontal eye (E), head (H) and gaze (G) position. C and D: vertical and horizontal head and gaze velocity. G: two-dimensional representation of eye, head and gaze position, during the movement. Dots correspond to positions 2 ms apart and their respective distance gives an idea of the velocity. The gaze movement on the left has an amplitude of 35°; gaze movement on the right has the same amplitude, but crosses the midline. Filled triangles show target first position and open squares, the second position.

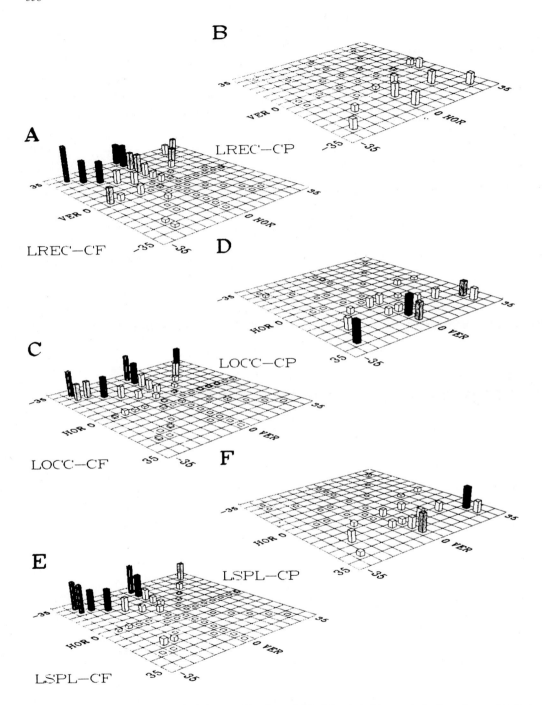

Fig. 5. Relationship between vertical (Ver) and horizontal (Hor) head position and phasic early agonist discharge of 3 left muscles (rectus capitis, obliquus capitis and splenius). In this case, EMG intensity is in arbitrary units. A, C and E correspond to centrifugal head movements, B, D and F to centripetal movements. Negative head positions correspond to left and down deviations. See comments in text.

these movements are visually guided. For centrifugal movements, the mean burst intensity has been plotted at the XY coordinates of the endpoint of the movement; whereas, for centripetal ones, the mean burst intensity has been plotted at the coordinates of the starting point. In centrifugal movements, a "preferential" direction clearly appears for the three muscles, corresponding quite well to the one observed in head fixed conditions. Moreover, the intensity of the discharge increases with the amplitude. Centripetal movements reveal the same preferential direction but also, as mean discharges are lower, illustrate the fact that, for a given direction and amplitude, the initial position influences muscle discharge: the more the muscle is stretched, the smaller the burst.

For a given muscle, not only does burst intensity depend on direction but also burst latency. This is illustrated in Fig. 6 for the right biventer and splenius. This figure shows the latency of the burst with respect to the onset of the head movement, as a function of various movement directions. For the right biventer, the latency of the burst is negative or null in the preferential direction of the muscle; it is largely positive (up to 300 ms after movement onset) for movements directed downward. The phenomenon is similar, though less marked, for the right splenius. The observed late bursts often occur around the time of maximum head velocity, slightly before (about 20 ms) the end of the eye saccade and probably reflect an active braking of the head. These bursts may also occur during the first phase of the head movement, especially when the direction is intermediate (between "on" and "off" directions): the muscle then probably plays a role of support or of control of trajectory.

Tonic or sustained activity, in head free condition, can be observed in certain muscles such as

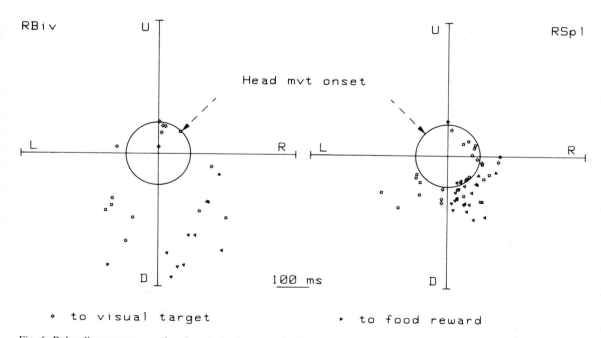

Fig. 6. Polar diagram representing the relation between the latency of the phasic discharge, with respect to head movement onset, and head movement direction, for two right muscles (biventer and splenius), in head free cats. Symbols inside the circle represent negative latencies.

biventer, rectus and complexus. This type of activity is especially visible when the head is eccentric to the preferential direction of the muscle. Phasic inhibitions may then be observed. Fig. 4, left, shows the left complexus: before (30 ms) and during the head movement, directed to the right, the sustained activity of the muscle is suppressed until the end of the saccade; then, a large and short pulse appears, just before the final deceleration of the head movement, followed again by a tonic discharge.

Discussion

Methodological aspects

The experimental paradigm used in these observations entails several distortions or errors in the measurement of some variables. They must be borne in mind for a correct interpretation of the results.

A first distortion concerns head movements: the coil method does not permit the detection of translations nor roll about the head antero-posterior axis. Observation reveals that these components are relatively minor in gaze orienting behaviour; they are more important in the feeding behaviour that occurs after each successful trial, which has not been considered here.

A second problem is related to possible and uncontrolled changes of posture of the cat within his box. During sessions, the cat is usually very quiet and attentive to the visual surround; moreover, the size of the restraining box is such that very little movement is permitted.

The trajectories of head movements are often rather complex and their speed varies: this is due to the fact that cats have been trained to orient their gaze towards visual targets, not to execute precise head movements. This paradigm, however is close to natural conditions and the aim of these experiments was the study of orienting and eye-head coordination mechanisms.

A large number of neck muscles participate in the orientation of the head: we only recorded six pairs of them, however. Moreover, due to technical constraints, only four pairs could be recorded

simultaneously, together with eye, head and target position. The interpretation of certain patterns of activity is thus sometimes difficult.

One last technical problem concerns the location of recording electrodes in the muscles: only one small part of the muscles is monitored and pairs of muscles may not be exactly symmetrically implanted. It has been shown, however (Wilson et al., 1983), that all compartments of splenius behave similarly in alert fixed head cats during different types of oculomotor activity. Moreover, an effort was made to calibrate the EMG (see Methods), in order to compare different muscles and different conditions.

Head fixed – head free comparison

When the head is fixed, neck muscle activity is characterized by a high and tonic level of discharge, proportional to eye position. The pattern of activity is coherent with the muscle function that may be derived from its anatomy. Variations of discharge rates very often precede saccades: this suggests mechanisms other than pure extraocular proprioception. The tonic level, especially during long fixations, may fluctuate significantly.

When the head is free, the tonic activity is difficult to assess. The head is almost never at rest and some phasic discharges are always present. In addition, the tonic level is low and is only present in those muscles that contain a fairly large percentage of slow fibres, acting against gravity, such as the biventer, complexus and rectus; these muscles are inhibited when the head moves downward. The phasic activity, related to head movement, is important and present in all the muscles. A preferential direction may be determined, which corresponds to that observed with head fixed. The temporal sequencing of this phasic activity is quite complex and depends on the different parameters of the trajectory, particularly on the direction.

It is surprising that, when the head is fixed, no phasic component can be observed and that the level of discharge is so high. This level is about as high as the maximum phasic discharge observed with head free. A possible explanation could be that, due to a neck-neck proprioceptive feedback loop, an initial phasic burst would immediately be followed by a rapidly rising activity, which would mask it. The fluctuations of the tonic level might be caused by variations of the gain in this loop, variations that also lead to a temporary decoupling of eye and head, as observed in head orientations towards food or in other tasks not requiring foveal vision.

Comparison between eye and head motor signals

Eye and head motor plants probably share some common control signals. Grantyn and Berthoz (1987) showed that the activity of reticulo-spinal neurones during a saccade, when the head is fixed, consists of a burst followed by a progressively decaying sustained discharge. The most striking difference between eye and neck motor signals is the absence, in most muscles, of a clear tonic activity related to head position, in the head free condition. Only anti-gravity, slow fibre muscles seem to receive this tonic component. It may be hypothesized that this component would not be necessary in the muscles mainly implicated in rotation, for biomechanical reasons: the inertia of the head is large and, at least for not too eccentric positions, the passive elastic components do not play a major role.

Comparison between head and limb motor signals

Neck EMG, in head orienting movements, shares many characteristics with limb muscle activity.

(A) The neck muscle agonist initial burst intensity is related to the amplitude of the movement: the larger the amplitude, the longer the burst. A long burst is made up of 2 or 3 successive components, as described by Brown and Cooke (1984) for visually guided arm movements. Initial position, however, does seem to influence neck and arm EMG differently. In Brown and Cooke's work (1986), the magnitude of the initial agonist burst associated with flexion movements increased as starting position became more extended. We observed that a neck muscle discharges more when the head is initially turned in the preferential direction of that muscle.

(B) The agonist burst, in the neck, in the case of fast head movements requiring a final precision, or directed along the gravity vector, is followed by a burst in the antagonist. It occurs just before the maximal velocity of the head and the end of the gaze movement. This was observed in the case of small amplitude, or centripetal, or downward gaze shifts, as well as for head movements aimed at food. In these cases, the passive visco-elastic forces and probably insufficient to help stop the movement and an active braking is needed. In some cases, the pattern is triphasic, as also demonstrated by Hannaford et al. (1984). This characteristic has been repeatedly shown for limbs (Hallett et al., 1975, Lestienne, 1979; Wadman et al., 1979; Marsden et al., 1983).

(C) The neck is driven by many muscles; when the direction of the movement progressively changes, the timing of the burst in a given muscle also changes: from a pure agonist role, this muscle becomes a "supporter" of the movement and finally an antagonist. A similar phenomenon has been shown for the shoulder, also an articulation moved by many muscles (Wadman et al., 1980).

(D) When the head movements are slow, neck muscles involved discharge in small, repeated bursts, alternating in agonist and antagonist muscles. This is also a characteristic of slow limb movement control (Hallett et al., 1975).

Conclusion

The EMG activity of neck muscles, in gaze orientation, reflects a highly specialized behaviour in which an excellent coordination between eye and head is required. Not only do the biomechanical constraints of the head motor apparatus determine their activity patterns but also their particular function: the control of gaze. In this respect, the neck muscle behaviour in gaze orientation constitutes an interesting example of multi-segmental control and coordination.

362

Acknowledgements

We wish to thank Drs A. Al-Ansari and J. Crémieux for their help in training animals and analysing part of the results.

References

Bizzi, E., Kalil, R.E., Morasso, P. and Tagliasco, V. (1972) Central programming and peripheral feedback during eye-head coordination in monkey. *Bibl. Ophthal.*, 82: 220 – 232.

Bizzi, E., Polit, A. and Morasso, P. (1976) Mechanisms underlying achievement of final head position. *J. Neurophysiol.*, 39: 435 – 444.

Brown, S.H. and Cooke, J.D. (1984) Initial agonist burst duration depends on movement amplitude. *Exp. Brain Res.*, 55: 523 – 527.

Brown, S.H. and Cooke, J.D. (1986) Movement-related EMG activity compensates for position-dependant changes in limb properties. *J. Hum. Movem. Studies*, 12: 297 – 3123.

Crommelinck, M., Roucoux, A. and Veraart, C. (1982) The relation of neck muscles activity to horizontal eye position in the alert cat. II: Head free. In A. Roucoux and M. Crommelinck (Eds.), *Physiological and Pathological Aspects of Eye Movements*, Dr W. Junk Publishers, The Hague, pp. 379 – 384.

Grantyn, A. and Berthoz, A. (1987) Reticulo-spinal neurons participating in the control of synergic eye and head movements during orienting in the cat. I. Behavioral properties. *Exp. Brain Res.*, 66: 339 – 354.

Hallett, M., Shahani, B.T. and Young, R.R. (1975) EMG analysis of stereotyped voluntary movements in man. *J. Neurol. Neurosurg. Psychiatry*, 38: 1154 – 1162.

Hannaford, B., Lakshminarayanan, V., Stark, L. and Nam, M.H. (1984) Electromyographic evidence of neurological controller signals with viscous load. *J. Motor Behav.*, 16: 255 – 274.

Lestienne, F. (1979) Effects of inertial load and velocity on the braking process of voluntary limb movements. *Exp. Brain Res.*, 35: 407 – 418.

Lestienne, F., Vidal, P.P. and Berthoz, A. (1984) Gaze changing behaviour in head restrained monkey. *Exp. Brain Res.*, 53: 349 – 356.

Loeb, G.E. and Richmond, F.J.R. (1986) Synchronization of motor units in and among diverse neck muscles during slow movements in intact cats. *Soc. Neurosci. Abstr., Vol. 12, Part 1*, p. 687.

Marsden, C.D., Obeso, J.A. and Rothwell, J.C. (1983) The function of the antagonist muscle during fast limb movements in man. *J. Physiol. (London)*, 335: 1 – 13.

Richmond, F.J.R., Loeb, G.E. and Reesor, D. (1985) Electromyographic activity in neck muscles during head movement in the alert, unrestrained cat. *Soc. Neurosci. Abstr., Vol. 11, Part 1*, p. 83.

Roucoux, A. and Crommelinck, M. (1988) Control of head movement during visual orientation. In B.W. Peterson and F.J. Richmond (Eds.), *Control of Head Movement*, Oxford University Press, New York, pp. 208 – 223.

Roucoux, A., Crommelinck, M., Decostre, M.F. Cremieux, J. and Al-Ansari, A. (1985) Gaze shift related neck muscle activity in trained cats. *Soc. Neurosci. Abstr., Vol. 11, Part 1*, p. 83.

Roucoux, A., Crommelinck, M. and Guitton, D. (1981) The role of Superior Colliculus in the generation of gaze shifts. In A.F. Fuchs and W. Becker (Eds.), *Progress in Oculomotor Research*, Elsevier North Holland, Amsterdam, pp. 129 – 135.

Roucoux, A., Vidal, P.P., Veraart, C., Crommelinck, M. and Berthoz, A. (1982) The relation of neck muscles activity to horizontal eye position in the alert cat. I: Head fixed. In A. Roucoux and M. Crommelinck (Eds.), *Physiological and Pathological Aspects of Eye Movements*, Dr W. Junk Publishers, The Hague, pp. 371 – 378.

Vidal, P.P., Roucoux, A. and Berthoz, A. (1982) Horizontal eye position-related activity in neck muscles of the alert cat. *Exp. Brain Res.*, 46: 448 – 453.

Wadman, W.J., Denier van der Gon, J.J., Geuze, R.H. and Mol, C.R. (1979) Control of fast goal-directed arm movements. *J. Hum. Movem. Studies*, 5: 3 – 17.

Wadman, W.J., Denier van der Gon, J.J. and Derksen, R.J.A. (1980) Muscle activation patterns for fast goal-direction arm movements. *J. Hum. Movem. Studies*, 6: 19 – 37.

Wilson, V.J., Precht, W. and Dieringer, N. (1983) Responses of different compartments of cat's splenius muscle to optokinetic stimulation. *Exp. Brain Res.*, 50: 153 – 156.

J.H.J. Allum and M. Hulliger (Eds.)
Progress in Brain Research, Vol. 80
© 1989 Elsevier Science Publishers B.V. (Biomedical Division)

CHAPTER 29

Comparison of neck muscle activation patterns during head stabilization and voluntary movements

B.W. Peterson, E.A. Keshner and J. Banovetz

Department of Physiology, Northwestern University Medical School, Chicago, IL 60611, U.S.A.

The motor system that controls the neck musculature serves two major functions: stabilization of the head in the face of external perturbations or body movements, and generation of voluntary or orientating head movements. Typically the latter are thought to be mediated by complex pathways involving cerebral cortex and superior colliculus while stabilization is thought to be mediated by simple short-loop pathways that generate vestibulocollic and cervicocollic reflexes (VCR and CCR). Our work has been directed towards evaluating the extent to which the VCR and CCR are in fact responsible for head stabilization, and to determining how the motor patterns produced by these reflexes compare with those produced by the voluntary head movement system. To address these questions we have analysed the dynamic and spatial (kinematic) properties of the head movement system in cats and humans.

Key words: Vestibulocollic reflex; Cervicocollic reflex; Voluntary movement; Neck muscle; Head stabilization; Activation pattern; Dynamics; Kinematics; Tensorial model; Electromyography

Dynamics of head stabilization

Initial studies of head stabilization focused on responses of the head – neck system to rotations in the earth-horizontal plane. Rotating the body together with the head generates an open-loop vestibulocollic reflex (VCR), which can be studied by recording neck muscle electromyographic (EMG) activity or horizontal head torque. In the decerebrate cat, the EMG shows a characteristic dynamic behaviour in which output lags the angular acceleration sensed by the horizontal semicircular canals (HSCCs) by nearly 180° at 0.1 – 0.2 Hz and then advances until it lags by only ~ 40° at 4 Hz (Berthoz and Anderson, 1971; Ezure and Sasaki, 1978; Bilotto et al., 1981). This place and gain behaviour indicates that VCR output is related to head angular position at lower frequencies, and to head angular acceleration at higher frequencies. Head torque exhibits less phase advance and gain increase with frequency, indicating that part of the high frequency phase advance serves to compensate for the low pass properties of the neck muscles (Goldberg and Peterson, 1986). The rest of the high frequency phase advance presumably helps the system compensate for the inertial load presented by the massive head.

If the high frequency dynamic properties of the VCR were indeed intended to compensate for biomechanical properties of the head – neck system, we would expect to observe similar dynamics in the cervicocollic reflex (CCR). In their study of the CCR elicited in decerebrate cats by rotating the body about an earth-fixed head, Peterson et al. (1985) showed that this is the case. In fact, the time constants of the lead terms modelling the transition from low frequency position-like to high frequency acceleration-like behaviour were highly correlated in individual cats, suggesting that the dynamics were adaptively matched to the physical properties of each animal. Furthermore, EMG outputs produced by the VCR and CCR were shown to sum linearly when the reflexes were evoked together by rotating the head on the trunk or by allowing the animal to move its head to compensate for rotation of the body. In the former case the reflexes added to oppose head rotation but in the latter (closed-loop VCR) case, the CCR acted to oppose the compensatory head rotations generated by the VCR.

Whereas our EMG studies of the VCR and CCR in decerebrate cats suggested that both reflexes play an important role in head stabilization, Bizzi et al. (1978) reported that the CCR was negligible in the alert, labyrinthectomized monkey and stressed that passive biomechanical properties of the head and neck might play the dominant role in head stabilization in this species. Goldberg and Peterson (1986) examined this possibility in the alert cat by recording both neck EMG and head movements when the animal's body was rotated with the head either fixed to the rotating platform (open-loop VCR), fixed in space (open-loop CCR) or allowed to counter-rotate (closed-loop VCR). Rotations consisting of a pseudo-random sum of 10 sinusoids were applied in total darkness to prevent animals from using visual cues or predictive movements to stabilize their heads. Data in Fig. 1A were obtained when weights had been added to the head to increase its inertia thereby enhancing the biomechanical contribution to head stability. This

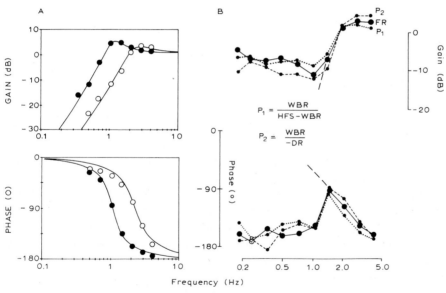

Fig. 1. Head movements elicited by pseudorandom horizontal rotations in the cat. A: head movements observed in a deeply anaesthetized cat where only passive biomechanical mechanisms were involved. Filled circles are data collected with weights added to increase head inertia. Open symbols are data without weights. A perfectly compensatory head-on-body rotation would have a gain of 0 dB and a phase of −180°. This occurs at high frequencies where inertia causes head to stand still in space. At low frequencies neck muscle viscoelasticity causes head to move with body so that gain of head-on-body rotation has a low gain and phase close to 0°. Between two extremes, head goes through a resonance point where gain peaks and phase is −90°. B: head movements with head weighted and cat alert. Resonant peak and high frequency compensatory response can still be observed although frequencies are shifted upwards due to greater stiffness of muscles in alert cat. At lower frequencies, rather than continuing along dashed lines that indicate the estimated passive mechanical response, head movements have compensatory −180° phase and gain of 0.5 (−6 dB). (Modified from Goldberg and Peterson, 1986.)

contribution appears as gain that rises sharply from 1 Hz to a peak at 2 Hz while phase jumps from $-180°$ to $-90°$ and then returns to $-180°$, which corresponds to the desired compensatory direction. Without added weights the behaviour was similar except that the cross-over frequency at which head stabilization became dominated by mechanical factors shifted to > 3 Hz. Below the cross-over frequency the biomechanical response would fall off steeply as shown by the dashed line in Fig. 1B. However, stabilizing head movements had a constant gain of ~ 0.5 from $0.1 - 2$ Hz. The driving force for these movements must therefore be of neural origin. Insight into the possible origins of this low frequency stabilizing behaviour can be obtained by examining the overall transfer function of the closed-loop VCR. As described by Goldberg and Peterson (1986), this transfer function can be expressed in Laplace form as:

$$N/\Theta = -[Is^2 + VCR(s)]/Is^2 + Bs + K + VCR(s) + CCR(s)$$

where N is the compensatory neck rotation, Θ is the platform rotation, I is head inertia, B and K are the neck muscle viscosity and elasticity, s is the Laplace operator and $VCR(s)$ and $CCR(s)$ represent the torques produced by these reflexes. The two driving terms in this transfer function are the torques produced by the VCR and by head inertia (Is^2). The s^2 in the latter term indicates that inertial force will vary as the square of frequency. For lower frequencies where Is^2 is $<<$ $VCR(s)$, the transfer function reduces to:

$$N/\Theta = -VCR(s)/VCR(s) + Bs + K + CCR(s).$$

Then if $VCR(s) \approx CCR(s) + Bs + K,$
$N/\Theta \approx -1/2.$

Thus the necessary and sufficient condition for low frequency stabilization with a gain of 0.5 is that torques produced by the CCR and neck viscoelasticity must match those produced by the VCR. While Goldberg and Peterson (1986) sug-

gested that the former might be produced primarily by the CCR, our more recent studies (Banovetz et al., 1987) have revealed that the CCR is often suppressed in alert cats. Although this question needs to be examined further, data at present suggest that head stabilization at frequencies < 1.0 Hz in the cat is dominated by the VCR and neck viscoelasticity.

An alternative possibility arises from recent observations of human head stabilization during pseudorandom horizontal body rotations (Guitton et al., 1987). These revealed that head stabilization was only present when subjects were instructed to keep their head aligned with a fixed point. When subjects were distracted with mental arithmetic, they made no compensatory movements. Futhermore, as illustrated in Fig. 2, time-domain analysis indicated that the latency of the effective head

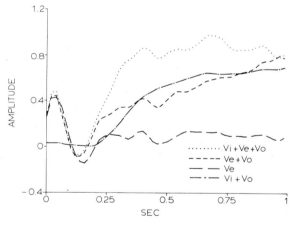

Fig. 2. Time domain analysis of head stabilization in humans. Subjects were exposed to pseudorandom chair rotations under 3 conditions: instructed to hold their heads aligned with a visible stationary target (Vi + Ve + Vo), instructed to hold their heads aligned with target while blindfolded (Ve + Vo) and performing mental arithmetic (Ve). In a fourth test they followed a pseudorandom moving visual target (Vi + Vo). Data were analysed to estimate the head's response to a rotation step. In Ve condition, no net compensatory movement was produced and after an initial transient the step was ≈ 0. Excellent and good compensation were observed in Vi + Ve + Vo and Ve + Vo where the step responses depart from that for Ve at 150 ms, the estimated latency of the compensatory response. For visual tracking, the step response has a latency of 250 ms. (From Schor et al., 1988.)

stabilizing movements was on the order of 150 ms, which is much longer than the latency expected for the relatively direct VCR pathway. It thus appears that humans use reaction-time movements that are under voluntary control to stabilize their heads. More recently we have found signs of involuntary reflex head stabilization when subjects performing mental arithmetic are rotated at frequencies above the 1 Hz cutoff of the Guitton et al. (1987) study (Keshner and Peterson, 1988a). These only appear at frequencies close to the resonant point (~ 2 Hz in humans) where head mechanics are beginning to play a significant role as well. They therefore do not relate to the lower frequency behaviour observed in the cat. Until we have latency measurements or better behavioural control in the cat, we cannot be sure whether cats also employ longer latency reaction time processes in this frequency range, or whether humans and cats employ different head stabilizing strategies.

Spatial properties of the VCR and CCR

Another method of determining the relative influence of the head stabilizing mechanisms is to measure their spatial parameters. In order to produce compensatory head movements, the VCR and CCR must precisely coordinate activation of 30 neck muscles inserting on the head (Baker and Wickland, 1988). Net torque resulting from their combined actions must produce the desired direction of head movement in 3-dimensional space. Since the head can move in, at most, 6 degrees of freedom (3 angular, 3 linear), the number of available muscles far exceeds the number of degrees of freedom of the object that they control. As a result, many different patterns of muscle activation could be used to make any particular head movement. We can then ask whether the neck is controlled in different ways by different systems (eg VCR, CCR, voluntary movement system) or even in different ways by the same system in different animals.

Spatial properties of the VCR and CCR have been studied in both decerebrate and alert cats

(Baker et al., 1985; Banovetz et al., 1987). To determine the spatial properties of these reflexes, neck muscle EMGs were recorded while cats were rotated at 0.25 Hz and ± 36° about 22 axes passing through the C1 – C2 and C1 – skull joints. These axes are in one of three planes: sagittal, frontal, or horizontal. Although the head – neck system involves 8 joints (from C7 – T1 to C1 – skull), fluoroscopic analysis of a variety of human and animal subjects suggests that the majority of movement occurs at the two ends of the cervical spine (Vidal et al., 1986). To study the neck reflexes, we concentrated on head-on-neck movements about the two aforementioned joints: C1 – C2 primarily allows yaw movements, and C1 – skull pitch and roll movements, so that there are essentially 3 rotational degrees of freedom of the head about the upper cervical spinal column. For the VCR task the whole body was rotated; in the CCR task the body was rotated while the head was held fixed in space.

Spatial properties of the muscle EMG responses are represented by maximal activation directions, or MADs. These are normalized vectors in 3-dimensional space showing the axes and directions of rotation which produce maximal activation of the muscles. These MADs are determined from the experiment above by plotting the gain of the response against the axis of rotation for axes in the same plane in each of three series of rotations. A sine wave is then fit to the points, and the values at 0° and 90° give two components of the MAD vector (e.g., the first series yields pitch and yaw, the second yields pitch and roll, and the third, yaw and roll). An example of one such fit is shown in Fig. 3. Rotations in three planes thus give two estimates of each of the three components necessary to characterize the MAD in space. Directional comparisons of vectors from an individual muscle in different animals or paradigms reveals the degree of variability of VCR or CCR kinematics. In decerebrate cats, the VCR and CCR produce well defined, and essentially identical spatial patterns of muscle activity in all animals. Fig. 3 shows the gains of a decerebrate cat's VCR

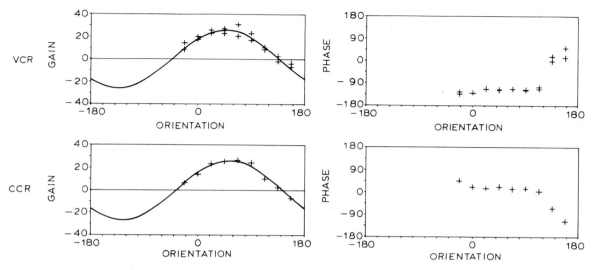

Fig. 3. Response of the biventer cervicis muscle to vestibulo-collic reflex (VCR) and cervico-collic reflex (CCR) stimulation. Rotations were at 0.24 Hz and ± 36° about axes in the horizontal (yaw-pitch) plane, such that 0° corresponds to yaw and 90° to pitch rotations. The sine curve is a least squares fit to the data, with negative values being assigned to points with a phase that differed by more than 180° from the phase at 0°. The spatial characteristics of the two reflexes, i.e. the pattern of gain variation with orientation, is quite similar for the two reflexes.

and CCR obtained from rotations about nine axes in the horizontal plane. The similarity of the fitted curves indicates the close spatial agreement between the reflexes. While the CCR is too variable to study in alert cats, the VCR is reliable and exhibits a spatial pattern indistinguishable from that in the decerebrate cat (Banovetz et al., 1987).

What principles govern the choice by the VCR and CCR systems of a single motor pattern from among the many that could be employed to produce the required compensatory head movements? The most parsimonious explanation is that each muscle would be activated most strongly in the direction of its best mechanical advantage. However, it can be readily shown that such a choice of muscle activation directions will not work when the muscle pulling directions are non-orthogonal (Pellionisz and Peterson, 1988). Furthermore, the pulling directions, which have been determined from the origins and insertions of the various muscles, their cross-sectional area, and their distance from and angle to the rotation axes (Baker and Wickland, 1988), do not align with the

neck muscle MADs observed during the VCR and CCR. Therefore this hypothesis must be rejected.

A more likely possibility, from a control standpoint, is that the selected motor patterns are chosen on the basis of some minimization criteria. Dul and colleagues (1984) have reviewed a number of suggested criteria, such as minimization of muscle forces, stress, or energy consumption. Pellionisz and Peterson (1988) have proposed a tensorial model that minimizes the sum of squares of neck muscle activation. Their model is attractive because it specifically predicts the spatial properties of the muscles, and involves a series of calculations of how the sensory afferent signals could conceivably be converted into motor commands by reflex control systems. Neural correlates for these mathematical processes have yet to be demonstrated, but the concept that in the typical sensorimotor system, where sensors and effectors are not arranged in an orthogonal Cartesian coordinate system, a transformation from a covariant sensory input to a contravariant motor command must occur is fundamental. Comparison of MAD vectors shown

368

in Fig. 4 for the VCR with those predicted by the tensorial model indicates that the spatial predictions of this model are quite good. A further review of the concepts of tensorial modelling can be found in Pellionisz and Llinas (1979, 1980).

Do kinematics of reflex and voluntary head movements differ?

To see whether the spatial patterns predicted by the tensorial model are also utilized by the voluntary movement system, we compared patterns of neck muscle activation by the VCR in alert cats with patterns used when the same animals made voluntary movements in the same 24 planes in space (Keshner et al., 1986). The animals were trained to

follow a water spout as it rotated sinusoidally (0.25 Hz), and neck muscle EMG responses were recorded. Results indicate that movements generated in a particular direction by the voluntary motor system use different muscle patterns than the same movements generated by the VCR or CCR. Correspondingly, the maximal responses of individual muscles occur at different orientations for the two tasks. VCR responses demonstrate the phase advance expected in a response related to stimulus velocity, whereas the phase of the response during tracking is related to the position of the head as it tracks the water spout.

Since muscle activity during the VCR serves to compensate for or oppose head movement, whereas activity during voluntary motion assists the movement of the head, we would expect the response vectors for matched head movements to occur in equal and opposite directions. This hypothesis is supported by the response vectors of the biventer cervicis muscle (see Fig. 4). Not all of the muscles behave in this fashion, however. For some of the muscles, reflex and voluntary activity occurs as a more orthogonal relationship (e.g., complexus). Thus, although the tensorial model reliably predicts reflex patterns in the alert cats, it does not accurately predict voluntary patterns of activation (Keshner and Peterson, 1988b). One explanation for the lack of fit by the model is the increased complexity of sensory inputs during the tracking movements. Unlike the VCR which occurs purely as a result of canal inputs, the tracking responses can be organized by retinal somatosensory, vestibular and descending inputs.

While response patterns for each muscle during voluntary head movement are quite consistent for an individual cat over several months of testing, they differ much more from animal to animal than the reflex muscle patterns. For example, one cat uses the splenius muscle to produce roll and occipitoscapularis for yaw during voluntary tracking, while in another cat the preferred directions of these two muscles are reversed. This reversal was never observed in the reflex-activated EMG responses. These observations suggest that kine-

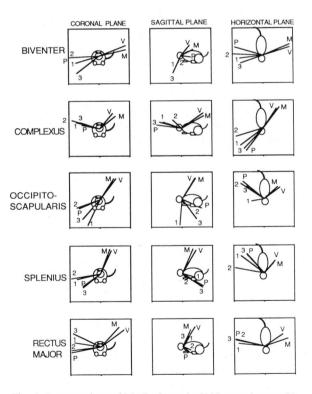

Fig. 4. A comparison of MADs from the VCR experiments (V), tracking experiments (1, 2, 3), pulling directions (P), and model predictions of VCR response (M) for five muscles. The 1, 2, and 3 refer to the three different cats in the tracking study; they were not averaged due to the variable nature of their responses.

matics of voluntary head movements may depend more upon learned motor strategies than do those of the head stabilizing reflexes (Keshner and Peterson, 1988b).

Kinematics of voluntary head stabilization in humans

Results from our experiments with cats suggest that the CNS programmes the neck muscles in a particular animal to respond in a unique fashion for each task, but that the direction of motion associated with maximal muscle activation may vary between animals. To see whether such variation between individuals occurs in humans, we have used surface electrodes to record the activity of four right sided neck muscles, including semispinalis capitis (SEMI), splenius capitis (SPL), trapezius (TRAP), and sternocleidomastoid (SCM) as subjects resisted forces applied to their heads (Keshner et al., 1988). Surface electrode placements were verified with bipolar intramuscular electrode recordings. Subjects were seated and received visual feedback of head position at all times. They were instructed to counteract a moderate horizontal force applied to the head at 22° intervals via a weight and pulley system attached to a specially adapted helmet. At 0°, the force was applied in a direction requiring neck extension to stabilize the head. A force at 90° required rightward lateral rotation (or rightward roll) of the head, and −90° required left roll. Placing the pulley directly behind the subject resulted in pure forward flexion of the head (180°). Average amplitudes of the EMG response for each muscle were calculated for each direction of applied force.

The mean percentage of maximum activation across all of the subjects ± one S.D. is plotted on a polar plot to determine the spatial activation for that muscle. Each muscle presents a restricted range of excitation with a consistent direction of maximal activation. Null responses of each muscle in directions opposite to the maximum indicate that muscles are reciprocally activated during this task (see Fig. 5 for an example of responses in one

subject). As predicted in standard anatomy and kinesiology textbooks (Lockhart et al., 1972), SEMI is maximally activated in pitch extension with some lateral rotation (0° to 45°), and SCM in flexion with lateral rotation (90° to 180°). SPL, however, has always been described as exhibiting a lateral rotation and extension action. Yet half of our subjects produce a strong rightward roll response with flexion (135°) rather than extension (45°). TRAP presents a somewhat confusing picture, probably due to the low levels of activation of this muscle in all of the tested directions (see Fig. 5). Upper TRAP fibres responded primarily in leftward roll with extension (−45°), suggesting that TRAP was actually performing scapular depression in order to stabilize the scapular during head movements. Intramuscular recordings confirmed that this muscle was much more strongly activated during isolated shoulder elevation than during head movements. It appears that each subject does

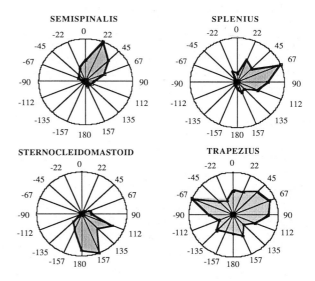

Fig. 5. Responses of four muscles in a human subject to forces applied to the head in 16 horizontal directions. EMG activation is normalized relative to maximum response and plotted against direction of force application (0° = head extension; 180° = head flexion; 90° = right roll; −90° = left roll). Except for trapezius, which is related primarily to shoulder movement, all muscles demonstrate a clear maximum activation direction in this isometric stabilization task.

use a consistent muscle activation pattern when opposing applied forces, but different subjects can use the same muscle in a different fashion.

In three subjects, we tested the robustness of the relationship between direction and activation level by gradually increasing the amount of force applied to the head. A linear relationship between increased force and the EMG response was observed only in the preferred directions of activation for each muscle. In non-preferred directions, each subject produced either a non-linear increase or decrease in EMG activation suggesting a shift from the centrally programmed reciprocal activation. Inter-subject variability is expected in this task since the voluntary response is complexly organized to respond to multiple sensory inputs. The division in splenius maximal activation directions, and variable shifts in the level of muscle activation with increases in force suggest, however, that differences between voluntary movement patterns and reflex responses are not solely the result of the available afferent information. Central motor programmes elicited by voluntary motor generators must also depend upon the biomechanical constraints of each subject's head-neck motor system, the mechanical constraints of the task, and the motor learning history of that individual.

Conclusions

The work described above provides preliminary indications of the roles of the VCR, CCR and voluntary systems in head stabilization and of the dynamic and spatial (kinematic) properties of the three systems. In the cat the VCR is reliably present and appears to play a key role in stabilizing the head at frequencies below about 3 Hz. In humans it is seen only at frequencies above 1 Hz where reflex and mechanical forces interact in controlling the head. Below this frequency head stabilization is produced by reaction time movements. This contrast would appear to be a species difference between cats, who rely on rapid reflex control and humans, who tend to favour predictive, voluntary control.

Properties of the cat's VCR have been well characterized. It exhibits second-order lead dynamics and activates the neck muscles in a kinematic pattern that can be predicted by least squares minimization (the Moore-Penrose generalized inverse) that is incorporated in the tensorial model developed by Pellionisz and Peterson (1988). This inverse is a logical choice both because it minimizes unnecessary muscle co-contractions and because it can be readily developed and implemented in a neuronal network. While it is usually active in the decerebrate cat, the CCR may frequently be suppressed by voluntary control in alert cats. Data of Bizzi et al. (1978) suggest that it is also suppressed in alert primates. In decerebrate cats it has dynamics and kinematics identical to those of the VCR. Since the VCR and CCR sum linearly, their common properties greatly simplify the control problem of the head stabilization system.

Voluntary head movements are mediated by a system that uses spatial patterns of muscle activation that vary from individual to individual and do not correspond to those predicted by tensorial models based on the Moore-Penrose generalized inverse. Their variability suggests that these voluntary movements are learned responses whose properties reflect the motor learning history of each individual.

References

Baker, J., Goldberg, J. and Peterson, B. (1985) Spatial and temporal response properties of the vestibulocollic reflex in decerebrate cats. *J. Neurophysiol.,* 54: 735–756.

Baker, J. and Wickland, C. (1988) Kinematic properties of the vestibulocollic reflex. In B.W. Peterson and F.J.R. Richmond (Eds.), *Control of Head Movement,* Oxford Univ. Press, New York, pp. 167–177.

Banovetz, J.M., Rude, S.A., Perlmutter, S.I., Peterson, B.W. and Baker, J.F. (1987) A comparison of neck reflexes in alert and decerebrate cats. *Soc. Neurosci. Abstr.,* 13: 1312.

Berthoz, A. and Anderson, J.H. (1971) Frequency analysis of vestibular influence on extensor motoneurons. II. Relationship between neck and forelimb extensors. *Brain Res.,* 34: 376–380.

Bilotto, G., Goldberg, J., Peterson, B.W. and Wilson, V.J. (1982) Dynamic properties of vestibular reflexes in the decerebrate cat. *Exp. Brain Res.,* 47: 343 – 352.

Bizzi, E., Dev, P., Morasso, P. and Polit, A. (1978) Effect of load disturbances during centrally initiated movements. *J. Neurophysiol.,* 41: 542 – 556.

Dul, J., Townsend, M., Shiavi, R. and Johnson, G. (1984) Muscle synergism. I. On the criteria for load sharing between synergistic muscles. *J. Biomech.,* 17: 663 – 673.

Ezure, K. and Sasaki, S. (1978) Frequency-response analysis of vestibular-induced neck reflex in cat. I. Characteristics of neural transmission from horizontal semicircular canal to neck motoneurons. *J. Neurophysiol.,* 41: 445 – 458.

Goldberg, J. and Peterson, B.W. (1986) Reflex and mechanical contributions to head stabilization in alert cats. *J. Neurophysiol.,* 56: 857 – 875.

Guitton, D., Kearney, R.E., Wereley, N. and Peterson, B.W. (1989) Visual, vestibular and voluntary contributions to human head stabilization. *Exp. Brain Res.,* 64: 59 – 69.

Keshner, E.A., Baker, J., Banovetz, J., Peterson, B.W., Wickland, C., Robinson, F.R. and Tomko, D.L. (1986) Neck muscles demonstrate preferential activation during voluntary and reflex head movements in the cat. *Soc. Neurosci. Abstr.,* 12: 684.

Keshner, E.A., Campbell, D., Katz, R. and Peterson, B.W. (1989) Neck muscle activation patterns in humans during isometric head stabilization. *Exp. Brain Res.,* 75: 335 – 344.

Keshner, E.A. and Peterson, B.W. (1988a) Mechanisms of human head stabilization during random sinusoidal rotations. *Soc. Neurosci. Abstr.,* 14: 1235.

Keshner, E.A. and Peterson, B.W. (1988b) Motor control strategies underlying head stabilization and voluntary head movements in humans and cats. In: O. Pompeiano and J.H.J. Allum (Eds.), *Vestibulospinal Control of Posture and Movement, Prog. Brain Res., Vol. 76,* Elsevier, North Holland, pp. 329 – 339.

Lockhart R.D., Hamilton G.F. and Fyfe F.W. (1972) *Anatomy of the Human Body,* J.B. Lippincott Co., Philadelphia, pp. 153 – 172.

Pellionisz, A.J. and Llinas, R. (1980) Tensorial approach to the geometry of brain frunction. Cerebellar coordination via a metric tensor. *Neuroscience,* 5: 1761 – 1770.

Pellionisz, A.J. and Peterson, B.W. (1988) A tensorial model of neck motor activation. In B.W. Peterson and F.J. Richmond (Eds.), *Control of Head Movement,* Oxford Univ. Press, New York, pp. 178 – 186.

Peterson, B.W., Goldberg, J., Bilotto, G. and Fuller, J.H. (1985) Cervicocollic reflex: its dynamic properties and interaction with vestibular reflexes. *J. Neurophysiol.,* 54: 90 – 109.

Schor, R.H., Kearney, R.E. and Dieringer, N. (1988) Reflex stabilization of the head. In B.W. Peterson and F.J. Richmond (Eds.), *Control of Head Movement,* Oxford Univ. Press, New York, pp. 141 – 166.

Vidal, P.P., Graf, W. and Berthoz, A. (1986) The orientation of the cervical vertebral column in unrestrained awake animals. I. Resting position. *Exp. Brain Res.,* 61: 549 – 559.

J.H.J. Allum and M. Hulliger (Eds.)
Progress in Brain Research, Vol. 80
© 1989 Elsevier Science Publishers B.V. (Biomedical Division)

Overview and critique of Chapters 30 and 31

H. Collewijn

Rotterdam, The Netherlands

Both of these papers are concerned with the stabilization of the head in space during motion of the body. Whereas *Pozzo et al.* have studied behavioural aspects of head-stability during locomotor activities in man, *Lacour and Borel* have taken the analytical approach, and have measured EMG activity in the neck muscles of the cat during passive, linear, vertical motion of the animal or its visual surroundings. These approaches are important, because they extend the classical ways of studying visual and vestibular stabilization in the direction of more complex and behaviourally relevant stimulus – response relations.

As pointed out elsewhere in this volume (see Chapter 17), the tendency in the past has been to treat the oculomotor responses to vestibular and other sensory stimuli as stereotyped, automatic reflexes. I argued that such a view is much too simplistic, and that meaningful control of gaze has to be programmed in the appropriate manner for a specific visual goal that is selected out of the many potential goals that are present in a natural environment. Berthoz expresses a similar idea with regard to posture, when he states that posture is regulated according to an internally specified set of goals, related to the motor task. One can agree with Pozzo et al. that posture, integrated with movement, cannot be studied within the theoretical framework of systems analysis, concerned with the control of motor output by sensory input. The same is true for the control of gaze.

Nevertheless, there may be some simplifying principles in the control of posture and gaze. One of these appears to be the stabilization of the angular head-position in the sagittal plane during locomotor activities, within a range with a standard deviation of 3 to 6 degrees. When larger head movements do occur, they appear to consist of steps, separated by intervals in which the head is relatively stable. Although all of us know intuitively that the head of a moving person is not moving erratically, the degree of stability documented by Berthoz is surprisingly good. Also, the stabilization in different angular positions in sequential intervals reminds us very much of saccadic eye movements, separated by intervals in which gaze is relatively stable.

Pozzo et al. did not measure gaze in any precise way, but we may combine their findings with those of Ferman et al. (1987), who found that, on average, about 2.5% of voluntary head movements in the vertical and horizontal directions remained uncompensated by eye movements. This would predict that the standard deviation of gaze-position, associated with the head rotations during locomotion, would be on the order of 7.5 min arc (2.5% of 5 deg arc). The small value of this figure suggests that rotational instability of the head during locomotion is unlikely to disturb gaze-stability, or visual acuity, to a significant extent.

One simplification in Pozzo and coworkers' analysis is the neglect of translational instability of the head, which is bound to be prominent in such activities as jumping. Except for targets at optical infinity, head translation requires additional compensatory eye movements. It would be interesting to study gaze control during locomotion more directly in future work, by means of reliable techniques for recording gaze such as the scleral sensor coil. In that way, one could establish whether moving humans and animals look preferentially at some particular point in space, for instance the centre of the optic flow-field created by their own motion, or whether they look in arbitrary directions.

The well-maintained angular orientation of the head in space requires exquisite control of the neck-extensors, and it is this aspect which is addressed by the work of Lacour and Borel. Their present paper is part of a series of investigations on the coding of vertical linear head motion (signalled by the otolith organs and visual motion detection processes) in the activity of vestibular nuclear neurones and neck muscles.

The specific aspect treated in Lacour and Borel's paper is the interaction of visual and vestibular information in the modulation of neck-extensor activity in the alert cat. It is shown that vestibular input is especially effective in the higher frequency range (>0.25 Hz), whereas visual stimuli dominate the response at lower frequencies (<0.25 Hz). A linear systems analysis showed a relatively constant gain of the EMG response (referred to peak velocity of the stimulus) throughout the frequency range tested ($0.05-1.39$ Hz) when vestibular and visual stimuli acted in synergy. In this situation, the EMG responses were also rather well in phase with stimulus velocity, such that neck extensors were activated when the animal moved downard (or the visual surroundings moved upward, relative to the animal). Responses of this type would tend to stabilize the head in space. Although passive vertical translation of the head, as isolated in these experiments, would be rare in natural conditions, the responses as such seem to be functionally meaningful. However, the coupling of such reflexes with gaze seems to be far from simple. First of all, vertical translation in darkness does not elicit any vertical eye movement (Lacour et al., 1987). Furthermore, the movements of the head on the trunk and the eye in the head are rotations, not translations; therefore, they have not the same dimension as the stimuli used. It is not clear whether visual motion-

detection processes in the cat can differentiate between linear and rotatory motion of the visual environment, a feature which would be important to create the visual complements to the detection of linear and rotatory accelerations by the otoliths and semicircular canals. It would be interesting to investigate this aspect of visual motion detection in the future, especially as the visual stimuli used in experiments of this type are often less than full field size, and the protection techniques used often result in motions that are neither pure rotations nor pure translations.

In any case, compensatory gaze movements, associated with linear head motion, would be effective only for a target at some specific distance because there is no constant relation between linear displacement and angular displacement. Therefore, it is probably very significant that linear translations do not elicit compensatory gaze movements unless a visual target is present. Interestingly, Lacour and Borel suggest that the weighting process of otolith and visual inputs takes into account the degree of coherency between converging and covariant inputs, and that evaluation of each sensory input is made on the basis of the internal relevance of the covariant cues with respect to the behavioural context. This is an important concept, which is applicable to sensorimotor coordination in general. It is strongly related to Pozzo et al.'s statement on the significance of internally specified goals. Such a way of functioning is essentially non-linear, and even non-stationary. As rightly observed by Pozzo and colleagues, it follows that it cannot be studied within the theoretical framework of traditional systems-analysis.

There is clearly a discrepancy between this insight and the use of simple frequency responses to characterize input – output relations. Although the traditional systems-approach to sensorimotor function has been very useful in promoting quantitative analysis and thinking in terms of models (cf. Robinson, 1986), it is also clear that linear systems models are in many ways inadequate and that another class of models will have to be developed in order to understand sensorimotor control (see Steinman, 1986, for further elaboration).

The challenge for the future seems to be in the development of new models, that account for the selection of goals, the selection of the relevant sensory information, and the programming of the behaviourally appropriate motor response.

References

Ferman, L., Collewijn, H., Jansen, T.C., and Van den Berg, A.V. (1987) Human gaze stability in the horizontal, vertical and torsional direction during voluntary head movements, evaluated with a three-dimensional scleral induction coil technique. *Vision Res.,* 27: 811 – 828.

Lacour, M., Borel, L., Barthelemy, J., Harlay, F. and Xerri, C. (1987) Dynamic properties of the vertical otolith neck reflexes in the alert cat. *Exp. Brain Res.,* 65: 559 – 569.

Robinson, D.A. (1986) The systems approach to the oculomotor system. *Vision Res.,* 26: 91 – 99.

Steinman, R.M. (1986) The need for an eclectic, rather than systems, approach to the study of the primate oculomotor system. *Vision Res.,* 26: 101 – 112.

J.H.J. Allum and M. Hulliger (Eds.)
Progress in Brain Research, Vol. 80
© 1989 Elsevier Science Publishers B.V. (Biomedical Division)

CHAPTER 30

Head kinematic during various motor tasks in humans

T. Pozzo, A. Berthoz and L. Lefort

Laboratoire de Physiologie Neurosensorielle du CNRS, F-75270 Paris cedex 06, France

Head kinematic during various motor tasks was studied in ten subjects. The movement of the body was recorded with a video system (E.L.I.T.E.) which allows a computer reconstruction of three-dimensional motion of selected points on the body. Analysis is focused on head rotation in the horizontal and vertical planes. The results demonstrate that the amplitude and the maximum velocity do not exceed respectively 38 deg/s and 185 deg/s. However the head is intermittently stabilized and the angle of this stabilization is dependent upon the task and related to the direction of gaze. Darkness had no significant effect on head rotational velocity during walking but caused a decrease in velocity during running and hopping. The results suggest that head stabilization (1) is related to an ocular fixation point in the direction of gaze in space and (2) is probably regulated on the basis of a predictive mode of sensory motor control

Key words: Kinematics; Head stabilization; Locomotion; Visuo-vestibular interaction; Motor coordination; Gravity; Gaze

Introduction

The control of head position is a complex process that integrates information from a variety of sources to generate functionally appropriate motor commands. When the body moves, head position can be adjusted by vestibulocollic (VCR), cervicocollic (CCR) and visual reflexes which have been studied separately as individual subsystems. In static condition head position is dependent upon the direction of gaze as well as upon the general setting of posture.

In a previous study (Berthoz and Pozzo, 1988) we have shown that, during walking, the angular rotation of the head in the sagittal plane is minimized in an intermittent fashion with a precision of a few degrees. It is important to note that what has been demonstrated is not a complete stabilization of the head in space but its intermittent positioning in discrete particular planes.

The aim of the current study was to extend our previous results by investigating head stabilization in the sagittal and horizontal planes during free movements.

Methods

We asked ten normal subjects (1 female, 9 males) to perform several locomotor tasks. Age was 20 – 45 years; heights ranged from 152 to 183 cm and weight ranged from 51 to 82 kg. The kinematics of the movement were analysed by means of an optical automatic TV-image processor (E.L.I.T.E. system) (Ferrigno and Pedotti, 1985). Ten hemispherical retroflective markers (8 mm in diameter), which determined nine "body segments" were placed on:
– the head; two of these markers defined the line between the canthus of the eye and the meatus of the ear which gave us an approximative evaluation of the plane of the horizontal semi-circular canal and its orientation with respect to the gravity;

– the upper limb, at shoulder level on the acromial process and on the lateral condyle of the elbow and wrist;

– the trunk on the tubercle of the iliac crest;

– the lower limb on the lateral condyle of the knee and on the lateral malleolus of the foot.

The sampling rate of successive images was 50 images per second. The accuracy of the measuring system and its computer processing was about 1/2500. Under the present condition in which the explored field of view was 3 metres by 3 metres the accuracy was in the order of 1 to 1.5 mm for linear displacement and 1.5 degrees for angular position. The recorded positions were processed on line by a PDP 11/73 computer. The computer provided several sets of data; at first it constructed stick figures of the human body in motion. Each picture was then translated in order to superimpose the points taken as the auditory meatus (this method was described in our previous paper: Berthoz and Pozzo, 1988). The angle between the head and the earth vertical was not changed by this translation which allowed us to visualize the angular rotations of the head with respect to the vertical. In addition numerical values of several parameters were calculated in sagittal and horizontal planes of the body: (1) the angle of the "cantho-meatic" line, with the earth vertical (or direction of gravity); (2) head linear and angular velocity. Kinematics measurements were taken during (a) free walking, (b) walking in place, (c) running, (d) hopping, and (e) jumping down (from a stool 50 cm in height). These conditions have been chosen because they represent three groups of motor tasks:

– natural and simulated locomotion (free walking and walking and running in place);

– dynamic equilibrium (hopping);

– visually guided jumping (jumping down).

In the first condition (a) the subjects were instructed to walk a distance of approximately 6 m in their normal style. The conditions b, c and d were performed at a rate chosen by the subject as his natural one and began just before the recording session. During free walking and jumping down the computer programme was triggered when the

subject began to move his head. Subjects were bare-foot. Following a brief explanation of the tasks, subjects underwent training periods with normal visual surround. The experiments, however, were performed in the light though some were repeated in darkness. Each trial repeated 5 times. Rest periods were permitted. Among all the examined subjects, the variation in the kinematic parameters related to each experimental condition decreased from trial to trial fairly consistently. For these experiments, there were only small changes in subject pattern performance.

Results

General characteristics of head rotation during jumping and running

Fig. 1 gives an example of the analysis which was performed on one subject during jumping down from a 50 cm stool. Fig. 1A shows the stick figures reconstructed by the computer from the various markers placed on the body. In Fig. 1B the same representation is shown with only three markers, two on the head and one on the shoulder. This enlarged view shows that, in spite of the large range of variation of head translation (70 cm ver-

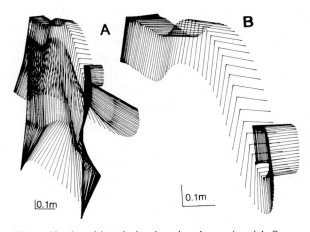

Fig. 1. Head position during jumping down. A: stick figures reconstructed by the computer during jumping down. Eight markers have been placed on body segments. B: enlarged view of the same movement with only two markers placed on the head and one on the shoulder.

tically and 50 cm horizontally), head angular position in the sagittal plane varies only slightly.

In Fig. 2, for the same experimental condition (A) and running in place (B), the computer has translated the stick figures in order to superimpose the different positions of the markers located near the auditory meatus. Figs. 2A and B give an enhanced illustration of the head-shoulder segment angular position during the 2 experimental conditions. The best stabilization is obtained during running. During jumping down we can observe a distribution of sticks representing cantho-meatic line around two main angular positions: in the upper one, the more horizontal angular position has a total spread of 13 degrees whereas in the lower one the spread is only of 4.5 degrees with an angular vertical mean axis at 15 degrees below the horizontal. The total range of head rotation is 19 degrees.

A similar distribution around two main angular positions is also visible for the head-shoulder link (vertical sticks) corresponding to arm movements from a backward rest position to a forward movement which takes place in synergy with the take off of the jump. These two resting zones have a mean value of 6 degrees and the total angular displacement is 22 degrees. During running the head is stabilized around the earth horizontal with a spread about of 7 degrees. The mean angular displacement of head-shoulder link is 25 degrees.

Body kinematics during jumping down

Typical raw data from one subject, illustrating head motor strategy during jumping down, are shown in Fig. 3. To further evaluate the relationship between head rotation and translation of the whole body, we have drawn on the same plot: (a) the linear displacement along the vertical (Z) and antero-posterior (X) axis of the markers placed on the foot and the meatus of the ear, and (b) the amplitude and the angular velocity of head rotation in the sagittal plane. The onset of the jump begins with a downward rotation of the head which corresponds probably to an orientation of the subject's gaze toward the landing surface. Then the subjects bend their head forward and downward. At take off time the head moves upward (Fig. 3C) together with the feet (Fig. 3A). Upward translation is associated with a downward rotation of the head (ventroflexion) (Fig. 3D). This compensatory rotation is slowed down at the end

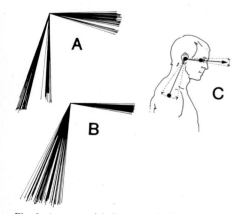

Fig. 2. A: same stick figures as in Fig. 1B but moved by translation so as to superimpose the markers on the auditory meatus. B: same editing for running in place. C: anatomic localization of the three markers placed at the head level (1) on the outer canthus of the eye, (2) near the auditory meatus, and at the shoulder level (3) on acromial process.

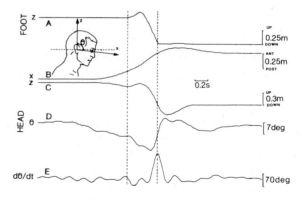

Fig. 3. Kinematic parameters during jumping down. A: translation along vertical axis of the marker placed on the lateral malleolus of the foot. B, C: translation of the marker placed on the meatus of the ear respectively along horizontal and vertical axis. D, E: rotation of the head and angular head velocity in sagittal plane. The onset of the take-off and the landing of the jump are given by the two vertical dotted lines. The space between the two dotted lines corresponds to the time duration of the weightlessness period.

of the ascending phase of the jump. The amount of head ventroflexion is 15 degrees for a duration of 1.3 s. Later, 100 ms before landing, the subject's head rotates rapidly in the opposite direction. Peak-to-peak amplitude and duration of this head saccade are respectively 19 degrees and 200 ms. This rapid rotation is compensatory with a downward head translation and resets the head near its initial horizontal position after a slight overshoot (2 degrees).

Landing, which occurred in the middle of head dorsiflexion, is synchronous to angular peak velocity (Fig. 3E). It is worth observing that the impact between foot and floor has no effect on (1) head translation along the vertical axis and (2) head upward resetting rotation. This shows that head motion may be independent of mechanical vibrations elicited by reaction forces during the impact between foot and floor.

Quantitative values of head amplitude and velocity angular displacement in the sagittal and horizontal planes (Table 1)

Amplitude of head rotation. For all the conditions, the maximum amplitude of head rotation in horizontal and vertical planes is less than 23 degrees except during jumping down, for which mean amplitude is 22 degrees and maximum amplitude is 38 degrees in vertical plane. The mean amplitude is always greater in the vertical than in the horizontal plane, except during walking in place (respectively 7 degrees and 12 degrees) and during free walking (respectively 8 degrees and 11 degrees). The mean value and standard deviation of the angle delimited by the earth vertical and the cantho-meatic line, averaged in the ten subjects when they stood quietly is 87 ± 6 degrees.

Angular velocity. The mean value of horizontal and vertical rotational velocities increases from locomotion tasks to dynamic equilibrium task and are maximum during the visually guided jumping task without exceeding 185 deg/s. During free walking these two parameters, which are less than 50 deg/s, have similar mean values. In contrast,

during walking in place, mean maximal horizontal velocity is increased by a factor of 2.25 compared to vertical velocity. These results are consistent with these of Grossman et al. (1988) obtained with a different recording system.

In comparing walking in place and running, mean maximal velocity in horizontal plane is the same whereas in vertical plane mean maximal velocity increases by a factor of 2.7. Vertical velocities obtained during hopping are near those obtained during running; in horizontal plane, mean value is halved, probably because of head swinging during running.

We have observed an up-down asymmetry of maximum vertical head velocities; during free walking, 64% of the values are oriented upward (i.e during dorsiflexion of the head); during running in place, 65% downward (i.e during ventroflex-

TABLE 1

Summary of group data from ten normal subjects in the different experimental conditions

Test condition	Amplitude (deg)	Maximum velocity (deg/s)
Walking in Place		
Horizontal	12 ± 2.5	68 ± 24
Vertical	7 ± 2.4	30 ± 18
Free Walking		
Horizontal	11 ± 5	25 ± 12
Vertical	8 ± 2	28 ± 7
Running		
Horizontal	12 ± 5	60 ± 23
Vertical	14 ± 4	81 ± 23
Hopping		
Horizontal	10 ± 3	31 ± 15
Vertical	14 ± 4.5	75 ± 25
Jumping down		
Horizontal	14 ± 5	30 ± 15
Vertical	22 ± 10	97 ± 25

Mean values of vertical and horizontal amplitudes of head rotation and maximum head rotational velocity are given with their standard deviations.

ion of the head); during hopping, 66% downward; during jumping down, 90% upward.

Kinematic data allowed us to calculated the fundamental frequency of head rotation in sagittal plane during the situations which provide pseudo-periodic head movements along vertical axis. The calculated values range between: 0.2 – 1 Hz for free walking; 0.2 – 1 Hz for walking in place; 2.5 – 3.5 Hz for running; 1.5 – 2.5 Hz for hopping.

Influence of vision on head stability

The role of vision in the control of head stability in the sagittal plane was investigated during four situations: free walking, walking in place, running in place and hopping. Compared to normal vision, darkness has no significant effect on mean amplitude and maximum velocity of head rotation in sagittal plane (see Fig. 4). In spite of this, we can note the tendency of maximum rotational velocity to decrease in darkness. This decrease is stronger during hopping and running which are more dynamic situations.

Comparing the kinematic data in the three axes of whole body movement obtained in darkness or in light, during any of the experimental conditions, did not reveal a significant modification of amplitude and velocity translational components. This observation indicates that the decrease of

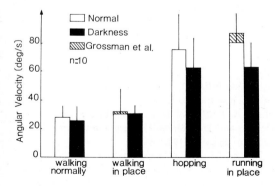

Fig. 4. Effect of vision upon maximum head angular velocity in sagittal plane during free walking, walking in place, running and hopping. The data from Grossman et al. (1988), have been inserted for comparison, for running and walking in place.

maximum vertical rotational velocity is not the result of a modification of whole body movement which might occur during abnormal input conditions.

Discussion

In this study we have extended the observations that human subjects exhibit an angular stabilization of head position in space with a precision which varies with the motor task. In spite of the differences in the tasks (visual task requiring gaze stabilization or dynamic task with a large linear acceleration component) the head angular position remains within small limits of variations.

We found that the range of predominant vertical head oscillation frequencies in rotation and translation during walking, running and hopping was 0.2 – 3.5 Hz. Because Rozendal (1986) and Guitton et al. (1986) speculated that the theoretical frequency at which inertial effects are important in head stabilization lies between about 2 and 4 Hz, we can estimate the same for these motor tasks. (head inertia does not play an important role in stabilizing the head in the sagittal plane.) The exception is during running for which the predominant frequency of vertical oscillation is within a 2.5 – 3.5 Hz range (and also probably during jumping down which has greater translational and rotational acceleration components). Darkness did not significantly affect head position in space and rotational velocities during free walking and walking in place, but caused a slight decrease of maximum head rotational velocity during hopping and running in place. It has been postulated that although vision plays a role in the correction of rapid postural perturbations (Nasher and Berthoz, 1978; Soechting and Berthoz, 1979), closing the eyes induces a reorganization of the postural control system (Vidal et al., 1982). Lack of visual input and more complex mechanisms of head stabilization during dynamic locomotory tasks could therefore involve a simplified strategy of stabilizing the head, illustrated here by the decrease of maximum head angular velocity. In this way reducing the complexity of head movement simplifies central processing of multimodal sensory information and provides a stable vestibular gravitational reference (Nasher, 1985). Our results do not match those of Shuppert et al. (1988) who find that head position is maintained closer to initial head position, and head velocity and acceleration were lower with eyes open than with eyes closed. These differences could be explained by the difference in the experimental conditions. Motor strategies may differ for disturbance of static posture on an uneven ground in comparison to actively initiated motor activity. However, our results indicate that systems of controlling head movements can work without visual information, presumably on the basis of a "projective mode" of sensory motor control (Droulez and Berthoz, 1986). Recent studies (Nasher et al., 1986; Keshner et al., 1988) support this idea, by assuming that head stabilization is not only the expression of vestibular reflexes but can be accomplished on a feed-forward basis. In the same way Guitton et al. (1986) suggest that the mechanisms influencing head stability during horizontal whole body rotation was strictly dependent on "voluntary" control. Indeed these authors showed that short latency VCR (vestibulocollic reflexes) and CCR (cervicocollic reflexes) are under "voluntary" control and are superseded by alternative, longer latency, visual and vestibular tracking mechanisms when the requirement is to stabilize the head in space.

Data obtained during jumping down (Figs. 2 and 3) illustrate the mechanisms of head control during a complex motor task. In this situation the subject receives precise visual information about the height and the orientation of the jump to plan his motor activity. The direction of the head is determined by the initial direction of gaze. In order to prepare landing phase the subject needs absolute and precise determination of distance, angle and timing. The head must therefore be stabilized with a precision compatible with the dynamic properties of visual and vestibular systems. The comparison of head translation along the vertical axis and head rotation in sagittal plane during the jump (Fig. 3C, D) indicates a compensatory movement of head rotation providing head anchoring to an earth-fixed target probably located on the landing surface.

Another interesting fact observed during jumping down is the unbroken trajectory of head rotation in sagittal plane during landing in spite of the impact between foot and floor. In our study the subjects trigger the fall themselves and know the height of fall (about 50 cm). For these reasons we think that the rapid dorsiflexion which brings the head back to its initial position is not disrupted by the impact between foot and floor because of a voluntary muscular prelanding activity.

This suggests a capacity to predict mechanical constraints resulting from physical contact and to reproduce the same smooth and regular head trajectory in space. This geometrical invariance and the intermittent stabilization of the head in particular planes may relate to the segmentation of three-dimensional movements demonstrated by Soechting and Lacquaniti (1981). This segmentation could be controlled by an internal representation of subject's goal in space.

Acknowledgements

Mr Lefort was supported by a grant from Centre National d'Etudes Spatiales (CNES). We acknowledge the contribution of the CNES to the equipment for this research.

References

Berthoz, A. and Pozzo, T. (1988) Intermittent head stabilization during postural and locomotory tasks in humans. In B. Amblard, A. Berthoz and F. Clarac (Eds.), *Development, Adaptation and Modulation of Posture and Gait,* Elsevier, Amsterdam, pp. 189 – 198.

Droulez, J. and Berthoz, A. (1986) Servo-controlled (conservative) versus topological (projective) mode of sensory motor control. In W. Bles and T. Brandt (Eds.), *Disorders of Posture and Gait,* Elsevier, Amsterdam, pp. 83 – 97.

Ferrigno, G. and Pedotti, A. (1985) Elite: a digital dedicated hardware system for movement analysis via real time TV-signal processing. *IEEE Trans. Biomed. Eng.,* 32: 943 – 950.

Guitton, D., Kearney, R.E., Wereley, N. and Peterson, B.W. (1986) Visual, vestibular and volontary contribution to human head stabilization. *Exp. Brain Res.,* 64: 59 – 69.

Grossman, G.E., Leigh, R.J., Abel, L.A., Lanska, D.J. and Thurston, S.E. (1988) Frequency and velocity of rotational head perturbation during locomotion. *Exp. Brain Res.,* 70: 470 – 476.

Keshner, E.A., Woollacott, M.H. and Debu, B. (1988) Neck, trunk and limb muscle responses during postural perturbations in humans. *Exp. Brain Res.,* 71: 455 – 466.

Nasher, L.W. and Berthoz, A. (1978) Visual contribution to rapid motor responses during postural control. *Brain Res.,* 150: 403 – 407.

Nasher, L.W. (1985) Strategies for organization of human posture. In M. Igarashi and F.O. Black (Eds.), *Vestibular and Visual Control of Posture and Locomotor Equilibrium,* Karger, Basel, pp. 1 – 8.

Nasher, L.M., Shupert, C.L. and Horak, F.B. (1986) Head trunk movement coordination in the standing posture. In O. Pompeiano and J. Allum (Eds.), *Vestibulospinal Control of Posture and Movement, Prog. Brain Res. Vol. 76,* Elsevier, Amsterdam pp. 243 – 251.

Rozendal, R.H. (1986) Biomechanics of standing and walking. In W. Bles and T. Brandt (Eds.), *Disorders of Posture and Gait,* Elsevier, Amsterdam, pp. 3 – 16.

Shupert, C.L., Black, O., Horak, F.B. and Nasher, L.M. (1988) Coordination of the head and body in response to support surface translations in normals and patients with bilaterally reduced vestibular function. In B. Amblard, A. Berthoz and F. Clarac (Eds.), *Development, Adaptation and Modulation of Posture and Gait,* Elsevier, Amsterdam, pp. 281 – 289.

Soechting, J.F. and Berthoz, A. (1979) Role of vision in the dynamic control of posture. Direction-specific effect of moving visual surrounds on the reaction to postural disturbance. *Exp. Brain Res.,* 20: 1 – 11.

Soechting, J.F. and Lacquaniti, F. (1981) Invariant characteristics of a pointing movement in man. *J. Neurosci.,* 1: 710 – 720.

Vidal, P.P., Berthoz, A. and Millanvoye, M. (1982) Difference between eye closure and visual stabilization in the control of posture in man. *Aviat. Space Envron. Med.,* 53(2): 166 – 170.

J.H.J. Allum and M. Hulliger (Eds.)
Progress in Brain Research, Vol. 80
© 1989 Elsevier Science Publishers B.V. (Biomedical Division)

CHAPTER 31

Functional coupling of the stabilizing gaze reflexes during vertical linear motion in the alert cat

M. Lacour and L. Borel

Université de Provence, Laboratoire de Psychophysiologie (UA CNRS 372), Centre de St Jérôme, 13397 Marseille Cedex 13, France

Eye – head coordination is mainly achieved by means of stabilizing reflexes (VOR, VCR, OKR) and orienting movements (eye – neck synergy) underlying the close cooperation of the visual and vestibular systems in gaze stabilization. The functional coupling of these different sensorimotor subsystems has been principally analysed using rotatory stimulation of the whole body and/or of the visual surround. The aim of the present study was to investigate the dynamic properties of these stabilizing gaze reflexes and their coupling during linear motion in the vertical plane. These investigations were performed in the alert cat under open-loop conditions (head fixed). Otolith stimulation consisted of vertically translating the cat in total darkness using sinusoidal linear motion (0.025 Hz – 1.39 Hz; 290 mm peak-to-peak amplitude). Optokinetic stimulation was provided by sinusoidally moving a pseudo-random visual pattern in front of the cat and in the vertical plane, with identical kinematic parameters. Normal visual – otolith interaction was performed by translating the cat in front of the stationary visual surround while conflicting interaction was provided by moving the animal and the visual pattern in phase and at the same velocity (visual stabilization). Results showed that the vertical otolith – neck reflex is very poorly developed or absent in the low frequency range of motion (0.025 Hz – 0.25 Hz) while consistent EMG activity is found during pure optokinetic stimulation. EMG responses are in phase with the visual surround velocity in the upward direction and with the upward OKR velocity. A close correlation is observed between the EMG gain and the OKR gain, which both decrease in this low frequency range, indicating that gaze stabilization would be mainly ensured by the OKR and a functional oculo-collic coupling or eye – neck synergy in the vertical plane. On the contrary, gaze stabilization is principally achieved by way of the otolith – neck reflex in the higher frequency range of motion (above 0.25 Hz). EMG responses recorded during otolith stimulation exhibit a relatively constant gain and a phase lead with respect to motion velocity which progressively reduces as the stimulus frequency increases up to 1.39 Hz. When present, EMG responses evoked during the optokinetic stimulation show strong gain attenuation and phase lag. Normal visual – otolith interaction induces neck muscle activity which parallels the optokinetic and the otolith responses in the low and high frequency ranges, respectively. The motor responses are however improved in terms of gain and phase values in the whole frequency range when both sensory inputs are combined. Conflicting visual – otolith interaction totally suppresses the OKR and the neck muscle responses in the low range of motion. It also considerably reduces the otolith – neck reflex at frequencies up to 0.5 Hz. No significant changes are observed at higher frequencies. The present experiments clearly point to the tight coupling between the visual and vestibular systems in head postural control and gaze stabilization during vertical linear motion. They show stimulus frequency-dependent strategies, with predominance of OKR and eye – neck coupling in the low range of motion, and of the stabilizing otolith – neck reflex in the higher range.

Key words: Optokinetic reflex (OKR); Eye – head synergy; Otolith – neck reflex (ONR); Alert cat; Vertical linear motion; Electromyography (EMG); Visual – vestibular interaction

Introduction

Stabilization of gaze in space occurs both when moving the visual surround around a stationary animal and when moving the animal in total darkness or in front of a stationary visual surround. Head acceleration induced by self-motion of the animal elicits vestibular reflexes which strongly participate in eye (vestibulo-ocular reflex, VOR) and head (vestibulo-collic reflex, VCR) stabilization. On the other hand, an optokinetic stimulation can produce eye (optokinetic reflex, OKR) and head (optocollic reflex, OCR) movements allowing gaze stabilization during visual world and/or animal motion.

The dynamic properties of these different sensorimotor subsystems involved in eye – head coordination have been extensively studied in various species (frog, rabbit, cat, monkey and man: see review in Berthoz, 1985). Most of these investigations have been performed by using angular acceleration of the head, which gives rise to canal-vestibular reflexes, and/or rotatory visual stimulation. It was demonstrated that visual – vestibular interaction improved gaze stabilization when congruent optokinetic and vestibular inputs were combined. The VOR gain (Godaux et al., 1983: cat) and the OKR gain (Koenig et al., 1978; Boehmer and Pfaltz, 1979: man) were increased during yaw rotatory visual – vestibular interaction. Head reflexes were also found to compensate more perfectly whole body sinusoidal rotation when performed in the light as compared to total darkness (Grestly, 1975: guinea pig). All these experiments also support the general statement that visual cues dominate in the low range of motion while vestibular inputs are predominant at higher frequencies.

The better gaze stabilization observed in a more extended domain when both eye and head reflexes are simultaneously triggered reflects their functional coupling. However, this coupling can vary according to the experimental conditions, suggesting thereby that different stabilizing strategies may develop by using different combinations of preexisting subsystems included in the sensorimotor repertoire. For instance, preponderance of head reflex (OCR) observed in the pigeon in closed-loop situation (head free) can be replaced by a strong OKR in open-loop condition with its head fixed (Gioanni, 1988). Such changes related to the behavioural context have also been reported in the guinea pig (Gresty, 1975), the rabbit (Fuller, 1981), the frog (Dieringer and Precht, 1982) and in the cat (Crommelinck et al., 1982). Variations in this coupling are also found depending on the species, with well developed optokinetic head nystagmus in the salamander (Kopp and Manteuffel, 1984), the frog (Dieringer et al., 1983) and the pigeon (Gioanni, 1988). In these animals, preponderance of head movements is associated with a rather weak OKR. On the contrary, the lack of head nystagmus reflex seems to be compensated for by strong OKR in most mammals (Fuller, 1985: rat; Grestly, 1975: guinea pig; Fuller, 1987: rabbit; Crommelinck et al., 1982: cat).

This tight coupling and coordination of eye and head reflexes in gaze stabilization is also supported by recent experiments which demonstrate the presence of an oculo-collic coupling subserving an orienting behaviour. This eye – neck coupling mechanism is illustrated by the presence of modulations of the dorsal neck muscles activity in relation with eye position signals. It was described in the horizontal plane in the alert cat (Vidal et al., 1982; Roucoux et al., 1982; Darlot et al., 1985) and monkey (Lestienne et al., 1984), and in the vertical plane in the cat (Al Ansari et al., 1985; Denise et al., 1987). It was found in both free-head (Crommelinck et al., 1982) and fixed-head (Vidal et al., 1982) conditions, associated with all types of eye movements (fixation, vestibular nystagmus, optokinetic nystagmus).

Eye – head coordination during linear motion of the animal and/or its visual surround is considerably less documented. However, a perfect gaze stabilization is required in most daily activities giving rise to an activation of the utricular and saccular otolith receptors (walking, running, jumping, etc.). The influence of otolith stimulation upon eye movements (see review in Young, 1985) as well as on head and limbs postural control (Lacour et al., 1978: monkey; Melvill Jones and Watt, 1971; Greenwood and Hopkins, 1976: man) has been recognized for many years. On the other hand, a dynamic effect of vision was observed in both low frequency (Lestienne et al., 1977: man) and rapid (Nasher and Berthoz, 1978; Vidal et al., 1978: man; Vidal et al., 1979; Lacour et al., 1981: monkey) postural perturbations. Using linear horizontal motion in man, Buizza et al. (1980) showed an enhanced effect of vestibular stimulation on the oculomotor function when it was combined with an optokinetic input.

We have provided in a previous paper (Lacour et al., 1987) the first description of the dynamic properties of the vertical otolith neck reflex (VONR). This investigation was performed in the alert cat submitted to sinusoidal vertical linear acceleration, in open-loop condition (head fixed) and in total darkness. The aim of the present study was to analyse stabilizing gaze reflexes (VONR, OCR, OKR) and their functional coupling during vertical optokinetic and otolith stimulation applied separately and in combination, in both congruent and conflicting visual-otolith interaction modes.

Methods

Experiments were performed on eight adult cats prepared for chronic EMG and EOG recordings (alert cats, non-anaesthetized and non-paralysed), in head fixed conditions.

Animal preparation

EMG electrodes were implanted under anaesthesia (pentobarbital sodium: 40 mg/kg) and aseptic conditions in the splenius capitus muscles on both sides. Neck muscle responses were recorded by means of bipolar intramuscular electrodes made of teflon-insulated silver wire (0.5 mm diameter), the insulation of which was removed for 2 or 3 mm at the tip. These electrodes were inserted and sutured in each muscle, and separated by 1 cm. Wires were tunnelled subcutaneously to a connector located on the head of the cat. A metal implant was stereotaxically fixed onto the skull with dental acrylic anchored by stainless steel screws. Three bolts fixing the implant to the head-holder ensured head immobilization during the recording sessions. Vertical eye movements were recorded using Ag – AgCl electrodes chronically implanted above and below one eye in a vertical plane.

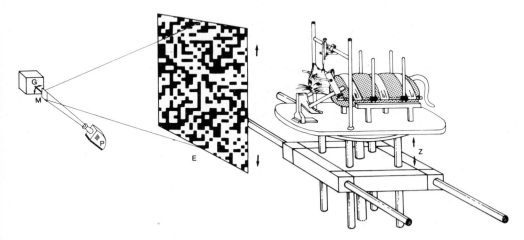

Fig. 1. Experimental set-up. The cat was placed on a platform with its head fixed in a stereotaxic frame and its body wrapped in a hammock. Otolith stimulation is elicited by submitting the animal to sinusoidal linear acceleration along the vertical Z axis, in total darkness. Optokinetic stimulation consisted of sinusoidally moving a pseudo-random pattern in the vertical plane on a screen located in front of the cat. Normal visual – otolith interaction was obtained by translating the animal in front of the stationary visual surround. Conflicting visual – otolith stimulation was performed by translating the cat together with the visual surround, in phase and at the same velocity.

Experimental procedures

The cat was placed in a stereotaxic frame rigidly attached to the platform of the linear accelerator (Fig. 1). Its head was fixed to a holder locked in the frame and bent forward by 23 degrees, its trunk was wrapped in a hammock.

Otolith stimulation was performed by sinusoidally moving the platform along the vertical Z axis in the 0.05 Hz – 1.39 Hz frequency range, with a 290 mm peak-to-peak amplitude (corresponding acceleration range: 0.0015 g to 1.12 g). Vertical translation of the cat was done in total darkness. *Optokinetic stimulation* was provided by sinusoidal vertical linear motion of a pseudo-random visual pattern, deflected by a mirror (M) driven by an optical scanner (G), and projected (P) onto a translucent screen (1.5 m × 1.5 m) located 0.5 m in front of the cat. The angular motion of the visual pattern on the screen was 32.3 degrees peak-to-peak, in the same frequency range (0.05 Hz – 1.39 Hz: corresponding velocity peaks: 5.05 deg/s to 140.4 deg/s). *Normal visual-otolith interaction* was obtained by translating the animal in front of the stationary visual surround. *Conflicting visual-otolith stimulation* was performed by translating the cat together with the visual surround, in phase and at the same velocity. In this visual stabilization condition, all visual motion cues were suppressed and no OKR was elicited.

Data analysis

The polyunitary EMG activity of splenius muscles was recorded on both sides through a band pass filter (50 – 5000 Hz), amplified, rectified and integrated (time constant: 20 ms), and fed to a computer which displayed the sequential histograms submitted to a Fast Fourier Transform (cf. Lacour et al., 1987). The gain of the EMG response was expressed as the ratio of muscular amplitude to velocity peak of animal or visual surround motion. The phase was defined as the difference in degrees between the peak of animal or visual scene velocity and the peak of the fundamental component of the motor output. Data collected from both muscles were averaged since no significant difference was observed between left and right splenius muscle EMG activity in all the tested cats.

Calibration of the EOG occurred at the beginning and at the end of each experimental session (cf. Barthelemy et al., 1988). Vertical eye movement and eye velocity (differentiated eye position signal) were stored on a paper chart recorder. Analysis of the OKR elicited during optokinetic and visual-otolith interaction was performed by constructing the slow cumulative eye position curve. The OKR gain and phase values were expressed relative to the velocity peak of the animal or visual surround motion.

Results

Sinusoidal vertical motion of the cat performed in total darkness (otolith stimulation) never evoked any modulation of splenius muscle EMG activity at frequencies lower than 0.05 Hz (corresponding to an acceleration amplitude zero to peak of 0.0015 g). In one cat, neck muscle responses consisting of a second harmonic with a frequency double that of the input signal were observed in the low frequency range (0.05 Hz – 0.25 Hz). This inconstant H2 EMG pattern already described in a previous paper (Lacour et al., 1987) will not be considered here.

As a rule, typical vertical otolith neck reflexes (VONR) were recorded in all tested cats in the higher frequency range (0.25 Hz – 1.39 Hz). In this frequency domain, the motor output is composed only of the fundamental frequency equal to that of the input frequency (H1 EMG pattern: cf. Lacour et al., 1987). It consists of bilateral and synchronous EMG modulations on both sides.

In contrast, consistent neck muscle responses are recorded in the low frequency range during sinusoidal vertical motion of the visual surround (optokinetic stimulation). In this low range of motion (up to 0.5 Hz), the visually-induced EMG modulations develop synchronously and bilaterally in the left and right splenius muscles as H1 EMG patterns. The muscular responses appear to be strongly correlated with the OKR slow phase

389

velocity in the upward direction, i.e. with the upward vertical component of eye velocity. This suggests a tight coupling between eye and head during vertical linear motion of the visual surround, which is also observed during normal visual-otolith interaction in the same frequency range.

The dynamic properties of these neck muscle responses have been investigated in the 0.25 Hz – 1.39 Hz frequency range in the three main experimental conditions where the visual and

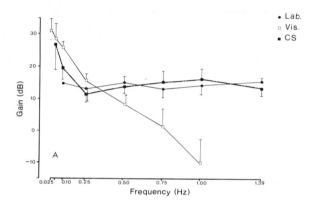

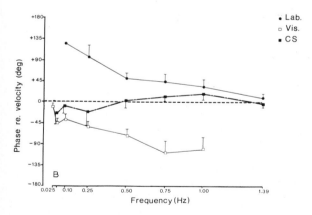

Fig. 2. Dynamic properties of the neck muscle responses in the different experimental situations. Bode diagrams showing the gain (A, upper) and the phase (B, lower) of the motor response recorded during otolith (filled circles), optokinetic (open squares) and visual – otolith (filled squares) stimulation. Gain is expressed in dB and phase is calculated in degrees re. velocity (ordinates) as a function of the stimulus frequency in Hz (abscissae). Confidence intervals are plotted as vertical bars (P < 0.05).

vestibular inputs are given independently (optokinetic and otolith stimulations) or in combination (normal visual-otolith interaction). The Bode diagrams showing the gain and the phase of the EMG responses are plotted in Fig. 2A and B, respectively.

The amplitude of the EMG modulation recorded during otolith stimulation progressively increases as the stimulus frequency increases from 0.25 Hz to 1.39 Hz. This results in a relatively stable gain of the motor response in the whole frequency range, as illustrated by the flat gain curve in Fig. 2A. The phase curve of the VONR shows a progressive phase shift from acceleration to velocity. At the 0.25 Hz stimulus frequency, the mean phase angle is closely distributed around the downward acceleration peak ($+6.72 \pm 25.15°$, S.D.). Increasing the stimulus frequency induces a significant phase lag which reaches on average $-40.03 \pm 11°$ at 0.5 Hz. Finally, neck muscle activity is closely distributed around the downward velocity peak at the highest frequency ($+8.03 \pm 10.2°$ at 1.39 Hz).

The visually-induced EMG modulations recorded during pure vertical optokinetic stimulation are only found in the low frequency range (0.025 Hz – 0.5 Hz). Above the 0.5 Hz stimulus frequency, neck muscle responses are very poorly developed or absent. Mean gain values calculated with respect to velocity of the visual surround point to a strong drop in gain (42 dB) between 0.025 Hz and 1 Hz. It is interesting to note that this EMG gain curve closely parallels that concerning the OKR gain. Evaluation of the OKR gain by dividing the amplitude of the electronically differentiated eye position (eye velocity) by the visual surround velocity gives mean gain values close to unity at the lowest frequencies (0.78 ± 0.15 at 0.025 Hz; 0.72 ± 0.1 at 0.05 Hz). Increasing the frequency induces a strong drop in gain (0.5 ± 0.10 at 0.010 Hz; 0.28 ± 0.09 at 0.25 Hz), with mean value close to zero at the highest frequency (0.07 ± 0.06 at 0.5 Hz). The EMG responses are centred around the upward visual surround velocity peak at low frequency

$(-10.28 \pm 7.65°$ at 0.025 Hz). A phase lag appears at higher frequencies which progressively increases up to 0.75 Hz $(-107.3 \pm 9.9°)$. A similar but less pronounced phase lag was also observed for the OKR velocity.

Interestingly, when both visual and vestibular inputs are combined in a congruent way, i.e. during normal visual-otolith interaction, neck muscle responses are present in the whole frequency range and exhibit more stable phase and gain values. A slight gain attenuation is found only in the low range of motion (15 dB between 0.05 Hz and 0.25 Hz), while stable or even increasing gain values are observed in the upper range. As far as phase is concerned, data collected in this experimental condition show a very flat curve, with EMG responses closely distrubuted around the downward velocity peak of the animal motion in the whole frequency range $(-24.93° \pm 23.49°$ at 0.05 Hz and $-4.12 \pm 7.68°$ at 1.39 Hz). These results indicate that the motor output is comparable to that induced by the optokinetic stimulation in the low frequency range $(< 0.25$ Hz) and to that obtained during the otolith stimulation in the high range $(>0.25$ Hz). However, combined visual-otolith stimulation produces an improvement of both gain and phase values of the neck muscle responses.

Conflicting visual-otolith interactions were performed using the visual stabilization method (VS). The total lack of OKR in this condition constitutes a good index of visual stabilization. Fig. 3 shows the data collected in one cat submitted to such a conflicting situation. A total suppression of the neck muscle responses is observed in the low range of motion, up to 0.25 Hz, when all visual motion cues and eye movements are eliminated (cf. Fig. 3A). It must be mentioned here that this motor reduction is not only found when comparing the VS to the optokinetic and visual-otolith stimulations, but also to the pure otolith stimulation. This suggests that the weight of the otolith input is modified, i.e. reduced, when this sensory information about self-motion is not associated with congruent visual motion cues. Modifications of the phase of the neck muscle responses is also evident

during visual stabilization, as illustrated in the Fig. 3B. When present, EMG responses in VS exhibit a strong phase lead as compared to those obtained in the normal visual-otolith costimulation, leading therefore to motor responses with phase angles closer to those found during pure otolith stimulation. In contrast, visual stabilization drastically

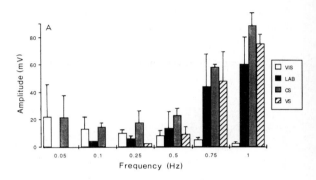

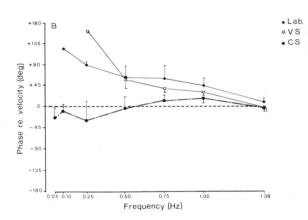

Fig. 3. Effects of visual stabilization on the dynamic properties of the neck muscle responses recorded during vertical linear motion. A (upper graph): comparison of the amplitude (in mV: ordinates) of the motor response as a function of the stimulus frequency (in Hz: abscissae) during optokinetic stimulation (open diagrams), otolith stimulation (filled diagrams), normal visual-otolith interaction (heavy dots) and conflicting costimulation (visual stabilization: strips). B (lower graph): comparison of the phase re. velocity (in degrees: ordinates) of the EMG response as a function of the stimulus frequency (in Hz: abscissae) during otolith stimulation (filled circles), normal (filled squares) and conflicting (open stars) visual-otolith interaction. Results from one cat; confidence intervals calculated at $P < 0.05$.

changes neither the amplitude nor the phase of the neck muscle responses in the high range of motion (0.75 Hz – 1.39 Hz: cf. Fig. 3B). Only slight phase advance and amplitude reduction are noticed as compared to the normal co-stimulation.

Discussion

As recently reviewed by Berthoz (1985), eye – head coordination in the cat may be achieved by using at least two different strategies. The compensatory mode utilizes a combination of stabilizing gaze reflexes like the VOR, the OKR and the VCR which can be complemented in closed-loop conditions by other reflexes (CCR, COR) triggered by neck proprioception. The second mode, or orienting strategy, refers to an eye-head coupling mechanism by which eye position signals influence the head control loop by synergistically activating the neck muscles. These two eye – head coordination modes probably do not operate independently of one another, since a rather linear algebraic summation of the VCR and horizontal ipsilateral eye position signal was found by Darlot et al. (1985) during passive head rotations in the alert cat.

The present experiments clearly demonstrate that the tight coupling between the visual and vestibular systems in head postural control and gaze stabilization operates also during linear motion in the vertical plane. Stimulus frequency-dependent strategies are particularly evidenced here. In the low range of motion (< 0.25 Hz), gaze stabilization would be mainly ensured by the optokinetic reflex and an eye – neck synergy. In contrast, gaze stabilization would be principally achieved by means of the stabilizing otolith-neck reflex in the high range of motion (> 0.25 Hz). These results are in agreement with the general statement that vision contributes to postural stabilization in the low frequency range of body movements (cf. Berthoz et al., 1979) while the vestibular system dominates at higher frequencies. They also point to an improvement of eye – head coordination when both sensory inputs are combined according to a congruent interaction mode.

Eye – head coordination in the low range of motion

Visually-induced EMG responses were recorded during the vertical optokinetic stimulation. These neck muscle responses were found in the low frequency range of motion (up to 0.5 Hz) where the OKR is present. Such an oculo-neck coupling mechanism has been previously described in the horizontal plane in the cat (Vidal et al., 1982; Roucoux et al., 1982) and in the monkey (Lestienne et al., 1984). It has also been described in the vertical plane in the cat (Al Ansari et al., 1985; Denise et al., 1987). In these investigations, dorsal neck muscle activity was found to be modulated by eye position signals, and it was proposed that second order vestibular neurones projecting to the contralateral abducens nucleus (VOR arc) also project down to the spinal cord (Mc Crea et al., 1980; Berthoz et al., 1981; Isu and Yokota, 1983). This eye – head coupling would be mediated by reticulospinal neurones reaching the neck motoneurones (Berthoz et al., 1982; Vidal et al., 1983).

The present study clearly demonstrates that dorsal neck muscle responses are closely correlated with the OKN slow phase velocity in the upward direction, i.e. with the upward vertical component of eye velocity. Interestingly, recent investigations we have performed by recording the extracellular activity of neurones located within the Deiters nucleus in the same experimental conditions showed two different patterns of neuronal modulation (Barthélémy et al., 1988). 43% of the tested cells exhibited an increase in their firing rate during motion of the visual surround in the upward direction while 57% showed the opposite behaviour. The firing rate modulation was only found at low frequencies (up to 0.5 Hz) and also closely correlated with the velocity peaks of visual scene motion and OKR slow phase velocity. This suggests that the lateral vestibulospinal system, which is well known to heavily project to the neck motoneurones (Wilson and Yoshida, 1969; Wilson et al., 1977), could be a good candidate and could constitute an alternative pathway for mediating the oculo-neck coupling during vertical linear translations. According to this hypothesis, EMG modulations from neck flexor muscles are expected to be associated with the OKN slow phase velocity in the downward direction. Recordings from these muscles remain to be done but, if true, such flexor responses should mainly depend on the second cell population we encountered within the Deiter's vestibular nucleus.

Eye – head coordination in the high range of motion

We have provided in a previous paper (Lacour et al., 1987) the first description of the vertical otolith-neck reflex (VONR). This study confirms its dynamic properties in a wider frequency range. In our open-loop conditions, with the head of the cat fixed, the VONR behaves like a stabilizing reflex. It appears to be implicated in the dynamic compensation of passive head displacement due to inertia. However, it does not perfectly compensate for the effects of inertia since head movement would be lagging the input acceleration by only 120° at the highest frequency, if taking into account the supplementary 30° phase lag induced by the muscle biomechanical properties. A more complete compensation may be expected in closed-loop conditions, with the head free, where the neck proprioception can trigger cervicocollic and cervico-ocular reflexes (Peterson and Goldberg, 1982). Moreover, gaze stabilization could be more perfectly performed with additional compensatory eye movements. In fact, no VOR was observed during otolith stimulation at frequencies up to 0.5 Hz, but we recorded a typical vertical VOR in the highest frequency range (0.75 Hz – 1.39 Hz). The gain of this VOR was relatively low but it improved as the stimulus frequency was increased (paper in preparation).

Functional coupling of the stabilization gaze reflexes

Eye – neck and otolith – neck reflexes appear to act in an agonistic way when elicited separately. During normal visual – otolith interaction, when these sensorimotor systems are combined, neck muscle responses reflect the predominance of the eye – neck coupling at low frequencies and of the VONR at higher frequencies. However, the amplitude of the EMG modulations are increased during normal co-stimulation, and a phase improvement is observed as shown by the phase shift towards the maximum downward velocity peak in the whole frequency range. This corroborates recent findings showing that motion velocity neuronal coding in vestibular cells was improved in terms of input – output phase relationship and response sensitivity when visual and otolith signals were combined (Xerri et al., 1988). Such correlation between neuronal activity of Deiters cells and EMG responses from dorsal neck muscles also support the above suggestion that the lateral vestibulospinal system could mediate both eye – neck synergy and otolith – neck compensatory reflex.

Conflicting visual – otolith interaction performed by using the visual stabilization method results in a total suppression of the OKR in the low frequency range of motion. This lack of vertical eye movements is associated with a complete motor suppression. On the contrary, visual stabilization does not greatly modify the VONR which develops at higher frequencies. Furthermore, the otolith component of the motor responses is strongly reduced at low frequencies when no relative movement between the animal and the visual environment is detected by the visual system. This result suggests that the weighting process of otolith and visual inputs takes into account the degree of coherency between converging and covariant inputs. It confirms that the CNS relies on the dominant and heavily weighted information: the visual and vestibular cues in the low and high velocity range of motion, respectively. It also suggests that evaluation of each sensory input is made on the basis of the internal relevance of the covariant cues with respect to the behavioural context.

Acknowledgements

This work was supported by UA-CNRS 372. The

authors wish to thank Mrs M.R. Ibrahim for typing the manuscript.

References

Al Ansari, A., Crémieux, J., Decostre, M.F., Crommelinck, M. and Roucoux, A. (1985) Eye position-related activity in different neck muscles in the head-fixed cat. *Arch. Int. Physiol. Biochim.*, 93: 12 – 14.

Anderson, J.H., Soechting, J.F. and Terzuolo, C.A. (1977) Dynamic relations between natural vestibular inputs and activity of forelimb extensor muscles in the decerebrate cat. I. Motor output during sinusoidal linear accelerations. *Brain Res.*, 120: 1 – 16.

Barthélémy, J., Xerri, C., Borel, L. and Lacour, M. (1988) Neuronal coding of linear motion in the vestibular nuclei of the alert cat. II. Response characteristics to vertical optokinetic stimulation. *Exp. Brain Res.*, 70: 287 – 298.

Berthoz, A., Lacour, M., Soechting, J.F. and Vidal, P.P. (1979) The role of vision in the control of posture during linear motion. In R. Granit and O. Pompeiano (Eds.). *Reflex Control of Posture and Movement, Prog. Brain Res., Vol. 50,* Elsevier/North Holland Biomed. Press, pp. 197 – 209.

Berthoz, A. (1985) Adaptive mechanisms in eye-head coordination. In A. Berthoz and G. Melvill Jones (Eds.), *Review in Oculomotor Research, Vol. I, Adaptative Mechanisms in Gaze Control, Facts and Theories,* Elsevier Science Publ. BV (Biomed Div.), pp. 177 – 201.

Berthoz, A., Yoshida, K. and Vidal, P.P. (1981) Horizontal eye movement signals in second-order vestibular nuclei neurons in the cat. In B. Cohen (Ed.), *Vestibular and Oculomotor Physiology, Ann. NY Acad. Sci.,* 374: 144 – 156.

Berthoz, A., Vidal, P.P. and Corvisier, J. (1982) Brain stem neurons mediating horizontal eye position signals to dorsal neck muscles of the alert cat. In A. Roucoux and M. Crommelinck (Eds.), *Physiological and Pathological Aspects of Eye Movements,* Dr W Junk, The Hague, pp. 385 – 398.

Boehmer, A. and Pfaltz, C.R. (1979) On the interaction of vestibular and optokinetic nystagmus in man. *Otorhinolaryngology,* 41: 121 – 128.

Buizza, A., Léger, A., Droulez, J., Berthoz, A. and Schmid, R. (1980) Influence of otolith stimulation by horizontal linear acceleration on optokinetic nystagmus and visual motion perception. *Exp. Brain Res.*, 39: 165 – 176.

Crommelinck, M., Roucoux, A. and Veraart, C. (1982) The relation of neck muscles activity to horizontal eye position in the alert cat. II. Head free. In A. Roucoux and M. Crommelinck (Eds.), *Physiological and Pathological Aspects of Eye Movements,* Dr W Junk, The Hague, pp. 379 – 384.

Darlot, C., Denise, P. and Droulez, J. (1985) Modulation by horizontal eye position of the vestibulo-collic reflex induced by tilting in the frontal plane in the alert cat. *Exp. Brain Res.*, 58: 510 – 519.

Denise, P., Darlot, C., Wilson, V.J. and Berthoz, A. (1987) Modulation by eye position of neck muscle contraction evoked by electrical labyrinthine stimulation in the alert cat. *Exp. Brain Res.*, 67: 411 – 419.

Dieringer, N. and Precht, W. (1982) Compensatory head and eye movements in the frog and their contribution to stabilization of gaze. *Exp. Brain Res.*, 47: 394 – 406.

Dieringer, N., Cochran, S.L. and Precht, W. (1983) Differences in the central organization of gaze stabilizing reflexes between frog and turtle. *J. Comp. Physiol.*, 153: 495 – 508.

Fuller, J.H. (1981) Eye and head movements during vestibular stimulation in the alert rabbit. *Brain Res.*, 205: 363 – 381.

Fuller, J.H. (1985) Eye and head movements in the pigmented rat. *Vision Res.*, 25: 1121 – 1128.

Fuller, J.H. (1987) Head movements during optokinetic stimulation in the alert rabbit. *Exp. Brain Res.*, 65: 593 – 604.

Gioanni, H. (1988) Stabilizing gaze reflexes in the pigeon. I. Horizontal and vertical optokinetic eye (OKN) and head (OCR) reflexes. *Exp. Brain Res.*, 69: 567 – 582.

Gioanni, H. (1988) Stabilizing gaze reflexes in the pigeon (*Columbia livia*). II. Vestibulo-ocular (VOR) and vestibulo-collic (closed-loop VCR) reflexes. *Exp. Brain Res.*, 69: 583 – 593.

Godaux, E., Gobert, C. and Halleux, J. (1983) Vestibulo-ocular reflex, optokinetic response, and their interactions in the alert cat. *Exp. Neurol.*, 80: 42 – 54.

Greenwood, R.J. and Hopkins, A. (1976) Muscle responses during sudden falls in man. *J. Physiol. (London),* 254: 507 – 518.

Gresty, M.A. (1975) Eye, head and body movements of the guinea pig in response to optokinetic stimulation and sinusoidal oscillation in yaw. *Pflügers Arch.*, 353: 201 – 214.

Isu, N. and Yokota, J. (1983) Morphological study on the divergent projection of axon collaterals of medial vestibular nucleus neurons in the cat. *Exp. Brain Res.*, 53: 151 – 162.

Koenig, E., Allum, J.H.J. and Dichgans, J. (1978) Visual-vestibular interaction upon nystagmus slow phase velocity in man. *Acta Oto-Laryngol.*, 85: 397 – 410.

Kopp, J. and Manteuffel, G. (1984) Quantitative analysis of salamander horizontal head nystagmus. *Brain Behav. Evol.,* 25: 187 – 196.

Lacour, M., Xerri, C. and Hugon, M. (1978) Muscle responses and monosynaptic reflexes in the falling monkey: role of the vestibular system. *J. Physiol. (Paris),* 74: 427 – 438.

Lacour, M., Vidal, P.P. and Xerri, C. (1981) Visual influences on vestibulospinal reflexes during vertical linear motion in normal and hemilabyrinthectomized monkeys. *Exp. Brain Res.*, 43: 383 – 394.

Lacour, M., Borel, L., Barthélémy, J., Harlay, F. and Xerri, C. (1987) Dynamic properties of the vertical otolith neck reflexes in the alert cat. *Exp. Brain Res.*, 65: 559 – 568.

Lestienne, F., Soechting, J.F. and Berthoz, A. (1977) Postural readjustments induced by linear motion of visual scenes. *Exp. Brain Res.*, 28: 363 – 384.

Lestienne, F., Vidal, P.P. and Berthoz, A. (1984) Gaze changing behaviour in head restrained monkey. *Exp. Brain Res.,* 53: 349–356.

McCrea, R.A., Yoshida, K., Berthoz, A. and Baker, R. (1980) Eye movement related activity and morphology of second order vestibular neurons terminating in the cat abducens nucleus. *Exp. Brain Res.,* 40: 468–473.

Melvill Jones, G. and Milsum, J.H. (1969) Neural response of the vestibular system to translational acceleration. In *Supplement to Conference on Systems Analysis, Approach to Neurophysiological Problems,* Brainerd, MN, pp. 8–20.

Melvill Jones, G. and Watt, D.G.D. (1971) Muscular control of landing from unexpected falls in man. *J Physiol. (London), 219:* 729–737.

Melvill Jones, G., Watt, D.G.D. and Rossignol, S. (1973) Eight nerve contributions to the synthesis of locomotor control. In R.S. Stein, K.G. Pearson, R.S. Smith and J.B. Redford (Eds.), *Control of Posture and Locomotion,* Plenum, New York, pp. 579–597.

Nashner, L. and Berthoz, A. (1978) Visual contribution to rapid motor responses during postural control. *Brain Res.,* 150: 403–407.

Peterson, B.W. and Goldberg, J. (1982) Role of vestibular and neck reflexes in controlling eye and head position. In A. Roucoux and M. Crommelinck (Eds.), *Physiological and Pathological Aspects of Eye Movements,* Dr W Junk, The Hague, pp. 351–364.

Roucoux, A., Guitton, D. and Crommelinck, M. (1980) Stimulation of the superior colliculus in the alert cat. II. Eye and head movements evoked when the head is unrestrained. *Exp. Brain Res.,* 39: 75–85.

Roucoux, A., Vidal, P.P., Veraart, C., Crommelinck, M. and Berthoz, A. (1982) The relation of neck muscles activity to horizontal eye position in the alert cat. I. Head free. In A. Roucoux and M. Crommelinck (Eds.), *Physiological and Pathological Aspects of Eye Movement,* Dr W. Junk, The Hague, pp. 371–378.

Vidal, P.P., Gouny, M. and Berthoz, A. (1978) Role de la vision dans le déclenchement de réactions posturales rapides. *Arch. Ital. Biol.,* 116: 281–291.

Vidal, P.P., Lacour, M. and Berthoz, A. (1979) Contribution of vision to muscle responses in monkey during free-fall: visual stabilization decreases vestibular-dependent responses. *Exp. Brain Res.,* 37: 241–252.

Vidal, P.P., Roucoux, A. and Berthoz, A. (1982) Horizontal eye position related activity in neck muscles of the alert cat. *Exp. Brain Res.,* 46: 448–453.

Vidal, P.P., Corvisier, J. and Berthoz, A. (1983) Eye and neck motor signals in periabducens reticular neurons of the alert cat. *Exp. Brain Res.,* 53: 16–28.

Wilson, V.J. and Yoshida, M. (1969) Comparison of effects of stimulation of Deiters' nucleus and medial longitudinal fasciculus on neck, forelimb, hindlimb motoneurons. *J. Neurophysiol.,* 32: 743–758.

Wilson, V.J., Gacek, R.R., Maeda, M. and Uchino, Y. (1977) Saccular and utricular input to cat neck motoneurons. *J. Neurophysiol.,* 40: 63–73.

Wilson, V.J., Precht, W. and Dieringer, N. (1983) Responses of different compartments of cat's splenius muscle to optokinetic stimulation: *Exp. Brain Res.,* 50: 153–156.

Xerri, C., Barthélémy, J., Harlay, F., Borel, L. and Lacour, M. (1987) Neuronal coding of linear motion in the vestibular nuclei of the alert cat. I. Response characteristics to vertical otolith stimulation. *Exp. Brain Res.,* 65: 569–581.

Xerri, C., Barthélémy, J., Borel, L. and Lacour, M. (1988) Neuronal coding of linear motion in the vestibular nuclei of the alert cat. III. Dynamic characteristics of visual-otolith interactions. *Exp. Brain Res.,* 70: 299–309.

Young, L.R. (1985) Adaptation to modified otolith input. In A. Berthoz and G. Melvill Jones (Eds.), *Adaptative Mechanisms in Gaze Control, Facts and Theories. Reviews in Oculomotor Research Vol. 1,* Elsevier Sci. Publ. (Biomed. Div.), pp. 155–162.

J.H.J. Allum and M. Hulliger (Eds.)
Progress in Brain Research, Vol. 80
© 1989 Elsevier Science Publishers B.V. (Biomedical Division)

Overview and critique of Chapters 32 – 34

B.W. Peterson

Chicago, U.S.A.

Prior to the Rhienfelden Meeting the participants in this session and others in the field of postural stabilizing mechanisms were involved in a vigorous debate concerning the relative roles of vestibular and proprioceptive signals in generating responses to postural perturbations. The three presentations at this meeting made a substantial contribution to resolving this dispute.

Historically the debate over relative roles of vestibular and proprioceptive contributions to postural responses dates back to studies by Nashner (1977) and Nashner et al. (1979), who studied responses of leg muscles to relatively small translations of the support surface and reported that proprioceptive inputs dominated the generation of these responses except where experimental conditions rendered proprioception inaccurate. These findings were supported by the work of Diener et al. (1984). However, the early work of Melvill-Jones and Watt (1971) and Watt (1976) had shown that vestibular receptors could generate substantial responses of leg muscles to vertical accelerations. More recently Allum and colleagues (Allum and Pfaltz, 1985; Keshner et al., 1987) have amassed several lines of evidence that vestibular input plays an important role in generating responses to relatively fast rotations of the support surface. Data described by Bussel et al. (1980) led them to a similar conclusion.

In their paper *Dietz et al.* present data on responses to uni- and bidirectional translations of the support surface which illustrate the good correspondence of muscle activation patterns with changes in ankle angle thus corroborating the likely role of proprioceptive signals in generating short latency responses to translations. They interpret the relatively less clear correspondence of response with head movements as evidence that vestibular signals are unlikely to contribute to the responses but the scale on which the data are plotted makes this difficult to verify. In any case, one cannot use data such as this to prove that vestibular signals do *not* contribute.

Allum et al. on the other hand, use a clever strategy to obtain evidence that vestibular responses *do* play a role in the responses they observe. They match translations and rotations so that they produce nearly identical ankle deflections and observe that the two types of stimulus produce quite different head movements and postural responses in leg, trunk and neck muscles. They thus obtain further strong evidence for a vestibular role in responses to *both* rotations and translations. It is important to note that the amplitude of their perturbations exceeds that typically employed by Nashner and his colleagues. Is is also not entirely clear that predictive mechanisms may not have contributed to the differences between rotations and translations although Allum claims that even the initial responses (not shown in the paper) differ.

Rather than a further exposition of experimental results, *Nashner et al.'s* paper is a theoretical analysis of how postural responses to both vestibular and proprioceptive input are likely to depend on stimulus parameters. It provides a framework for understanding how both Nashner and Allum could be correct under their particular experimental conditions. As shown in Nashner's Fig. 1, under conditions of quiet standing or small, slow translations, the head movements accompanying postural sway will be below semicircular canal threshold. While such sway will activate otolith organs, the signals that these receptors produce have an inherent ambiguity: as first pointed out by Nashner (1971, 1972), a given otolith signal can either indicate static tilt in one direction or dynamic falling in the opposite direction. It is therefore reasonable to believe that the central nervous system may not generate responses to otolith signals unless they are accompanied by other confirming inputs from other sensors. As the amplitude of perturbations increase, on the other hand, the diagram implicitly indicates that the vestibular signals arising from the head movements produced by these perturbations may generate postural responses once they are large enough to exceed semicircular canal threshold.

Allum's data indicate that his perturbations are indeed producing head movements that are sufficiently large to activate semicircular canal receptors. In the discussion, he and Nashner agreed that vestibular inputs were likely to be involved in the generation of the responses he reports. Thus the session led to the conclusion that vestibular signals are likely to contribute to postural responses except under conditions of minimal sway where head movements are too weak to activate semicircular canals.

It is worth pointing out in this review the aftershocks of an earlier dispute that was largely settled by a re-alignment of the positions of Nashner and Allum at the Barany Meeting in Bologna in 1987 (Pompeiano and Allum, 1988). Prior to that meeting, the publications of Nashner and colleagues (Nashner and McCollum, 1985; Horack and Nashner, 1986) had stressed two distinct patterns of response to translations, which they termed the ankle synergy and hip synergy. At the Barany Meeting, Nashner affirmed that the usual response to translation was in fact a mixture of the two synergies. In discussing differences between his responses and those reported by Allum to rota-

tions, he also pointed out that rotations would be expected to elicit an entirely different class of response. This clarification of the position of the Portland group helped to resolve the apparent differences between them and Allum on the issue of response synergies.

At this meeting Allum reported responses to translations for the first time. His "multilink strategy" would appear to correspond reasonably well with Nashner's mixed response, although the limited number of muscles studied by the Portland group make detailed comparisons difficult. Allum also found a very different pattern of response to rotations, which he called a "stiffening strategy". Nashner's earlier comments suggest that he would not be surprised by this difference. Still lacking is evidence by the Basel group for the pure ankle synergy described by Nashner (1976, 1977). This response, however, may only be seen in the small stimulus regime where head movements are subthreshold for semicircular canal activation. Recording responses over a wide range of translation amplitudes could resolve this remaining discrepancy.

In closing, I would like to indicate my satisfaction that many of the differences of opinion concerning postural responses to anterior – posterior perturbations are being resolved. Still to come is a more complete description of responses to a wide range of directions of perturbation. Also unresolved is the thorny issue of the role of predictive mechanisms in postural responses. Most studies thus far have employed perturbations whose parameters were either totally or partially predictable. The responses that they report may not be the simplest, most reflex-like responses of the system. Those will only be revealed when a study is done employing fully randomized perturbations. I think that it is not unlikely that such a study could reveal responses quite different from those heretofore described.

References

Allum, J.H.J. and Pfaltz, C.R. (1985) Visual and vestibular

contributions to pitch sway stabilization in the ankle muscles of normals and patients with bilateral peripheral vestibular deficits. *Exp. Brain Res.,* 58: 82–94.

Bussel, B., Katz, R., Pierrot-Deseilligny, E., Bergego, C. and Hayat, A. (1980) Vestibular and proprioceptive influences on the postural reactions to a sudden body displacement in man. In J.E. Desmedt (Ed.), *Spinal and Supraspinal Mechanisms of Voluntary Motor Control and Locomotion, Progress in Clinical Neurophysiology, Vol. 8,* Karger, Basel, pp. 310–322.

Diener, H.C. and Dichgans, J., Guschlbauer, B. and Mau, H. (1984) The significance of proprioception on postural stabilization as assessed by ischemia. *Brain Res.,* 296: 103–109.

Horak, F.B. and Nashner, L.M. (1986) Central program of postural movements: Adaptation to altered support-surface configurations. *J. Neurophysiol.,* 55: 1369–1381.

Keshner, E.A., Allum, J.H.J. and Pfaltz, C.R. (1987) Postural coactivation and adaptation in the sway stabilizing responses of normals and patients with bilateral peripheral vestibular deficit. *Exp. Brain Res.,* 69: 66–72.

Melvill Jones, G. and Watt, D.G.D. (1971) Observations on the control of stepping and hopping movements in man. *J. Physiol. (London),* 219: 709–727.

Nashner, L.M. (1971) A model describing vestibular detection of body sway motion. *Acta Otolaryngol. (Stockh).,* 72: 429–436.

Nashner, L.M. (1972) Vestibular postural control model. *Kybernetik,* 10: 106–110.

Nashner, L.M. (1976) Adapting reflexes controlling human posture. *Exp. Brain Res.,* 26: 59–72.

Nashner, L.M. (1977) Fixed patterns of rapid postural responses among leg muscles during stance. *Exp. Brain Res.,* 30: 13–24.

Nashner, L.M. and McCollum, G. (1985) The organization of human postural movements: A formal basis and experimental synthesis. *Brain Behav.,* 8: 135–172.

Nashner, L.M., Woollacott, M.H. and Tuma, G. (1979) Organization of rapid responses to postural and locomotor-like perturbations of standing man. *Exp. Brain Res.,* 36: 463–476.

Pompeiano, O., Allum, J.H.J. (Eds.) (1988) *Vestibulospinal Control of Posture and Locomotion, Prog. Brain Res., Vol. 76,* Elsevier, Amsterdam.

Watt, D.G.D. (1976) Response of cats to sudden falls: An otolith-originating reflex assisting landing. *J. Neurophysiol.,* 39: 257–265.

J.H.J. Allum and M. Hulliger (Eds.)
Progress in Brain Research, Vol. 80
© 1989 Elsevier Science Publishers B.V. (Biomedical Division)

CHAPTER 32

The role of stretch and vestibulo-spinal reflexes in the generation of human equilibriating reactions

J.H.J. Allum, F. Honegger and C.R. Pfaltz

Department of ORL, University Hospital, Basel, Switzerland

Equilibrating reactions in standing humans were examined for evidence that either vestibulo-spinal or proprioceptive long loop stretch reflexes from ankle muscles, or both, are responsible for the control and organization of rapid postural responses. Specifically, the hypothesis was tested that the same postural response could be evoked by rotation of the support surface that mimics the ankle rotation occurring during support surface translations. Rotation perturbations evoked postural responses in leg and trunk muscles that were different in strategy, synergy and coactivation from translation responses, even though the short-latency response in the stretched triceps surae muscles was equal in latency and size. Movement patterns consisted of a stiffening strategy and hardly any compensating ankle rotation for rotation stimuli, and a multi-link strategy with motion focused about the neck, hip and ankle joints for translation stimuli. Dorsiflexion rotations caused earlier and stronger responses in tibialis anterior and quadriceps muscles just post to the onset of paraspinal muscles, whereas rearward translation activated soleus and abdominals strongest, both just prior to hamstring muscles. Correlated activation strengths of agonist and antagonist activity was a common feature for both types of perturbation, albeit, only in the ankle muscles for rotations and only in the trunk muscles for translations. These data suggest that sensory inputs, other than those generated in the lower leg predominate, in the triggering and modulation of equilibrating reactions. Possible candidates are those of the vestibular system or proprioceptive inputs from the trunk.

Key words: Vestibulo-spinal reflex; Stretch reflex; Movement coordination; Postural control; Peripheral vestibular deficit; Head movement; Electromyographic activity

Introduction

When upright stance is disrupted a number of sensory systems, including those exciting vestibular and proprioceptive afferents, signal the onset and direction of the destabilizing forces. The equilibrating reactions that result could be controlled centrally in a number of ways. One possibility is that the timing and strength of muscular activity and the resulting movement coordination pattern between body segments (termed here "strategy", cf. Horak and Nashner, 1986) are highly dependent on features of the incoming sensory input. Another possibility is that both muscular activity and movement coordina-tion are centrally preprogrammed and only triggered by the sensory input. A common feature of these different types of motor command is the origin of the effector sensory input.

Several authors have suggested that the primary reflex pathway underlying equilibrating reactions in man is the long-loop stretch reflex originating in ankle muscles (Nashner, 1976; Diener et al., 1983; Dietz et al., 1987). Alternatives include vestibulo-spinal reflexes, as emphasized by Allum and Pfaltz (1985), or proprioceptive signals from the neck or trunk. If the pattern of muscle activation and resulting movement strategy re-establishing equilibrium is the result of sensory inputs originating in the lower leg, then the same postural response should be elicited by different categories of support surface movements which stretch the ankle muscles, rotate the ankle, and pressure load the sole of the foot similarly, regardless of resulting head and trunk motion. Such was the case in cat where the same linked activation of muscle responses (termed here the "synergy") was obtained under these stimulation conditions (Macpherson et al., 1986). These authors concluded that proprioceptive inputs from the lower leg triggered centrally preprogrammed postural responses to stance disturbances.

The present study sought to test in man whether stretch responses at the ankle joint are the effector signal for postural reactions. For this purpose, responses to rearward support surface translation which causes forward body sway and ankle dorsiflexion were compared with responses to direct rotation of the feet about the ankle joint. The two types of stimuli were adjusted to have equal amounts of ankle rotation and therefore triceps surae muscle stretch, though with oppositely directed, initial stimulus-related, head and trunk accelerations. Strategy and synergy observed in the responses was found to be fundamentally different for rotation and translation stimuli. Thus these data suggest that sensory inputs from the head and/or trunk are responsible for the control and organization of rapid postural responses in the standing human.

Methods

The techniques employed in this study expanded on those described in detail in previous publications (Allum and Pfaltz, 1985; Keshner et al., 1987). The developments specific for this project concerned the addition of linear translation of the support surface on which subjects stood, the direct measurement of lower leg rotation with respect to the support surface with a potentiometer system (lower leg angle in Fig. 1), and a change in the initial stance of subjects. In our previous research, subjects were asked to lean back slightly prior to each perturbation. In this study they were asked to stand in their "upright" position.

Since the aim of this study was to compare the responses to rearward translation and direct toe-up rotation of the support surface under identical conditions of ankle rotation, considerable care was taken to ensure that 3 degrees of rotation occurred with comparable stretch velocities. The linear translation amplitude, 4 cm, and velocity, 21 cm/s, produced changes of perturbation in lower leg angle higher in peak (40 cf. 34 deg/s) but lower in average velocity (21 cf. 25 deg/s) than the 3.4 degree 27 deg/s support surface rotations. Amplitudes of ankle rotation were, on average, equal to 3 degrees. A series of 11 rotations followed by 11 translations was presented to each subject first under eyes-open conditions, then repeated with eyes closed.

EMG activity of ankle, thigh, lower trunk and neck muscles was recorded from 7 normal subjects and 2 subjects with bilateral peripheral vestibular deficit and then analysed for specific patterns of muscular activity. In addition to standard recordings from tibialis anterior, soleus and trapezius (see Keshner et al., 1987), recordings were also taken from biceps femoris (hamstrings), rectus femoris (quadriceps), rectus abdominis and lumbar paraspinalis. The lower trunk surface EMG electrodes were placed just above the waistline, 4 cm apart.

Subjects were instructed to stand first in a comfortable upright position with knees locked and hands by the side. A reference torque signal measured with strain gauges imbedded in the support surface and displayed on an oscilloscope mounted at eye level 1 m from the subject provided a constant guide on deviations from the upright. The subjects were instructed to return quickly to upright on onset of a perturbation.

Offline, EMG responses were individually analysed for response latencies, referred to the time of the first inflexion in the ankle torque trace (see vertical dashed line in Figs. 1 and 3). Responses consistently occurring after 85 ms but before 200 ms were termed medium latency (ML) responses, whereas those whose onset was earlier were termed short latency (SL) responses. The area under a burst of ML EMG activity was calculated as the area between time of the average individual muscle and subject onset latency until 80 ms later. Average EMG activity over the 100 ms before the perturbation was subtracted prior to area calculations. Average values of response latencies and areas were computed for the first 3 and last 8 of a series of 11 trials with one type of perturbation in order to take adaptation effects into account (Keshner et al., 1987; Nashner et al., 1982).

Results

Multi-link and stiffening strategies

Rearward translation of the support surface causes from the very first perturbation a characteristic set of leg, trunk and head movements different from those induced by support surface rotation despite an equal angle of imposed ankle dorsiflexion. The resulting differences in biomechanical recordings are shown in Fig. 1. Those for rearward translation may be best understood by assuming the hips remain stationary in space for the first 100 ms, that is, are thrust forward relative to the support base. Thus, a dorsiflexion at the ankle and hip extension is induced. As the hips are thrust forward, the head and trunk pitch are accelerated backwards after a short pulse of forward-pitching head acceleration associated with the platform acceleration (see top two, acceleration traces, in Fig. 1). Fig. 1 also documents that relative movements of the head on the trunk are small over the first 100 ms following the support surface movement (third trace from top in Fig. 1).

Compensatory action opposing the stimulus induced body sway commences at approximately 150 ms from stimulus onset for both translation and rotation stimuli. For translation the changes in ankle torque and shear force (latter not shown in Fig. 1) resulting from the hips being thrust back coincide with fast trunk motion pitching forwards and a return of the lower leg angle to upright. As illustrated in Fig. 1, an overshoot, past upright, of

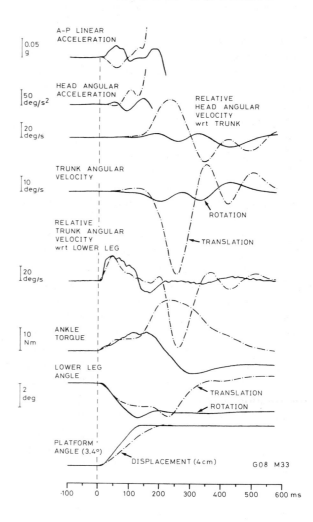

Fig. 1. Biomechanical changes and equilibriating movements induced by rotating (solid lines) and translating (interrupted line) the support surface. All traces are from one normal subject. Each trace is the average of the last 8 of a series of 11 trials. Head and trunk movements were measured with angular accelerometers, lower leg ankle with a potentiometer system. An upward deflection of the head, trunk and lower leg traces in the figure indicates backwards pitching. Increasing plantar flexion torque on the support surface is represented by an upward deflection of the ankle torque curve. Note that the compensating changes in ankle torque are different, and trunk angular velocity is considerably larger for translation compared to rotation responses, despite an equal amplitude and velocity of lower leg angle changes.

the initial lower leg inclination almost always occurs. Simultaneously, the head pitches backwards on the trunk, thus maintaining gaze direction, though the head is not stable in space. Because the equilibrating action compensating for support surface translation involves rotations about each of the principal rotation axes, ankle, hip and neck, we have termed it a "multi-link" strategy, though the term "ankle-hip" strategy would not be inappropriate.

Toe-up rotation of the support surface elicits a completely different movement strategy (see Fig. 1) which we have termed a "stiffening" strategy. Despite an equal amount of ankle dorsiflexion and equal, if oppositely directed head accelerations being imposed for rotation, the compensatory rotation velocities of body segments are an order of magnitude less than those for translation (see Fig. 2). Essentially, the rotation of the support surface is mostly absorbed at the ankle joint though it is evident from the traces of Fig. 1 that the hips are thrust backwards by the toe-up rotation. From these traces it can be observed that the trunk and head pitch forwards, after an initial stimulus-induced backwards pitching, and the lower legs rotate backwards. Two aspects of the lower leg angle trace confirm the assumption of rearward hip motion for rotation stimuli. Firstly, the lower leg angle displacement (the angle between the lower leg and support surface) is less than the total platform rotation, and secondly, the lower legs continue to rotate backwards on cessation of the stimulus rotation. A rapid change in plantar flexion torque at 150 ms arrests this rearward motion. Simultaneously forward pitch of the trunk terminates. No further correction for the induced ankle dorsiflexion occurs presumably because the body is held stable in an upright position.

The two movement strategies, multi-link and stiffening, are very different despite comparable changes imposed at the ankle joint. Fig. 2 documents peak-to-peak amplitudes of trunk velocity and head velocity, with respect to that of the trunk, which are much larger in response to translations. Since the translations followed a series of rotations, it might be argued that the stiffening strategy to rotation might be retained as a compensating action by central nervous structures for the first few trials of translation. The averaging techniques employed in this study, averaging responses to the first 3 trials separate from those of the succeeding 8 trials, were designed to reveal such adaptation effects. The data plotted in Fig. 2 include both averages. A clustering of the data points for the first 3 trials to translation near to the data for rotation trials, or even separate from those of the second 8 trials is not observed either for peak forward-pitching trunk velocity, or rearward pitch of the head on the trunk. In short, the appropriate strategy appears to be dependent on the direction of trunk and head acceleration, and is executed from the very first compensatory response.

Muscle synergies underlying multi-link and stiffening strategies

Muscle activation patterns recorded in the trunk and leg muscles were consistent with the intersegmental movements caused by the perturbation and the compensation strategy utilized to reestablish upright posture. Fig. 3 shows that in response to translation soleus, hamstrings, and abdominal muscles were the earliest and predominant muscles activated of the antagonist pair recorded at the lower leg, thigh and trunk. When the hips were thrust backward by toe-up rotation tibialis anterior (TA), quadriceps and paraspinal muscles provided the earliest and predominant responses. Excepted from these observations on latencies are the short latency (SL) stretch reflex responses in soleus, and the early 80 ms responses latencies seen in the quadriceps muscle of some subjects (see Fig. 3). As Fig. 3 illustrates, the soleus SL responses are common to rotation and translation. In Fig. 3 the increased EMG activity occurring in response to rotation, over that present for translation is shown in black. The excess response for translation is shown hatched.

As documented in Fig. 3, multi-link and stiffen-

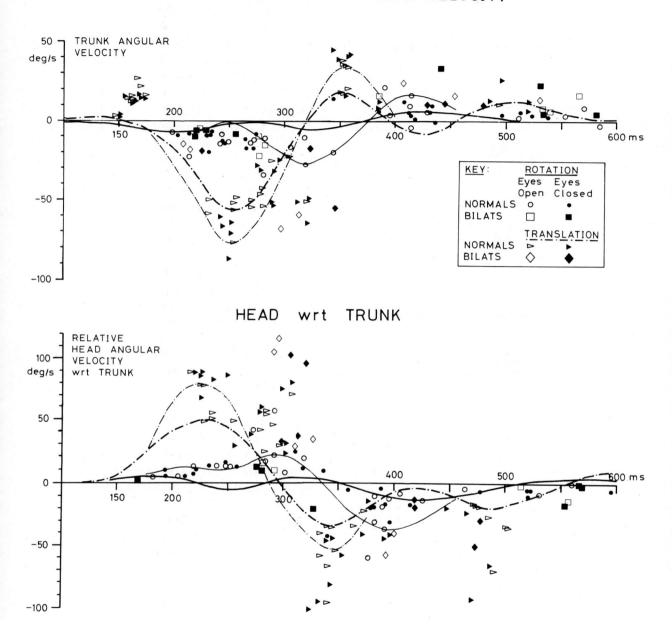

Fig. 2. Peak trunk and head-on-trunk angular velocities indicating different equilibriating strategies in response to rotations and translations of the support surface. The maximum and minimum velocities were calculated from average traces of the 1st 3 and 2nd 8 trials and plotted against the time when the maximum or minimum occurred. Typical examples of average traces for the 1st 3 and 2nd 8 trials are provided as guides. The traces with full lines are for rotation, the interrupted traces are translation. Of the two pairs of traces, the thinner trace with larger amplitudes is for the 1st 3 trials. The maximum absolute trunk and head on trunk velocities are approximately 10 deg/s for rotation and an order of magnitude larger for translation. Inset indicates visual conditions and subject category associated with each data point symbol.

404

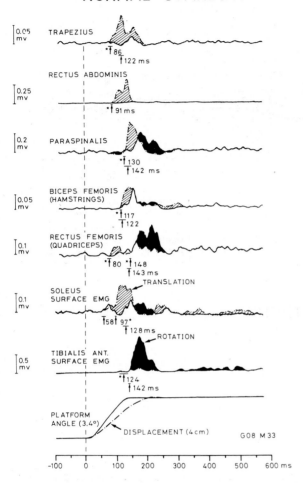

NORMAL-STANDING

Fig. 3. Muscle response patterns of a normal subject to rotations and translations. Same subject as in Fig. 1. The traces are average EMG responses for the 2nd 8 trials. Differences between the means of the EMG curves are shown as a filled area when the rotation response was larger, as a hatched area when the translation response was larger. The zero latency reference is given by a vertical dashed line, and corresponds to the first inflexion of ankle torque (see Fig. 1). Average values of EMG burst-onset latencies are marked by a vertical arrow, one standard deviation by a horizontal bar above the arrow. The upper set of latencies (marked with an asterisk) below each trace correspond to translation responses, the lower set for rotation responses, except for SL onset in soleus which was equal in latency for rotation and translation.

ing strategies are easily identified on the basis of activation synergies in the lower leg and trunk muscles. The differences in muscle synergies are less distinct in the quadriceps, hamstrings and neck extensor (trapezius) muscles. These latter muscles have overlapping periods of muscle activity in response to rotation and translation. Fig. 4 documents for all subjects tested the different activation patterns observed in response to rotation and translation as medium latency (ML) responses in lower leg muscles. The upper part of the figure plots the onset of the TA ML response against that of soleus. The lower part of Fig. 4 plots the ML response areas measured under the first 80 ms of each EMG response. The separation of the data points for rotation and translation in Fig. 4 indicate significant differences with respect to coactivation at the ankle joint for these stimuli. Translation responses consist of a sequential activation of soleus and then after 40 ms, or even later, TA. There is no significant covariation between response amplitudes as measured by EMG ML areas. Rotation responses, in contrast, appear, from both the onset latencies within one standard deviation of each other and the significant linear correlation between response areas, to be coactivated. The broken line in the upper part of Fig. 4 indicates exactly equal onset latencies. A similar coactivation effect, albeit with subjects initially leaning back slightly prior to onset of the support surface rotation, has been described previously (Keshner et al., 1987). Vision had no apparent effect on the ankle muscle synergies. The filled symbols representing eyes-closed responses in Fig. 4 are scattered among open symbols (for eyes open).

The subjects with vestibular deficits had reduced TA responses to rotation (see square symbols in Fig. 4) as reported previously (Keshner et al., 1987). If the soleus response to translation were assumed to be a vestibulo-spinal response to head accelerations opposite in direction to those occurring with support surface rotations, the soleus responses, like the TA responses, should also be depressed in vestibularly deficient subjects. Surprisingly, the soleus response in these subjects was not affected in area, only its onset was slightly delayed with respect to normal responses.

Fig. 3 shows a fundamental difference between the activation of trunk muscles for the two types of support surface perturbation. For rotation, the ab-

dominal muscle response is absent and that of paraspinalis, straightening the back, has a delayed response. This typical example is shown to be representative of the normal population by the data in Fig. 5. Fig. 5 presents the delays and coactivation between abdominals and paraspinalis for all translation responses as averages for the first 3 and second 8 trials. This data demonstrates that the trunk muscle synergy is constant from the very first response as noted above for the movement strategy. Otherwise, both the onset delays and EMG amplitudes of the ML responses depicted in Fig. 5 would consist of two separate clusters of

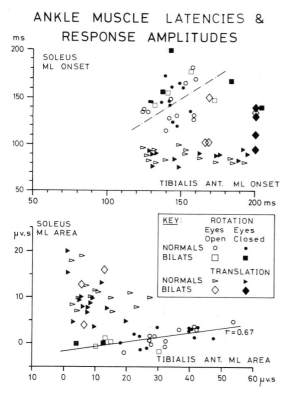

Fig. 4. Response amplitudes and latencies for soleus (SOL) and tibialis anterior (TA) muscles following a rotation or a translation perturbation to stance. In the upper part of the figure SOL ML onset is plotted against TA ML onset, equal onset is marked by the dash-dot line. Several TA responses to translation for the vestibular deficit patients had onset latencies over 200 ms. These are plotted as 200 ms. The lower part of the figure shows plots of the area of the first 80 ms of the response. Rotation response areas had a significant linear correlation. The plots illustrate an earlier larger response in SOL for translation, a coactivated action of SOL and TA for rotation with TA the larger response. Inset indicates visual conditions and subject category associated with each data point symbol. Since for some subjects responses were absent in the less active, antagonist muscle of the two, less data points than subjects (9) × averages (4) are present.

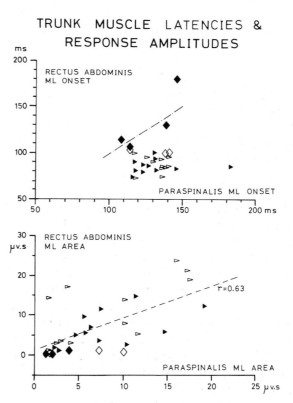

Fig. 5. Response amplitudes and latencies for rectus abdominis (ABDOM) and paraspinalis (PARAS) muscles after a translation. No responses were observed in ABDOM recordings for rotation. The dash-dot line in the upper part of the figure marks equal onset latencies. ABDOM responses are some 50 ms earlier than PARAS, though significantly correlated in EMG area as shown in the lower part of the figure. See Fig. 4 for explanation of symbols.

data, one for the first 3 trials, another for the second 8 trials.

A strong coactivation of the trunk muscles is suggested by the data in Fig. 5. Although abdominis occurs some 40 ms prior to paraspinalis, the range of both onset latencies is small suggesting a fixed coactivation delay. The concept of coactivation is further supported by the linear correlation between the trunk muscles' response areas shown in the lower part of Fig. 5. Such a covariation is conspicuously absent from the ankle muscle response to translation (see Fig. 4).

Under eyes-closed conditions, which eliminates visual feedback, vestibularly deficient subjects could cope with translation perturbations relatively easier than with rotations. The magnitude of their compensating trunk rotations, thrusting the hips backward, was not less than those of normals but only delayed (see Fig. 2). Assuming that the abdominal muscles generate the forward trunk rotation, Fig. 5 presents two possible causes for this delay. Firstly, the abdominal responses are delayed with respect to normals, so that the response begins when that of paraspinalis commences. Secondly, the abdominal muscle response is reduced in these subjects.

Synergies across body segments were examined by calculating the difference between the onset delays of the major muscles involved with each strategy: soleus, hamstrings, abdominals for the multi-link or ankle-hip strategy; and TA, quadriceps and paraspinalis in the stiffening strategy. Fig. 6 plots these differences with the more distal muscle onset subtracted from the more proximal onset. If muscle contractions commenced in the lower leg and then radiated in a distal to proximal sequence to the thigh and trunk muscles as proposed by Horak and Nashner (1986), then the delays depicted in Fig. 6 should be positive. The lower part of Fig. 6 reveals that for the main activators of the multi-link strategy, the intersegmental delays are near zero and indicate a simultaneous activation of soleus and abdominal muscles, followed shortly thereafter by hamstring muscles. A similar result has been established by Keshner et

al. (1988). The scatter away from near zero intersegmental delay was provided almost exclusively by vestibularly deficient subjects.

For rotations, fixed intersegmental activation delays across subjects were not observed to underlie the stiffening strategy. Both normal and vestibularly deficient subjects had activation delays in a proximal to distal order. TA and quadriceps were active simultaneously at an interval after the onset of paraspinalis. As indicated by the regression line in the upper part of Fig. 6, this interval was fixed for one subject but varied between subjects. Interestingly, the intersegmental

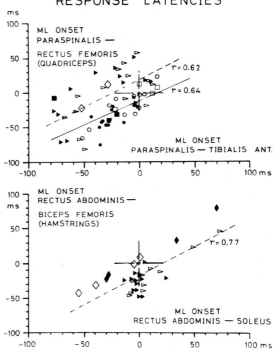

Fig. 6. Synergy of onset latencies across body segments. Differences in response latencies between muscles' primarily active during the stiffening strategy correcting a toe-up rotation perturbation are plotted in the upper part of the figure. In the lower part of the figure differences in response latencies are plotted for those muscles primarily active during the multi-link strategy correcting a rearward translation perturbation. Symbols as in Fig. 4.

delays changed only with respect to quadriceps when these muscles were active as antagonists during the multi-link strategy (dashed regression line in the upper part of Fig. 6). Although the onset of paraspinalis occurred earlier in response to support surface translation, its delay with respect to TA was not affected. A common feature of response strategies to both rotation and translation was an intersegmental synergy programmed as trunk before ankle muscle onset.

Discussion

This study indicates that rotation of the support surface which mimics the dorsiflexion ankle rotation occurring during rearward support surface translation is not sufficient to evoke the multi-link movement strategy and its underlying muscle synergy elicited during translation. The stiffening strategy evoked by rotation is so fundamentally different from the multi-link strategy that neither muscle spindle receptors in lower leg muscles, ankle joint receptors, nor pressure receptors at the sole of the foot appear to trigger or modulate human equilibriating reactions to a significant degree. The precise nature of the necessary and sufficient sensory inputs that trigger and/or modulate the underlying patterns of muscle activity is not yet clear. However, the biomechanical recordings shown in Figs. 1 and 2 highlight differences in stimulus-evoked movements that might lead to activation of different groups of muscles and ensuing compensatory reactions.

Before considering the stimulus-evoked movements, it is important to consider the patterns or "synergies" of muscle activity observed in this study. In previous studies, the onset times of EMG responses elicited by a support surface movement were grouped into three epochs of short, medium, and long latency (Allum and Pfaltz, 1985). The short latency (SL) responses were usually of brief duration and small amplitude. For the soleus and TA muscles these occurred in the period 40 to 120 ms from stimulus onset and could commence as early as 40 ms in soleus and 78 ms in TA depending

on the prior state of activation in each muscle. In the present study the SL response in soleus is common to both translation and rotation perturbations, but the SL TA response was seldom observed since TA is often not active when subjects stand in their perceived upright position. Though this early activity in soleus and TA does not appear to produce any measurable biomechanical effect, careful analysis can demonstrate an appreciable smoothing effect of the SL soleus response on the mechanical responses of stretched ankle muscles (Allum and Mauritz, 1984).

Medium latency (ML) responses occurred in many muscles following rotation or translation of the support surface. By comparing Figs. 1 and 3, it is evident that these responses are well-correlated in timing and amplitude (EMG area) with torques exerted on the support surface, and rotations at the ankle joint, trunk and head. Thus these responses, termed here "equilibriating" or "compensatory" responses, result in significant biomechanical consequences for the maintenance of stance. From observations of the biomechanical consequences and antagonist-agonist, pair-wise recordings of muscle activity at each joint we have concluded that the soleus, hamstring and abdominal muscles predominate in compensating for stance perturbations induced by rearward support surface translations, and TA, quadriceps and paraspinal muscles predominate in arresting body sway induced by toe-up support surface rotations. In our previous work on rotation responses only those occurring after 120 ms were termed ML responses (Keshner et al., 1987). Clearly the observation of responses to translation commencing as early as 85 ms and lasting another 100 ms requires a revision of the 120 ms onset as the identifying characteristic of ML responses. Here this definition has been revised so that the first muscle response causing significant biomechanical consequences for the maintenance of stance is termed the ML response. The previous description of long latency (LL) responses, as those occurring after 200 ms, need not be altered on the basis of the current work. The effect of LL responses is not as easily quantified from biomechanical recordings as ML responses, though the soleus LL EMG response in ankle muscles has been postulated to underlie braking movements which follow the initial postural response (Keshner et al., 1987).

Differences in the ML response synergies of pairs of agonist-antagonist muscles acting across the ankle joint and at the trunk were observed. Soleus and TA responses demonstrated several characteristics of coactivation for rotation, linked onsets, covariation of amplitudes, and none at all for translation (Fig. 4). In contrast abdominals and paraspinals were coactivated in response to translation, but no abdominal response to rotation, i.e. a complete lack of coactivation, was observed (Fig. 5). The aforementioned differences in the predominant muscle synergies and coactivation patterns, noted for the multi-link and stiffening strategies elicited by translation and rotation perturbations respectively, provide the strongest evidence for the hypothesis that sensory inputs other than those generated in the lower legs determine the organization of the equilibrating strategy.

If one can exclude proprioceptive inputs from the lower legs, what then are the necessary and sufficient sensory inputs to trigger and/or modulate the appropriate synergy and movement strategy? The most effective receptors must rapidly detect the occurrence and direction of body movements. Thus sensory systems registering differences in polarity and having early onsets, such as those registering stimulus-related accelerations, would be the best candidates to trigger the multi-link, translation-evoked and the stiffening, rotation-evoked strategies. Visual inputs can be excluded as a candidate since these have no measurable effect on the responses of normals. Also sensory inputs from the neck are not a likely candidate since relative motion of the head on the neck changes little during the first 100 ms after stimulus onset (see Fig. 1). Reviewing Fig. 1, it appears that the vestibular system registering head accelerations is an ideal candidate because vestibular afferents have early onsets (20 ms) and receive oppositely

directed changes for translation and rotation perturbations. Indeed our previous work, comparing the responses of normals and vestibularly deficient subjects has suggested that vestibular afferents excited by head angular accelerations play a major role in the control and organization of equilibrating reactions to rotation perturbations (Allum et al., 1988). Whether or not these latter results can be extended to translation perturbations requires further investigation. The number of vestibularly deficient subjects examined in this study was too small to permit definitive conclusions. A tendency for reduced abdominal responses was observed. In contrast, soleus responses to translation were only marginally affected by a vestibular deficit. Trunk angular accelerations could also excite a number of proprioceptive sensory systems appropriate to generate the correct compensating reaction. Among the sensory systems transducing these accelerations are stretch receptors in the hip and trunk muscles as well as joint receptors at the hip joint and in the spinal column. At this point it would be useful to conduct experiments distinguishing between the contributions of sensory systems excited by trunk and head accelerations.

Once the question of the reflexogenic sensory input (or inputs) underlying equilibrating responses is answered, future research could be targeted towards examining the number of centrally organized strategies, and the extent to which the associated muscle synergies are modulated by incoming sensory signals. Whether or not the strategies are limited in number as suggested by Horak and Nashner (1986) or can be modulated on a continuous scale by sensory inputs could then be investigated more directly. In conclusion, this study has described two equilibrating strategies appropriate to correct for induced body sway following two types of support surface perturbations. These perturbations had an equal effect on ankle angle, but opposite effects on head and trunk accelerations. It was demonstrated that the reflex circuitry responsible for controlling equilibrium attaches a greater weighting to sensory signals excited by trunk and head accelerations when forming the appropriate strength and synergy of muscle commands. Specifically, sensory signals generated by ankle rotation appear to have a minor role to play in equilibriating reactions.

Acknowledgement

This research was supported by Swiss National Science Foundation grant 3.148-0.85.

References

Allum, J.H.J. and Mauritz, K.H. (1984) Compensation for intrinsic muscle stiffness by short-latency reflexes in human triceps surae muscles. *J. Neurophysiol.,* 52: 797 – 818.

Allum, J.H.J. and Pfaltz, C.R. (1985) Visual and vestibular contributions to pitch sway stabilization in the ankle muscles of normals and patients with bilateral peripheral vestibular deficits. *Exp. Brain Res.,* 58: 82 – 94.

Allum, J.H.J., Keshner, E.A., Honegger, F. and Pfaltz, C.R. (1988) Indicators of the influence a peripheral vestibular deficit has on vestibulo-spinal reflex responses controlling postural stability. *Acta Otolaryngol. (Stockh.),* 106: 252 – 263.

Diener, H.C., Bootz, F., Dichgans, J. and Bruzek, W. (1983) Variability of postural reflexes in humans. *Exp. Brain Res.,* 52: 423 – 428.

Dietz, V., Quintern, J. and Sillen, M. (1987) Stumbling reactions in man: significance of proprioceptive and preprogrammed mechanisms. *J. Physiol. (London),* 386: 149 – 163.

Horak, F.B. and Nashner, L.M. (1986) Central programming of postural movements: adaptation to altered support-surface configuration. *J. Neurophysiol.,* 55: 1369 – 1381.

Keshner, E.A., Allum, J.H.J. and Pfaltz, C.R. (1987) Postural coactivation and adaptation in the sway stabilizing responses of normals and patients with bilateral vestibular deficit. *Exp. Brain Res.,* 69: 77 – 92.

Keshner, E.A., Woollacott, M.H. and Debu, B. (1988) Neck and trunk muscle responses during postural perturbations in humans. *Exp. Brain Res.,* 71: 455 – 466.

Macpherson, J.M., Rushmer, D.S. and Dunbar, D.C. (1986) Postural responses in the cat to unexpected rotation of the support surface: evidence for a centrally generated synergic organization. *Exp. Brain Res.,* 62: 152 – 160.

Nashner, L.M. (1976) Adapting reflexes controlling the human posture. *Exp. Brain Res.,* 26: 59 – 72.

Nashner, L.M., Black, F.O. and Wall, III C. (1982) Adaptation to altered support and visual conditions during stance: patients with vestibular deficits. *J. Neurosci.,* 2: 536 – 544.

J.H.J. Allum and M. Hulliger (Eds.)
Progress in Brain Research, Vol. 80
© 1989 Elsevier Science Publishers B.V. (Biomedical Division)

CHAPTER 33

Organization of posture controls: an analysis of sensory and mechanical constraints

L.M. Nashner, C.L. Shupert, F.B. Horak and F.O. Black

The R.S. Dow Neurological Sciences Institute and the Department of Neuro-otology of Good Samaritan Hospital and Medical Center, 1120 N.W. 20th Ave. Portland, OR 97209, U.S.A.

We analyse two components of posture control in standing human subjects: (1) the mechanical properties which constrain the body's ability to execute stabilizing postural movements and (2) the mechanical and neural properties which constrain the ability of the vestibular system to sense changes in body orientation. Rules are then proposed to describe the central organization of posture controls within the sensory and mechanical constraints. The organizational rules and knowledge of constraints are combined to predict the effects of selective semicircular canal and utricular otolith lesions on postural stability and the patterns of body and head movements used to maintain balance. Our analysis leads to the prediction that semicircular canal and otolith deficits destabilize patients at different frequencies, and force them to use different patterns of body and head movements. These predictions are compared to posture controls observed in patients with different types of vestibular deficits. The additional steps required to prove or disprove the theory are discussed.

Key words: Posture; Vestibular system; Biomechanics; Vestibular deficit; Movement coordination

Introduction

The central neural mechanisms responsible for maintaining the body centre of gravity over the base of support during stance are constrained by two external factors. Ability to detect errors in position of the body's centre of gravity is limited by the transductive properties of the visual, vestibular, and somatosensory inputs to posture. Mechanical properties of the body and configuration of the support surface limit ability to move the body centre of gravity in response to the detected errors in position. In the present chapter, we analyse the sensory and mechanical constraints on posture and develop a formalism for predicting the effects of these constraints on the neural mechanisms of posture control. While the primary forcus of this chapter is the organization of vestibular inputs, the formalism can be expanded to include visual and somatosensory inputs.

The contribution of the vestibular system to balance is constrained by the threshold properties and the dynamic characteristics of the semicircular canals and utricular otoliths. Canal acceleration thresholds as low as 0.05 deg/s^2 were reported for the oculogyral illusion during very low frequency stimulation (Clark and Stewart, 1969; Doty, 1969). Threshold for otolith perception of horizontal linear accelerations below 0.015 Hz averaged 0.005 g (Meiry, 1966). Nashner (1971) combined the above minimum threshold values with second order models of canal and otolith dynamics to calculate the minimum sway angles detectable by the canals and otoliths as functions of the sway frequency.

Previous theoretical (Nashner and McCollum, 1985) and experimental (Horak and Nashner, 1986) studies suggested that the automatic postural movements supporting erect stance are organized using one or a combination of two basic patterns. The "ankle" pattern relies on large torsional moments about the ankle joints to accelerate the body centre of gravity forward and backward. When the ankle pattern is used, the amplitude and frequency of the centre of gravity motions are constrained by mechanical limits on the ankle torque. The ankle pattern is effective for maintaining forward and backward leaning positions and for moving the centre of gravity within an arc of approximately 12 degrees. Centre of gravity movements within this region of stability, however, are constrained to low frequencies because the moment of body inertia about the ankles is large.

The "hip" pattern relies on torsional movements about the hips to rotate the ankle and hip joints in opposite directions. Because this pattern uses transient inertial forces to move the centre of gravity, it cannot maintain forward and backward leaning positions or move the centre of gravity over large distances. Hip movements, however, move the centre of gravity rapidly. And, they are effective when standing on small support surface areas and when the centre of gravity is positioned near the limits of stability (Moore et al., 1986).

In the present chapter, we develop a formal approach to the study of posture control which incorporates the mechanics of body sway, and the threshold and dynamic characteristics of the vestibular organs. Four rules define how the neural controls are organized in relation to these constraints. The formalism and organizational rules are then combined to predict how normal subjects detect and control sway motions of the body in a variety of sensory conditions. The validity of these predictions is tested by comparing them with experimental observations. Finally, the formalism is used to predict how selective canal and otolith deficits might alter stability and patterns of body and head movement. These predictions are compared to previous clinical observations, and issues for future research are discussed.

Analysis of sensory and mechanical constraints

Simplifying assumptions

Mathematical calculations to define constraints on the ability to sense body sway motions and move the body centre of gravity over the base of support are based on two simplifying assumptions. First, body sway is sinusoidal and confined to the antero-posterior plane. This assumption allows variations in sway amplitudes and frequencies, and gives results which generalize to all types of oscillatory motion. Second, postural movements are limited to the ankle and hip joints. This assumption simplifies the mechanical analysis. It is justified by experimental observations showing that automatic postural movements are normally executed with little if any knee joint motion (Nashner and McCollum, 1985; Horak and Nashner, 1986; Nashner, 1986).

Interactions between the sensory and mechanical constraints are analysed by graphing constraint boundaries in amplitude-frequency space (Figs. 1–3). The vertical axis of the space represents the peak to peak (P-P) amplitude of sway motions with respect to vertical. The horizontal axis represents the frequency of sway motions.

Mechanical constraints on ankle sway

Constraints on the amplitudes and frequencies of centre of gravity sway using the pure ankle pattern are illustrated in Fig. 1. The solid line shows regions of the amplitude-frequency space within which the centre of gravity can be moved with the ankle pattern. This constraint results from the upper limit on ankle torque. Ankle torque is limited, in turn, by the length of the feet in relation to the body height and total mass. Torque during postural sway is not limited by the ankle muscle strength, as the forces produced during running and jumping are much larger (Cavanagh and LaFortune, 1980; Valiant and Cavanagh, 1984).

For sway frequencies below 0.2 Hz the maximum sway angle is limited by the torque necessary

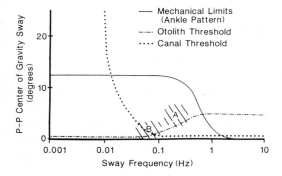

Fig. 1. The mechanical and sensory constraints on the ankle pattern of sway. The vertical axis shows the amplitude of sway. The horizontal axis shows the frequency of sway. The solid line shows the limits of stability for sway at the body centre of gravity. Dotted and dashed lines show the threshold boundaries for sensing sway with the canals and otoliths, respectively. Area A shows amplitudes and frequencies typical of sway in the absence of useful visual and somatosensory inputs. Area B shows typical sway with normal visual and somatosensory inputs.

to resist the destabilizing effects of gravity. As the rate of sway increases, the additional torque required to overcome the inertia of the body rapidly reduces the maximum sway amplitude (Gurfinkel and Osevets, 1972).

Mechanical constraints on hip sway

The solid line in Fig. 2 illustrates upper limits on the amplitudes and frequencies of centre of gravity sway when the pure hip movement pattern is used. The maximum amplitude of the centre of gravity sway is approximately 3 degrees. This limit depends on the range of hip joint motion and the relative inertial properties of the trunk and legs.

Centre of gravity sway motions with the hip pattern are constrained to a range of frequencies between approximately 0.5 and 2.5 Hz. Stable hip sway is not possible below approximately 0.5 Hz, because the hip pattern relies on transient inertial forces which at low frequencies cannot resist the low frequency destabilizing effects of gravity. High frequency hip sway is limited by the strength of hip joint muscles in relation to the inertial properties of the trunk and legs. Experimental obser-

vations and mechanical analysis suggest that the natural frequency of hip sway is approximately 1.5 Hz (McCollum and Leen, 1989).

Constraints on combined ankle and hip sway

The ankle and hip movement patterns can be combined to expand the limits of stability up to 3 degrees beyond the ankle sway stability limits. This is because hip movements are equally effective with the body centred over the feet, or leaning forward or backward to the limits of stability (Moore et al, 1986; Nashner and McCollum, 1985). And, because the frequencies of the combined ankle and hip components can differ, the additional 3 degrees of stability can be added at any point along the limits of stability boundary.

Constraints on sensing sway

Threshold boundaries for the vertical semicircular canals and utricular otoliths were based on the following assumptions. The head is fixed to the trunk. The input acceleration signal of each receptor is transformed into an output by passing through a second order dynamic filter and then through a threshold. Parameter values for the dynamic and threshold characteristics were taken from the literature cited in the Introduction. Final-

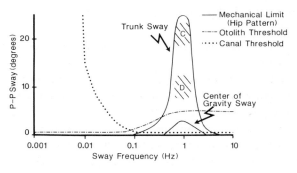

Fig. 2. The mechanical and sensory constraints on the hip pattern of sway. The two solid lines show the limits of stability for sway measured at the body centre of gravity and at the trunk. The dotted and dashed lines show the threshold boundaries for sensing sway with the canals and otoliths, respectively. Shaded area C shows typical trunk sway during the hip pattern. Shaded area D shows typical amplitudes and frequencies of head rotation during hip sway.

ly, we assumed that the resulting output signals must be above threshold during one-quarter of each cycle to be useful as feedback signals. The resulting canal and otolith threshold constraints are plotted in relation to the ankle sway constraints in the amplitude-frequency space of Fig. 1.

The response characteristics of the canals limit the use of angular acceleration as a feedback signal to sway frequencies above 0.1 Hz. The otolith constraint, in contrast, limits the use of linear acceleration as a feedback signal to low sway frequencies. Otolith information at sway frequencies above 0.5 Hz is available but ambiguous. This is because the otolith signal does not distinguish between tangential acceleration of the head in one direction and head tilt in the opposite direction (Nashner, 1971).

During hip sway, linear and angular motions of the head (fixed to the trunk) are approximately 10-times larger than those of the centre of gravity, although the movement frequencies of the two components are the same. To analyse the effects of sensory constraints on feedback control of the hip pattern, the mechanical limits are graphed in terms of the trunk sway amplitudes and frequencies (second solid line in Fig. 2). Dotted and dashed lines identical to those in Fig. 1 show the canal and otolith threshold constraints relative to the angle and frequency of the trunk motions.

Sensory constraints on coordinated head movements

During ankle sway, hip sway, or combinations of the two patterns the head can rotate in relation to the trunk to decrease (or increase) its amplitude of rotation in relation to gravity. Decreasing head rotation in relation to gravity, however, reduces the angular acceleration inputs to the vertical semicircular canals and the gravity component of linear acceleration to the otoliths. Thus, ability to stabilize the head in space is subject to sensory constraints similar to those affecting feedback control of the centre of gravity sway.

Rules for organization of neural controls

Rule 1

Amplitudes and frequencies of sway must be above the threshold boundaries for the sensory systems controlling sway. This rule is based on a fundamental principle governing feedback control systems. To maintain stability, an error feedback signal is required. When applied to the vestibular system, this hypothesis states that the combined signals from the canals and otoliths must be sufficient to control sway at all points along the boundary defining the limits of stability.

Rule 2

The amplitudes and frequencies of sway are controlled to maximize distances to the limits of stability and to minimize head rotations in relation to gravity. Minimizing error is a second fundamental property of feedback control systems. In functional terms, this hypothesis states that the nervous system minimizes the risk of losing balance. Current experimental evidence indicates that head rotations in relation to gravity are also minimized during hip sway (Shupert et al., 1988a).

Rule 3

Ability to stabilize the rotational position of the head in space is limited to head amplitudes and frequencies above the canal threshold boundary. This rule is an expansion of the first. It is based on the assumption that head rotations are stabilized with canal feedback signals. Otolith information is assumed inappropriate due to the ambiguities between tilt and tangential acceleration inputs. Neck proprioceptive information is assumed insufficient, because this input does not distinguish head rotations in relation to a fixed trunk from the converse.

Rule 4

If there exists one or more frequencies at which the threshold for sensing sway lies above the mechanical stability limits of sway, loss of balance will occur at these sway frequencies. A fundamental property of feedback control systems is that undetected errors continue to grow.

Supporting experimental evidence

Rules 1 and 2

A combination of rules 1 and 2 predict that, for a given set of sensory conditions, subjects will sway near the threshold boundaries of the senses being used to control the sway.

When useful visual and somatosensory inputs were eliminated by eye closure and sway-referencing of the support surface (Nashner, 1970; Nashner et al., 1982), the maximum sway energy occurred between 0.1 and 0.3 Hz, and peak to peak amplitudes ranged between 3 and 6 degrees. This region of the amplitude-frequency space (shaded area A in Fig. 1) is above the canal and otolith threshold boundaries. With the support surface fixed and eyes open to restore normal somatosensory and visual inputs, sway frequencies were reduced to regions below the canal threshold boundary (shaded area B in Fig. 1). While precise threshold boundaries for visual and somatosensory inputs are not known, it is generally believed that somatosensory inputs provide high frequency sway information more sensitive than that from the canals (Diener et al., 1984).

Rule 3

This rule predicts that the amplitudes of head rotations will be slightly above the canal threshold boundary, regardless of the amplitudes and frequencies of the associated body sway. Because body sway motions were already near or below the canal threshold boundary during eyes open stance on a fixed support surface (shaded areas A and B of Fig. 1), additional head stabilization should not occur in this case. During hip sway, in contrast, stabilizing head movements should occur because the trunk rotations are much greater than the canal threshold (Fig. 2).

Predictions about head stabilization based on

rule 3 are supported by experimental observations (Shupert et al., 1988a). During ankle sway, head–trunk motions were uncorrelated. During hip sway, coordinated head movements reduced head rotations in relation to gravity to approximately 8 to 12 degrees (shaded area D of Fig. 2), compared to the much larger 20 to 30 degree trunk rotations (shaded area C).

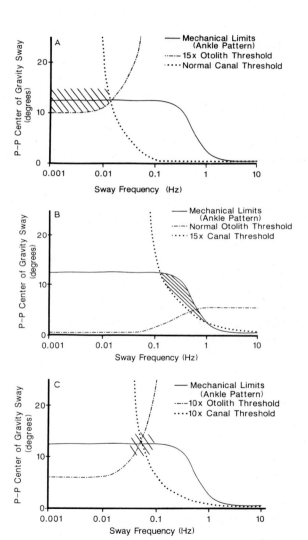

Fig. 3. Changes in sensory constraints with selective vestibular deficits. A: effects of selective increases in otolith threshold. B: effects of selective increases in vertical canal threshold. C: effect of combined otolith and canal threshold increases.

Predictions with selective vestibular deficits

Rule 4 applied to selective otolith deficits

Fig. 3A shows the sensory threshold boundaries for a hypothetical patient with a 15-times increase in otolith threshold. According to our theory, this threshold increase is the minimum necessary to cause significant balance impairment. As a consequence of rule 4, such a patient would show large sway oscillations or instability at frequencies below 0.5 Hz whenever useful visual and somatosensory inputs are disrupted. Ability to control higher frequency sway and to use the hip pattern near the limits of stability, in contrast, would be intact in this patient, because higher frequency feedback signals are normal. Thus, the theory predicts that otolith patients would drift towards a fall and then make frequent use of the high frequency hip movements to regain balance.

Rule 4 applied to selective canal deficits

Fig. 3B shows the sensory threshold boundaries for a patient with a 15-times increase in canal threshold, the minimum necessary to produce significant balance impairment. According to rule 4, a patient with an increased canal threshold would be unstable at high frequencies and low amplitudes of sway. Ability to use hip motions at the limits of stability would not be impaired with a 15-times threshold increase, since motions of the head during hip sway would still be above the increased threshold boundary. Patients with more profound threshold increases, however, would be restricted to the ankle sway pattern due to lack of the required high frequency feedback information.

Rule 4 applied to mixed canal and otolith deficits

As suggested in Fig. 3C, combinations of smaller canal and otolith threshold increases could produce instability in very narrow frequency bands. These focused instabilities could occur at any frequency between 0.01 and 0.5 Hz, depending on the relative magnitudes of the canal and otolith threshold increases.

Discussion

We have combined basic knowledge of body mechanics and sensory transduction with simple rules of feedback control to predict how information from the vertical semicircular canals and utricular otoliths is used to control antero-posterior sway in normal subjects and patients with vestibular deficits. The approach, however, can be expanded to include dynamic and threshold models for vision and somatosensory inputs. Lateral sway can be incorporated by including a model of body mechanics in this plane of motion.

The predictions provided by the formalism are robust, because they do not depend on precise knowledge of the canal and otolith dynamic and threshold characteristics. The values selected from the literature must increase by 5 to 15 times to produce substantive changes in balance control. Insensitivity to minor fluctuations in dynamic and threshold properties means that the predictions are also relatively insensitive to passive and active movements of the head in relation to the trunk.

The most useful predictions to evolve from the theory concern the effects of selective vestibular system deficits on posture. The theory predicts that different types of vestibular deficits will destabilize vestibular patients at all sway frequencies or selectively at low, high, or in narrow frequency bands. The theory also predicts which patients will use the hip pattern to maintain balance near the limits of stability, and which will be confined to using the ankle pattern. If true, these predictions could expand the value of posturography as a clinical test of vestibular dysfunction. Because current clinical methods for vestibular assessment do not allow precise separation of the vertical canal and otolith abnormalities, further research is required to test the validity of these predictions.

Black and Nashner (1984, 1985) used posturography to categorize patients into those thought to have vestibular "losses", vestibular "distortions", and combinations of the two abnormalities. The hypothesis proposed in these earlier studies was that patients in the vestibular loss category had increased thresholds and decreased dynamic range of vestibular function. Based on patient histories and other test results, patients classified with distortions were presumed to have a vertical canal abnormally sensitive to linear accelerations and gravity (see also Shuknecht, 1974).

Patients classified as having vestibular losses did not make use of vestibular inputs to control balance, and they fell freely when deprived of useful visual and somatosensory inputs. In agreement with the present theory, those patients with profound bilateral losses also did not make use of the hip pattern, even when provided with normal somatosensory and visual inputs (Shupert et al., 1987, 1988a).

The abnormal sway patterns of patients thought to have distorted vestibular inputs (Black et al., 1988; Shupert et al., 1988a) resembled the sway patterns predicted by the current theory for patients with selective increases in otolith thresholds. Although an amplitude-frequency analysis of sway was not performed in the earlier studies, the impression was that patients thought to have distorted inputs drifted forward and backward and then used hip motions to regain stability. Recently, Shupert et al. (1988b) found that a majority of patients exhibiting this abnormal sway pattern had normal findings on caloric and high frequency rotary chair vestibulo-ocular tests. Thus, while we have no further evidence for selective abnormalities in linear motion detection, clinical evidence supports the prediction that patients in this category detect angular accelerations approximately as well as normals.

In conclusion, a formal analysis of sensory and mechanical constraints has led to predictions about the posture control behaviours of normal subjects and vestibular deficit patients performing under a variety of conditions. The predictions reinforce the earlier hypothesis that patients previously classified as having vestibular "distortions" may have selective abnormalities in the senses of linear acceleration and gravity. With currently available information, however, we cannot isolate this abnormality to altered otolith thresholds, abnormal canal sensitivity to gravity, or central vestibular mechanisms. The goal of future research, therefore, will be to test these predictions in groups of patients with clinically documented otolith and canal deficits, and to expand the formalism to include the influences of visual and somatosensory inputs.

Acknowledgements

This research has been supported by the National Institutes of Health grants NS-12661 and NS-19221.

References

Black, F.O. and Nashner, L.M. (1984) Vestibulo-spinal control differs in patients with reduced versus distorted vestibular function. *Acta Otolaryngol. Suppl.,* 406: 110 – 114.

Black, F.O. and Nashner, L.M. (1985) Posture control in four classes of vestibular abnormalities. In M. Igarashi and F.O. Black (Eds.), *Vestibular and Visual Control of Posture and Locomotor Equilibrium,* Karger, Basel, pp. 271 – 281.

Black F.O., Shupert, C.L., Horak, F.B., and Nashner, L.M. (1988) Abnormal posture control associated with peripheral vestibular disorders. In O. Pompeiano and J. Allum (Eds.), *Vestibulo-spinal Control of Posture and Movement: Prog. Brain Res., Vol. 76,* Elsevier, Amsterdam, pp. 263 – 275.

Cavanagh, P. and LaFortune, M. (1980) Ground reaction forces in distance running. *J. Biomechanics,* 13: 397 – 406.

Clark, B. and Stewart, J.D. (1969) Effects of angular acceleration on man: Threshold for perception of rotation and the oculogyral illusion. *Aerospace Med.,* 40: 952 – 956.

Diener, H.C., Dichgans, J. Guschlbauer, B., and Mau, H. (1984) The significance of proprioception on postural stabilization as assessed by ischemia. *Brain Res.,* 296: 103 – 109.

Doty, R.L. (1969) Effect of duration of stimulus presentation on the angular acceleration threshold. *J. Exp. Psychol.,* 80: 317 – 321.

Gurfinkel, V.S. and Osevets, M. (1972) Dynamics of the vertical posture in man. *Biophysics,* 17: 496 – 506.

Horak, F.B. and Nashner, L.M. (1986) Central programming of postural movements: Adaptation to altered support surface configurations. *J. Neurophysiol.,* 55: 1369 – 1381.

McCollum, G. and Leen, T.K. (1989) Form and exploration of mechanical stability limits in erect stance. *J. Motor Behav.,* 21: 225 – 244.

Moore, S., Horak, F.B. and Nashner, L.M. (1986) Influence of initial stance position on human postural response. *Soc. Neurosci. Abstr.,* 12: 1301.

Nashner, L.M. (1970) *Sensory Feedback in Human Posture Control,* Massachusetts Institute of Technology Report MVT-70-3.

Nashner, L.M. (1971) A model describing vestibular detection of body sway motion. *Acta Otolaryngol.,* 72: 429 – 436.

Nashner, L.M. (1986) Organization of human postural movements during standing and walking. In S. Grillner, P.S.G. Stein, D.G. Stewart, H. Forssberg and R. Herman (Eds.), *Neurobiology of Posture and Locomotion,* Mac-Millan Press, London, pp. 637 – 648.

Nashner, L.M., Black, F.O. and Wall III, C. (1982) Adaptation to altered support surface and visual conditions during stance: Patients with vestibular deficits. *J. Neurosci.,* 2: 536 – 544.

Nashner, L.M. and McCollum, G. (1985) The organization of human postural movements: A formal basis and experimental synthesis. *Behav. Brain Sci.,* 8: 135 – 172.

Schuknecht, H.F. (1974) *Pathology of the Ear,* Harvard Univ. Press, Cambridge, pp. 475 – 478.

Shupert, C.L., Nashner, L.M., Horak, F.B. and Black, F.O. (1987) Coordination of the head and body in standing posture in normals and patients with bilaterally reduced vestibular function. *Soc. Neurosci. Abstr.,* 13: 352.

Shupert, C.L., Black, F.O., Horak, F.B. and Nashner, L.M. (1988a) Coordination of the head and body in response to support surface translations in normals and patients with bilaterally reduced vestibular function. In B. Amblard, A. Berthoz and F. Clarac (Eds.), *Posture and Gait: Development, Adaptation and Modulation,* Elsevier, Amsterdam, pp. 281 – 289.

Shupert, C.L., Horak, F.B. and Black, F.O. (1988b) Abnormal postural coordination in patients with distorted vestibular function. *Soc. Neurosci. Abstr.,* 14: 65.

Valiant, G.A. and Cavanagh, P.R. (1984) A study of landing from a jump: Implications for the design of a basketball shoe. In E. Fredrick (Ed.), *Sport Shoes and Playing Surfaces,* Human Kinetics Publishers, Champaign, pp. 24 – 46.

Young, L.R. and Meiry, J.L. (1968) A revised dynamic otolith model. *Aerospace Med.,* 39: 606 – 616.

J.H.J. Allum and M. Hulliger (Eds.)
Progress in Brain Research, Vol. 80
© 1989 Elsevier Science Publishers B.V. (Biomedical Division)

CHAPTER 34

Significance of proprioceptive mechanisms in the regulation of stance

V. Dietz, G.A. Horstmann and W. Berger

Department of Clinical Neurology and Neurophysiology, University of Freiburg, Freiburg, F.R.G.

Compensatory electromyographic (EMG) responses and several biomechanical parameters were studied following impulsive disturbance of the limbs during stance of human volunteers on a treadmill. Treadmill acceleration impulses were backwards or forwards directed, or their initial direction was reversed after 30 ms. Backwards directed impulses were followed by gastrocnemius, forwards directed ones by tibialis anterior EMG responses (latency 65 to 75 ms) whose durations depended on impulse duration. When the direction of the impulse was reversed, the respective antagonistic leg muscles were activated again with a delay of 68 to 75 ms after onset of stretch of these muscles. The behaviour of the EMG responses could best be correlated to the displacement at the ankle joint and may be described in terms of a stretch reflex response. The results indicate that these stretch reflex responses help control of the body's centre of gravity thereby preventing falling. Head movements induced by the impulses showed little correlation with the appearance of the EMG responses, suggesting that the vestibular system is unlikely to be directly involved in the generation of these responses. Vestibular signals may, however, significantly contribute to slow body sway stabilizaton.

Key words: Vestibulo-spinal reflex; Spinal stretch reflex; Muscle stretch; Muscle receptor; Muscle activity; Joint movement; Motor control; Human posture; Electromyogram; Head movement; Centre of gravity

Introduction

Perturbations of gait automatically evoke functionally directed complex responses in the leg muscles in order to compensate for body imbalance. The reactions adapt quickly to a given mode of perturbation (Nashner, 1976; Nashner et al., 1979; Forssberg and Nashner, 1982; Quintern et al., 1985) and cannot, therefore, be explained in terms of a simple stimulus – response relationship. Recent observations following impulsive disturbance of stance on a treadmill indicate that functionally directed EMG responses are mediated by stretch reflexes and incorporated into a complex EMG pattern controlled by central mechanisms (Dietz et al., 1987). Other experiments, using dorsiflexing rotations of the support surface have in-

dicated an involvement of the vestibular system in the stabilization of body sway (cf. Allum and Keshner, 1986; Keshner et al., 1987).

The aim of this study was to further clarify which receptors and mechanisms are involved in the regulation of posture. This was achieved by the analysis of changes in several biomechanical parameters affected by stance perturbations and their correlation with the behaviour of the EMG responses evoked in the leg muscles.

Methods

The general technique for recording the EMG responses of leg muscles to unexpected perturbations has been fully described in an earlier paper (Berger et al., 1984). The experiments were per-

420

formed on 11 normal subjects with a mean age of 24 years (S.D. ± 1.8 years). In addition, two patients with a loss of labyrinthine function (one after a meningitis, the other after surgery of a bilateral acoustic neurofibroma) were investigated. EMG was recorded, using surface electrodes, from the medial gastrocnemius and tibialis anterior muscles. Ankle and knee joint angles were indicated by mechanical goniometers fixed at the lateral aspect of the leg. The acceleration of the head in space induced by the treadmill impulses was recorded by two accelerometers (Kistler Piezobeam; range + 50 g; sensitivity 100 mV/g; time constant 0.5 s) fixed on the forehead: the difference of the signals of the two accelerometers indicated the linear acceleration of the head in space. The treadmill belt was placed over a force measuring platform (Kistler). The antero-posterior sway exerted by the subject was measured in terms of the centre of foot pressure (CFP, cf. Diener et al., 1983) or ankle torque (torque$_{CM}$ in the figures) calculated from the output of 4 Piezo-elements fixed at the corners of the platform. An additional antero-posterior shift of the torque signal for backward accelerations, or postero-anterior shift for forward accelerations induced by the belt displacement has to be considered in the following figures (see dotted lines in Fig. 1).

Acceleration impulses were unexpectedly applied during stance on a treadmill (Woodway MTR 250-40). Four different types of impulses were randomly delivered by a microcomputer-based impulse generator. The onset of the impulses was used as trigger to average the rectified EMG responses and biomechanical data. The leg muscle EMG responses evoked by the externally induced perturbations were analysed using methods described earlier (Berger et al., 1984).

Results

Fig. 1A, B shows the mean values of the leg muscle EMG responses following a backwards (A) and forwards (B) directed treadmill acceleration impulse (rate 12.4 m/s², duration 90 ms) obtained in 11 subjects. The backwards directed impulse (A) induced a dorsiflexion movement at the ankle joint

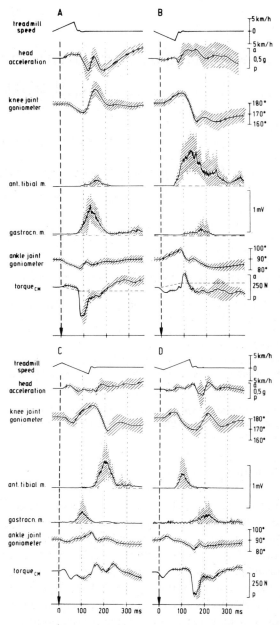

Fig. 1. Mean values (with S.D.) of the rectified and averaged (n = 10) leg muscle EMG responses together with the ankle and knee joint movements as well as the signal of the accelerometers fixed at the head and the torque of centre of gravity (torque$_{CM}$) following backwards (A) and forwards (B) directed treadmill accelerations (rate 12.4 m/s², duration 90 ms) in 11 subjects during stance. The interrupted line indicates the shift in the torque signal induced by the passive displacement of body's mass. In C and D the initially backwards (C) or forwards (D) directed impulses were inverted after 30 ms and continued, with the same acceleration rate, over 100 ms.

($t = 0$ ms) and, 25 ms later, knee flexion. The displacement shifted the centre of gravity forwards and, after a delay of 25 to 30 ms (i.e. 45 ms before the onset of the EMG response), the head was accelerated in the same direction. This impulse evoked a gastrocnemius response (mean latency 75 ms, half amplitude duration 75 ms), followed by a weak tibialis anterior activation.

The forwards directed impulse (Fig. 1B) induced a plantarflexion movement at the ankle joint, followed 20 ms later by knee extension. Compared to condition A, the shift of the centre of gravity (backwards, in this case) was larger (about 2.5 times) but the head was less accelerated in this direction. This impulse evoked a tibialis anterior response (mean latency 68 ms, half amplitude duration 90 ms), followed by a weak gastrocnemius activation.

Fig. 1C, D shows the leg muscle EMG responses following impulses with the same acceleration rate as in A and B, but in which the direction of the impulses was inverted after 30 ms (over a period of 100 ms). The impulses were initially directed backwards (C) or forwards (D). The impulse depicted in Fig. 1C evoked a gastrocnemius response (mean latency 74 ms, half amplitude duration 45 ms) followed by a stronger tibialis anterior response (latency from onset of foot dorsiflexion (90 degrees) 75 ms; half amplitude duration 70 ms). The centre of gravity shifted briefly (15 ms) forwards, then backwards (duration 120 ms). The head acceleration signal indicated oscillatory movements, initially in an anterior direction.

The impulse shown in Fig. 1D evoked a strong tibialis anterior response (mean latency 73 ms; half amplitude duration 40 ms), followed by a smaller gastrocnemius response (latency from onset of foot plantarflexion (90 degrees) 75 ms; half amplitude duration 75 ms). The brief, initial backward shift in the centre of gravity was larger and the second, forward one, smaller than in condition C. The head acceleration signal again indicated oscillatory head movements. In neither condition C nor in D was a clear-cut acceleration signal observed which could be correlated with the onset and duration of the EMG responses detected.

The two patients with a loss of labyrinthine function in the electrophysiological tests showed EMG responses which were within the normal range.

Discussion

The results obtained in the different experimental conditions showed a close correlation between foot displacement and appearance of the impulse directed EMG responses. This is in agreement with earlier observations demonstrating that stretch velocity and amplitude are closely correlated with the amplitude and duration of the leg muscle EMG response during gait perturbations (Dietz et al., 1987). Neither head acceleration nor shifts of the centre of gravity induced by the perturbations could easily be correlated with the appearance of the response pattern. In addition, the delay between onset of movements of the head or knee joint and the appearance of the EMG responses (about 45 ms) seems too short to allow a direct involvement of these biomechanical parameters in the generation of the early part of the EMG responses. This suggests that stretch reflex mechanisms predominate in the generation of the leg muscle EMG responses involved in the maintenance of posture.

Nevertheless, muscle stretch per se is unlikely to be solely responsible for the EMG responses observed here: stretching the gastrocnemius muscle by a torque motor (Gottlieb and Agarwal, 1979) or by dorsiflexing rotations during stance on a force measuring platform (Diener et al., 1983; Allum and Keshner, 1986), (i.e. in conditions which did not require a functionally essential gastrocnemius EMG response), only small single monosynaptic reflex responses were elicited in this muscle. These responses were negligible in this study and have previously been shown to be reduced during stance (Dietz et al., 1984) and inhibited during gait (Morin et al., 1982; Berger et al., 1984; Capaday and Stein, 1986). It is, therefore, suggested that the stretch reflex responses described here are due to a different mechanism: on the basis of earlier experiments (Berger et al., 1984) it is suggested that they may be mediated predominantly by peripheral information from group II afferents at a spinal level which would be in accordance with animal experiments (Lundberg et al., 1987).

The purpose of the compensatory EMG responses is to prevent falling, i.e. to control the centre of gravity. Therefore, the presence and functional significance of the stretch reflex activity observed here may be connected with the shift of the body's centre of gravity. The observation that the tibialis anterior responses were generally larger than the gastrocnemius responses, corresponds to the observation that the shifts in the centre of gravity were larger when forwards directed perturbations were induced, i.e. the tibialis anterior muscle became activated. Such a combination of signals from muscle stretch receptors and from receptors monitoring shifts in the centre of gravity (foot pressure receptors for example) might be expected to lead to the generation of functionally meaningful EMG responses directed to regulate posture.

The vestibular system in our opinion is suggested to be involved mainly in the stabilization of slow body sway, which is achieved by a much lower level of leg muscle activation (Mauritz and Dietz, 1980; Horstmann and Dietz, 1988). Indeed, the adequate stimulus to evoke the compensatory reaction following a toe-up displacement standing on a moveable platform was shown to be represented not by the stretching of ankle muscles but by the body sway induced by the toe-up movement (Berger et al., 1988).

In the experiments presented here the EMG activity induced by the vestibular system may be a part of the overall response pattern, though not easily quantified because of its small amplitude. This suggestion is in line with recent experiments showing that head movements as well as head tilts have only a minor effect on compensatory reactions during stance and gait perturbations (Dietz et al., 1988).

Acknowledgements

We are grateful to Dr. S. Fellows for reading and correcting the English text and Mrs. U. Römmelt and U. Möllinger for technical assistance. This work was supported by the Deutsche Forschungsgemeinschaft (SFB 325).

References

Allum, J.H.J. and Keshner, E.A. (1986) Vestibular and proprioceptive control of sway stabilization. In W. Bles and T. Brandt (Eds.), *Disorders of Posture and Gait,* Elsevier, Amsterdam, pp. 19 – 40.

Berger, W., Dietz, V. and Horstmann, G. (1988) Are "long loop" reflexes involved in the stabilization of posture? *Eur. J. Physiol.,* 411 (Suppl.): R 138.

Berger, W., Dietz, V. and Quintern, J. (1984) Corrective reactions to stumbling in man: neuronal co-ordination of bilateral leg muscle activity during gait. *J. Physiol. (London),* 357: 109 – 125.

Capaday, C. and Stein, R.B. (1986) Amplitude modulation of the soleus H-reflex in the human during walking and standing. *J. Neurosci.,* 6: 1308 – 1313.

Diener, H.C., Bootz, F., Dichgans, J. and Bruzek, W. (1983) Variability of postural "reflexes" in humans. *Brain Res.,* 52: 423 – 428.

Dietz, V., Horstmann, G. and Berger, W. (1988) Fast head tilt has only a minor effect on quick compensatory reactions during the regulation of stance and gait. *Exp. Brain Res.,* 73: 470 – 476.

Dietz, V., Quintern, J. and Berger, W. (1984) Corrective reactions to stumbling in man: functional significance of spinal and transcortical reflexes. *Neurosci. Lett.,* 44: 131 – 135.

Dietz, W., Quintern, J. and Sillem, M. (1987) Stumbling reactions in man: significance of proprioceptive and preprogrammed mechanisms. *J. Physiol. (London),* 386: 149 – 163.

Forssberg, H. and Nashner, L.M. (1982) Ontogenetic development of postural control in man: adaptation to altered support and visual conditions during stance. *J. Neurosci.,* 2: 545 – 552.

Gottlieb, G.L. and Agarwal, G.C. (1979) Response to sudden torques about ankle in man: myotatic reflex. *J. Neurophysiol.,* 42: 91 – 106.

Horstmann, G.A. and Dietz, V. (1988) The contribution of vestibular input to the stabilization of human posture: a new experimental approach. *Neurosci. Lett.,* 95: 179 – 184.

Keshner, E.A., Allum, J.H.J. and Pfaltz, C.R. (1987) Postural coactivation and adaptation in the sway stabilizing responses of normals and patients with bilateral vestibular deficit. *Exp. Brain Res.,* 69: 77 – 92.

Lundberg, A., Malmgren, K. and Schomburg, E.D. (1987)

Reflex pathway from group II muscle afferents. 3. Secondary spindle afferents and the FRA: a new hypothesis. *Exp. Brain Res.*, 65: 294 – 306.

Mauritz, K.H. and Dietz, V. (1980) Characteristics of postural instability induced by ischemic blocking of leg afferents. *Exp. Brain Res.*, 38: 117 – 119.

Morin, O., Katz, R., Mazieres, L. and Pierrot-Deseilligny, E. (1982) Comparison on soleus H-reflex facilitation at the onset of soleus contractions produced voluntarily and during the stance phase of human gait. *Neurosci. Lett.*, 33: 47 – 53.

Nashner, L.M. (1976) Adapting reflexes controlling the human posture. *Exp. Brain Res.*, 26: 59 – 72.

Nashner, L.M., Woollacott, M. and Tuma, G. (1979) Organization of rapid response to postural and locomotor-like perturbations of standing man. *Exp. Brain Res.*, 36: 463 – 476.

Quintern, J., Berger, W. and Dietz, V. (1985) Compensatory reactions to gait perturbations: short and long term effects of neuronal adaptation. *Neurosci. Lett.*, 62: 371 – 376.

Higher Order Control of Posture and Locomotion

J.H.J. Allum and M. Hulliger (Eds.)
Progress in Brain Research, Vol. 80
© 1989 Elsevier Science Publishers B.V. (Biomedical Division)

Overview and critique of Chapters 35 – 37

Inferring functional roles of cortical neurones from their activity during movement

J.A. Hoffer

Calgary, Canada

The three studies presented in this session were aimed at understanding the function of motor cortical regions, on the basis of the activity of single neurones recorded in awake monkeys during the execution of well-learned upper limb motor tasks. Interestingly, each study included a comparison of the activity of motor cortical cells with the activity of cells from one other brain area. I will first discuss the studies by Hyland et al. and Hepp-Reymond et al., that share many aspects of experimental design. The paper by Fetz et al. introduces a novel strategy and computational approach to quantify the functional involvement of corticospinal and rubrospinal neurones. I will conclude this critique by assessing how the experimental approach used by Fetz et al. may be applied to the study of other cortical control centres.

Hyland et al. pose the question of whether the supplementary motor area (SMA) is indeed a "hierarchically superior" structure with respect to the primary motor cortex (MI), as was implied from several recent works (e.g., Mann et al., 1988; Tanji et al., 1988) that found SMA neurone activity to be better related to movement "preparation" than to movement "execution".

From their data on the timing of burst activity of "task-related" SMA and MI neurones with respect to the initiation of visually triggered arm movements, Hyland et al. note that a large percentage of SMA neurones could be classified as "short-lead" neurones and were indistinguishable, in this respect, from the majority of task-related

MI neurones. From this evidence, Hyland et al. argue against a strictly hierarchical relation and support the original conclusion of Woolsey et al. (1952), that the SMA and MI regions also function "in parallel".

In critically reviewing this paper I must query the appropriateness of using the timing of neural activity bursts as sole criterion for "parallel" vs "hierarchical" organization in this system. There exist abundant reciprocal interconnections between SMA and MI and, as was already pointed out in a more general context by Fetz (1981), the duration of bursts from "short-lead" SMA and MI neurones is long enough that there could be sufficient time for one- or two-way transfer of information between these two areas during the course of bursting activity. Thus, the timing argument is not sufficient to disprove that SMA neurones (even the "short-lead" ones that burst at the same times as MI neurones) could still be "hierarchically superior" with respect to the MI neurones. What is missing in Hyland et al.'s argumentation is evidence, either for or against, any causal linkage between the individually recorded SMA and MI neurones that would allow them to interpret the recorded discharge patterns within the context of proven synaptic action.

In answer to the question in the title of their paper, Hyland et al. propose that the relation between the SMA and MI regions is probably neither exclusively hierarchic nor exclusively parallel, thus leaving behind previous arguments that tended to focus on an "either/or" dichotomy (e.g., Wiesen-danger, 1985; see also Macpherson et al., 1982; Mitz and Wise, 1987). Hyland et al. suggest that in both the SMA and MI regions there may be a range of cell classes represented. Although the authors do not comment on how the internal organization and role assignment among these cell classes might be further investigated, they do indicate that in future research a main objective must be to iden-tify the targets of recorded SMA neurones. This is a central point of my critique, to which I will return.

Hepp-Reymond et al. seek to understand whether the somatosensory cortex has a mainly "motor" or a mainly "sensory" involvement dur-ing the execution of skilled hand movements. In this paper the authors compare the discharge pat-terns of primary motor (MI) and somatosensory (SI) cortical neurones during precision grip. They describe six "very clear contrasting properties" that, in their view, ". . . strongly suggest that SI neurones are mainly, or even exclusively, involved in processing sensory information from the digits rather than participating in the generation of motor output."

The authors' observation that qualitative or quantitative differences exist in the firing patterns and sources of sensory input of SI and MI neurones need not be challenged. It is not clear, however, how significant these differences are, nor what is the logical basis from which the authors concluded that SI neurones may be exclusively in-volved in processing sensory information rather than participating in the generation of motor out-put. In particular, the finding that during force in-creases, SI neurones increase their firing later than MI neurones suggests that SI may have a minor role in movement initiation, but does not take away from it potentially having an important role in the shaping of ongoing movements. The com-parison of force sensitivities of SI and MI neurones is interesting, but its significance in terms of an "active" vs "passive" role of SI neurones toward force generation is obscure. Microstimulation results should always be interpreted keeping in

mind that it is unlikely that the recorded neuron will be the only stimulated cell (viz., Lemon, 1988). The difference in modality of dominant afferent input to MI and SI neurones (viz., Dykes, 1983) provides no clear clue on the nature of the par-ticipation of SI in movement execution. And the observed differences in visually evoked responses of MI and SI neurones are intriguing but do not solve the puzzle of the role of SI in movement ex-ecution.

As was the case with work presented by Hyland et al., it is unfortunate that Hepp-Reymond et al. did not identify the targets of the recorded cells, since this information could have shed further light on their comparisons. It might also have helped in-terpret the apparent disagreement with previous studies that reported similarities between MI and SI neurones that were shown to project along the pyramidal tract (e.g., Fromm and Evarts, 1982).

Fetz et al., in the third paper of this set, obtain a quantitative estimation of the time-varying in-fluence that populations of corticomotoneuronal (CM) and rubromotoneuronal (RM) cells have on the activity of spinal motoneurones during the ex-ecution of voluntary movement. With this method they estimate that the aggregate CM and RM cell activity contributes at least half of the tonic drive received by wrist extensor motoneurones during the static "hold" phase of ramp-and-hold changes in wrist torque.

Fetz et al. were able to carry out their quan-titative estimation because CM and RM cells have demonstrable effects on motoneurone firing, shown by the technique of spike-triggered averag-ing. It was also possible to derive the dependence of motoneurone firing probability on EPSP, at least for Ia inputs.

Inevitably, Fetz et al. had to make a number of simplifying assumptions in order to proceed with their calculations. Most of these assumptions are quite reasonable but some assumptions may be challenged either because of the absence of any supporting data, as in the estimation of number of CM cells projecting onto each motoneurone, or because some data do exist that could have been considered. For example, in their Relation 2, Fetz et al. assume that the increment in motoneurone firing rate is independent of the firing rates of the presynaptic cell as well as the motoneurone. However, Ia EPSP amplitude has been shown to vary during high-frequency afferent activity (Collins et al., 1986), and facilitation, depression and potentiation have all been shown to contribute to Ia EPSP amplitude modulation (Collins et al., 1988). It remains to be determined whether the instantaneous frequency and activation history of CM and/or RM neurones may also affect their EPSP amplitude and so influence the firing probability of spinal motoneurones. A reduction in EPSP amplitude at higher CM or RM firing frequencies, if present, could partially account for the saturation of motoneurone firing that occurs in spite of continued increase in the firing rates of CM and RM neurones.

An instantaneous, dynamic estimation was not attempted by Fetz et al.; their estimation applies to the static "hold" phases of movement. Nevertheless, their approach has provided a quantitative estimation of corticomotoneuronal and rubromotoneuronal cell population effects on spinal cord output that is causally based and takes into account a larger number of physiological parameters than previous efforts, and their result is quite important.

General comments

For some 25 years now, microelectrode recordings in awake monkeys have provided considerable data on the activity patterns of individual neurones from various cortical areas during the execution of voluntary movements. In spite of this information, the specific functional roles of the several areas involved in the control of limb movements have largely remained unclear. The work of Fetz et al. demonstrates that it is possible to begin to assemble a quantitative picture of time-varying, causal relationships involving populations of identified neurones. The same approach should be applicable to study several supraspinal descending control systems.

In order to obtain the necessary information, it is essential to identify the target areas of each recorded neurone. For example, corticospinal neurones arising from SMA, MI or SI should be routinely identified with chronically implanted stimulating electrodes (viz., Evarts, 1964; Fetz et al., 1976; Lemon, 1984). To test for a causal hierarchical relation between SMA and MI neurones, it will be necessary to conclusively identify cortico-cortical neurones projecting from SMA to MI or vice-versa, even if this kind of data are technically difficult to obtain in behaving monkeys (viz., Weinreich, 1985). Once each cortical neurone is so classified at the time of recording its activity, and the action of populations of such neurones is taken into account, it is likely that much of the current uncertainty or controversy regarding the activity patterns and roles of SMA, MI or SI neurones will be overcome.

References

Collins, W.F., III, Davis, B.M. and Mendell, L.M. (1986) Amplitude modulation of EPSPs in motoneurons in response to a frequency modulated train in single Ia afferent fibers. *J. Neurosci.,* 5: 1463 – 1468.

Collins, W.F., III, Davis, B.M. and Mendell, L.M. (1988) Modulation of EPSP amplitude during high frequency stimulation depends on the correlation between potentiation, depression and facilitation. *Brain Res.,* 442: 161 – 165.

Dykes, R.W. (1983) Parallel processing of somatosensory information: a theory. *Brain Res. Rev.,* 6: 47 – 115.

Evarts, E.V. (1964) Temporal patterns of discharge of pyramidal tract neurons during sleep and waking in the monkey. *J. Neurophysiol.,* 27: 152 – 171.

Fetz, E.E. (1981) Neuronal activity associated with conditioned limb movements. In: A.L. Towe and E.S. Luschei (Eds.), *Motor Coordination, Handbook Behav. Neurobiol.,* 5, Plenum, New York, pp. 493 – 526.

Fetz, E.E., Cheney, P.D. and German, D.C. (1976) Corticomotoneuronal connections of precentral cells detected by post-spike averages of EMG activity in behaving monkeys. *Brain Res.,* 114: 505 – 510.

Fetz, E.E., Cheney, P.D., Mewes, K. and Palmer, S. Control of forelimb muscle activity by populations of corticomotoneuronal and rubromotoneuronal cells. *Prog. Brain Res., Vol. 80,* Elsevier, Amsterdam, pp. 437 – 449.

Fromm, C. and Evarts, E.V. (1982) Pyramidal tract neurons in somatosensory cortex: central and peripheral inputs during voluntary movements. *Brain Res.,* 238: 186 – 191.

Hepp-Reymond, M.C., Wannier, T.M.J., Maier, M.A. and Rufener E.A. Sensorimotor cortical control of isometric force in the monkey. *Prog. Brain Res., Vol. 80,* Elsevier, Amsterdam, pp. 451 – 463.

Hyland, B., Chen, D.F., Maier, V., Palmeri, A. and Wiesendanger, M. What is the role of the supplementary motor area in movement initiation? *Prog. Brain Res., Vol. 80,* Elsevier, Amsterdam, pp. 431 – 436.

Lemon, R. (1984) Methods for Neuronal Recording in Conscious Animals. *IBRO Handbook Series: Methods in the Neurosciences, Vol. 4,* 162 pp.

Lemon, R. (1988) The output map of the primate motor cortex. *Trends Neurosci.,* 11: 501 – 506.

Macpherson, J.M., Wiesendanger, M., Marangoz, C. and Miles, T.S. (1982) Corticospinal neurones of the supplementary motor area of monkeys. A single unit study. *Exp. Brain Res.,* 48: 81 – 88.

Mann, S.E., Thau, R. and Schiller, P.H. (1988) Conditional task-related responses in monkey dorsomedial frontal cortex. *Exp. Brain Res.,* 69: 460 – 468.

Mitz, A.R. and Wise, S.P. (1987) The somatotopic organiza-tion of the supplementary motor area: intracortical microstimulation mapping. *J. Neurosci.,* 7: 1010 – 1021.

Tanji, J., Okano, K. and Sato, K.C. (1988) Neuronal activity in cortical motor areas related to ipsilateral, contralateral and bilateral digit movements of the monkey. *J. Neurophysiol.,* 60: 325 – 343.

Weinreich, M. (1985) Medial versus lateral motor control. A commentary on a target article by Goldberg, G., (1985) Supplementary motor area structure and function: Review and hypotheses. *Behav. Brain Sci.,* 8: 567 – 616.

Wiesendanger, M. (1985), The SMA: A "supplementary motor" or a "supramotor" area? A commentary on a target article by Goldberg, G., (1985), Supplementary motor area structure and function: Review and hypotheses. *Behav. Brain Sci.,* 8: 567 – 616.

Woolsey, C.N., Settlage, P.H., Meyer, D.R., Spencer, W., Hamuy, T.P. and Travis, A.M. (1952) Patterns of localiza-tion in precentral and supplementary motor areas and their relation to the concept of a premotor area. *Res. Publ. Ass. Res. Nerv. Ment. Dis.,* 30: 238 – 264.

J.H.J. Allum and M. Hulliger (Eds.)
Progress in Brain Research, Vol. 80
© 1989 Elsevier Science Publishers B.V. (Biomedical Division)

CHAPTER 35

What is the role of the supplementary motor area in movement initiation?

B. Hyland, D.-F. Chen, V. Maier, A. Palmeri and M. Wiesendanger

Institut de Physiologie, Université de Fribourg, CH-1700 Fribourg, Switzerland

The hierarchical position of the supplementary motor area (SMA) relative to the primary motor cortex is discussed on the basis of neurological observations and of animal experiments. In the last 10 years evidence has accumulated, especially from studies on the human brain, that the supplementary motor area is a hierarchically superior structure involved in the processes of movement initiation. Single unit studies in subhuman primates also revealed neuronal populations related to aspects of movement preparation rather than to the movement per se. However, we report that a surprisingly large subpopulation of SMA neurones has features classically found in the primary motor cortex (MI). These MI-like neurones precede movement onset by a relatively short interval. The occurrence of such "short-lead neurones" was somewhat higher in MI, but the histograms of lead-times were completely overlapping in the two areas. Taken together with the fact that the SMA is microexcitable and is part of the origin of the pyramidal tract, these findings suggest that the SMA functions also in parallel with MI as concluded by Woolsey and coworkers (1952). Finally, the SMA and MI are reciprocally interconnected, a situation which is not unlike that of the cortical visual areas.

Key words: Supplementary motor area; Motor cortex; Monkey; Reaction time; Hierarchy; Cortico-cortical connection; Microstimulation

Introduction

Recent studies on motor cortical areas of the human brain led to the proposition that the supplementary motor area (SMA), situated in front of area 4 on the mesial surface, is involved in movement initiation at a hierarchically higher level than the precentral motor strip (MI), considered to be intimately involved in the process of movement execution. This assumption is based on neurological symptoms in patients with SMA lesions, on measurements of cerebral blood flow and on the recordings of slow potentials accompanying voluntary movements (for recent reviews see Goldberg, 1985; Wiesendanger, 1986). This is a remarkable departure from the original interpretation of

Woolsey and coworkers (1952) that the SMA is a somatotopically organized motor area controlling the motor apparatus directly and independently, i.e. in parallel to the primary motor cortex. This opinion was based mainly on results of repetitive surface stimulation of the motor cortical fields.

In recent years, many new investigations in subhuman primates were performed to further analyse the role and the hierarchical position of the SMA in the control of movements. A brief summary of experimental data which favour the "hierarchic" or "upstream" model is presented, followed by a discussion of our own data which suggest that many features of the SMA support the older notion of a parallel motor cortical system. It will then be argued that the parallel hypothesis is not exclusive of a serial "upstream" hypothesis and that the areal classification into distinct hierarchic levels is too simple to account for the massive reciprocal interconnections of the two areas and for the complex functional attributes found in neurones of both areas.

Evidence for hierarchically superior functions of the SMA

Studies on the human brain

Lesions within the territory of the SMA have been shown to result in a general reduction of self-initiated voluntary movements including spontaneous speech (e.g. Laplane et al., 1977). Cerebral blood flow studies revealed local increases within the medial frontal cortex in subjects performing a complex sequence of finger movements and even when subjects simply imagined the finger sequence (Roland et al., 1980). Finally, it was found that the largest amplitudes of readiness potentials preceding self-initiated finger movements were recorded with highest amplitude over the vertex and were therefore believed to originate in the SMA (Deecke et al., 1969). These relatively novel observations are of great interest and importance, but some caution as to the exact localization of the phenomena is appropriate, as discussed previously in more detail (Wiesendanger, 1986). In brief, an exact delimitation of presumed SMA lesions (often infarcts of the anterior cerebral artery) was rarely possible or was found to extend beyond the SMA. Similarly, the premovement potentials have been recorded from a wide area of the cerebral cortex suggesting that areas outside the SMA territory (as originally defined by cytoarchitecture and electrical stimulation) contribute as well. With regard to cerebral blood flow measurements, a close temporal association of its changes with the task is not possible and it appears from several published charts that the movement-associated changes may occur over wider regions than the SMA.

Results from animal experiments

The effects of lesions of the SMA on motor behaviour appear to be discrete and may not readily be appreciated by "clinical" observations. In contrast to precentral lesions, SMA lesions do not result in a paresis of the contralateral limb and the use of the hand in grasping seem hardly affected (forced grasping in SMA-lesioned monkeys was observed transiently by Smith et al., 1981, but this was not confirmed by Brinkman, 1984). Only refined tasks with a modified Klüver board revealed subtle changes in the strategy used by the monkey to retrieve food morsels from the slots of the board: the trajectories were more erratic as compared to the orderly sequential preoperative performance. A unilateral (but not a bilateral) SMA lesion led to an incoordination of both hands in a bimanual food-retrieving task (Brinkman, 1984). Grasping an object in a constant location deteriorated when a SMA-lesioned animal had to perform the task in the dark (Passingham, 1987). It was suggested that this deficit could be explained by the SMA normally controlling movements that depend on proprioceptive feedback signals (rather than on visual signals).

Single unit recordings are more revealing as to the possible "higher" functions of the SMA. Thus, experiments by Tanji and collaborators (Tanji and Kurata, 1983) have shown convincingly that some populations of SMA cells have features which seem more remote from the direct control aspects of movements. Thus, a considerable number of SMA neurones covary with instruction signals or exhibit set-dependency during the waiting period. Perhaps the most intriguing properties of SMA neurones which so far have only been found in this area, are covariations that are specific for either the right, or the left, or for both hands working together (Tanji et al., 1988). If a neurone is activated in a bimanual task but not with the component movements of either hand, one might speculate that this neurone encodes a "higher-order" command for a bimanual act. Also recently reported are somewhat similar findings of Mann et al. (1988) showing that SMA neurones may be effector independent, in that the activity of the same neurone could covary either with goal-directed saccades or with hand movements directed towards the same goal.

From this brief summary it is tempting to suggest that the SMA has complex features which appear to be more related to higher-order commands and, in a general sense, to movement preparation.

Evidence for parallel functions of the SMA and MI

Anatomical criteria

The SMA and MI are both within the agranular frontal cortex; both areas are occupied by corticospinal neurones and share the property of producing movements with either surface stimulation or intracortical microstimulation (Wiesendanger, 1986). Both areas receive inputs from somatosensory pathways (Hummelsheim et al., 1988) and from afferents from the motor nuclear complex of the thalamus, although from different subdivisions (Schell and Strick, 1984; Wiesendanger and Wiesendanger, 1985). Most importantly, the cortico-cortical connections between MI and the SMA are reciprocal, with the terminal pattern of SMA-to-MI fibres being different from that of MI-to-SMA fibres (Primrose and Strick, 1985).

Following similar reasoning as in work on the visual cortical areas (Maunsell and Van Essen, 1983), Primrose and Strick suggested that the primary motor cortex has feedforward connections with the secondary motor areas, whereas these areas in turn feedback to MI. Given that such a hypothetical interpretation of anatomical data holds also for the interconnections of motor areas, it would mean that MI is "upstream" of the SMA which is the reverse from what is usually assumed (see above).

Criteria from single unit recordings

Although the presence of "higher-order" neurones in the SMA has been well documented, neurones with "MI-like" activity relation to movements were also observed by all investigators of the SMA. Such SMA cells could function in parallel with similar neurones in MI; alternatively they could transmit "instructions" to MI. An argument which has often been used in discussions about serial processing in motor centres has been the timing of neural activity changes relative to movement onset (e.g. Thach, 1978; Weinrich et al., 1984; but see also Fetz, 1981). We have addressed this question by recording from single unit from the two areas in the same two monkeys performing visually-triggered arm movements in a choice-reaction paradigm. The results from this study will be published in detail elsewhere. We here summarize some of the features which are relevant to the question of hierarchies.

Comparison of lead-times of MI neurones and SMA neurones

Neurones with activity changes occurring in the interval between the go-signal (which also contained the instruction of desired movement direction) and movement onset were termed short-lead neurones. These were 290 out of all 431 task-related neurones (67%), and 303 out of 353 task-related MI neurones (86%). In order to extract neurones clearly related with movement execution, dot rasters were constructed in which the individual trials were displayed in order not of their occurrence during recording, but of increasing reaction time. Activity changes associated with movements then shift progressively further away from the time of the go-signal (time 0). Examples of such short-lead neurones from the SMA and from MI are shown in Fig. 1. Neurones were also extracted which were in, or nearby, tracks from which well-defined microstimulation effects were obtained, in order to compare neurones from somatotopically equivalent areas. Whether the entire population or any of the subpopulations were compared (including subpopulations from either monkey and from separate movement directions), we failed to detect consistent differences in the lead-time distributions between MI and SMA neurones. In fact, the lead-time distributions of the entire populations of short-lead neurones in the two areas were completely overlapping.

This thus means that there are subpopulations of neurones in the SMA that are temporally active

434

fairly much in parallel with MI, and with similar patterns of activity. This is also reflected in the average lead-times of electromyographic activity (EMG) and of neuronal activity when comparing the two movement directions. Both monkeys performed the inward rotations of the arm more rapidly than the outward rotations and this resulted in shorter EMG lead-times for the more rapid movement as compared to the slower movement. This was paralleled in a similar difference in neuronal lead-times not only for MI short-lead cells, but also for those of the SMA. This is additional support for our contention that the sub-populations of short-lead neurones of both areas

are clearly linked with movement execution. Finally, it is worth mentioning that most of the antidromically identified pyramidal tract neurones were of the short-lead type, including those of the SMA.

Conclusion

A number of results briefly reviewed above indicate that the SMA has many anatomical and electrophysiological features in common with MI. Of special importance is the now well established presence of corticospinal neurones and of positive microstimulation effects in the SMA. To this we

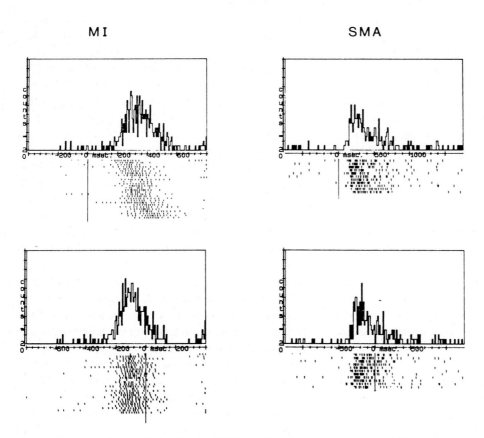

Fig. 1. Examples of short-lead cells recorded from the primary motor cortex (MI) and from the supplementary motor area in a monkey performing arm movements in a choice reaction-time paradigm. The peri-event time histograms and the rasters are aligned to the "go-signal" in the upper two panels. The trials in the raster are ordered with reaction time increasing from top to bottom. Note that the burst of discharges moves with the reaction time. In the lower two panels the histogram and the raster is aligned to movement onset.

add recent results of single unit recordings in monkeys trained to perform arm movements in a choice-reaction paradigm. A surprisingly large subpopulation of SMA neurones was found to have "MI-like" properties, i.e. displaying activity-changes being clearly linked with movement execution. We therefore suggest that the parallel model of the SMA, as proposed by Woolsey, cannot be discarded (cf. Introduction). On the other hand, it is also obvious that many neurones of the SMA have properties that are compatible with the "upstream-model" of the SMA. For example, we confirmed the presence of neurones that covaried better with the visual signals and the preparatory phase rather than with the movement per se.

From the available data it appears that the proportion of clearly movement-related cells is higher in MI (in our sample 71% of the task-related neurones) than in the SMA (41% of all task-related neurones). Conversely, it is our impression that signal-related and set-related neurones (as exemplified in Fig. 2) exist in higher proportions in the SMA as compared to MI. Effector-independent neurones, referred to above, have so far been observed exclusively in the SMA (Mann et al., 1988; Tanji et al., 1988). On the whole, we would concur with the opinion of Kubota (1985) that the premotor and motor cortical areas mainly differ in terms of their proportions of the different cell classes represented. In this context, it is interesting to note that even one and the same neurone may code aspects of both movement preparation and execution. As exemplified in Fig. 2, the activity changes of the illustrated MI neurone consisted of a small signal-related peak, some gradual increase shortly before the "go-signal", merging into a sharp peak related to the conditioned arm movement as demonstrated in the shift of the dot display.

In conclusion, single unit recordings in monkeys trained to perform a motor task have clearly demonstrated that in both motor areas there is a rich repertoire of different cell classes, partly rather complex and encoding different aspects of movement preparation and execution. This pro-

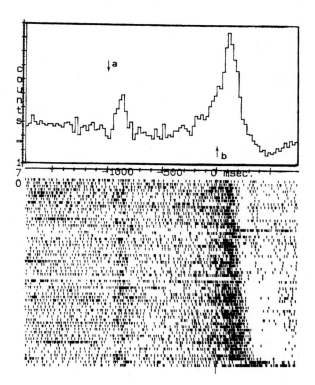

Fig. 2. Example of a neurone recorded in area 4 of MI. Arrow a indicates time of the "ready-signal"; arrow b the time of the "go-signal" to which the activity is aligned. Note small peak following the visual ready-signal, the build-up of activity occurring before the go-signal, and the movement-related sharp peak of activity.

bably reflects the fact that the two areas are reciprocally interconnected. The pattern and the functional significance of the physiological interactions of the interconnected neuronal populations in MI and the SMA are virtually unknown. One main objective in future research must be to determine the targets of the various classes of SMA neurones.

Acknowledgements

The work in our laboratory was supported by the Swiss National Science Foundation (Grant 3.509-0.86) and the Thomas Stanley Johnson Foundation. B.H. was supported by the New Zealand

MRC and the Neurological Foundation. D.-F. C is an IBRO fellow.

References

Brinkman, C. (1984) Supplementary motor area of the monkey's cerebral cortex: short- and longterm deficits after unilateral ablation, and the effects of subsequent callosal section. *J. Neurosci.,* 4: 918 – 929.

Deecke, L., Scheid P. and Kornhuber, H. (1969) Distribution of readiness potentials, pre-motion positivity, and motor potential of the human cerebral cortex preceding voluntary finger movements. *Exp. Brain Res.,* 7: 158 – 168.

Fetz, E.E. (1981) Neuronal activity associated with conditioned limb movements. In A.L. Towe and E.S. Luschei (Eds.), *Motor Coordination, Vol. 5, Handbook Behavioral Neurobiology,* Plenum Press, New York, London, pp. 493 – 526.

Goldberg, G. (1985) Supplementary motor area structure and function: Review and Hypotheses. *Behav. Brain Sci.,* 8: 567 – 616.

Hummelsheim, H., Bianchetti, M., Wiesendanger, M. and Wiesendanger, R. (1988) Sensory inputs to the agranular motor fields: a comparison between precentral, supplementary-motor and premotor areas. *Exp. Brain Res.,* 69: 289 – 298.

Kubota, K. (1985) Prefrontal and premotor contributions to the voluntary movement in learned tests. In *The Cerebral Events in Voluntary Movement: The Supplementary Motor and Premotor Areas. Proc. Ringberg Symp., Exp. Brain Res.,* 58: A8.

Laplane, D., Talairach, J., Meininger, V., Bancaud, J. and Orgogozo, J.M. (1977) Clinical consequences of corticectomies involving the supplementary motor area in man. *J. Neurol. Sci.,* 34: 301 – 314.

Mann, S.E., Thau, R. and Schiller, P.H. (1988) Conditional task-related responses in monkey dorsomedial frontal cortex. *Exp. Brain Res.,* 69: 460 – 468.

Maunsell, J.H.R. and Van Essen, D.C. (1983) The connections of the middle temporal visual area (MT) and their relationship to a cortical hierarchy in the Macaque monkey. *J. Neurosci.,* 3: 2563 – 2586.

Passingham, R.E. (1987) Two cortical systems for directing movement. In *Motor Areas of the Cerebral Cortex, Ciba Foundation Symposium,* 132: 151 – 161.

Primrose, D.C. and Strick, P.L. (1985) The organization of interconnections between the premotor areas in the primate frontal lobe and the arm area of primary motor cortex. *Soc. Neurosci. Abstr.,* II: 1274.

Roland, P.E., Larsen, B., Lassen, N.A. and Skinhoj, E. (1980) Supplementary motor area and other cortical areas in organization of voluntary movements in man. *J. Neurophysiol.,* 43: 118 – 136.

Schell, G.R. and Strick, P.L. (1984) The origin of thalamic inputs to the arcuate premotor and supplementary motor area. *J. Neurosci.,* 4: 539 – 560.

Smith, A.M., Bourbonnais, D. and Blanchette, G. (1981) Interaction between forced grasping and a learned precision grip after ablation of the supplementary motor area. *Brain Res.,* 222: 395 – 400.

Tanji, J. and Kurata, K. (1983) Functional organization of the supplementary motor area. In J.E. Desmedt (Ed.), *Motor Control Mechanisms in Health and Disease,* Raven Press, New York, pp. 421 – 431.

Tanji, J., Okano, K. and Sato, K.C. (1988) Neuronal activity in cortical motor areas related to ipsilateral, contralateral and bilateral digit movements of the monkey. *J. Neurophysiol.,* 60: 325 – 343.

Thach, W.T. (1978) Correlation of neural discharge with pattern and force of muscular activity, joint position, and direction of intended next movement in motor cortex and cerebellum. *J. Neurophysiol.,* 41: 654 – 676.

Weinrich, M., Wise, S.P. and Mauritz, K.H. (1984) A neurophysiological study of the premotor cortex in the Rhesus monkey. *Brain,* 107: 385 – 414.

Wiesendanger, M. (1986) Recent developments in studies of the supplementary motor area of primates. *Rev. Physiol. Pharmacol. Biochem.,* 103: 1 – 59.

Wiesendanger, R. and Wiesendanger, M. (1985) The thalamic connections with medial area 6 (supplementary motor cortex) in the monkey (Macaca fascicularis). *Exp. Brain Res.,* 59: 91 – 104.

Woolsey, C.N., Settlage, P.H., Meyer, D.R., Spencer, W., Hamuy, T.P. and Travis, A.M. (1952) Patterns of localization in precentral and supplementary motor areas and their relation to the concept of a premotor area. *Res. Publ. Ass. Res. Nerv. Ment. Dis.,* 30: 238 – 264.

J.H.J. Allum and M. Hulliger (Eds.)
Progress in Brain Research, Vol. 80
© 1989 Elsevier Science Publishers B.V. (Biomedical Division)

CHAPTER 36

Control of forelimb muscle activity by populations of corticomotoneuronal and rubromotoneuronal cells

E.E. Fetz[1], P.D. Cheney[2], K. Mewes[2] and S. Palmer[1]

[1]Department of Physiology and Biophysics and Regional Primate Research Center, University of Washington, Seattle, WA 98195 and [2]Department of Physiology, University of Kansas, Kansas City, KS 66103, U.S.A.

We review and synthesize evidence on the activity of corticomotoneuronal (CM) and rubromotoneuronal (RM) cells and single motor units in forearm muscles in monkeys performing alternating wrist movements. The CM and RM cells were identified by post-spike facilitation of rectified forelimb EMG activity. RM cells facilitated more muscles per cell (mean: 3.0 of 6 synergist muscles) than CM cells (2.4/6). Both groups had "reciprocal" cells which also suppressed antagonists of their facilitated target muscles. Unlike CM cells, some RM cells co-facilitated flexor and extensor muscles (5.8 of 12 muscles). During performance of a standard ramp-and-hold force tracking task the firing patterns of CM and RM cells, as well as single motor units, fell into distinct response types. Each population had phasic-tonic and tonic cells. Unique to the CM population were cells whose discharge increased during the static hold period; unique to RM cells were bidirectionally responsive and unmodulated neurons. Many motor units showed decrementing discharge. To estimate the ensemble activities of these populations the response histograms of different cells were summed (with force ramps aligned) in proportion to the relative frequency of each cell type. The population response histogram of CM cells was phasic-tonic, consistent with the predominant response type. The population response of RM cells was also phasic-tonic, but showed a shallower phasic modulation relative to discharge that was sustained during both directions of movement. The population histogram of motor units of a muscle was proportional to the average of rectified multiunit EMG, and typically exhibited decrementing activity during the static hold. The effects of excitatory postsynaptic potentials (EPSPs) on firing probability of motoneurons previously documented in intracellular studies are combined with the mean firing rates in the population histograms and the known amplitudes of CM-EPSPs and RM-EPSPs to infer the relative contributions of the supraspinal cells to tonic discharge of active motoneurons. This analysis suggests that for intermediate levels of force, the CM cells would increment motoneuron discharge by about 9 impulses/second (i.p.s.) and RM cells by about 2.4 i.p.s. The analysis also reveals differences in the population activity of CM and RM cells compared to their target motoneurons, which may be due to other input cells and to recruitment properties of motoneurons.

Key words: Muscle; Motor cortex; Red nucleus; Spike triggered average; Neuropopulation; Primate

Introduction

The relations between firing patterns of neurons in the motor system and parameters of voluntary movement are commonly used to infer which movement parameters are "coded" by central neurons. A causal explanation of the neural mechanisms that generate voluntary movement should ultimately provide a quantitative account of how populations of cells control activity of spinal motoneurons. It is not enough to contend that certain response patterns observed in particular cells *could* underlie the programming and execution of movements. A causal explanation also requires demonstration that the responses of these cells *do* contribute to the movement. Proving causality is usually difficult, but is possible for premotoneuronal cells that have demonstrable post-spike effects on motoneurone firing.

Investigators have recently found that the activities of populations of cells can provide functions that match movement parameters more closely than the firing patterns of any single neurones. Humphrey et al. (1970) first showed that the smoothed activity of a population of motor cortex neurones could be used to match several different movement parameters. Weighted averages of the cells' firing rates could match the force trajectories and wrist displacements, as well as their temporal derivatives, if the weighting factors for each cell could be optimally chosen for each trajectory. Moreover, the match between the cells' weighted activities and the mechanical parameters improved with the number of cells included. The ability to freely optimize the weighting coefficients, of course, helped to assure convergence on the movement trajectories; closer matches are obtained with larger populations because each additional nonredundant cell could only serve to further reduce the remaining difference.

More recently, Georgopoulos et al. (1984) have shown that populations of motor cortex cells could be used to match the direction of limb movement by invoking the "vector hypothesis" to sum the activity of directionally tuned cells. For a given movement direction each cell is assumed to make a vector contribution pointing in the direction of its maximal activity, and by an amount proportional to its mean rate during the given movement. The vector sum of the population then approximates the direction of arm displacement. Again, the match improved as more cells with diverse directional preferences were included. This match with movement direction could be taken to suggest that arm *displacement* is coded in motor cortex populations rather than muscle force, as previously proposed (e.g., Evarts, 1968; Cheney and Fetz, 1980). The direct match between the population function and arm displacement is appealing because it conveniently avoids the intervening complexities of synaptic connections and limb mechanics, which present formidable obstacles to a causal explanation. Indeed, the vector hypothesis will produce a match with movement direction whether the directionally "tuned" cells have any output effects on muscles or not.

Although one can find good *descriptive* matches between functions of the activity of neuronal populations and particular movement parameters, this correspondence is no proof of neuronal coding in the *causal* sense. To demonstrate that the candidate cells actually make a causal contribution requires additional evidence that they have appropriate output effects. Evidence for synaptic linkages of cells recorded in behaving animals can be obtained by cross-correlation techniques, and evidence for direct effects on muscle activity can be demonstrated by spike-triggered averaging of EMG. Here we synthesize information on cells in the primate motor system that have demonstrable effects on muscles, namely, corticomotoneuronal (CM) and rubromotoneuronal (RM) cells. The activity of these supraspinal premotoneuronal cells and forelimb motor units was documented under behavioural conditions which were sufficiently similar across different experiments to compare their activity. The cells were recorded in monkeys performing a step-tracking task, and generating ramp-and-hold wrist torques, consisting of a change of force between flexion and extension zones followed by a static hold in a force zone. The monkeys typically performed the responses with similar timing across experiments, allowing comparisons of the cells' response patterns.

The synaptic connections of the cortical and rubral cells to motoneurones was inferred from post-spike effects observed in spike-triggered averages of forelimb EMG activity. This correlational linkage identifies these output cells and their target muscles, and also implies that the premotoneuronal cells affect their target muscles in proportion to their firing rates. Other studies have provided quantitative evidence on the magnitude of correlational effects of single cells synapsing on motoneurones (Cope et al., 1987). These observations can be combined into a quantitative picture of the time-varying interactions between populations of connected cells in the primate motor system during voluntary wrist movements.

Correlational linkages obtained by spike-triggered averaging

The spike-triggered averaging (STA) technique can best be understood by examining the expected effects of a single input cell to a motoneurone. Fig. 1 illustrates a hypothetical CM cell synapsing on a motoneurone. The illustrated EPSP is taken from a STA of intracellularly recorded membrane potential in a cat motoneurone at rest, triggered from a single Ia afferent fibre (Cope et al., 1987). When the motoneurone was induced to fire rhythmically, this unitary EPSP transiently increased the motoneurone firing probability, as measured by the peak in the cross-correlation histogram between the spikes of the Ia fibre and

the motoneurone. In these experiments, the measure of the cross-correlogram peak that was most strongly related to the EPSP was the peak area, i.e., the number of motoneurone action potentials above baseline triggered by each EPSP. This peak area (N_p) was proportional to the EPSP amplitude (h), and is given by the following relation:

$$N_p = 1.1 \times 10^{-4} \, h \, \mu V \qquad (1)$$

Thus, the effect of unitary EPSPs of 100 μV is to trigger about one firing per 100 EPSPs. This suggests that if the unitary EPSPs of height h arrive at a rate of f per second, the mean increment in motoneurone firing would be approximately:

$$df_m \cong 10^{-4} * h * f \qquad (2)$$

Relation 2 assumes that the increment in firing given by Relation 1 is independent of the firing rates of the presynaptic cell and the motoneurone; this assumption seems reasonable in light of preliminary evidence, but requires further investigation. The relation also assumes that the correlogram peak is followed by a negligible trough below baseline. Under these conditions, Relation 2 provides the proportionality between the firing rate of the premotoneuronal cell (f) and its effect on the motoneurone firing rate.

In chronic recording studies, one can compile spike-triggered averages of multi-unit EMG (Fetz and Cheney, 1980; Buys et al., 1986) more readily than correlograms with single motor units — although the latter have also been documented (Mantel and Lemon, 1987; Smith and Fetz, 1989). The typical effect observed in STA of coactivated muscles was a post-spike facilitation (PSF), which rose above baseline after some onset latency, reached a peak and declined again. This post-spike facilitation represents the summed effects of all the motor units in the EMG record that were facilitated. The contribution of a single facilitated motor unit would be the convolution of its correlogram peak with its rectified motor unit poten-

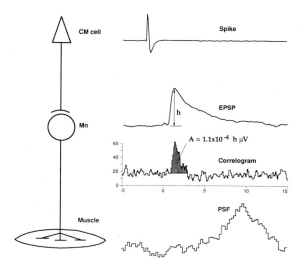

Fig. 1. Events mediating the post-spike effects of a premotoneuronal cell. The monosynaptic connection produces an EPSP and increased motoneurone firing probability — represented here by STA of a Ia EPSP and the associated correlogram (data from Cope et al., 1987). The area (A) of the correlogram peak was found to be proportional to the height (h) of the EPSP. STA of multiunit EMG produces post-spike facilitation (PSF), representing the contribution of all facilitated motor units.

tial. Since the EMG includes the activity of multiple units with unknown and variable relative timing, the net PSF is some nonlinear function of the contribution of the underlying motor units. Although the shape and size of the PSF have limited quantitative significance, they serve to identify those cortical and rubral cells that have output effects on their target muscles, and also identify their muscle fields.

The magnitude of PSF was measured as a mean percent increase (MPI) above baseline. CM cells produced a somewhat greater facilitation of their target muscles (MPI = 7.0%) than RM cells (5.1%). The mean onset latency of PSF was longer for CM cells (6.3 ms) than RM cells (5.2 ms); this difference probably reflects the difference in conduction distance, although conduction velocities of descending cells and motoneurones could add considerable variance.

In addition to the excitatory effects in the PSF, spike-triggered averaging has also demonstrated inhibitory linkages from cells to muscles, usually to antagonists of the coactivated target muscles. Such inhibitory linkages were first deduced from stimulus-triggered averages obtained by single-pulse microstimulation applied during both flexion and extension (Cheney et al., 1985). At about one-third of the sites of CM cells that facilitated target muscles, microstimulation produced a post-stimulus suppression in their antagonists. Post-spike inhibitory effects from single CM cells were directly demonstrated from action potentials evoked by glutamate during the antagonist phase of movement, when the CM cell would normally be inactive (Kasser and Cheney, 1985). The mean percent decrease below baseline for post-spike suppression (PSS) was −4.1% for CM cells and −4.5% for RM cells. The latencies of PSS tended to be about 3 ms greater than the latencies of PSF for the same cells (i.e., 9.3 ms for CM cells and 8.4 ms for RM cells).

Muscle fields

In our experiments spike-triggered averages were typically compiled simultaneously for six coactivated synergistic muscles. The muscles that were coactivated with the cell are referred to as agonists, and those facilitated by the cell are its target muscles. The number of facilitated target muscles ranged from one to all six of the coactivated agonist muscles. The mean number of facilitated muscles per cell was somewhat larger for RM cells (3.0 of 6 muscles) than for CM cells (2.4/6). In both groups the excitatory muscle fields tended to be slightly larger for extension cells than for flexion cells. Buys et al. (1986) found that the proportion of facilitated muscles was larger for intrinsic hand muscles than forearm muscles.

Some of the supraspinal cells that facilitated their coactivated agonist muscles also exhibited post-spike effects on antagonists of their target muscles. The patterns of post-spike effects produced in agonist and antagonist muscles are summarized in Fig. 2. About 59% of CM cells and 39% of RM cells produced a *pure facilitation* of agonists, without any detectable effect on the recorded antagonist muscles. About 30% of both

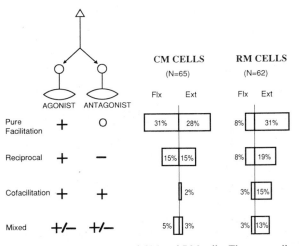

Fig. 2. Projection patterns of CM and RM cells. The post-spike effects on coactivated agonist muscles and their antagonists include facilitation (+), suppression (−), or no effect (0). The mixed category includes cells which facilitated and suppressed agonist muscles, and some "pure suppression" cells. The proportions of each type of projection pattern are given separately for cells which facilitated flexor and extensor muscles.

CM and RM cells produced post-spike suppression in antagonists of their target muscles. The activity of these *reciprocal* cells simultaneously facilitated agonists and inhibited antagonists. The magnitude of inhibition tended to be stronger in flexor than extensor muscles.

A third type of cell produced post-spike facilitation in both flexor and extensor muscles. Such *co-facilitation* cells were common among RM cells, but were relatively rare in the CM cell population. Most of these co-facilitation cells produced greater post-spike facilitation of extensor than flexor muscles. RM co-facilitation cells were often active during both flexion and extension movements (like other RM cells), suggesting that their output might function to raise the excitability of motoneurons, independent of the direction of movement.

Finally, a miscellaneous category of cells produced *mixed* effects on their target muscles. Most of these facilitated particular agonist muscles and suppressed other agonists. A few exerted no measured effect on their coactivated muscles, but only suppressed the antagonist muscles (so-called "pure suppression" cells). Still other cells exhibited stronger modulation with antagonists of their facilitated muscles. These miscellaneous types are combined in the "mixed" group.

Discharge properties during active movements

The response patterns of CM and RM cells, as well as motor units, fell into several distinct categories on the basis of their discharge during the dynamic and static phase of the torque trajectory. Fig. 3 illustrates these patterns and tabulates the relative proportion of cells within each population exhibiting these patterns.

A common response pattern in all three groups was *phasic-tonic,* consisting of a phasic discharge at onset of movement, followed by a tonic firing during the static hold period. This represented the predominant type for both CM and RM cells. Another category observed in all three groups were *tonic* cells, which discharged with a steady firing rate during the hold period, with a time course

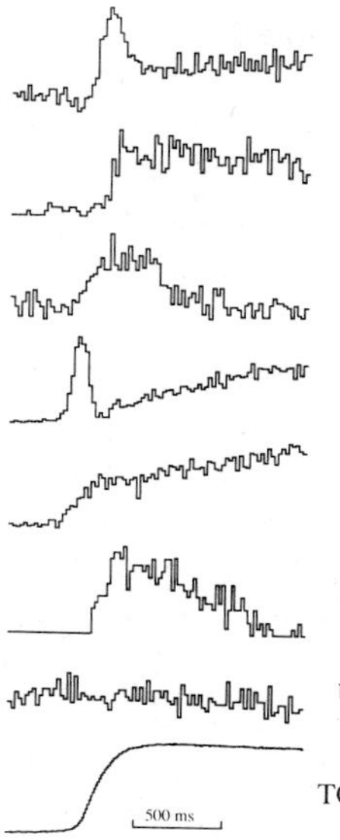

RESPONSE TYPE	POPULATION		
	CM	RM	MU
PHASIC-TONIC	48%	46%	23%
TONIC	28	8	33
PHASIC	2	20	5
PHASIC-RAMP	10	0	0
RAMP	6	0	0
DECREMENTING	5	3	39
UNMODULATED	0	23	0
TORQUE N =	211	61	86

Fig. 3. Response patterns of CM and RM cells and motor units during ramp-and-hold wrist responses. Examples of each type of discharge pattern are shown at left, and the proportions of cells in each population are tabulated on the right.

resembling the torque trajectory. The tonic firing rate of cells in all groups (CM, RM and motor units) was an increasing function of the static force exerted by the monkey.

The remaining categories of firing patterns appeared predominantly in one or another of the three populations. Many RM cells and some motor units exhibited a purely *phasic* discharge pattern at onset of movement, with no sustained increase in activity during the hold period. Unique to the cortical population were CM cells that exhibited a gradually increasing *"ramp"* discharge during the static hold period; some of these also had a phasic discharge at onset of movements. A *decrementing* discharge during the hold period was characteristic of many motor units, but was seen more rarely in the supraspinal premotor populations. This decrementing discharge dropped steadily at a rate exceeding any change in static torque.

Remarkably, many RM cells were *unmodulated* during alternating movements. These cells exhibited strong PSF and were located within the region of the magnocellular red nucleus. All of these cells showed a higher continuous discharge during movement of 6 – 20 Hz; this allowed spike-triggered averages to be computed for both flexor and extensor muscles.

These response categories encompass the patterns seen at intermediate force levels. A few motor units showed a transition from one type of pattern to another. For example, some phasic motor units exhibited phasic-tonic or decrementing discharge at the highest force levels. The proportions of these discharge patterns given in Fig. 3 are representative for intermediate load levels.

Whether particular types of supraspinal cells preferentially affect specific types of motor units remains to be determined. In microstimulation experiments all types of motor units were facilitated by S-ICMS applied at a single cortical site (Palmer and Fetz, 1985b). Cross-correlations between CM cells and motor units indicate that most of the motor units in a facilitated muscle were affected by a CM cell (Mantel and Lemon, 1987). This would suggest that CM cells, like Ia afferent fibers, probably send divergent terminals to most, if not all motoneurons of their target muscles.

The variety of response patterns seen for individual CM and RM cells, and the differences between these responses and those of their target muscles, indicates that these response patterns alone provide no reliable guide to inferring causal linkages. A clear example is the phasic-ramp CM cells, whose sharply modulated discharge pattern is radically different from that of its target muscles. At the other extreme, the steady discharge of the unmodulated RM cells would make them unlikely candidates for causal involvement in the task, although such contribution is revealed by their post-spike effects. Given the PSF as evidence that these different types of cells *do* have synaptic linkages to motoneurons, one could infer a rationale for their observed discharge patterns. For example, the prominent phasic discharge at movement onset exhibited by many premotoneuronal cells appears necessary to activate the target muscles; in the case of reciprocal cells, this phasic activity would simultaneously inhibit the antagonist muscles. In contrast to the unidirectional activation of CM cells with either flexion or extension, many RM cells fired during both movements; those bidirectional cells which also cofacilitate both sets of muscles may be more involved in sustaining motoneuron excitability than controlling the movement direction.

The ramp discharge in CM cells may be viewed as a mechanism for overcoming the tendency of motoneurons to adapt during the hold period; a steady increase in synaptic input would help to sustain motoneuron firing during the static hold period. It may be significant that a phasic-ramp pattern can be obtained by subtracting the decrementing discharge of motor units from the common phasic-tonic pattern of CM cells. This would suggest that phasic-ramp cells may represent a difference between a phasic-tonic command and the decrementing response of agonist motor units; such an "error signal" in CM cells would provide a proportional excitatory effect on their target muscles, reducing the difference between command and response.

Relation to active force

The activity of CM and RM cells clearly "encodes" active force, in the sense that this activity causally contributes to force through the correlational linkage with motor units. Yet the relation between neural activity and force is significantly different for these supraspinal cells compared to their target motor units. These differences are illustrated by graphs of the tonic firing rate observed during the static hold period plotted as a function of the active force for representative units from each group (Fig. 4). Both CM and RM cells showed some discharge during the hold period at even the lowest force levels. In contrast to motor units, the supraspinal premotoneuronal cells were not sequentially recruited into activity at higher forces. However, it should be noted that although the external load was off at the origin of the abscissa, a small amount of force was required to overcome internal loads, such as stretch of the antagonist muscles. Above these minimal force levels, CM and RM cells increased their firing rates rapidly. In contrast, motor units contribute to increasing force by two mechanisms: recruitment of new motor units at successively higher force levels, and increases in firing rate as a function of force. In addition, the discharge of motor units typically saturated at rates well below those which supraspinal cells attained.

The rate – torque slope, namely, the increase in firing rate per increase in static force over the linear range, was higher for extensor cells than flexor cells, for both CM and RM populations. The average rate – torque slope for all extensor CM cells (480 Hz/Nm) was about twice that of flexor CM cells (250 Hz/Nm). Similarly, the average rate – torque slope for all extensor RM cells (128 Hz/Nm) was larger than that of flexor RM cells (22 Hz/Nm). In contrast, motor units showed no statistically significant difference in the

mean rate – torque slopes of extensor and flexor motor units (260 and 410 Hz/Nm, respectively). This suggests that the difference exhibited by supraspinal populations is not simply related to the mechanical advantage of flexion over extension, but represents an intrinsic asymmetry in their relation to flexor and extensor muscles.

Population responses

Since the monkeys performed the ramp-and-hold responses similarly across different recording sessions, it is possible not only to compare the response patterns of these cells, but also to combine the individual contributions to obtain a more complete picture of the ensemble activity. Summing the individual response histograms can provide a more comprehensive population average.

Such a summation has been performed previously for motor units recorded in forearm muscles (Palmer and Fetz, 1985a). As shown in Fig. 5, adding the response histograms of seven motor units (left) yielded a population histogram which matched the rectified EMG activity of their parent muscle quite well (right). This suggests that the response averages of target muscle EMG obtained with CM and RM cells can be taken as representative of the activity of their target motoneurone pool.

The response histograms of the supraspinal cells were added in a similar manner, as illustrated in Fig. 6. Selecting cells associated with comparable force ramps, we calculated population histograms by aligning the force ramps and summing the response histograms of the units. We also summed the average EMG of their target muscles and the torque trajectories, and normalized by the number of cells. Subpopulation averages were first compiled for cells of each response type (Fig. 6, middle). Then these averages were combined in proportion to the relative frequency of each response type to get the overall population average (Fig. 6, right).

The overall population histograms of CM and RM cells both exhibited a phasic-tonic discharge pattern, as shown in Fig. 7. However, the CM

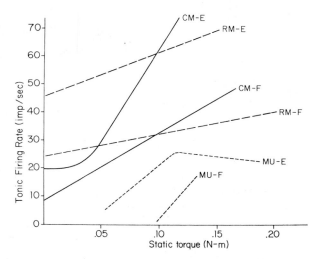

Fig. 4. Firing rates of CM and RM cells and motor units as function of static torque. The tonic rates during the static hold period were measured from response averages compiled at different force levels. Representative curves are shown for flexor and extensor cells.

population showed greater depth of modulation with the task: the difference between tonic rates during agonist and antagonist hold period was larger, and so was the relative height of the phasic burst.

The activity of these supraspinal populations began well before their target muscle activity, and clearly differed from their target muscles. Since these cells facilitated their target motor units, one can interpret their activity as representing the direct synaptic influence of these cells on motoneurons. Any motoneuron receiving converging input from the supraspinal populations would receive a time-varying current proportional to the population histogram, and displaced by a conduction delay of several milliseconds (considerably less than the histogram bin width). The difference between the ensemble discharge of these pre-

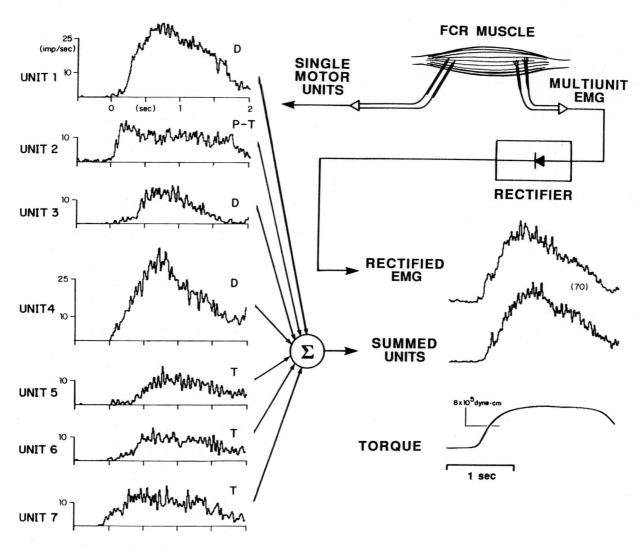

Fig. 5. Response histograms of 7 single motor units (left) recorded in the same flexor carpi radialis muscle. The sum of the response histograms gives a good approximation to the average of multi-unit EMG recorded with wire electrodes (modified from Palmer and Fetz, 1985a).

motoneuronal populations and their target motoneuron pools is illustrated in the bottom traces of Fig. 7. The initial phasic peak in this difference trace indicates that synaptic input from CM and RM cells precedes the overt activity of motor unit by several hundred milliseconds. This initial input would bring the motoneurons to threshold; it could also counter any inhibitory effects from antagonist input cells producing reciprocal inhibition on these motoneurons.

The profile of EMG activity in these response averages can also be interpreted as a measure of the net excitatory drive that the motoneurons are receiving from *all* their inputs. This can be concluded from the experiments of Hoffer et al. (1987), who reported that intracellular injection of current proportional to EMG activity that had been recorded previously in moving animals could generate motoneuron discharge mimicking activity of motor units recorded in the active muscles. Thus, the difference between the synaptic drive from premotoneuronal cells (reflected in their population histograms) and the net synaptic excitation in their target muscles (reflected by the EMG averages) suggests the presence of other inputs during the dynamic phase of movement. Analysis of

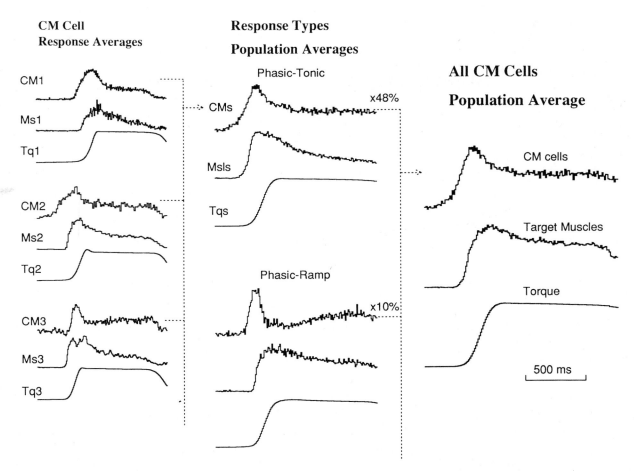

Fig. 6. Derivation of the population histograms of CM cells. The response averages of individual cells in each category were summed, along with their target muscle and the corresponding torque trajectories. The population averages for each response type were then weighted in proportion to the relative number of cells in each type. This provided the net population average of the CM cells.

the neural mechanisms involved in the transition between flexion and extension zones is complicated by many unknown variables, including the changing activity of inhibitory interneurons, the currents required to bring motoneurons to threshold, and potential inputs from many other premotoneuronal cells whose discharge patterns are not known.

In contrast to the complex factors during the dynamic phase of movement, the activity during the static hold period presents a steady-state situation in which activities of the input populations and motoneurons may be quantitatively compared. In particular, the firing rates of CM and RM cells at specific force levels can be used to infer their effect on the activity of motoneurons. Given the correlational effect of unitary EPSPs in motoneurons (Relation 1), we can estimate the contribution of the colony of CM cells to the tonic firing of a motoneuron as the sum of Relation 2 over the population:

$$\mathrm{d}f_{\mathrm{m;\,c}} \cong \Sigma\ 10^{-4}\ h_{\mathrm{i}}f_{\mathrm{i}}$$

where $\mathrm{d}f_{\mathrm{m;c}}$ is the increment in firing rate of a

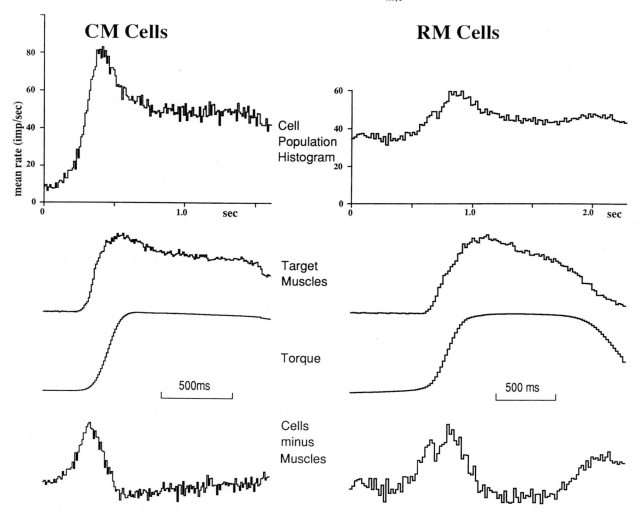

Fig. 7. Population averages for CM and RM cells, with corresponding target muscles and torque trajectories. The difference between the population activity and their target muscle activity is plotted at the bottom. This shows the net surplus of descending activity at movement onset and the incrementing difference during the static hold.

motoneurone caused by its colony of CM cells; h_i is the height of the CM-EPSP of the ith CM cell and f_i is its firing rate. If h_i and f_i are not correlated, we can estimate the summation over the population by using their mean values. In this case the sum is equal to the number of CM cells converging onto the motoneurone (N_c), times the mean amplitude of the unitary CM-EPSP (h_c), times the mean firing rate of a CM cell (f_c):

$$\sum_{i=1}^{N_c} 10^{-4}\, h_i f_i \cong 10^{-4}\, N_c h_c f_c$$

The first two terms on the right — the number of CM cells in the colony and the mean height of their unitary CM-EPSPs — are generally unknown; however, their product is the maximal CM-EPSP H_c, which has been experimentally measured. Thus,

$$df_{m;c} = 10^{-4}\, H_c f_c$$

Note that the use of H_c in this expression does *not* imply that the CM cells are firing synchronously. The derivation is valid for asynchronous firing, but leads to the product of two terms, N_c and h_c, whose product is equal to the measured quantity H_c. When measured in cervical motoneurones of barbiturate-anaesthetized baboons, the value of H_c ranged from 1 to 3 mV (Clough et al., 1968; Phillips and Porter, 1977). In hindlimb motoneurones of barbiturate-anaesthetized macaques, Shapovalov et al. (1971) found the mean H_c evoked from cortex to be 1.0 mV. In forearm motoneurones of chloralose-anaesthetized macaques, Fritz et al. (1985) found the mean H_c evoked from the pyramidal tract to be 2.0 mV. Taking the latter estimate for the behaving monkey, the contribution of the CM population with a mean firing rate of f_c would be

$$df_{m;c} = 10^{-4} * 2000\ \mu V * f_c = 0.2\, f_c$$

Given the mean static firing rate of 45 Hz for the CM population (Fig. 7), the CM cells would increment motor unit activity by about 9 impulses/second (i.p.s.).

A comparable analysis applies for the RM population. The maximal RM-EPSPs obtained in macaques by Shapovalov averaged to 0.6 mV. This suggests that the population of RM cells would increment the motoneurone firing by:

$$df_{m;r} = 0.06\, f_r$$

where f_r is the mean firing rate of RM cells. For an $f_r = 40$ i.p.s., the contribution of RM cells to motor unit firing is about 2.4 i.p.s.

Finally, the sum of these terms would represent the estimated contribution of both CM and RM populations to motoneurone activity. For example, at an intermediate extension load level of 0.1 Nm, we have, from Fig. 4, $f_c = 45$ i.p.s. and $f_r = 40$ i.p.s., giving a net $df_m = 9 + 2.4 = 11.4$ i.p.s. This represents over half of the maximal firing rate of the extensor motor unit illustrated in Fig. 4.

Of course this estimate is qualified by several major assumptions. One significant assumption is that the population average reflects the mean input to the motoneurone; it may well turn out that each motoneurone receives inputs preferentially from particular types of premotoneuronal cells. Another assumption is that the ratio between EPSP amplitude and the increase in motoneuron firing probability (Relation 2) applies across experimental conditions and is independent of motoneurone firing rate. Until more information is available these assumptions appear reasonable, and provide the best quantitative inference from the existing evidence.

The curves in Fig. 4 indicate that additional mechanisms must come into play at higher force levels, which limit the increase in motoneurone firing rates. While the supraspinal populations continue to increase their firing, the motor unit rates saturate, and sometimes begin to decline. Since these levels are well below the maximal rates obtained by intracellular stimulation, these results would suggest the presence of some inhibitory control to restrict their rates, perhaps mediated by Renshaw or other inhibitory interneurones.

Concluding comments

Our analysis of population effects on motoneurons from identified premotoneuronal cells can be compared to previous studies of population coding in motor cortex cells. The vector hypothesis of Georgopoulos et al. (1984) is based on unit vectors derived from the cells' net neural activity over the entire movement, whereas the present approach provides a quantitative picture of the time-varying drive on motoneurons. The study of Georgopoulos et al. (1984) also illustrates a time-varying population histogram of cortical unit activity, analogous to ours; this net population histogram is presumably quite similar for each direction of movement. A time-varying population vector can also be generated from the sum of unit vectors whose lengths are proportional to the cells' instantaneous activity. This function can be calculated whether the cells have any output effects or not. In contrast, we are utilizing cells whose contribution to muscle activity is confirmed by spike-triggered averaging, and so are dealing with a population of premotor cells whose activity causally codes muscle force, and whose population histogram is proportional to their synaptic drive on their target motoneurons. The population study of Humphrey et al. (1970) computed matches between weighted averages of neural activity and movement parameters by calculating the coefficients required to optimize the match. In contrast, our model incorporates a weighting factor derived from physiological experiments on motoneurons, and calculates the estimated contributions to motoneuron activity.

This analysis may be extended eventually to include other populations of cells affecting motoneurones. It may also be applied to other types of repetitive responses; the study of Prochazka et al. (1989, this volume) calculates population histograms of afferent fibers during the hindlimb step cycle. Afferent fibers can also be recorded in the behaving primate in cervical dorsal root ganglia (Schieber and Thach, 1985). Preliminary evidence from monkeys performing our ramp-and-hold task indicates that afferent fibres in the C8 root can produce strong post-spike effects in multiple muscles and that these have response patterns similar to supraspinal premotoneuronal cells (Flament and Fetz, in press). Other sources of premotoneuronal inputs include various spinal interneurons; the activity of inhibitory interneurons would be of particular interest in resolving the difference between the excitatory input from supraspinal cells and the net excitation reflected in muscle activity. The effects of these different populations may eventually be synthesized into a quantitative picture of the neural mechanisms underlying execution of voluntary movement.

Acknowledgements

We thank colleagues whose efforts contributed to this report, particularly Rick Kasser and Wade Smith for additional information on CM cells, and Larry Shupe for developing the requisite software. This work was supported by NIH grants NS12542, RR00166 and NSF grant BNS 82-16608.

References

Buys, E.R., Lemon, R.N., Mantel, G.W.B. and Muir, R.B. (1986) Selective facilitation of different hand muscles by single corticospinal neurones in the conscious monkey. *J. Physiol. (London)*, 381: 529 – 549.

Cheney, P.D. and Fetz, E.E. (1980) Functional classes of primate corticomotoneuronal cells and their relation to active force. *J. Neurophysiol.*, 44: 773 – 791.

Cheney, P.D. and Fetz, E.E. (1985) Comparable patterns of muscle facilitation evoked by individual corticomotoneuronal (CM) cells and by single intracortical microstimuli in primates: Evidence for functional groups of CM cells. *J. Neurophysiol.*, 53: 786 – 804.

Cheney, P.D. and Fetz, E.E. (1984) Corticomotoneuronal cells contribute to long-latency stretch reflexes in the rhesus monkey. *J. Physiol. (London)*, 349: 249 – 272.

Cheney, P.D., Fetz, E.E. and Palmer, S.S. (1985) Patterns of facilitation and suppression of antagonist forelimb muscles from motor cortex sites in the awake monkey. *J. Neurophysiol.*, 53: 805 – 820.

Cheney, P.D., Kasser, R.J. and Fetz, E.E. (1985) Motor and sensory properties of primate corticomotoneuronal cells.

Exp. Brain Res., Suppl. 10: 211–231.

Cheney, P.D., Mewes, K. and Fetz, E.E. (1988) Encoding of motor parameters by corticomotoneuronal (CM) and rubromotoneuronal (RM) cells identified by spike-triggered averaging in the awake monkey. *Behav. Brain Res.,* 28: 181–191.

Clough, J.F.M., Kernell, D. and Phillips, C.G. (1968) The distribution of monosynaptic excitation from the pyramidal tract and from primary spindle afferents to motoneurons of the baboon's hand and forearm. *J. Physiol. (London),* 198: 145–166.

Cope, T.C., Fetz, E.E. and Matsumura, M. (1987) Cross-correlation assessment of the synaptic strength of single Ia fibre connections with lumbar motoneurones in the cat. *J. Physiol. (London),* 390: 161–188.

Evarts, E.V. (1968) Relation of pyramidal tract activity to force exerted during voluntary movement. *J. Neurophysiol.,* 31: 14–27.

Fetz, E.E. and Cheney, P.D. (1980) Postspike facilitation of forelimb muscle activity by primate corticomotoneuronal cells. *J. Neurophysiol.,* 44: 751–772.

Fetz, E.E. and Gustafsson, B. (1983) Relation between shapes of postsynaptic potentials and changes in firing probability of cat motoneurones. *J. Physiol. (London),* 341: 387–410.

Flament, D. and Fetz, E.E. (1989) Response patterns of peripheral afferent fibers producing post-spike facilitation of forelimb muscles in the behaving monkey. *Can. J. Physiol. Pharmacol.,* 67: Axi.

Fritz, N., Illert, M., Kolb, F.P., Lemon, R.N., Muir, R.B., van der Burg, J., Wiedemann, E. and Yamaguchi, T. (1985) The cortico-motoneuronal input to hand and forearm motoneurones in the anesthetized monkey. *J. Physiol. (London),* 366: 20P.

Georgopoulos, A.P., Kalaska, J.F., Crutcher, M.D., Caminin, R. and Massey, J.T. (1984) The representation of movement direction in the motor cortex: single cell and population studies. In G.E. Edelman, W.E. Gall and W.M. Cowan (Eds.), *Dynamic Aspects of Neocortical Function,* John Wiley, New York, pp. 501–524.

Henneman, E. and Mendell, L.M. (1981) Functional organization of the motoneuron pool and its inputs, In V.B. Brooks (Ed.), *Handbook of Physiology, Vol. II, Part 1,* pp. 423–507.

Hoffer, J.A., Sugano, N., Loeb, G.E., Marks, W.B., O'Donovan, M.J. and Pratt, C.A. (1987) Cat hindlimb motoneurons during locomotion. II. Normal activity patterns. *J. Neurophysiol.,* 57: 530–553.

Humphrey, D.R., Schmidt, E.M. and Thompson, W.D. (1970) Predicting measures of motor performance from multiple spike trains. *Science,* 170: 758–762.

Jankowska, E., Padel, Y. and Tanaka, P. (1975) Disynaptic inhibition of spinal motoneurones from the motor cortex in the monkey. *J. Physiol. (London),* 258: 467–487.

Kasser, R.J. and Cheney, P.D. (1985) Characteristics of corticomotoneuronal postspike facilitation and reciprocal suppression of EMG activity in the monkey. *J. Neurophysiol.,* 53: 959–978.

Lemon, R.N., Mantel, G.W.H. and Muir, R.B. (1986) Corticospinal facilitation of hand muscles during voluntary movement in the conscious monkey. *J. Physiol. (London),* 381: 497–527.

Mantel, G.W.H. and Lemon, R.N. (1987) Cross-correlation reveals facilitation of single motor units in thenar muscles by single corticospinal neurons in the conscious monkey. *Neurosci. Lett.,* 77: 113–118.

Muir, R.B. and Lemon, R.N. (1983) Corticospinal neurons with a special role in precision grip. *Brain Res.,* 261: 312–316.

Palmer, S.S. and Fetz, E.E. (1985a) Discharge properties of primate forearm motor units during isometric muscle activity. *J. Neurophysiol.,* 54: 1178–1193.

Palmer, S.S. and Fetz, E.E. (1985b) Effects of single intracortical microstimuli in motor cortex on activity of identified forearm motor units in behaving monkeys. *J. Neurophysiol.,* 54: 1194–1212.

Phillips, C.G. and Porter, R. (1977) *Corticospinal Neurones. Their Role in Movement.* Monographs of the Physiological Society, Academic Press, London.

Prochazka, A., Trend, P., Hulliger, M. and Vincent, S. (1990) Ensemble proprioceptive activity in the cat step cycle: towards a representative look-up chart. In J.H.J. Allum and M. Hulliger (Eds.), *Afferent Control of Posture and Locomotion, Prog. Brain Res., Vol. 80,* Elsevier, Amsterdam, pp. 61–74.

Schieber, M.A. and Thach, W.T. (1985) Trained slow tracking II. Bidirectional discharge patterns of cerebellar nuclear, motor cortex, and spindle afferent neurons. *J. Neurophysiol.,* 55: 1228–1270.

Shapovalov, A.I., Karamjen, O.A., Kurchavyi, G.G. and Repina, Z.A. (1971) Synaptic actions evoked from the red nucleus on the spinal alpha-motoneurones in the rhesus monkey. *Brain Res.,* 32: 325–348.

Smith, W.S. and Fetz, E.E. (1989) Effects of synchrony between corticomotoneuronal cells on post-spike facilitation of muscles and motor units. *Neurosci. Lett.,* 96: 76–81.

J.H.J. Allum and M. Hulliger (Eds.)
Progress in Brain Research, Vol. 80
© 1989 Elsevier Science Publishers B.V. (Biomedical Division)

CHAPTER 37

Sensorimotor cortical control of isometric force in the monkey

M.-C. Hepp-Reymond, T.M.J. Wannier, M.A. Maier and E.A. Rufener

Brain Research Institute, University of Zurich, CH-8029 Zurich, Switzerland

Recordings from single neurones in the primary somatosensory (SI) and motor (MI) cortex of monkeys trained to precisely regulate force between thumb and index finger have disclosed the following contrasting properties between neurones in these two cortical regions: (1) the existence of neurones with similar discharge patterns within MI and SI but, between these regions, significantly different distributions of the classes of discharge patterns; (2) a late onset of activity change in SI neurones in relation to force increase as compared to significantly earlier changes in MI neurones; (3) linear relations between firing rate and isometric force for SI and MI neurones, however with a larger range of rate-force slopes in SI as compared to MI; (4) infrequent motor reactions to intracortical microstimulation in SI but frequent reactions in MI; (5) a majority of SI neurones with cutaneous afferent input in contrast to predominant input from deep tissues to MI neurones; and (6) context independent visually evoked activity observed exclusively in MI neurones. These major differences suggest that SI neuronal activity most likely reflects the input from peripheral receptors rather than, as postulated for MI neurones, the participation in movement initiation and the control of muscular contractions.

Key words: Monkey; Single cell recording; Isometric force; Precision grip; Motor cortex; Somatosensory cortex; Hand; Microstimulation; Somatic afferent input; Visually responsive neuron

Introduction

The control of force in prehension relies both on the synergy of a large number of intrinsic and extrinsic finger muscles and on the integration of afferent inputs from the digits. The contribution of the primary motor cortex (MI) neurones during active force generation has been repeatedly confirmed by various investigators for different tasks (Evarts, 1968, 1969; Schmidt et al., 1975; Smith et al., 1975; Hepp-Reymond et al., 1978; Hoffman and Luschei, 1980). In addition, Cheney and Fetz (1980) were able to demonstrate that the tonic discharge of corticomotoneuronal neurones increased with the force exerted by their target muscles. The close relation between MI neuronal activity and force has been so far demonstrated for movements of the distal, proximal and jaw musculature, and under isotonic, auxotonic (spring-like) and isometric conditions.

The participation of the somatosensory cortex (SI) in the control of movement and in the specification of movement parameters is, in contrast to MI, still unclear and controversial. Lesion experiments have shown that SI is involved in the execution of skilled hand movements but is not indispensable (Asanuma and Arissian, 1984; Brinkman et al., 1985). At the single cell level some investigations stress similarities between SI and MI neurones (Soso and Fetz, 1980), in particular for

452

PT neurones (Fromm and Evarts, 1982). Others, in contrast, emphasize the role of SI neurones in processing information from the peripheral receptors and in movement perception (Evarts, 1974; Bioulac and Lamarre, 1979; Jennings et al., 1983; Darian-Smith et al., 1984).

In view of the close anatomical relation of the postcentral and parietal cortex with the motor areas, in particular the projections of Brodmann areas 2 and 5 onto area 4 (Strick and Kim, 1978; Jones et al., 1978; Pons and Kaas, 1986), it is of interest to compare the behaviour of postcentral with that of precentral neurones under the same experimental conditions and in the same monkeys. We have thus investigated input and output properties of neurones in SI and MI and their relative participation in the generation and control of fine-graded isometric force between thumb and index finger. Preliminary results have been the subject of a short communication (Wannier et al., 1986).

Methods

The details of the experimental paradigm have been described previously (Hepp-Reymond et al., 1978; Hepp-Reymond, 1988), as well as the force transducer, its fixation and calibration (Smith et al., 1975). Briefly, three monkeys *(Macaca fascicularis)* were trained to generate and control force isometrically on a transducer held between thumb and index finger. Signals on a screen 40 cm in front of the monkey indicated the required and exerted force (Fig. 1). The task consisted in generating a force (displayed as a small moving bar) to reach a force window (indicated by two horizontal lines) and maintaining it for 1.5 s. At the end of this period a displacement of the two lines instructed the monkey to increase force to a higher level and maintain it for one more second. The forces required were between 0.1 and 0.4 N for the low level and between 0.4 and 1.0 N for the higher one (Fig. 1). A correct sequence was rewarded with syrup. Auditory feedback could also be provided.

At the end of the training period a recording

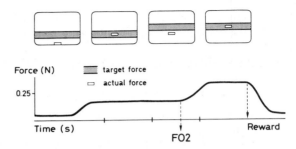

Fig. 1. Experimental paradigm. Above: screen with required (target) and exerted (actual) force. Below: time course of an idealized force curve in a successful trial. FO2: onset of force increase from the lower to the upper force window. Reward: time of occurrence of the reward.

chamber was implanted under general anaesthesia (pentobarbital sodium after induction with ketamine hydrochloride) over the central sulcus contralaterally to the trained hand. Single cells were recorded using varnished tungsten microelectrodes (0.1 – 1.6 MΩ measured at 1000 Hz). Neuronal activity showing some relation to the task was digitized on-line with a PDP 11/73 laboratory computer or recorded on magnetic tape. Intracortical microstimulation (60 ms train of cathodal pulses at 300 Hz, pulse width 0.2 ms, 5 – 30 μA) was applied through the microelectrode close to the recorded neurones. Receptive field properties of the neurones were assessed by manipulating skin, muscles and joints. In two monkeys, electromyographic activity was recorded with percutaneously implanted bipolar wire electrodes, stored on magnetic tape and analysed off-line (Rufener and Hepp-Reymond, 1988). Muscles were identified by the movement or muscular contraction elicited by stimulation applied through the electrodes.

At the end of the experimental period, small electrolytic lesions were made to provide landmarks for the localization of the electrode tracks. The animals were perfused following a lethal dose of pentobarbital. The brains were cut parasagittally, parallel to the electrode penetrations, and the sections stained with Cresyl violet. The cytoarchitectural areas of SI were defined following the description given by Powell and Mountcastle (1959). According to their Fig. 5 we located the controversial caudal border of area 2 in the lower part of the rostral bank of the intraparietal sulcus. The frontier between area 3a and 4 was based on the criteria of Sessle and Wiesendanger (1982). Two-dimensional reconstructions of the recorded regions were made from the histological sections using the method of van Essen and Maunsell (1980).

Results

Muscles involved in the precision grip

Analysis of EMG activity was made for 21 muscles in one monkey and for 18 in the other. One main observation was that in both animals all the finger muscles were coactivated during the task (Rufener and Hepp-Reymond, 1988). This confirms reports of Smith (1981) and Buys et al. (1986) in slightly different paradigms. In contrast elbow and shoulder muscles were irregularly active with clear differences between the two monkeys (Fig. 2, left part).

The mean temporal differences between EMG activity changes and onset of force increase from the low to the high level (FO2) is displayed for 10 representative muscles in Fig. 2 (right) on an enlarged time scale. For each muscle the onset of activity change was determined trial by trial from the first derivative of the rectified and integrated EMG traces, as the first point departing from the zero line in positive direction. In all the intrinsic and extrinsic finger muscles the activity increase occurred almost in synchrony at latencies of 10 to 55 ms prior to FO2. The proximal muscles showing some relation to the task had activity changes occurring much later, either during or after the force ramp (35 ms after FO2 for the triceps, Fig. 2) or even later, at the end of the hold period.

A clear rise of activity with force increase was found in all intrinsic and extrinsic finger muscles, with some individual variations in the activity patterns (Fig. 2). One group of muscles showed a strong tonic activity increase as force increased

(FDP, FDS, EDC), whereas another group showed phasic-tonic activity during the ramp and hold force changes (OPP, APBr, ADD, ID1). The assignment of these EMG patterns to phasic, phasic-tonic and tonic classes was not similar for all the muscles in the two monkeys. This observation suggests that the specific contribution of each muscle to the generated force had a more central origin, depending on the motor strategy used by each monkey, rather than being peripherally determined.

A final striking result was the apparent absence of reciprocal inhibition in the functional antagonists EDC, APL and APBr which also increas-

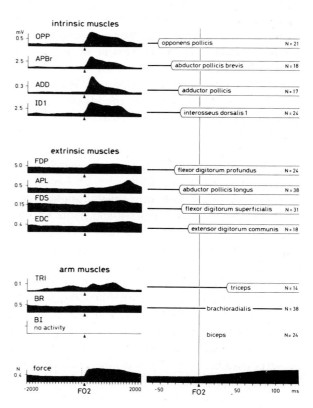

Fig. 2. Muscle coactivation patterns and latencies (one animal). Left: mean full wave rectified and integrated EMG activity aligned on FO2 (one experimental session per muscle). Underneath: representative mean force curve. Display time: 2 s before and after FO2. Right: mean latencies of EMG activity increase with respect to FO2 displayed on an enlarged time scale. FO2: see Fig. 1. (From Rufener and Hepp-Reymond, 1988.)

ed activity with force. Correlations between EMG activity and static force suggested some minor differences between the functional agonists and their antagonists. In intrinsic and extrinsic agonists, like ADD, OPP, FPBr, ID1, FDP, the correlation coefficients were in general quite high (up to 0.92). In the other muscles (APL, EDC, and APBr in one monkey), moderate (around 0.5) or weak (0.21) correlation coefficients were found. This last finding could be explained by the main stabilizing function of these muscles in the precision grip.

Neuronal sample

In three monkeys we recorded a total of 555 neurones showing some relation to the task. From those, 506 neurones were clearly located in the hand region of the sensorimotor cortex, within the region extending from the rostral lip of the intraparietal sulcus to 3 – 4 mm rostral to the central sulcus. Two-dimensional reconstructions of the recorded sites on the basis of the histological sections allowed assignment of each neurone to one of the following areas of Brodmann: 4, 3a, 3b, 1 or 2.

Low current microstimulation applied in close proximity to the recorded neurones elicited motor reactions restricted to one or several digits. Occasionally movements of the wrist and hand, even of the whole arm were observed (21.5%). In 181 of the 207 tested points in MI clear motor responses were observed, the majority (88%) at currents lower than 15 μA. In SI, in contrast, microstimulation could elicit movements only in 25% of the 77 sites tested with half of the positive points in area 3a. The small number of sites from which motor responses could be elicited probably reflects the poverty or lack of direct projections from SI to the motoneuronal pool in the spinal cord.

Somatosensory input

For 172 MI neurones and 120 SI neurones with afferent inputs from the digits and hand the receptive field characteristics were carefully tested.

In MI, the location of the receptive fields was, for the majority of the neurones (85%), closely related to those body parts (here mainly fingers) which showed motor reactions on application of microstimulation through the recording electrode. Only 18% of our MI sample were activated by stimulation of glabrous skin or hair, whereas more than 73% of the neurones responded to joint movements and taps on muscles. There was a significant decrease in number of neurones with cutaneous afferent input towards the rostral part of the recorded region. The importance of deep afferent input (from joints and muscles) to MI neurones is in accordance with early observations of Lemon and Porter (1976) and Wong et al. (1978). It contrasts however with later reports by Lemon (1981) who recorded mainly from the bank of the sulcus and identified more than 46% of the neurones as receiving cutaneous afferent inputs. Lemon (1981) interpreted this divergence from his previous findings as a specialization of the MI hand region. In our investigation the predominant afferent input from the deep tissues may be caused by a bias in the neuronal population, since most neurones tested were related to force exerted between the fingers.

In SI the receptive field characteristics presented a gradient of far more complex and larger receptive fields towards the caudal part of area 2 (rostral bank of the intraparietal sulcus). Only 18% area 2 neurones had receptive fields located only on one finger in contrast to 51% in area 3b and 49% in area 1. Many area 2 neurones have discontinuous receptive fields located on several fingers (Hyvärinen and Poranen, 1978; Iwamura et al., 1980; Darian-Smith et al., 1984). A second important observation is the predominance (68%) of neurones responding to stimulation of the skin and hair throughout SI. Although area 2 did not contain a majority of neurones with afferent inputs from deep tissues as should be expected according to Powell and Mountcastle (1959), the proportion of neurones with cutaneous receptive fields was significantly less in this area compared to area 1 (60.5% vs 85%).

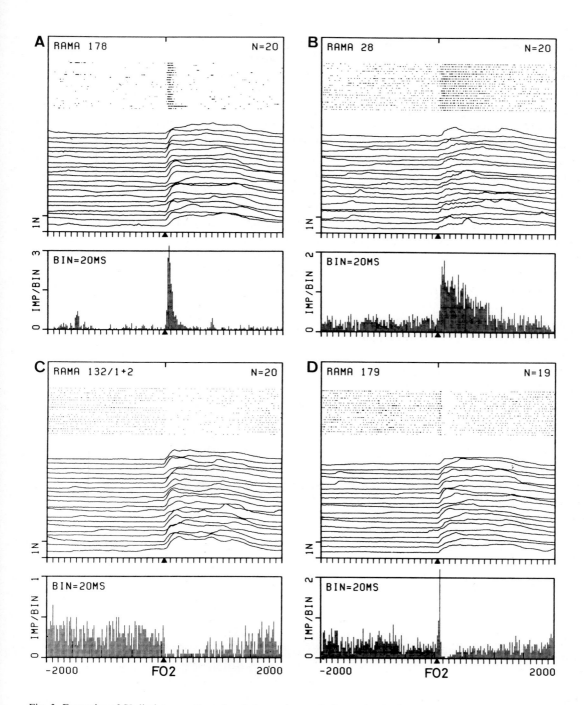

Fig. 3. Examples of SI discharge patterns in relation to isometric force. A: phasic (p +) neurone; B: phasic-tonic (p + t +) neurone; C: decreasing (D) neurone; D: neurone with mixed discharge pattern, e.g. p + and D. For each neurone the upper part of the display is a raster of unit activity with the corresponding force traces aligned on FO2 (see Fig. 1) and organized in chronological order from bottom to top. Below: the peri-response time histogram constructed from the raster (bin width: 20 ms). Display time: 2 s before and after FO2. (From Wannier et al., 1986.)

Characterization of discharge patterns and regional distribution

191 MI neurones and 109 SI neurones with activity related to the motor task had clear and stable discharge patterns over 10 or more trials. The analysis disclosed very similar activity patterns for SI and MI neurones: phasic neurones (p +) active during force increase, phasic-tonic neurones (p + t +) active during both ramp- and hold phases of the task, tonic neurones (t +) with increase in firing rate during the hold periods only, neurones with decreasing firing rate with force (D) and mixed neurones with complex discharge patterns not corresponding to EMG patterns observed in the hand and arm muscles (p + t − in Fig. 3). Fig. 3 displays four of the five patterns recorded in several SI areas.

These 5 classes of firing patterns were differentially distributed between SI and MI in a highly significant manner, with a stronger occurrence of p + and p + t + neurones and a smaller number of D neurones in SI (Table 1). Neurones sensitive to transients like p + and p + t + were found in all somatosensory areas, except 3a, with a slight increasing gradient towards area 1 and 2. In area 2 the neurones with steady discharge during the hold period (t +), though less frequent than expected in this area (Powell and Mountcastle, 1959; Hyvärinen and Poränen, 1978), represented 30% of the whole population.

TABLE 1

Distribution in percent of the various cell types in the cortical areas

		p +	p + t +	t +	D	M
MI	(n = 191)	19.4	7.9	19.4	41.9	11.5
SI	(n = 109)	33.0	27.5	19.3	16.5	3.7
Area 3a	(n = 7)	0.0	28.6	42.9	28.6	0.0
Area 3b	(n = 34)	20.6	29.4	17.6	23.5	8.8
Area 1	(n = 31)	41.9	35.5	3.2	19.4	0.0
Area 2	(n = 32)	43.2	18.9	29.7	5.4	2.7

Note the small population in area 3a. (p +, phasic; p + t +, phasic-tonic; t +, tonic; D, decrease; M, mixed).

Timing of activity changes

The latencies of changes in firing rate were assessed with respect to the onset of force increase from the low to the high force level (FO2, Fig. 1). They were measured from peri-response time histograms as those displayed in Fig. 3, using a 20 ms bin width and following the criteria of Smith et al. (1975). The onset of force increase was determined trial by trial as the point where the first derivative of the force trace departed from the zero line in the positive direction.

The latency histograms of MI and SI neurones (Fig. 4) disclosed important differences between the two neuronal populations. Firstly, the activity changes occurred relatively late in SI neurones, i.e. for 13% just before and for the rest after FO2, whereas more than 56% of the MI neurones had

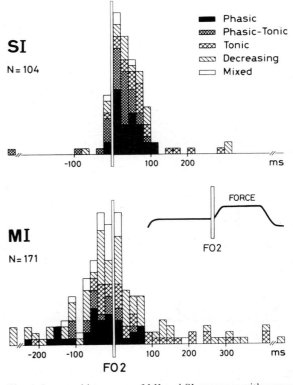

Fig. 4. Latency histograms of MI and SI neurones with respect to the onset of force increase from the low to the higher force level (FO2). Each square represents mean value for one neurone with the type of its discharge pattern.

457

changes in firing rate preceding FO2. These differences in latency are statistically significant for the 3 classes of neurones with activation during the force ramps (phasic and phasic-tonic $P < 0.0001$, mixed $P < 0.05$ in Kruskal – Wallis test). The late activation of SI neurones supports earlier observations (Evarts, 1974) and extends them to the finger muscles and the control of isometric force.

According to the hierarchical organization of the cortico-cortical connections within SI, regional differences in latency should be found between the cytoarchitectural areas. The latency histograms for neurones located within area 3b, 1 and 2 do not differ significantly, but a trend towards slightly delayed activity changes in area 1 and 2 neurones could be in accordance with the concept of serial processing within SI.

Relation between neuronal activity and force
The relation between firing rate and static force

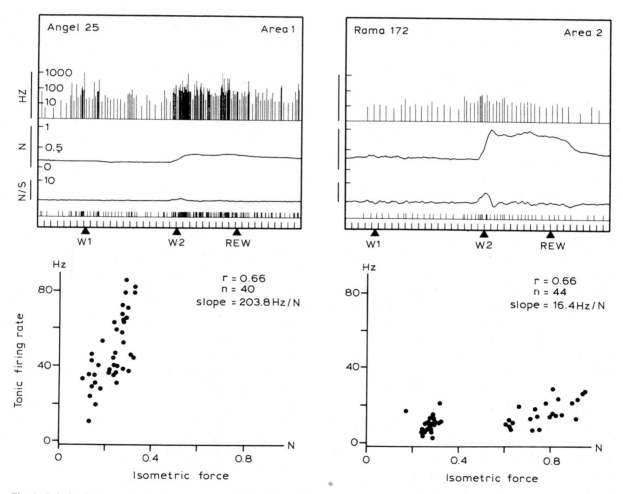

Fig. 5. Relation between discharge frequency and force for two SI neurones with phasic-tonic discharge patterns. On the top: single trial computer generated displays of instantaneous frequency (on logarithmic scale), force, rate of force change (dF/dt) and spike train (from top to bottom). W1 and W2: time at which the force reached the lower and upper force window respectively. REW: reward. Display time: 4 s. Below: scatter diagram displaying the relation between mean force and mean discharge rate. *r*, linear regression coefficient; *n*, number of measurements; *slope,* rate – force slope.

was evaluated for 78 tonic and phasic-tonic neurones, i.e. 37 SI and 41 MI neurones. Time segments of stable force during both hold periods at lower and higher force were chosen in individual rewarded trials (Fig. 5) and linear correlation coefficients calculated between mean instantaneous frequency and mean force in these intervals (Hepp-Reymond et al., 1978). Only 46 neurones were finally retained after rejection of 10 neurones activated mainly on the second force level only, 17 with non-significant correlation coefficients and 5 with too few data points. For 23 SI and 23 MI phasic-tonic and tonic neurones the regression coefficients were statistically significant ($P < 0.001$, Student t-test).

The force-related neurones in SI differ however in many respects from those in MI. Their rate – force slopes, i.e. the increase in firing rate per unit of force increase, calculated from the regression lines, had quite a wide range extending from 14.4 to 212.6 Hz/N, even after rejection of 5 neurones with a large scatter of data points due to high frequency bursts. From the remaining 18 rate-force slopes, two main groups can be arbitrarily built, one with shallow (mean 31 Hz/N, $n = 11$) and one with steep slopes (mean 155 Hz/N, $n = 7$). Examples of these two neuronal groups are displayed in Fig. 5. These findings for SI strongly contrast with those for 23 MI neurones which rarely had rate – force slope values above 100 Hz/N. Mean rate – force slope for these neurones was 68 Hz/N, i.e. quite similar to data previously recorded in other monkeys (Hepp-Reymond and Diener, 1983).

Responses to visual stimuli

During several recording sessions we observed that some neurones modified their firing rate in close relation to objects moving across the visual field of the monkey. Various strategies of visual stimulation were developed in order to characterize the properties of these neurones. Briefly, the experimenter moved his hand up and down ca. 40 cm

in front of the monkey or in other directions. These tests were occasionally repeated with a small blinking light emitting diode (LED) attached to a stick. To assess the relation between changes in firing rate and the visual stimulation a manual trigger was activated in synchrony with the start of the moving stimuli. Parameters such as velocity, position and acceleration were not controlled.

In 3 monkeys 36 visually triggered neurones could be isolated which showed clear modulation of activity in close relation to the visual stimuli. These neurones were distributed throughout the MI hand region explored, and microstimulation in their close vicinity elicited motor reactions in the hand or forelimb. No visually activated cell could be detected in SI.

The analysis of the visually evoked neuronal activity disclosed a number of interesting characteristics. The neurones responded preferentially to visual stimuli moving with high velocity and several neurones had a clear direction sensitivity. In Fig. 6, for example, the firing rate of the neurone increased when the stimulus moved downwards and decreased with upward movement along the same trajectory. As to the latencies of these visually evoked responses, manual triggering did not permit precise determination of the onset of the activity changes with respect to stimulus movement. No relation was found between the visually evoked activity and the monkeys' horizontal eye movements recorded using standard electrooculogram techniques.

Half of the visually activated neurones were also tested in the motor task. 50% clearly modulated their firing rate in close relation to force and were assigned to one of the 5 neuronal classes described above. The majority of these neurones showed a decrease in firing rate with force increase. Finally, no EMG activity could be detected in 13 distal, proximal and axial muscles during the presentation of the visual tests.

These observations strongly support the existence of area 4 neurones activated by context in-

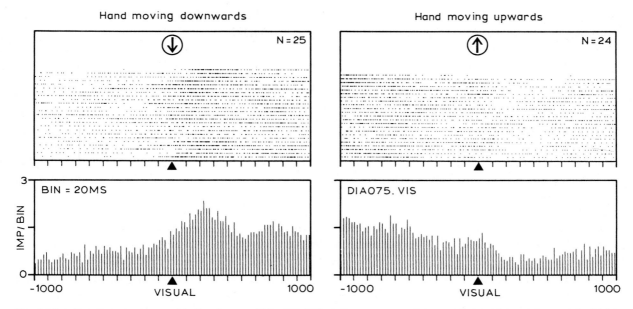

Fig. 6. Visually activated neurone with direction specificity (Dia075). Left: movements of the experimenter's hand downwards. Right: movements upwards. The upper parts of the displays are rasters of unit activity aligned on the activation of the manual trigger. Below the same activity is shown in peri-response time histogram form (bin width: 20 ms). Display time: 1 s before and 1 s after the trigger.

dependent visual stimuli, i.e. without an apparent relation to the learned motor task. They support and extend earlier findings in the motor cortex of anaesthetized or curarized cats (Buser and Imbert, 1961; Garcia-Rill and Dubrovsky, 1974).

Discussion

The results of this investigation indicate that MI and SI neuronal populations active in the control of isometric force in the precision grip have very clear contrasting properties. The changes in activity relative to force increase occur much later in SI than in MI neurones. The distribution of the discharge patterns reveals a larger population of neurones activated during force transients in SI. Moreover the force-sensitivity of the SI neurones has a much wider range extending from very low to high values never found in MI. Responses to low current microstimulation are quite rare in SI and the afferent input to SI neurones active in the precision grip comes predominantly from cutane-

ous receptors, in contrast to an important input from deep tissue receptors to MI neurones. Finally, visually evoked activity discovered in some precentral neurones was never found in postcentral ones.

These six major findings strongly suggest that SI neurones are mainly, if not exclusively, involved in processing sensory information from the digits rather than participating in the generation of motor output. This conclusion differs from that reached by other investigators who, on the basis of timing and relation to force, proposed a centrally originating input to postcentral neurones during active movement (Soso and Fetz, 1980; Fromm and Evarts, 1982).

One piece of evidence which supports our assumption of sensory processing by SI neurones is the very late change in activity of these neurones as force increases from the low to the high level. The changes occurred *after* the increase of EMG activity in the force generating intrinsic and extrinsic finger muscles and for most neurones after the onset of force increase. The activity of MI phasic neurones clearly preceded FO2 by 38.8 ms whereas SI phasic neurones were later, on average 39.4 ms after FO2. In a pioneering investigation on neuronal activity in SI during visually triggered movements, Evarts (1974) reported that very few postcentral cells were activated before rapid forelimb movements. Later Soso and Fetz (1980) found for self-paced forearm movements that a group of neurones located in areas 1 and 2 had early latencies, up to 100 ms before movement onset. According to Fromm and Evarts (1983) firing in area 3a and area 2/5 PT neurones related to a supination-pronation movement of the forearm precedes movement onset with values almost comparable to that in area 4. The discrepancies reported here may be due to the type of movements investigated, in particular to basic differences between the control of the distal and proximal parts of the forelimb.

A second line of evidence that supports a predominantly sensory role for SI in the control of isometric force in the precision grip is established by properties of neurones responding to active mechanical transients on the skin. These are phasic and phasic-tonic SI neurones which are strongly activated during the force ramps. These discharge patterns are also to be found in MI but are significantly less numerous and qualitatively different. Phasic and phasic-tonic SI neurones are characterized by high frequency bursts and higher dynamic sensitivity than MI neurones. In many respects they have properties similar to those of peripheral afferent units recently described by Westling and Johansson (1987) in human subjects during the control of force in precision grip. Although their motor task differs from ours in some aspects, the firing patterns of phasic and phasic-tonic SI neurones show a remarkable resemblance to the behaviour of afferents from rapidly adapting (RAI) and slow adapting (SAI) receptors. Several investigations have identified in macaques 3 major types of cutaneous afferent fibres, i.e. SA, RA and Pacinian-like (Darian-Smith et al., 1984; Phillips et al., 1988). Further-

more it has been demonstrated in primate that inputs from SA, RA and Pacini-like are relayed to SI areas through parallel channels (Paul et al., 1972; Hyvärinen and Poranen, 1978; Dykes, 1983; Phillips et al., 1988). In our investigation a small number of SI tonic neurones, active during the force holding periods, showed properties similar to SA type II receptors with lower frequency and saturation at low force levels. It is however not yet clear whether several sets of RA and SA receptor types exist in the primate hand (Darian-Smith, 1984).

Our data do not confirm the predominant presence of tonic and kinesthetic neurones in area 2 as compared to 3b and 1 (Powell and Mountcastle, 1959), although a slightly larger number of the tonic neurones was found in this area. This finding is not unexpected in view of the major cutaneous input to neurones in all 3 areas, even in the most caudal portion of SI. Only 25% of the whole SI and area 2 population were activated by passive manipulation. This small percentage is at variance with previous investigations in primates proposing that area 2 mainly receives input from deep tissues, in particular joints (Powell and Mountcastle, 1959; Hyvärinen and Poranen, 1978; Sur et al., 1981). However, Mountcastle stresses in a recent review (1984) that the segregation of submodality types to the 4 SI areas is only partial and that their differential distribution varies within the representation of the various body parts. In fact there is strong evidence that the hand region receives a larger input from cutaneous rather than deep receptors (McKenna et al., 1982; Darian-Smith et al., 1984).

Additional evidence stresses the close resemblance of SI neurones and peripheral receptors and their differences with MI neurones in the control of active force. The force-sensitivity of SI neurones is, on average, either quite low (31 Hz/N) or very high (155 Hz/N) with the tendency towards a large scatter, and it can be compared with that of slow adapting units in human hand afferents (Westling and Johansson, 1978). In contrast, the MI neurones recorded in the same monkeys have similar rate – force slopes to those found earlier

(Hepp-Reymond and Diener, 1983). The mean value of 68 Hz/N for MI neurones is also much closer to the mean rate – force slopes reported for neurones in the motor nuclei of the thalamus and in the globus pallidus (Allum et al., 1983; Anner-Baratti et al., 1986), than those of SI neurones. These results thus suggest much closer interactions between subcortical motor regions and MI than between SI and MI. Fromm and Evarts (1982) reported rate – force slopes similar and even higher than those of MI neurones for PTNs located in areas 2 and 3a respectively. These trends were not observed in the present investigation. Different input submodalities to SI cells related to either proximal or distal parts of the forelimb may account for these divergent findings (Soso and Fetz, 1980; Jennings et al., 1983).

The data discussed above emphasize the sensory properties of the SI neurones active in force regulation during the precision grip, but they do not answer the question as to whether SI neurones participate in movement control and in which manner. In view of the strong projection from area 2 or junction 2/5 to the hand region of area 4 (Jones et al., 1978; Strick and Kim, 1978) this question has been repeatedly asked. The somatosensory cortex, in particular area 2, has been proposed as the most obvious candidate for the pathway forwarding information from the mechanoreceptors to precentral neurones. In the present investigation the differences between pre- and postcentral neurones, in particular the differential distribution of submodality classes with predominant cutaneous input to SI and deep receptor input to MI, is difficult to reconcile with this assumption. Our findings rather suggest that the neuronal activity recorded in SI during the precision grip mainly reflects the properties of peripheral receptors processing information about the on-going movement. They support the conclusions reached after ablation (Asanuma and Arissian, 1984) and reversible deactivation of SI (Sasaki and Gemba, 1984; Brinkman et al., 1985; Hikosaka et al., 1985), or on deafferented monkeys (Bioulac and Lamarre, 1979), according to which SI participates in active movement but is not indispensable to it. In view of the importance of the afferent inputs from the digits during manipulation of objects (Hikosaka et al., 1985; Darian-Smith et al., 1984), additional pathways are required to forward sensory information to the motor cortex and perform the sensorimotor integration (Asanuma and Arissian, 1984; Sakata and Iwamura, 1978; Burton and Robinson, 1981). Our evidence that not only somatosensory but also visual input reaches motor cortex suggests that the convergence and integration of various parallel inputs into this region provides the substrate for fine finger manipulation as well as for visuomotor behaviour such as manual reaching.

Acknowledgements

This research was supported by the Swiss National Science Foundation Grants 3.441.83 and 3.549.86 and the Dr Eric Slack-Gyr Foundation.

References

Allum, J.H.J., Anner-Baratti, R.E.C. and Hepp-Reymond, M.-C. (1983) Activity of neurones in the "motor" thalamus and globus pallidus during the control of isometric finger force in the monkey. Exp. Brain Res., Suppl. 7: 194 – 203.

Anner-Baratti, R., Allum, J.H.J. and Hepp-Reymond, M.-C. (1986) Neural correlates of isometric force in the "motor" thalamus. Exp. Brain Res., 63: 567 – 580.

Asanuma, H. and Arissian, K. (1984) Experiments on functional role of peripheral input to motor cortex during voluntary movements in the monkey. J. Neurophysiol., 52: 212 – 227.

Bioulac, B. and Lamarre, Y. (1979) Activity of postcentral cortical neurons of the monkey during conditioned movements of a deafferented limb. Brain Res., 172: 427 – 437.

Brinkman, J., Colebatch, J.G., Porter, R. and York, D.H. (1985) Responses of precentral cells during cooling of postcentral cortex in concious monkeys. J. Physiol. (London), 368: 611 – 625.

Burton, H. and Robinson, C.J. (1981) Organization of the SII parietal cortex. Multiple sensory representations within and near the second somatic area of cynomolgus monkeys. In C.N. Woolsey (Ed.), Cortical Sensory Organization. Multiple Somatic Areas, Humana, Clifton, pp. 67 – 119.

Buser, P. and Imbert, M. (1961) Sensory projections to the motor cortex in cats: a microelectrode study. In W.A.

462

Rosenblith (Ed.), *Sensory Communication,* Wiley, New York. pp. 607 – 626.

Buys, E.J., Lemon, R.N., Mantel, G.W.H. and Muir, R.B. (1986) Selective facilitation of different hand muscles by single corticospinal neurones in the conscious monkey. *J. Physiol. (London),* 381: 529 – 549.

Cheney, P.D. and Fetz, E.E. (1980) Functional classes of primate corticomotoneuronal cells and their relation to active force. *J. Neurophysiol.,* 44: 773 – 791.

Darian-Smith, I. (1984) The sense of touch: performance and peripheral neural processes. In I. Darian-Smith (Ed.), *Handbook of Physiology. The Nervous System III, Part 2,* American Physiological Society, Bethesda, Maryland. pp. 739 – 788.

Darian-Smith, I., Goodwin, A., Sugitani, M. and Heywood, J. (1984) The tangible features of textured surfaces: their representation in the monkey's somatosensory cortex. In G.M. Edelman, W.E. Gall and W.M. Cowan (Eds.), *Dynamic Aspects of Neocortical Function,* Wiley, New York. pp. 475 – 500.

Dykes, R.W. (1983) Parallel processing of somatosensory information: a theory. *Brain Res. Rev.,* 6: 47 – 115.

Evarts, E.V. (1968) Relation of pyramidal tract activity to force exerted during voluntary movements. *J. Neurophysiol.,* 31: 14 – 27.

Evarts, E.V. (1969) Activity of pyramidal tract neurons during postural fixation. *J. Neurophysiol.,* 32: 375 – 385.

Evarts, E.V. (1974) Precentral and postcentral cortical activity in association with visually triggered movement. *J. Neurophysiol.,* 37: 373 – 381.

Fromm, C. and Evarts, E.V. (1982) Pyramidal tract neurons in somatosensory cortex: central and peripheral inputs during voluntary movements. *Brain Res.,* 238: 186 – 191.

Garcia-Rill, E. and Dubrovsky, B. (1974) Responses of motor cortex cells to visual stimuli. *Brain Res.,* 82: 185 – 194.

Hepp-Reymond, M.-C. and Diener, R. (1983) Neural coding of force and of rate of force change in the precentral finger region of the monkey. *Exp. Brain Res.,* Suppl. 7: 315 – 326.

Hepp-Reymond, M.-C., Wyss, U.R. and Anner, R. (1978) Neuronal coding of static force in the primate motor cortex. *J. Physiol. (Paris),* 74: 287 – 291.

Hikosaka, O., Tanaka, M., Sakamoto, M. and Iwamura, Y. (1985) Deficits in manipulative behaviors induced by local injections of muscimol in the first somatosensory cortex of the conscious monkey. *Brain Res.,* 325: 375 – 380.

Hoffman, D.S. and Luschei, E.S. (1980) Responses of monkey precentral cortical cells during a controlled jaw bite task. *J. Neurophysiol.,* 44: 333 – 348.

Hyvärinen, J. and Poranen, A. (1978) Receptive field integration and submodality convergence in the hand area of postcentral gyrus of the alert monkey. *J. Physiol. (London),* 283: 539 – 556.

Iwamura, Y., Tanaka, M. and Hikosaka, O. (1980) Overlapping representation of fingers in the somatosensory cortex (area 2) of the concious monkey. *Brain Res.,* 197: 516 – 520.

Jennings, A., Lamour, Y., Solis, H. and Fromm, C. (1983) Somatosensory cortex activity related to position and force. *J. Neurophysiol.,* 49: 1216 – 1229.

Jones, E.G., Coulter, J.D. and Hendry, S.H.C. (1978) Intracortical connectivity of architectonic fields in the somatic sensory, motor and parietal cortex. *J. Comp. Neurol.,* 181: 291 – 347.

Lemon, R.N. (1981) Functional properties of monkey motor cortex neurones receiving afferent input from the hand and fingers. *J. Physiol. (London),* 311: 497 – 519.

Lemon, R.N. and Porter, R. (1976) Afferent input to movement related precentral neurons in concious monkeys. *Proc. R. Soc. Lond. B.,* 194: 313 – 339.

McKenna, T.M., Whitsel, B.L. and Dreyer, D.A. (1982) Anterior parietal cortical topographic organization in macaque monkey: a reevaluation. *J. Neurophysiol.,* 48: 289 – 317.

Mountcastle, V.B. (1984) Central nervous mechanisms in mechanoreceptive sensibility. In I. Darian-Smith (Ed.), *Handbook of Physiology. The Nervous System III, Part 2,* American Physiological Society, Bethesda, Maryland, pp. 789 – 878.

Paul, R.L., Merzenich, M. and Goodman, H. (1972) Representation of slowly adapting and rapidly adapting cutaneous mechanoreceptors of the hand in Brodmann's areas 3 and 1 of Macaca mulatta. *Brain Res.,* 36: 229 – 249.

Phillips, J.R., Johnson, K.O. and Hsiao, S.S. (1988) Spatial pattern representation and transformation in monkey somatosensory cortex. *Proc. Natl. Acad. Sci. U.S.A.,* 85: 1317 – 1321.

Pons, T.P. and Kaas, J.H. (1986) Corticocortical connections of area 2 of somatosensory cortex in macaque monkeys: a correlative anatomical and electrophysiological study. *J. Comp. Neurol.,* 248: 313 – 335.

Powell, T.P.S. and Mountcastle, V.B. (1959) Some aspects of the functional organization of the cortex of the postcentral gyrus of the monkey: a correlation of findings obtained in a single unit analysis with cytoarchitecture. *Bull. Johns Hopkins Hosp.,* 105: 133 – 162.

Rufener, E.A. and Hepp-Reymond, M.-C. (1988) Muscle coactivation patterns in the precision grip. *Advances in the Biosciences, Vol. 70,* pp. 169 – 172.

Sakata, H. and Iwamura, Y. (1978) Cortical processing of tactile information in the first somatosensory and parietal association areas in the monkey. In G. Gordon (Ed.), *Active Touch,* Pergamon Press, Oxford, pp. 55 – 72.

Sasaki, K. and Gemba, H. (1984) Compensatory motor function of the somatosensory cortex for the motor cortex temporarily impaired by cooling in the monkey. *Exp. Brain Res.,* 55: 60 – 68.

Schmidt, E.M., Jost, R.G. and Davis, K.K. (1975) Reexamination of the force relationship of cortical cell discharge patterns with conditioned wrist movements. *Brain Res.,* 83: 213 – 223.

Sessle, B.J. and Wiesendanger, M. (1982) Structural and functional definition of the motor cortex in the monkey *(Macaca fascicularis)*. *J. Physiol. (London)*, 323: 245 – 265.

Smith, A.M. (1981) The coactivation of antagonist muscles. *Can. J. Physiol. Pharmacol.*, 59: 733 – 747.

Smith, A.M., Hepp-Reymond, M.-C. and Wyss, U.R. (1975) Relation of activity in precentral cortical neurones to force and rate of force change during isometric contractions of finger muscles. *Exp. Brain Res.*, 23: 315 – 332.

Soso, M.J. and Fetz, E.E. (1980) Responses of identified cells in postcentral cortex of awake monkeys during comparable active and passive joint movements. *J. Neurophysiol.*, 43: 1090 – 1110.

Strick, P.L. and Kim, C.C. (1978) Input to primate motor cortex from posterior parietal cortex (area 5). I. Demonstration by retrograde transport. *Brain Res.*, 157: 325 – 330.

Sur, M., Wall, J.T. and Kaas, J.H. (1981) Modular segregation of functional cell classes within the postcentral somatosensory cortex of monkeys. *Science*, 212: 1059 – 1061.

Van Essen, D.C. and Maunsell, J.H.R. (1980) Two-dimensional maps of the cerebral cortex. *J. Comp. Neurol.*, 191: 255 – 281.

Wannier, T.M.J., Töltl, M. and Hepp-Reymond, M.-C. (1986) Neuronal activity in the postcentral cortex related to force regulation during a precision grip task. *Brain Res.*, 382: 427 – 432.

Westling, G. and Johansson, R.S. (1987) Responses in glabrous skin mechanoreceptors during precision grip in humans. *Exp. Brain Res.*, 66: 128 – 140.

Wong, Y.C., Kwan, H.C., MacKay, W.A. and Murphy, J.T. (1978) Spatial organization of precentral cortex in awake primates. I. Somatosensory inputs. *J. Neurophysiol.*, 41: 1107 – 1119.

J.H.J. Allum and M. Hulliger (Eds.)
Progress in Brain Research, Vol. 80
© 1989 Elsevier Science Publishers B.V. (Biomedical Division)

Overview and critique of Chapters 38 and 39

H.-C. Diener

Tübingen, F.R.G.

The paper by *Rothwell et al.* is very important for the discussion of the concept of a motor programme. This concept assumes that fast limb movements are executed through phasic EMG activity in antagonistic muscles. The typical triphasic EMG pattern is preprogrammed prior to the start of execution and not, or only to a limited amount, accessible to any kind of feedback. The study by Rothwell et al. shows that magnetic or electrical stimulation delivered to the cortex during the preparation phase of the movement leads to a delay of the motor sequence but not to changes in the structure of the motor programme (e.g. the triphasic EMG pattern). Additional experiments indicate that this phenomenon cannot be explained by a decreased excitability of spinal motoneurones or non-specific effects on perception or attention (startle). The methods employed and the results obtained in this study are not debatable, but some additional explanations for the phenomena observed could well be.

Movements of limbs are preceded and accompanied by postural activity which stabilizes proximal joints in space and prevents shifts of the body centre of gravity. Even relatively small movements like those of the wrist are preceded and accompanied by activity in elbow and shoulder muscles. Postural and executional EMG activity is closely related. Active movements are delayed in cases of changed postural requirements.

Magnetic stimulation of the cortex results in twitch contraction of all limb muscles including proximal muscles and the diaphragm. The feedback from these muscle twitches will have to be evaluated by the brain first, in order to determine if changes in limb or body posture have occurred. Until this evaluation has taken place, motor programmes will be delayed.

Another explanation for the observed delays concerns the role of the cerebellum and the basal ganglia in the generation of motor programmes. Lesions in these two structures are known to increase the reaction time to the onset of EMG activity, but not to affect the basic pattern of agonist-antagonist activity. Neuronal activity in the cerebellum, the dentate nucleus, and the striatum may precede neural activity in the motor cortex. The magnetic stimulus might increase the threshold of the motor cortex for these incoming start signals from the subcortical structure and therefore delay the execution of the motor programme.

One would, however, like to see recordings of the movements at the wrist joint in order to see whether the magnetic stimulus given prior to the movement affects wrist movement parameters such as velocity or acceleration, and the quality of the movement in terms of matching the target movement.

The paper by *Romo and Shultz* shows that dopaminergic neurones in the substantia nigra of the monkey were activated in specific behavioural contexts by somatosensory or visual stimuli. One of the predominant features of Parkinson's disease is a loss of dopaminergic neurones in the substantia nigra. Self-initiated movements as performed in the experiments of Romo and Shultz are slowed and delayed in latency in patients with Parkinson's disease. Sometimes, patients with Parkinson's disease are totally unable to initiate a movement (mostly trunk movements or step initiation). There are two mechanisms by which it is possible to overcome this deficit: An external stimulus can help the patient — either by pulling the patient at a finger of his hand, visually structuring the working path (steps), or by giving a verbal command ("go") one can initiate the behaviour. Patients with Parkinson's disease are able to perform all kinds of motor acts if under extreme stress like trying to run away from a fire or when experiencing strong pain. Some of the neurones investigated by Romo and Shultz could be responsible for this behaviour. Most of the neurones investigated, however, show a decrease of neural activity with painful stimuli. There is, however, sensory input to all structures within the basal ganglia especially in the striatum. These sensory inputs are mostly unspecific and have large receptive fields.

J.H.J. Allum and M. Hulliger (Eds.)
Progress in Brain Research, Vol. 80
© 1989 Elsevier Science Publishers B.V. (Biomedical Division)

CHAPTER 38

Interruption of motor programmes by electrical or magnetic brain stimulation in man

J.C. Rothwell, B.L. Day, P.D. Thompson and C.D. Marsden

MRC Human Movement and Balance Unit, Institute of Neurology, The National Hospital for Nervous Diseases, London WC1N 3BG, U.K.

These experiments describe the effect on voluntary movement of an electrical or magnetic stimulus delivered to the brain through the scalp. Subjects were trained to flex or extend their wrists as rapidly as possible in response to an auditory tone. A single brain stimulus delivered after the tone, and before the usual time of onset of the voluntary reaction, could delay the movement for up to 150 ms, without affecting the pattern of agonist and antagonist EMG bursts. Movement was not delayed when similar experiments were performed with supramaximal stimulation of the median nerve instead of the brain stimulus. The delay following a cortical shock was not due to spinal motoneurones being inaccessible to input during the delay, since H-reflexes given in the middle of the delay period were capable of activating the muscle. Neither could the delay be explained by the brain stimulus altering the time of the subject's intention to respond, since a stimulus delivered to one hemisphere prior to an attempted simultaneous bilateral wrist movement produced a far greater delay on the contralateral than the ipsilateral side. We suggest that the brain stimulus delayed movement by inhibiting a group of strategically placed neurones in the brain (probably in the motor cortex) which made them unresponsive for a brief period to the command signals which initiate agonist and antagonist muscle activity.

Key words: Motor cortex; Motor programme; Ballistic movement

Introduction

Electrical (Merton and Morton, 1980) and magnetic (Barker et al., 1985) stimulation of the brain through the scalp produces remarkably few positive effects. Muscle twitches, produced by stimulation over central scalp and visual phosphenes, from stimulation over occipital scalp are the only phenomena which have been described (e.g. Merton and Morton, 1980). If these were the only effects, then these methods would seem to have a relatively limited role in the investigation of normal brain function. However, it is well-known from neurosurgical accounts (e.g. Penfield and Jasper, 1954), that stimulation of the brain can produce negative as well as positive effects. For ex-ample, stimulation of the motor strip during surgery not only evokes muscle twitches, but may also induce a feeling of voluntary paralysis in the appropriate part of the body. Similarly, Amassian et al. (1988), using transcranial stimulation in normal volunteers, have described a transient loss of visual sensation when stimuli are applied at certain points over the occipital scalp. In this report, we describe an inhibitory effect on the motor system. The effects are more complex than those above. We show that a voluntary motor output is not simply inhibited by a scalp stimulus, it is delayed. It is as if a part of the brain, and the information contained within it had been "frozen" for a short period of time.

Methods

Eight normal volunteers participated in the experiments with the approval of the local ethical committee. They were trained to react as rapidly as possible to a tone delivered through headphones by flexing one (or both) wrists through an angle of about 30°. The angular position of the wrist and the surface EMG activities from the flexor and extensor muscle in the forearm was monitored. A visual warning signal was given 1 s before the reaction tone. After some practice, subjects were able to react to the tone with a relatively stable reaction time. At this point, we then introduced trials in which a stimulus was given over the central areas of scalp in the interval between the tone and the normal time of onset of voluntary EMG activity. Subjects were instructed to continue to respond to the auditory tone, ignoring as far as possible the shock to the head. Brain stimuli were randomized so that they occurred only in about 1 in every 3 trials. In one quarter of all trials, no auditory tone was given in order to prevent anticipation by the subjects.

Data from each single trial was collected and measured separately. The figures in this chapter are of average data. Stimuli were delivered to the scalp with either a Digitimer D180 high voltage electric stimulator or a Novametrix magstim 200 magnetic stimulator. In early experiments, prototypes of these two devices were used which were kindly constructed for us by Mr HB Morton and Dr AT Barker respectively. Further details of the experimental design can be found in the paper by Day et al. (1989).

Results

The principal finding is illustrated in the example in Fig. 1. This shows average rectified EMG traces from flexor and extensor muscles during the reaction task. The first pair of records shows activity in the trials in which no scalp stimulus was given. The reaction tone came at the start of the sweep and the subject responded by flexing the wrist

some 100 ms later. A typical triphasic pattern of agonist/antagonist EMG activity can be seen. The second pair of traces shows the average response of the subject in those trials in which a magnetic scalp shock was given about 30 ms before the expected time of onset of the voluntary reaction. The shock produced a stimulus artefact, which was followed some 20 ms later by a muscle twitch. This is the normal pattern of response to a supramotor threshold scalp shock. However, its effect on the subsequent voluntary reaction is unexpected. The whole reaction was delayed by some 40–50 ms. The timing and duration of the agonist and antagonist EMG bursts was preserved, but the onset

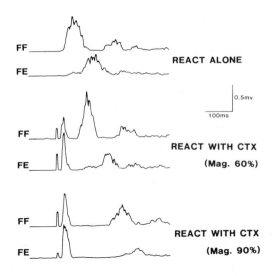

Fig. 1. Average rectified surface EMG responses from flexor (FF) and extensor (FE) muscles of the wrist during the wrist flexion reaction task. The top pair of traces are the control responses of the subject to a reaction tone given at the onset of the sweep. A typical triphasic ("ballistic") pattern of activity can be seen in agonist and antagonist muscles. The middle pair of traces show the responses in those trials in which a magnetic stimulus of 60% maximum was delivered over the scalp just before the expected time of onset of voluntary activity. A stimulus artefact can be seen, followed about 20 ms later by a cortically evoked muscle twitch. The triphasic voluntary response follows about 40 ms later. The bottom pair of records illustrates the effect of interposing a larger magnetic shock (90% maximum) at the same timing. The muscle twitch is larger and the voluntary response is delayed for longer.

of the triphasic pattern seems to have been shifted to the left.

The delay of the voluntary reaction was dependent upon stimulus intensity. The larger the shock, the longer the delay. In the bottom pair of traces of Fig. 1, a large magnetic stimulus of 90% maximum was given. In this case, the subject's reaction was delayed by more than 100 ms. However, it should be noted that the final reaction is not quite the same as in the control trials at the top of the figure. The bursts of EMG activity are smaller than expected. It may be that during such long

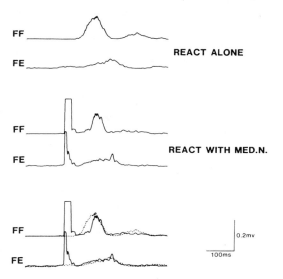

Fig. 2. The effect of an interposed supramaximal peripheral nerve stimulus given to the median and ulnar nerves in the axilla on the voluntary response to an auditory "go" signal. The upper pair of traces are average surface rectified EMG responses from wrist flexor (FF) and extensor (FE) muscles during control trials in which the subject reacted to a tone given at the start of the sweep by flexing his wrist as rapidly as possible. As in Fig. 1, a triphasic EMG pattern is visible. The middle pair of traces show the result of giving a supramaximal nerve shock just before the expected time of onset of voluntary activity. The shock produces a stimulus artefact which merges into a larger, saturated, M-wave. The voluntary reaction follows after a short silence. In the bottom pair of traces, the control trials (dotted lines) have been superimposed over the trials in which a nerve shock was given. The effect of the shock appears to have been to "eat away" at the onset of the first burst of flexor muscle activity. The timing of the remainder of the EMG pattern is unchanged.

delays, the intent of the subject may change and hence make interpretation of the results difficult. In the rest of this chapter we shall confine ourselves mostly to a discussion of stimuli giving delays of 60 ms or less.

It was surprising to find that the voluntary reaction was delayed by the scalp stimulus. We had expected that the silent period following the evoked muscle twitch would simply interact with the onset of the first agonist EMG burst and produce a relative silence at the start of the reaction. In fact, this is what happened when a supramaximal peripheral nerve stimulus was given instead of a scalp shock. In Fig. 2, a supramaximal shock was given in the axilla to the median and ulnar nerves in order to evoke a twitch and subsequent silent period in the EMG of the wrist flexor muscles. When this stimulus was given just before the onset of the voluntary reaction to an auditory stimulus, the voluntary response was not delayed. The silence following the twitch seemed to "eat away" at the start of the voluntary response, with the result that although the onset of the first agonist EMG burst occurred later, the offset of the burst and the timing of the antagonist activity was the same as in the control trials. Clearly, the effect of a peripheral nerve stimulus on the timing of a voluntary reaction was different from that of a scalp shock.

There are several possible reasons why the voluntary response was delayed by the scalp stimulus. One possibility is that the spinal cord is refractory following the directly evoked muscle twitch and that the spinal motoneurones are inaccessible to further input. In order to explore this, we interposed test H-reflexes into the apparently silent period between the cortically evoked twitch and the onset of voluntary activity. The results from one subject are shown in Fig. 3. A magnetic shock delayed the voluntary reaction to the auditory signal by about 100 ms. When H-reflexes were given 20 and 50 ms after the shock, the response was larger than that seen in the relaxed state. Only at intervals greater than 50 ms was the H-reflex reduced in size. Even so, the H-reflex was

470

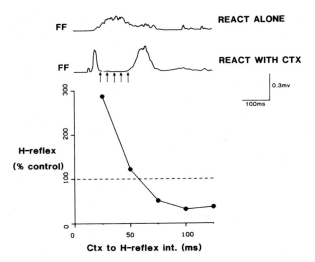

Fig. 3. Testing the excitability of the silent period following a cortical shock by giving H-reflex test stimuli at different times during the silence. The top rectified EMG trace shows the average control response in the wrist flexor (FF) following the reaction tone. The trace beneath shows the average response when a magnetic stimulus was given to the scalp just before the expected time of onset of the voluntary reaction. A stimulus artefact and a cortically evoked muscle twitch can be seen, followed by a silent period and then the voluntary response. The arrows beneath indicate times at which H-reflexes were given to probe spinal excitability during the silence. At each timing 10 H-reflexes were elicited and their peak-to-peak size expressed as a percentage of the size of control responses elicited in the relaxed muscle. The graph beneath shows the time course of the results. At 25 and 50 ms after the brain shock, the H-reflex was larger than its control value, whereas at 75, 100 and 125 ms, it was smaller.

never abolished, indicating that spinal moto-neurones are relatively accessible in the silent period following the evoked twitch. For some reason, they do not seem to be accessible to a voluntary command.

The same results can be seen if a second (electric) cortical shock is given as the test input to spinal motoneurones rather than an H-reflex. Again, this indicates that motoneurones may be accessed by a direct corticospinal input but not by a voluntary motor command.

A second possible reason for the delayed voluntary response is that the scalp stimulus has some relatively non-specific effect on the reaction pro-

cess. For example, it might interfere with the subjects' perception of the auditory signal, or change the intent of the subject as to how or when to react to the tone. In order to test this, we asked subjects to react by flexing both wrists simultaneously when they heard the tone. On random trials electrical stimuli were then applied to either the left or right hemisphere. (The anode was 7 cm lateral to the vertex, and the cathode at Fz. This arrangement minimizes current spread to the opposite hemisphere.) Fig. 4 shows that the stimulus delayed the voluntary response only on the side contralateral to the stimulated hemisphere. The ipsilateral reaction was virtually unaffected. This suggests that perception of the tone and the intent of the subject remained intact during stimulation:

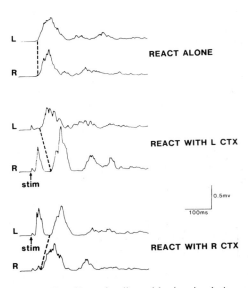

Fig. 4. The effect of unilateral brain stimulation on a bilateral reaction task. Traces are average surface rectified EMGs from the left (L), and right (B) wrist flexor muscles. The top pair of traces show the average voluntary reaction to an auditory tone given 20 ms before the start of the sweep. The middle pair of traces show the reaction when an electric stimulus was given to the left central scalp just before the expected time of onset of the voluntary response. A stimulus artefact can be seen in both EMG traces but the muscle twitch is only present in the right arm. The onset of the voluntary response is delayed on the right compared with left. The bottom pair of traces illustrate the effect of stimulating the right hemisphere. Voluntary activity is delayed on the left but not the right.

the effect of the scalp stimulus appeared to be limited to the processing of motor output.

Discussion

These results show that an appropriately timed scalp shock applied over the central regions of the cortex delays the onset of a voluntary reaction without affecting its form. The experiments in which an H-reflex or a second brain shock were used to probe spinal excitability after the initial scalp stimulus show that the spinal motoneurones are relatively accessible during the delay period. We conclude that the shock produces its effects by interfering with some mechanism within the brain. Since the delay occurs only in the arm contralateral to the stimulated hemisphere, and does not affect the perception of the reaction stimulus or the intent of the subject, it seems probable that the shock is affecting some aspect of motor processing.

As pointed out in the introduction, it is not surprising that such a gross stimulus as the electrical or magnetic scalp shocks, can disrupt normal brain activity. What is unexpected is that, at least in the present experiments, the subject's voluntary reaction was interrupted, but not disrupted, by the shock. It was as if the processes leading up to the voluntary reaction simply were halted for a short period and then continued from where they left off.

The experiments described above are incomplete in 2 major aspects. First, we do not know which part of the brain must be stimulated in order for a delay to be seen. The results so far suggest that the major effect is observed when stimuli activate motor cortical output and produce a direct muscle twitch in contralateral muscles. However, it is not clear whether a stimulus to motor cortex alone would be sufficient to give a delay, or whether stimulation of other, adjacent areas is also involved. The second fault is that there is no information on the time at which the stimulus has its effect. The shocks always were given just before the expected time of onset of movement. Are there, for example, times in the reaction period during which application of a shock would be ineffective?

Despite these limitations, some conclusions can be drawn from the data as they stand. The most important is that the brain must be able to store temporarily during the period of the delay at least some of the information necessary for voluntary reaction. If this is true then a further implication follows. The brain must have had some internal knowledge that the voluntary reaction had been interrupted in order to detect the failure to deliver a motor command at a specified time. The nature of the feedback cannot be deduced from the present work. The brain might, for example, check the progress of the motor command by some form of internal reafference, or check the readiness of downstream sites to respond to impending instructions. An example of how the latter possibility could be applied might go as follows. Assume (i) that the motor cortex receives the motor commands for the reaction movement from some other site in the brain, (ii) that the scalp stimulus produces its delay by activating elements within motor cortex, and (iii) that the signals are delivered to the motor strip only when it has signalled to the upstream brain areas that it is ready to respond. On receipt of a shock, the "ready" signal would be removed, and only reinstated when the motor cortex had recovered. The delivery of motor commands would be postponed until the "ready" signal was active again and the reaction would have been delayed.

References

Amassian, V.E., Cracco, J.B., Cracco, R.Q., Eberle, L., Maccabee, P.J. and Rudell, A. (1988) Suppression of human visual perception with the magnetic coil over occipital cortex. *J. Physiol. (London)*, 398: 40P.

Barker, A.J., Jalinous, R. and Freeston, I.L. (1985) Non-invasive magnetic stimulation of human motor cortex. *Lancet*, ii: 1106–1107.

Day, B.L., Rothwell, J.C., Thompson, P.D., Maertens de Noordhout, A., Nakashima, K., Shannon, K. and Marsden, C.D. (1989) Delay in the execution of voluntary movement by electrical or magnetic brain stimulation in intact man: evidence for the storage of motor programmes in the brain.

472

Brain, 112: 649 – 664.

Merton, P.A. and Morton, H.B. (1980) Stimulation of the cerebral cortex in the intact human subject. *Nature (Lon-* *don),* 285: 227.

Penfield, W. and Jasper, H. (1954) *Epilepsy and the Functional Anatomy of the Human Brain,* Churchill, London.

J.H.J. Allum and M. Hulliger (Eds.)
Progress in Brain Research, Vol. 80
© 1989 Elsevier Science Publishers B.V. (Biomedical Division)

CHAPTER 39

Somatosensory input to dopamine neurones of the monkey midbrain: responses to pain pinch under anaesthesia and to active touch in behavioural context

R. Romo and W. Schultz

Institut de Physiologie, Université de Fribourg, CH-1700 Fribourg, Switzerland

The somatosensory responses of single dopamine (DA) neurones were recorded in the pars compacta of substantia nigra and in neighbouring DA cell groups of four *Macaca fascicularis* monkeys. These neurones were electrophysiologically discriminated against other cells by their polyphasic, relatively long impulses (2.0 – 5.0 ms) occurring at low rates (mostly 1.0 – 5.0/s), by antidromic activation from caudate or putamen, and by reduction of impulse rate following subcutaneous injection of apomorphine (0.05 – 0.15 mg/kg). Of 140 DA neurones recorded in two monkeys under barbiturate anaesthesia, 51% showed reductions and 17% increases in impulse rate during intense noxious pinch stimulation. Neurones responded non-somatotopically to stimulation of the hand, foot, face, dorsum and tail on both sides of the body. Innocuous, even intense, surface or deep somatosensory stimuli were ineffective. Systemic injection of the DA receptor antagonist haloperidol (0.33 – 0.5 mg/kg) strongly reduced the pinch responses. Of 154 DA neurones recorded in two monkeys during self-initiated arm movements, 84% showed phasic activations with latencies of 65 ms when the monkey's hand touched a food morsel inside the target box. Responses were absent when touching other objects. Touch responses to food did not occur when the reaching movement into the same food box was performed in reaction to an external trigger stimulus. In conclusion, DA neurones were activated in specific behavioural contexts by somatosensory stimuli of low intensities while responding unconditionally to noxious input.

Key words: Dopamine; Monkey; Substantia nigra; Neuron; Behavior; Reactivity; Movement; Somatosensory; Pain; Parkinsonism

Introduction

Behavioural reactions to external stimuli are reduced in Parkinsonian patients and in animals with experimental lesions of the nigrostriatal dopamine (DA) system. Visual, auditory and somatosensory signals, normally capable of eliciting behavioural reactions, are largely neglected (Marshall et al., 1971; Ljunberg and Ungerstedt, 1976; Feeney and Wier, 1979). It appears that stimuli require higher intensities for eliciting behavioural reactions in subjects with a decreased number of DA neurones, while specific deficits in sensory recognition are lacking.

Dopamine neurones are synaptically more remote from peripheral input than primary sensory systems. Electrophysiological studies on sensory responses of midbrain DA neurones in anaesthetized rats revealed mainly depressant responses to high-intensity, often noxious somatosensory stimuli (Chiodo et al., 1980; Maeda and Mogenson, 1983; Tsai et al., 1980). Dopamine neurones also respond to electrical stimulation of peripheral nerves (Hommer and Bunney, 1980; Tsai et al., 1980) and the anterior olfactory nucleus (Tulloch and Arbuthnott, 1979).

The potential behavioural implications of stimuli tested in anaesthetized animals are difficult to evaluate, and the obtained results provide insufficient information pertaining to the sensory deficits in subjects with lesions of DA neurones. After having investigated somatosensory responses of DA neurones in anaesthetized monkeys (Schultz and Romo, 1987), we found that these neurones were activated when the awake animal touched specific objects in a behavioural context. The present report compares the nature of somatosensory responses of DA neurones between anaesthetized and awake, behaving monkeys.

Methods

This study employed four *Macaca fascicularis* monkeys. Two of them were conditioned in the behavioural tasks described below. Prior to neuronal recordings, animals were implanted under general anaesthesia with a microelectrode base on the skull and, for the behavioural study, with electromyographic (EMG) electrodes in muscles of the arm and oculographic electrodes in the canthi of the eyes. One of the untrained monkeys was implanted with electrical stimulation electrodes in the caudate and putamen (3 mediolaterally arranged electrodes in each structure on each side; outer diameter, 0.2 mm).

Using methods described previously (Schultz, 1986; Schultz and Romo, 1987), extracellular activity was recorded with moveable microelectrodes from single DA neurones in the ventroanterior midbrain. This was done in two monkeys for 10–14 h once or twice per week under pentobarbital anaesthesia (initial dose of 20–25 mg/kg intraperitoneally, with additional doses of 5 mg/kg whenever the animal reacted to somatosensory stimulation). These animals were mounted in the prone position and the head was fixed non-traumatically by chronically implanted holding cylinders. In the other two monkeys, neuronal activity and EMGs from the implanted or acutely inserted electrodes of arm, shoulder, dorsum and leg muscles on both sides were recorded each weekday during performance of behavioural tasks in a primate chair. Signals from

neuronal activity were conventionally amplified, filtered, displayed on oscilloscopes, passed through an adjustable Schmitt-trigger, and sampled, together with markers from behavioural performance, at a rate of 2 kHz on-line by a laboratory computer. EMGs were filtered (10–250 Hz band pass; −12 dB at 1 kHz), rectified and sampled at a rate of 2 kHz simultaneously with all neuronal signals after 12-bit analog-to-digital conversion or passage through an adjustable Schmitt-trigger. Following termination of data collection, sites of recorded neurones and of stimulation electrodes were reconstructed from small electrolytic marker lesions on Cresyl violet-stained, 50-μm thick, coronal sections of the brain.

Two of the monkeys were trained in two behavioural tasks. They were seated for 3–6 h each weekday in a completely enclosed experimental apparatus. In the first task, the animal released a touch-sensitive, immovable key, reached into a food box when its door opened (20–22 ms time for complete opening), and collected a small morsel of apple or cookie, or a raisin (Schultz, 1986). The box had a frontal opening of 40 × 40 mm and was positioned at 27° lateral to the midsagittal plane in front of the primate chair and at eye level. A cover could be mounted in front of it which prevented vision of the opening door and the interior of the box while permitting access by the hand from below. During waiting periods in the primate chair, monkeys occasionally released the resting key and reached into the food box. These self-initiated movements in the absence of external stimuli constituted the main task and were systematically reinforced by food reward as soon as animals were able to remain relaxed for several tens of seconds while their hand rested on the key. The door of the food box was kept open and the cover was mounted in front of it. Intervals between movements varied spontaneously between 5 and 30 s. The food inside the box was held by a rigid wire that was connected to an amplifier with high input impedance. Touching the food stuck to the other end of this wire produced an electric artifact, which was passed through an appropriately set Schmitt-trigger and sampled by the computer together with other behavioural markers. Animals performed stimulus-triggered and self-initiated movements in separate sessions each day.

Results

Histological reconstructions revealed that DA neurones were predominantly recorded in the cell-dense areas of pars compacta of substantia nigra (group A9), while a smaller number was found in adjoining DA cell groups A8 and A10. Dopamine neurones discharged initially negative or positive impulses at low frequencies (0.5 – 10.5 impulses/second) and with polyphasic waveforms of relatively long durations (1.5 – 5.0 ms), as documented in detail elsewhere (Aebischer and Schultz, 1984; Schultz, 1986; Schultz and Romo, 1987). In contrast, neurones of pars reticulata of substantia nigra discharged impulses of 0.5 – 1.1 ms duration at rates of 25 – 150/s. These neurones, as well as slowly discharging neurones with shorter impulses (0.5 – 1.0 ms) and presumptive fibres having very narrow impulses (0.1 – 0.3 ms), are not the subject of the present report. When tested with systemic injections of low doses of the DA receptor agonist apomorphine (0.05 – 0.15 mg/kg sub-cutaneously), DA neurones typically showed pronounced reductions or complete cessation of impulse activity for 5 – 20 min. Thus, the electrophysiological characteristics of DA neurones in monkeys were similar to those in cats (Steinfels et al., 1983), rats (Bunney et al., 1973; Ruffieux and Schultz, 1980) and mice (Sanghera et al., 1984; Studer and Schultz, 1987).

About half of DA neurones (65 of 145; 45%) were antidromically activated from the chronically implanted stimulating electrodes in caudate or putamen, as judged from collision with spontaneous impulses. Seventeen of them were driven from both structures. Latencies ranged from 3.0 to 7.8 ms. Conduction velocities of 0.7 – 2.5 m/s were calculated for neurones projecting to caudate or putamen by taking into account distances of 5.5 – 7.5 mm between striatal stimulating electrodes and sites of neuronal recordings. Neurones followed double shock stimulation with frequencies of 200 – 500 Hz, with the second impulse being frequently truncated to its initial portion.

Pinch responses under anaesthesia

The effective somatosensory stimulus for changing the impulse rate of DA neurones in anaesthetized monkeys was an intense, noxious pinch applied by a serrated forceps or the fingernails of an experimenter to the skin (Fig. 1). Innocuous but intense stimulation, such as rubbing of the skin, muscle taps and passive joint rotation, was ineffective, with the exception of one neurone being moderately activated. Pinch stimulation of the contralateral fingers depressed the impulse activity of 72 of 140 DA neurones (51%) while activating 24 neurones (17%). Most of the responses were maintained during the usual durations of 5 – 6 s of stimulation (56 of depressed and 23 of activated neurones). A subgroup of 62 DA neurones depressed by pinch stimulation was tested for antidromic activation. Of these, 22 projected to caudate, putamen or both structures. Of 14 DA neurones activated by pinch stimulation, 8 projected to the striatum.

Pinch responses of DA neurones showed a striking absence of somatotopy. Thus, neurones typically responded to pinch of the contralateral and ipsilateral fingers, toes, face, tail and dorsum. Convergent responses always occurred in the same direction from all effective loci. Responses from the fingers of both sides were frequently more pronounced than from other parts of the body.

The DA receptor antagonist haloperidol was injected intramuscularly in doses of 0.33 – 0.5 mg/kg while recording depressant pinch responses from a total of 7 DA neurones. The responses of all neurones were strongly reduced 10 – 80 min after drug injection while recovering thereafter. The pinch response during the initial 1 s of stimulation in each trial was often only partially blocked, while the following part of the response was almost entirely abolished. These data suggest an involvement of dopaminergic neurotransmission in pinch responses of DA neurones.

Touch responses during movements

During self-initiated movements, animals released the resting key and reached into the food box at a self-chosen moment. Inside the box, the animal's hand touched the morsel of food hidden behind the cover. Of 154 DA neurones tested in this task, 130 (84%) showed a short burst of activity when the contralateral hand touched the food morsel (Fig. 2A). Responses occurred without habituation over successive trials. They showed median onset latencies of 65 ms and lasted for 160 ms. Similar touch responses were seen during self-initiated movements on the ipsilateral side (38 of 41 DA neurones; 93%).

Being unable to see into the food box, animals occasionally entered it in the absence of food. They touched the wire normally holding the food and even pulled on it, and touched the interior walls of the empty box. Only four DA neurones were activated by the touch of non-food objects in these situations, while activity in the remaining neurones either remained unchanged (Fig. 2B) or

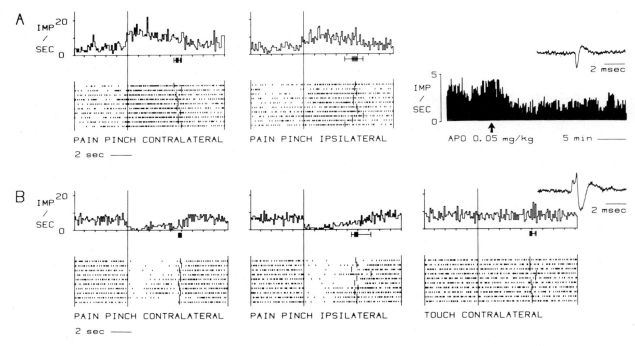

Fig. 1. Pinch responses of two DA neurones (A, B) in the monkey substantia nigra under pentobarbital anaesthesia. A: activation during pinch stimulation of the contralateral and ipsilateral fingers (left and middle, respectively). Right part shows impulse form of the same neurone (above, positivity upwards, 100 Hz lower cutoff filtering) and depression of its activity following subcutaneous injection of apomorphine (APO) into the dorsum. B: depression during contra- and ipsilateral pinch stimulation to the fingers. Right part shows lack of response to intense, innocuous touching of contralateral hand and fingers, and impulse form of the same neurone. Each of the peristimulus time histograms is composed of the impulses shown as dots in the raster displays underneath. Vertical lines represent the time of pinch or touch onset, short markers below histograms and in raster displays indicate stimulus offset. Onset and offset of stimulation were marked by aid of a simultaneously operated electric switch. Each line of dots represents neuronal activity from one trial, their original sequences being shown downward. Separate time scales apply to histograms and dot displays (2 s), to rate meter recording in relation to APO administration (5 min), and to impulse forms (2 ms). Bin width for histograms is 100 ms, short lines below histograms indicate 10 bins. IMP/SEC = impulses/second.

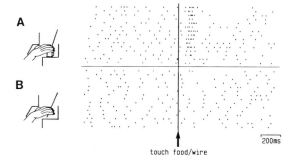

touch food/wire

200ms

Fig. 2. Context-dependent nature of touch responses of a DA neurone during self-initiated arm movements in monkey. A: response to active touch of a food morsel. B: lack of response when touching the bare wire normally holding the food. The two situations shown in A and B alternated randomly during experiments and were separated off-line. Apart from this, the original sequence of trials is preserved downward. Dots are referenced in time to the touch of the food morsel at the end of the wire (A), or to touching the bare wire (B).

showed decreases. Thus, the somatosensory responses of DA neurones depended on the object actively touched.

During stimulus-triggered movements, animals released the resting key and reached into the food box immediately after its door had opened. The majority of DA neurones responded with a short burst of impulses to door opening, in agreement with earlier data (Schultz, 1986). However, none of the DA neurones in this and the earlier study responded to the touch of food in this task, independent of the food being touched under visual control or invisibly (without or with the cover mounted in front of the box, respectively). Of 86 DA neurones tested in both tasks in separate sessions, 60 responded both to touch during self-initiated movements and to door opening during stimulus-triggered movements, while 14 responded exclusively to touch, 6 responded exclusively to door opening and 8 were unresponsive in both situations. This shows that, in individual neurones, the absence of touch response during stimulus-triggered movements was independent of their response to door opening. In sum, these data demonstrate that touch responses in DA neurones only occurred in a specific behavioural context.

Discussion

The present results demonstrate that DA neurones in barbiturate-anaesthetized monkeys respond to high-intensity, noxious somatosensory stimuli, while even intense but innocuous surface or deep stimulation is ineffective. The lack of somatotopy does not suggest a specific involvement of DA neurones in the spatial detection of noxious stimuli. Rather, DA neurones respond to stimuli that have the property to cause strong behavioural activation in awake subjects. In awake monkeys, DA neurones equally appear to be unresponsive to innocuous somatosensory input unless it represents a stimulus of specific behavioural significance. The context-dependent responses to the active touch of food suggest an involvement of impulse activity of DA neurones in particular behavioural reactions to external stimuli. Thus, DA neurones respond to somatosensory input in two ways: they are activated by stimuli of low intensity in specific behavioural situations while being unconditionally influenced by massive stimuli causing strong behavioural activation.

The depression of excitatory synaptic drive by the barbiturate used in one part of this study may have reduced the responsiveness of DA neurones and thus explain the high intensity of effective stimuli. This effect should not be specific for barbiturates, since other studies using chloralhydrate or urethane anaesthesia in rats report similar high intensities for effective somatosensory stimuli (Chiodo et al., 1980; Tsai et al., 1980; Maeda and Mogenson, 1982). Unconditional responses to somatosensory stimuli of moderate intensity were equally absent during limited testing with non-food objects in the two awake monkeys of this study and during more exhaustive somatosensory exploration in monkeys of an earlier study (Schultz et al., 1983). Thus, although it cannot be ruled out that anaesthetic agents raise the thresholds for somatosensory responses in DA neurones, it is unlikely that these neurones respond unconditionally to input of moderate intensity.

The presently described somatosensory input

forms a part of the responses of DA neurones to a wide range of external sensory stimuli. In anaesthetized animals, they also respond to activation of the olfactory system and to light flashes (Tulloch and Arbuthnott, 1979; Chiodo et al., 1980). Outside of behavioural contexts, DA neurones in awake cats are phasically activated by intense visual and auditory stimuli, such as light flashes and clicks (Steinfels et al., 1983). The present study, as well as earlier work (Schultz, 1986), showed responses to auditory and combined auditory-visual stimuli eliciting arm movements. Further analysis revealed that DA neurones react with similar latencies separately to all three major sensory modalities in specific behavioural contexts (Schultz and Romo, 1986).

The response of DA neurones to external stimuli correspond to the reduction in behavioural reactivity after lesions of the nigrostriatal DA system. Subjects with striatal DA depletions nevertheless react to particular environmental stimuli of sufficient intensity. In their character, these stimuli are comparable to those effective for activating DA neurones in monkeys (Schultz, 1986). It is conceivable that these stimuli activate the remaining DA neurones in lesioned subjects, lead to a short release of DA in the striatum and thus facilitate the behavioural reaction.

Acknowledgements

Technical aid was provided by F. Tinguely and P. Hübscher. The study is supported by the Swiss National Science Foundation (grants 3.533 − 0.83, 3.473 − 0.86).

References

Aebischer, P. and Schultz, W. (1984) The activity of pars compacta neurones of the monkey substantia nigra is depressed by apomorphine. Neurosci. Lett., 50: 25 − 29.

Bunney, B.S., Walters, J.R., Roth, R.H. and Aghajanian, G.K. (1973) Dopaminergic neurones: Effects of antipsychotic drugs and amphetamine on single cell activity. J. Pharmacol. Exp. Ther., 185: 560 − 571.

Chiodo, L.A., Antelman, S.M., Caggiula, R. and Lineberry, C.E. (1980) Sensory stimuli alter the discharge rate of dopamine (DA) neurons: evidence for two functional types of DA cells in the substantia nigra. Brain Res., 189: 544 − 549.

Feeney, D.M. and Wier, C.S. (1979) Sensory neglect after lesions of substantia nigra or lateral hypothalamus: differential severity and recovery of function. Brain Res., 178: 329 − 346.

Hommer, D.W. and Bunney, B.S. (1980) Effect of sensory stimuli on the activity of dopaminergic neurones: Involvement of non-dopaminergic nigral neurons and striatonigral pathways. Life Sci., 27: 377 − 386.

Ljungberg, T. and Ungerstedt, U. (1976) Sensory inattention produced by 6-hydroxydopamine-induced degeneration of ascending dopamine neurons in the brain. Exp. Neurol., 53: 585 − 600.

Maeda, H. and Mogenson, G.J. (1982) Effects of peripheral stimulation on the activity of neurons in the ventral tegmental area, substantia nigra and midbrain reticular formation. Brain Res. Bull., 8: 7 − 14.

Marshall, J.F., Turner, B.H. and Teitelbaum, P. (1971) Sensory neglect produced by lateral hypothalamic damage. Science, 174: 523 − 525.

Ruffieux, A. and Schultz, W. (1980) Dopaminergic activation of reticulata neurones in the substantia nigra. Nature (London), 285: 240 − 241.

Sanghera, M.K., Trulson, M.E. and German, D.C. (1984) Electrophysiological properties of mouse dopamine neurons: in vivo and in vitro studies. Neuroscience, 12: 793 − 801.

Schultz, W. (1986) Responses of midbrain dopamine neurons to behavioural trigger stimuli in the monkey. J. Neurophysiol., 56: 1439 − 1462.

Schultz, W. and Romo, R. (1986) Dopamine neurons of monkey midbrain discharge in response to sensory stimuli implicated in behavioural reactions. Soc. Neurosci. Abstr., 12: 207.

Schultz, W. and Romo, R. (1987) Responses of nigrostriatal dopamine neurons to high intensity somatosensory stimulation in the anesthetized monkey. J. Neurophysiol., 57: 201 − 217.

Schultz, W., Ruffieux, A. and Aebischer, P. (1983) The activity of pars compacta neurons of the monkey substantia nigra in relation to motor activation. Exp. Brain Res., 51: 377 − 387.

Steinfels, G.F., Heym, J., Strecker, R.E. and Jacobs, B.L. (1983) Behavioural correlates of dopaminergic unit activity in freely moving cats. Brain Res., 258: 217 − 228.

Studer, A. and Schultz, W. (1987) The catecholamine uptake inhibitor nomifensine depresses impulse activity of dopamine neurones in mouse substantia nigra. Neurosci. Lett., 80: 207 − 212.

Tsai, C.T., Nakamura, S. and Iwama, K. (1980) Inhibition of neuronal activity of the substantia nigra by noxious stimuli and its modification by the caudate nucleus. Brain Res., 195: 299 − 311.

Tulloch, I.F. and Arbuthnott, G.W. (1979) Electrophysiological evidence for an input from the anterior olfactory nucleus to substantia nigra. Exp. Neurol., 66: 16 − 29.

J.H.J. Allum and M. Hulliger (Eds.)
Progress in Brain Research, Vol. 80
© 1989 Elsevier Science Publishers B.V. (Biomedical Division)

Overview and critique of Chapters 40 and 41

J.C. Rothwell

London, England

With these last two papers we finally reach the apex of a pyramid of questions about mechanisms and actions of postural control. These are what happens when the postural mechanisms go wrong, and how should we go about looking after patients who are afflicted with such abnormalities?

Diener and colleagues' paper concers the preparatory activity in postural muscles which precedes the action of the prime mover. Their observations in normal subjects generally confirm those made by other workers, and they have gone on to demonstrate changes in the timing of these responses in patients with cerebellar disease but not in patients with Parkinson's disease. The observations are relatively straightforward, the problem comes in the interpretation. The first question to ask is what are these prior EMG responses doing? In older normals, the tibialis anterior is active first, then 20–30 ms later comes hamstrings and erector spinae, followed by the prime mover, anterior deltoid. Diener interprets the results in terms of an inverted pendulum of the body, with movement limited to the ankle. Backwards force on the shoulder caused by initiating the arm movements is thought to be counteracted by tibialis anterior activity pulling the body forwards. The later erector spinae and hamstring activity is said to be important in opposing the forward shift of the body in the second stage of movement, during and after the end of arm elevation. Now all this is reasonable, but I think that we need some measurement in order to decide whether it is true. The two assumptions on which the interpretation is based, i.e. the inverted

pendulum model, and the idea that early postural movement can be deduced from EMG activity of recorded muscles, are both questionable.

In young normals, Friedli et al. (1988) and Zattara and Bouisset (1988) have found that the inverted pendulum is not a particularly adequate model in these conditions. They have measured the body sway which precedes elevation of the forearm or arm, and describe a more complex strategy. Before any arm movement occurs, there is an anticipatory backwards movement of the hip and plantarflexion of the ankle. This is accompanied by flexion of the trunk, with the net result that the shoulders move forwards to counteract the backwards force produced by the forthcoming prime movement. Thus the anticipatory postural movement occurs at both the ankle and the hip, rather than just at the ankle, as predicted by the inverted pendulum model. A second point from these experiments is also of relevance: it was not possible to predict the direction of the anticipatory movement from examining the EMG pattern alone. Both Zattara and Bouisset (1988) and Friedli et al. (1988) found that the first anticipatory activity in their (young) normals was a decrease in soleus EMG. This would be expected to result in dorsiflexion of the ankle, whereas plantarflexion is the movement that actually occurs. The difference presumably arises because of forces transmitted to the ankle from more proximal body segments. Applying this data to the results of Diener et al., it may be that rather than the body behaving as an inverted pendulum, with the anticipatory tibialis anterior activity bringing the

480

pendulum forwards, the tibialis anterior activity simply limits the rate at which the hip moves *backwards* in the combined hip-ankle strategy. Without measurement of the actual movement that occurs, it is impossible to decide which is correct.

The question of knowing precisely what is going on has some practical implications if we wish to examine pathological data. For example, it may be that both postural models are true. If so, then different subjects (or perhaps more interestingly, different groups of subjects, such as young vs old normals) might use different strategies of postural maintenance. If different strategies are possible then it becomes almost impossible to interpret any pathological data without any direct measurement of body movement. The cerebellar patients in the present paper may be adopting a different strategy than normals, but this might be equally effective in producing anticipatory forwards force at the shoulder.

The paper by *Quintern et al.* has two main ingredients. One is how to solve the technological problems encountered in functional neural stimulation, and integrating a normal top half of the body with an abnormal lower half. The second is the physiological principles which become apparent when these techniques are applied. The main physiological conclusion is that control of standing is difficult in open-loop mode, and that feedback of some sort is necessary in order to regulate the contraction of the various muscles involved. Now there is no doubt that feedback can be a good thing, but can we deduce from these experiments that it is necessary in the normal control of sitting and standing?

Standing in the paraplegics was accomplished relatively well using functional neural stimulation in open-loop mode. A little more tinkering with the precise pattern of stimulation and its timing might improve it still further. Sitting down was the more difficult problem. That was because in order to initiate sitting, quadriceps stimulation had to be turned off completely so that the knee would begin to flex under the weight of the body. Unfortunately, it proved impossible in open-loop mode to reactivate quadriceps at the appropriate time so that the rate of knee flexion was adequately controlled. Feedback of position and velocity into the control circuit looked after this timing problem quite well.

These experiments in paraplegics are difficult to compare with the normal control of sitting in intact subjects. The reason is that in normals, sitting is initiated by silencing the triceps surae muscles and activating tibialis anterior. This causes the calf to move forwards, dorsiflexing the ankle and flexing the knee under the weight of the body. The advantage of this pattern of muscle activity is that the quadriceps need not be silenced, and presumably is much stiffer so that it can limit the rate of knee flexion in a more easily controlled fashion. The point is that this may be a system which is much more easily controlled in an open-loop mode than a system which relies only on controlling the level of quadriceps activity. Without testing it seems unfair to conclude that sitting in normal subjects relies on feedback control.

There is another reason for thinking that feedback control of sitting may not be as important in normal man as it is in the present experiments. Using FNS the *gain* of the feedback control was quite large, and could provide almost 50% of the applied force. To my knowledge, no one has measured the gain of muscle stretch reflexes in the legs of normal subjects during sitting. However, if we extrapolate from measurements made on arm muscles during voluntary movements, then the gain is likely to be quite low. After all, if there were, for example, strong position servo control, then attempting to sit down when someone has discretely removed the chair would not be as disastrous as it usually is.

References

Friedli, W.G., Cohen, L.G., Hallett, M., Stanhope, S. and Simon, S.R. (1988) Postural adjustments associated with rapid voluntary arm movement. II. Biomechanical analysis. *J. Neurol. Neurosurg. Psychiatry*, 51: 232–243.

Zattara, M. and Bouisset, S. (1988) Posturo-kinetic organisation during the early phase of voluntary upper limb movement. I. Normal subjects. *J. Neurol. Neurosurg. Psychiatry*, 51: 956–965.

J.H.J. Allum and M. Hulliger (Eds.)
Progress in Brain Research, Vol. 80
© 1989 Elsevier Science Publishers B.V. (Biomedical Division)

CHAPTER 40

Disturbances of motor preparation in basal ganglia and cerebellar disorders

H.C. Diener, J. Dichgans, B. Guschlbauer, M. Bacher and P. Langenbach

Department of Neurology, University of Tuebingen, D-7400 Tuebingen, F.R.G.

Movements of the arms (execution) in standing human subjects are preceded (preparation), accompanied, and followed (compensation) by muscular activity in postural trunk and leg muscles. Postural muscular activity compensates inertial forces acting on the body at the beginning and during arm movements and keeps the centre of gravity within the limits of stable upright standing. Standing normal subjects and patients performed bilateral arm elevations in response to an acoustic trigger. The beginning of EMG activity in the anterior deltoid muscle reflects the reaction time. Postural activity prior to the arm movement was observed in anterior tibialis, paraspinalis, and hamstring muscles. Compensatory muscular action occurred in the triceps surae. Motor preparation and compensation thus are an integral part of a motor programme. Muscles involved, latencies, and amount of EMG activity change with variations in the motor task (e.g. range of arm movement, changes in inertia of the arm, changes in initial body postition). Reaction times and the pattern of preparatory and compensatory postural EMG activity were normal in most of the patients with Parkinson's disease. Reaction times were significantly increased in patients with cerebellar atrophy. The most prominent pathological feature in cerebellar patients was the inadequate temporal sequence of motor preparation and execution. Our results indicate that the basal ganglia play a minor role in motor preparation, whereas the cerebellum seems to coordinate the relative timing between motor preparation and execution.

Key words: Motor preparation; Postural muscular activity; Reaction time; Parkinson's disease; Cerebellar atrophy

Introduction

Movements of the arms or the trunk in standing human subjects are preceded, accompanied, and followed by muscular activity in trunk and leg muscles (Massion, 1984). The underlying principle of motor coordination may be elucidated by the following example: Raising both arms as fast as possible to a horizontal position initially exerts inertial forces that result, if not counteracted by muscular activity, in a backward shift of the centre of gravity (COG) with respect to the support. Due to the subsequent change in mass distribution, the early phase of displacement is followed by a forward displacement of COG if not compensated by a matching muscular action. Feedforward preparatory postural adjustments anticipate and compensate the otherwise unbalancing early changes in body posture (Belen'kii et al., 1967; Gahéry and Massion, 1981).

In order to make the following section more comprehensible, we define some of the terms used in this chapter: premovement EMG activity occurs in postural muscles prior to that of the prime mover. Compensatory motor action occurs both during and immediately after the voluntary movement. Premovement activity must be and compensatory activity may be preparatory in nature, i.e. they represent an integral part of the feedforward programme. Feedback mechanisms only subserve compensatory activity in reaction to body displacement.

The task of keeping the body stable above its support has priority over all voluntary movements of the limbs or the trunk (Cordo and Nashner, 1982). Conceptually, this task could either be served by feedback-triggered activity or preprogrammed patterns of coordination. The former has the obvious disadvantage of being slower and possibly less efficient in maintaining stability, since displacements of the body must first lead to stretch of muscles before afferent information from spindle-, tendon-, and joint receptor afferents can in turn evoke postural reflexes (Nashner, 1977; Diener et al., 1984; Dietz et al., 1985). From the standpoint of saving energy, it is more economical to counteract a possible displacement of the body than to correct it afterwards. Residual deviations could still be corrected by feedback.

The aim of the present study was to investigate preparatory and compensatory reactions to various motor tasks with normal subjects and with patients having motor deficits due to diseases of the cerebellum and the basal ganglia (Parkinson's disease). We were interested in changes in the structure of the response pattern (which muscles are involved), the timing (latencies and intermuscle latencies), and the size of EMG activity in each muscle brought about by the different disorders investigated.

In order to compare our results with earlier reports, we used an experimental paradigm that has been extensively studied in normal subjects. Raising one or both arms in a standing subject leads to premotor activity in lower trunk muscles (sacrolumbar muscles) and leg muscles e.g. tibialis anterior and biceps femoris prior to the activation of the prime mover, deltoideus (Belen'kii et al., 1967; Bouisset and Zattara, 1981, 1983; Zattara and Bouisset, 1986; Lee, 1980; Lee et al., 1987; Friedli et al., 1984; Horak et al., 1984).

Our study indicates that the basic structure of motor preparation is preserved following the motor disturbances we investigated. The temporal pattern, however, is greatly and somewhat specifically disturbed in patients with cerebellar lesions.

Patients and Methods

Normal subjects and patients

(1) Twenty normal subjects aged from 20 to 28 years participated in the first part of this study.

(2) Ten older normal subjects aged 22 to 74 years and matched in age and sex to the population of patients were investigated. All were neurologically normal on examination and not under medication.

(3) The group of patients with basal ganglia dysfunction comprised ten patients with idiopathic Parkinson's disease. They mostly represented the akinetic-rigid type of the disease and showed little tremor. Patients with hemi-Parkinson or dementia were excluded. None of the patients was severely disabled.

(4) Eighteen patients with cerebellar atrophy were also investigated. Most patients suffered from degenerative cerebellar atrophy without involvement of the basal ganglia, central motor pathways, and cerebral cortex according to neurological, neurophysiological, and computer tomogram criteria. Four patients suffered from olivo-ponto-cerebellar atrophy in its early stages. Patients with multiple sclerosis, inflammatory central disorders, or toxic degeneration (alcohol) were excluded.

Informed consent was obtained from all normal subjects and patients.

Methods and evaluation

Normal subjects and patients stood upright and relaxed on a force measuring platform. Their weight was equally distributed on each foot. Initially, the arms were hanging along the body. Subjects were asked to raise the two arms as fast as possible into a horizontal position and keep them in this position for five seconds with the hands pronated. Normal subjects and patients reacted in a reaction time paradigm to an acoustic signal.

Five training trials were used to make the subject familiar with the task. They were followed by eight trials which were recorded and evaluated. In addition, the 20 young normal subjects performed the same task with changed initial position of the body. Prior to arm raising, they were asked to shift actively the centre of foot pressure forward or backward. This ± 3 cm shift of CFP was monitored on an oscilloscope by the experimenter.

EMG surface electrodes were attached to the anterior portion of the deltoid muscle (prime mover for arm elevation), the paraspinal lumbar muscle (erector spinae), hamstrings, quadriceps femoris, anterior tibialis, and triceps surae muscles.

Data evaluation

EMG signals were amplified, full wave rectified, high-pass filtered (15 Hz), and stored on a PDP 11/44 computer together with the output of the measuring platform reflecting the anterior-posterior displacement of the centre of foot pressure (CFP), and signals from a potentiometer attached to the shoulder. The sampling time was 500 ms. The sampling rate was 1 kHz. EMGs from single trials were evaluated in terms of latency, duration, and integral on an interactive terminal. We calculated mean values and standard deviations for single muscles within a particular experimental condition and a single subject. Intermuscle latency differences were calculated from the mean values.

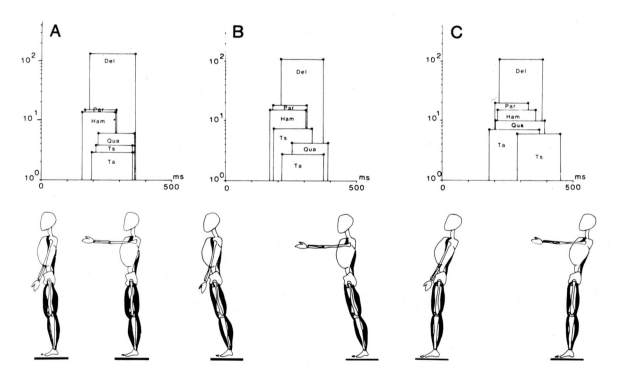

Fig. 1. Mean latencies and durations (abscissa) as well as integrals (ordinate, logarithmic scale) for the arm raising task. A: normal body position. B: leaning forward prior to arm movement. C: leaning backward prior to arm movement. Del, deltoideus; Par, paraspinalis; Ham, hamstring; Qua, quadriceps femoris; Ts, triceps surae; Ta, tibialis anterior. Note the shift of tibialis anterior and triceps surae respectively from compensatory to premovement activity according to functional demands.

Results

Arm elevation in young normals under different functional demands

The reaction time for deltoid muscle activity was 187 ± 63 ms. Premovement EMG activity in paraspinalis and hamstring started 20 to 30 ms prior to deltoid activity. Tibialis coincided with the prime mover. Compensatory EMG activity in triceps surae and quadriceps femoris started between 20 and 35 ms after activity in deltoid muscle (Fig. 1A). The duration of the EMG bursts lasted between 100 and 200 ms. The timing of muscle activity acting on the ankle joint was systematically altered in the experiments by modifying the initial position. When leaning forward, triceps surae changed to a premovement activity preceding deltoideus by 27 ms thus preventing the body from

TABLE 1

Mean latencies (A.M., ms), interindividual standard deviation (S.D., ms), and number of subjects who exhibit phasic EMG bursts within at least four of the eight trials (N)

		Age matched older normals N 10	Parkinson 10	Cerebellum 18
Deltoideus	A.M.	206.5	223.4	262.0
	S.D.	33.6	66.9	56.9
	N*	20.0	10.0	18.0
Tibialis	A.M.	159.1	150.9	174.3
anterior	S.D.	32.3	42.6	77.5
	N	13.0	8.0	14.0
Paraspinalis	A.M.	187.9	180.2	206.1
	S.D.	19.4	66.1	45.8
	N	20.0	8.0	11.0
Hamstring	A.M.	198.5	225.3	247.7
	S.D.	30.0	68.5	49.7
	N	19.0	10.0	13.0
Quadriceps	A.M.	204.9	179.1	315.0
	S.D.	46.3	41.0	
	N	12.0	4.0	2.0
Gastrocnemius	A.M.	239.9	276.9	270.9
	S.D.	40.1	58.9	51.1
	N	18.0	10.0	16.0

*N, normal subjects were recorded bilaterally.

moving further forward (Fig. 1B). In contrast, tibialis anterior was activated 37 ms prior to deltoid muscle when leaning backward (Fig. 1C). This result indicates that the change in functional requirements leads to a corresponding change in the coordinated pattern of preparatory and compensatory muscular activity. Activity of a given muscle may shift from compensatory to premovement activity.

Arm elevation in older normal subjects

EMG activity started in 65% of the older subjects in the anterior tibial muscle with a mean interval of 47 ms prior to the deltoid muscle (latency deltoideus: 206 ± 33 ms, Table 1). Paraspinalis followed and appeared 18.6 ms prior to deltoideus. Hamstrings and quadriceps were simultaneously active with the deltoid. Only the gastrocnemius exhibited a mean delay of 33.4 ms in relation to deltoid activation (Fig. 2). The activity in tibialis anterior counteracts the intertial forces at the beginning of the arm movement whereas the consecutive activity in paraspinalis, hamstrings, and gastrocnemius prevents the body from shifting forward during and after the end of arm elevation. This sequence of muscular activity results in stabilization first of the trunk, then thigh, and finally the ankle joint.

The nonparametric analysis of variance for related samples revealed significant differences in latencies between the muscles investigated. There was no statistical difference between the latencies of single muscles recorded from the right or left side of the body.

The electromechanic coupling time, i.e. the interval from the beginning of deltoid EMG activity to the first upward deflection of the arm measured by a potentiometer averaged 49.5 ms.

Arm elevation in patients with Parkinson's disease

The mean reaction time in these patients, measured by the latency to deltoid activity was only 17 ms longer than in normal subjects. This difference was not significant. The typical pattern of motor preparation was seen in eight of ten patients. Two, however, showed paraspinal after deltoid activity. As in normal subjects, the preparatory and compensatory activity travelled in a proximal to distal distribution from paraspinalis to hamstrings and gastrocnemius. The intersubject variability was increased in this population, whereas the variation within a particular patient across the eight trials was comparable to normals. The main difference between normals and patients with Parkinson's disease was the increase in inter-muscle latency between tibialis and deltoideus (47.4 ms in normals, 72.5 ms in patients), as well as paraspinalis and hamstring (10 ms in normals, 45 ms in patients) and hamstring and gastrocnemius (41 ms and 52 ms, respectively). No data on potentiometer tracings of arm movements were available for this patient population. Therefore, we were unable to correlate the speed of arm movement with EMG signals.

Arm elevation in cerebellar disorders

Reaction times of the deltoid muscle were significantly longer (+ 56 ms on average) than in normal subjects (Fig. 2). The basic structure of the motor sequence starting in tibialis anterior followed by paraspinalis, hamstring, and triceps surae was preserved in 11 of these patients. Seven had no premotor activity in paraspinalis, five a missing response in hamstrings, and four in tibialis anterior. Compared to normal subjects, the mean intraindividual variation between single trials was not increased for deltoid muscle and paraspinalis.

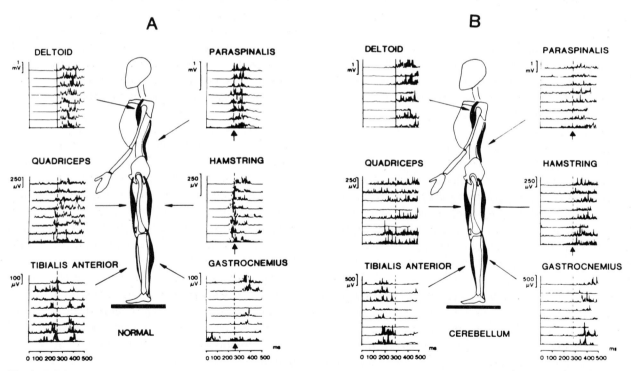

Fig. 2. Original recordings of rectified EMGs on a single trial basis prior to and during the task of elevating both arms. The single traces in the prime mover, the deltoid muscle, are aligned in time irrespective of their real latency (206 ± 33 ms). All the other muscles are accordingly shifted in time. The average latency of deltoid activity is marked in the remaining recordings by a broken vertical line. Note the start of premotor activity in tibialis anterior, later on in paraspinalis, hamstring, and compensatory activity in gastrocnemius in a normal older subject on the left (A). On the right (B), EMG recordings from a patient with cerebellar atrophy. Note the increased activity in tibialis anterior and the delay between preparatory activity in tibialis and start of the movement by deltoid activity.

The time intervals between the premotor action of the tibial muscle and paraspinalis and the arm movement (deltoid activity) were much longer than in normals (between 38 and 40 ms) and also more variable. The longest time interval between tibialis and deltoideus observed in normals was 80 ms, whereas two thirds of the cerebellar patients, who showed this response, presented a longer time interval. This prolonged time interval makes motor preparation partly less useful, since the activity of tibialis is terminated, when the arm begins to move. In a similar way, the compensatory action of gastrocnemius started at the moment of deltoid activity, too early to compensate forward body motion.

Discussion

The maintenance of upright stance in human subjects is provided by muscle tone and muscular action based on corrective sensory input from visual, vestibular, and proprioceptive receptors, but also by feedforward motor coordination. The task to keep the projection of the centre of gravity inside the area of stability delineated by the surface of the feet has priority over any other voluntary movement. This has been shown in our experiments with changed initial body position. Under these circumstances, muscle activity may shift from compensatory to premovement activity. With active movement of the extremities or the head postural adjustments must occur. Obviously, these postural adjustments are part of the programme to execute the movement.

Belen'kii et al. (1967) were the first to describe EMG activity in biceps femoris and sacrolumbar muscles prior to deltoid muscle activity in an arm raising task. In addition, they observed that both the composition and timing of muscle activation and inhibition were constant from trial to trial and from subject to subject. With our experimental design, we observe the earliest preparatory activity in tibialis anterior 50 ms prior to deltoid activity in the older group of normals. This activity counteracts the backwards force exerted on the

body by the beginning of arm movement upwards. The forward body sway induced during the arm movement is then compensated by a proximal to distal motor sequence beginning in the lumbar paraspinal muscles, followed by biceps femoris (hamstrings) and triceps surae. The upright standing body can be considered to represent a multilinked inverted pendulum (Cordo and Nashner, 1982). Activity in the lumbar muscles prevents the lumbar spine from flexing and stabilizes the pelvis together with the hamstrings. Triceps surae activity finally stabilizes the inverted pendulum at the level of the ankle joint.

Our study in patients with Parkinson's disease and cerebellar atrophy shows that the basic structure — the sequence — of premotor and compensatory muscle activity is preserved in these disease states. This observation favours the assumption that the pattern structure is not generated within the basal ganglia or in the cerebellum. The overall duration and the time interval between single components of the sequence, however, varies with these diseases. It is significantly prolonged in patients with cerebellar lesions.

As well as the significant increase in reaction time in patients with cerebellar disorders we were able to show specific variations in timing relative to the onset of activity of the prime mover with the largest dissociation from normals in these patients rather than in Parkinsonians. The increased standard deviations of deltoideus and paraspinalis latencies are mainly due to interindividual differences.

The reaction times of the prime mover in patients with Parkinson's disease was only slightly longer than in normals. The overall duration of the motor sequence measured from the beginning of premotor tibialis anterior to the beginning of compensatory gastrocnemius was increased (126 ms compared to 80 ms in normals). Rogers et al. (1987) observed no difference in onset latencies in Parkinsonians and normals in a visual reaction arm flexion task. Intact motor preparation was observed in 80% of their Parkinsonians. The time intervals between the reacting muscle and motor preparation were, however, increased.

A normal timing of associated postural adjustments was also observed by Dick et al. (1986) in fourteen patients with Parkinson's disease. In their experiment, patients had to pull a strap connected to a motor as fast as possible 15 – 20 cm forward. The amplitude of the EMG bursts and their frequency of occurrence were less in patients off-treatment than when on therapy with L-DOPA. This could be explained by slower movement velocities when not on medication, producing less momentum of the body. Bazalgette et al. (1986), however, reported that 95% of their 18 Parkinsonian patients showed no anticipatory postural movement with the same task.

Patients with cerebellar atrophy had the longest motor reaction times (Holmes, 1917; Hallett et al., 1975). The basic difference compared to normals was in the timing of the response sequence relative to the prime mover. The sequence of body adjustments was considerably advanced in relation to the start of arm movement. The sequence of postural adjustments although released was so poorly coordinated in time with the arm movement that it lost effectiveness and resulted in postural instability. The forward shift of timing to a smaller degree was also observed in Parkinson's disease.

One may ask why preparatory and compensatory muscle responses cannot be observed in all muscles and subjects investigated across all trials. Tibialis anterior activity was absent in four healthy subjects and followed deltoid activity in 60% of our young subjects. There are several possible answers. (1) We record with surface electrodes from restricted areas of a muscle and thereby may miss activity in other compartments of the muscle. (2) Subjects could have changed either tonic discharge in a particular muscle or initial body position prior to the ''go'' signal (Lee and Tang, 1985). Shifting body position slightly forward renders tibialis activity unnecessary. (3) The speed of arm movements could be slower in some subjects, again making compensatory activity less important (Lee et al., 1987). (4) The subject could use different strategies in motor preparation using muscle groups not recorded by us.

Our results cannot answer the question where in the central nervous system preparatory motor patterns are generated, but allow us to state where not, i.e. not in the cerebellum and basal ganglia. Another unanswered question is whether focal and preparatory motor activity are programmed as a unit and processed in parallel pathways or whether they reflect a hierarchically organized motor pattern. In the latter case, one would assume that a movement signal is generated in motor cortex, but can only be released if subcortical structures provide the additional postural activity necessary to stabilize the body on its support surface. The spinal cord is unlikely to generate premotor activity by itself.

The preparatory and compensatory postural activity is not strictly fixed in its temporal and spatial structure but depends on the parameters of the arm movement (Lee et al., 1987) as well as on the initial stance condition of the subject. The cerebellum participates in the temporal optimization of the preparatory and compensatory components of the feedforward pattern of postural stabilization in relation to volitional movements.

In conclusion, we have indicated that the basic structure of preparatory and compensatory motor activity associated with voluntary arm movements is preserved in lesions of the basal ganglia and the cerebellum. The role of the cerebellum seems to be that of coordinating the timing between single motor components.

Acknowledgements

Supported by the Deutsche Forschungsgemeinschaft, SFB 307: A3.

References

Bazalgette, D., Zattara, M., Bathien, N., Bouisset, S. and Rondot, P. (1986) Postural adjustments associated with rapid voluntary arm movements in patients with Parkinson's disease. In M.D. Yahr and K.J. Bergmann (Eds.), *Advances in Neurology, Vol. 45*, Raven Press, New York, pp. 371 – 374.

488

Belen'kii, V.Y., Gurfinkel, V.S. and Pal'tsev, Y.I. (1967) Elements of control in voluntary movements. *Biophysiology,* 12: 134 – 141.

Bouisset, S. and Zattara, M. (1981) A sequence of postural movements precedes voluntary movement. *Neurosci. Lett.,* 22: 263 – 270.

Bouisset, S. and Zattara, M. (1983) Anticipatory postural movements related to a voluntary movement. International Conference on Space Physiology (C.N.E.S.) Toulouse. In Cepadue (Ed.), *Space Physiology,* Toulouse, pp. 137 – 141.

Cordo, P.J. and Nashner, L.M. (1982) Properties of postural adjustments associated with rapid arm movement. *J. Neurophysiol.,* 47: 187 – 302.

Dick, J.P.R., Rothwell, J.C., Berardelli, A., Thompson, P.D., Gioux, M., Benecke, R., Day, B.L. and Marsden, C.B. (1986) Associated postural adjustments in Parkinson's disease. *J. Neurol. Neurosurg. Psychiatry,* 49: 1378 – 1385.

Diener, H.C., Dichgans, J., Bootz, F. and Bacher, M. (1984) Early stabilization of human posture after a sudden disturbance: influence of rate and amplitude of displacement. *Exp. Brain Res.,* 56: 126 – 134.

Dietz, V., Quintern, J. and Berger, W. (1985) Afferent control of human stance and gait: evidence for blocking of group I afferents during gait. *Exp. Brain Res.,* 61: 153 – 163.

Friedli, W.G., Hallett, M. and Simon, S.R. (1984) Postural adjustments associated with rapid voluntary arm movements. I: Electromyographic data. *J. Neurol. Neurosurg. Psychiatry,* 47: 611 – 622.

Gahéry, Y. and Massion, J. (1981) Coordination between posture and movement. *Trends Neurosci.,* 4: 199 – 202.

Hallett, M., Shahani, B.T. and Joung, R.R. (1975) EMG analysis of patients with cerebellar deficits. *J. Neurol. Neurosurg. Psychiatry,* 38: 1163 – 1169.

Holmes, G. (1917) The symptoms of acute cerebellar injuries due to gunshot injuries. *Brain,* 40: 461 – 535.

Horak, F.B., Esselman, P.E., Anderson, M.E. and Lynch, M.K. (1984) The effects of movement velocity, mass displaced and task certainty on associated postural adjustments made by normal and hemiplegic individuals. *J. Neurol. Neurosurg. Psychiatry,* 47: 1020 – 1028.

Lee, W.A. (1980) Anticipatory control of postural and task muscles during rapid arm flexion. *J. Motor Behav.,* 12: 185 – 196.

Lee, W.A. and Tang, S.H. (1985) Effects of initial posture on postural adjustments during rapid and slow voluntary arm movement. *Soc. Neurosci. Abstr.,* 15: 72.

Lee, W.A., Buchanan, T.S. and Rogers, M.W. (1987) Effects of arm acceleration and behavioural conditions on the organization of postural adjustments during arm flexion. *Exp. Brain Res.,* 66: 257 – 270.

Massion, J. (1984) Postural changes accompanying voluntary movement. Normal and pathological aspects. *Human Neurobiol.,* 2: 261 – 267.

Nashner, L.M. (1977) Fixed patterns of rapid postural responses among leg muscles during stance. *Exp. Brain Res.,* 30: 13 – 24.

Rogers, M.W., Kukulka, C.G. and Soderberg, G.L. (1987) Postural adjustments preceding rapid arm movements in parkinsonian subjects. *Neurosci. Lett.,* 75: 246 – 251.

Zattara, M. and Bouisset, S. (1986) Etude chronometrique du programme posturo-cinétique lié au mouvement volontaire. *J. Physiol. (Paris),* 81: 14 – 16.

J.H.J. Allum and M. Hulliger (Eds.)
Progress in Brain Research, Vol. 80
© 1989 Elsevier Science Publishers B.V. (Biomedical Division)

CHAPTER 41

Control mechanisms for restoring posture and movements in paraplegics

J. Quintern, P. Minwegen and K.-H. Mauritz

Institut für Rehabilitation und Behindertensport, Deutsche Sporthochschule Köln, D-5000 Köln 41, F.R.G.

The control mechanisms underlying undisturbed movements were analysed in two series of experiments: (1) normal physiological responses were investigated in neurologically intact subjects; (2) an artificial motor control system for paraplegic patients using functional neuromuscular stimulation (FNS) of the paralysed leg muscles was developed and tested. In both series of experiments standing-up from a chair and sitting-down were studied. A three-link model of the human body was used for recording and processing biomechanical data. In 5 normal subjects ground reaction forces and the surface electromyogram of different leg muscles were also recorded. Basic physiological aspects of FNS such as muscle force regulation and fatigue could be documented. For the standing-up and sitting-down experiments in 2 paraplegic patients the gluteal and quadriceps muscles were stimulated. The best results were achieved with a combination of open-loop and closed-loop stimulation with position and velocity feedback. The importance of feedforward and feedback control during undisturbed movements is discussed for natural and artificial motor control systems. It is concluded that the control of knee joint angle during standing-up and sitting-down represents an unstable system which cannot be controlled open-loop only. Different aspects of sensory feedback including the regulated variables, gain and stability of the system are discussed on the basis of the experimental data and the literature.

Key words: Electrical stimulation; Prosthesis; Motor control; Spinal cord injury; Computer; Afferent feedback; Joint angle; Muscle activity; Movement; Mechanoreceptor

Introduction

Functional neuromuscular stimulation (FNS) is a method for restoring lost motor functions in patients with central or spinal nervous lesions. A microcomputer controlled multichannel stimulator delivers impulses to the paralysed muscles and therefore replaces the input lacking from the central nervous system. FNS has two different aspects: first it is a method of great promise for patients severely disabled by central or spinal motor lesions. The second aspect of FNS concerns the scientist in the field of motor control. With FNS, theories about human motor control can be applied and tested in artifical motor control systems.

Although FNS was attempted almost 30 years ago (Kantrowitz, 1960), present FNS systems are still in an early stage of development. This is partly due to fundamental problems, like fatigue of the stimulated muscles, interactions with the intact part of the motor system and spinal reflexes, the complexity of the system and the number of channels needed to get a satisfactory performance, the high energy demand of implanted multichannel stimulators, the lack of appropriate sensors for feedback systems, and difficulties concerning the communication between the patient and the FNS system (Mauritz, 1986). Many of these problems can be solved by technical improvements, particularly the rapid progress in microelectronics and sensor technology. Further improvements in FNS systems and also in our understanding of human motor control can be expected from a better communication between scientists working in both fields: natural motor control and development of FNS systems.

To date, testing of control strategies in the field of human posture and locomotion has used mostly two different kinds of approach: experiments in normal subjects and patients with specific neurological lesions or computer simulations based on mathematical models. One major disadvantage of these experimental approaches is that only the resulting output of the system and not the internal signal processing can be measured. Especially for undisturbed movements, conclusions about the origin of muscle activation are almost impossible. On the other hand the major disadvantage of simulations is that too many variables are unknown or cannot be taken into account. A mathematical model of human posture has not only to include the reflex and central control by the nervous system but also muscle properties and biomechanical considerations. Within this framework FNS of paralysed individuals offers the possibility to simulate only one part of the system and otherwise to use real muscles and a real body. A similar approach, which is called "hardware-in-the-loop", is used by the industry when complex systems like airplanes and robots have to be developed.

To aim of this paper is to explore the role of feedforward and feedback control in two different types of undisturbed movements: shortening contraction of the knee extensor muscles during standing-up, and lengthening contraction during sitting-down. Both movements are investigated in neurologically intact subjects and in paraplegic patients using FNS.

Methods and Results

Standing-up and sitting-down in healthy subjects

This series of experiments was performed in five neurologically intact subjects. The subjects were

asked to stand up from a 47 cm high chair and to sit down slowly but as naturally as possible with the arms crossed in front of the chest. It was required that the whole sole of the foot was kept on the ground.

Measurements were based on a three-link model of the body. This model is restricted to movements in the anterior-posterior plane with the foot always on the ground and assumes symmetric movements of the left and right legs and arms. For this model the dimensions of the foot and body segment lengths (shank, thigh, trunk) have to be known. The trunk length was defined as the distance between the hip centre of rotation and the shoulder. The joint centres of rotation of the ankle, knee and hip joint were approximated by surface landmarks. The ankle was at a constant position in the middle of the force plate. In the experiments, the positions of the joint centres of rotation (knee and hip) and the shoulder of the trunk segment on the left side of the subject were measured with a mechanical device (Fig. 1). This device is very similar to the pulley system developed by the Pritzker Institute of Medical Engineering in Chicago (Jaeger et al., 1986) but modifications had to be made because of the large vertical displacements during standing-up and sitting-down. Two 10-turn precision servo potentiometers are used to measure

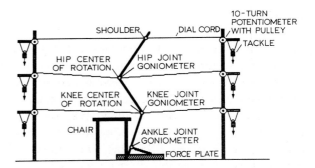

Fig. 1. Schematic diagram of three-link model and experimental arrangement. Non-elastic cord ("Dial cord") and pulleys are used to rotate the potentiometers for position measurement. On the other side of the body electrogoniometers were used for registration of the joint angles at the ankle, knee and hip. Notice that the chair was not standing on the force plate.

translation of each point of interest. By using simple geometric functions the net sagittal displacement can be separated from the vertical and lateral component. Tests proved that this pulley system is very accurate for position measurement during slow movements but because of inertia of the mechanical components fast movements are smoothed out. In order to increase the reliability of the data the angles of ankle, knee and hip joint on the right side of the subject were also measured using conventional electrogoniometers.

The ground reaction vector was measured with a force plate (Hentschel). The axis convention used was sagittal, y axis; lateral, x axis; vertical, z axis. Two forces (Fz and Fy) and one moment (Mx) are necessary to calculate the sagittal projection of the ground reaction vector. Because the chair was not standing on the force plate changes in the ground reaction vector indicated the moment the weight was shifted from the chair to the feet.

The electromyogram (EMG) of the anterior tibial, the medial part of the gastrocnemius, the rectus femoris, and the long head of the biceps femoris muscles was recorded using surface electrodes and transmitted by a Glonner 8-channel telemetric system. Because of the low sampling frequency (200 Hz) the EMG was full-wave rectified and low-pass filtered.

All data were digitized and displayed on-line by a Victor Sirius I computer system. The data for standing-up and sitting-down were averaged ($n = 10$) separately. The knee joint goniometer was used as a trigger to average the parameters, usually over a period of 4 s.

From the averaged data stick figure representations during different periods of the movements could be obtained and displayed together with the ground reaction vector. Data were rejected if there was a discrepancy between the stick figures calculated from goniometer data and from pulley system data.

The net joint torques were also calculated from both position and angle measurements. The mass distributions of body segments and the centre of mass for each segment were taken from an-

thropometric data (Dempster, 1955). In the biomechanical model used to calculate the net joint torques, only gravity and acceleration of the different segments were taken into account. The rotary moments of inertia could be neglected because the analysed movements were relatively slow. The force exerted on the chair and its reaction force, respectively, were not included in the model calculations. Therefore, the values of forces obtained when the subject had contact with the chair represent the torques which would hold this position without the chair.

Fig. 2 shows averaged data together with the stick figure representations from one subject during standing-up (left) and sitting-down (right). The stick figures and the net knee joint torque were calculated from position data recorded with the pulley system described above. The dotted line next to the stick figures indicates the ground reaction force exerted at the feet of the subject.

When a subject intends to stand up he first bends the hip and the trunk is moved forward. This is necessary in order to shift the centre of body mass over the supporting surface of the feet. As can be seen from the ankle joint torque calculations (second trace) this movement reduces the knee joint torque, needed to rise from the chair, by almost half. During the first period of the movement, the tibialis anterior muscle is highly active anticipating the general forward shift of body mass. The weight transfer from the chair to the feet of the subject (indicated by an increase of the ground reaction force) is initiated by a steep increase of quadriceps activity and coactivation of the hamstring muscles. At the moment when the subject rises from the chair the total amount of knee joint torque for both legs is in the range of 70 to 140 Nm depending on the weight and size of the subject and the individual movement characteristics. The following knee extension period is characterized by an almost linear reduction of knee joint torque and a continuous decrease of thigh muscle activity.

When the subject is standing with fully extended knees no knee extensor muscle activity is needed because the ground reaction vector is usually in front of the knees and only gastrocnemius/soleus need be active to prevent forward rotation of the body about its ankle joints (Quintern and Jaeger, 1987). When the subject intends to sit down (Fig. 2, right) a sudden decrease of triceps surae activity causes dorsiflexion at the ankle and bending at the knee due to the weight of the upper body segments. The ensuing sitting-down movement is almost the reversal of standing-up. Because the knee joint torque increases with decreasing knee joint angle, the knee extensor muscle activity also increases in the course of the movement. As in standing-up a coactivation of antagonistic thigh muscles can be seen. When the knee is half-bent tibialis anterior muscle prevents the body from falling backward. The

maximum torque values observed are in the same range as during standing-up.

The results of standing-up and sitting-down in neurologically intact subjects indicate that the torque provided by the muscles must be regulated within a wide range. The next section therefore reviews briefly the basis of force production and regulation of paralysed muscles using FNS.

Factors influencing muscle force output using FNS

The basis of FNS is that an action potential is elicited in the peripheral nerve by electrical current applied through surface, percutaneous wire or implanted electrodes. Therefore the technique will not work in patients with lower motor neurone damage.

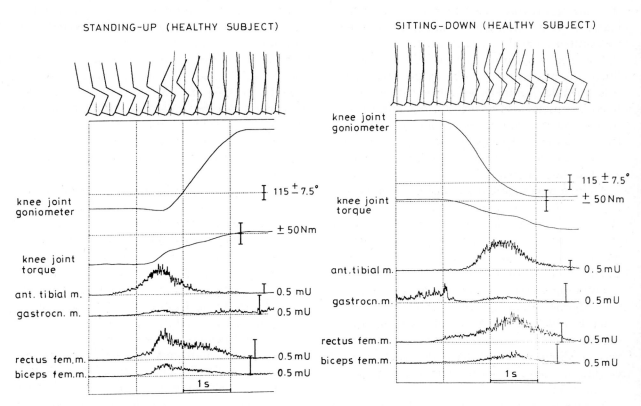

Fig. 2. Standing-up (left) and sitting-down (right) of a healthy subject, averaged data ($n = 10$). The stick figure representations and the knee joint torque were calculated from the joint positions. The dotted line among the stick figures is the ground reaction vector (see text). Curves from top to bottom: angle of knee joint, knee joint torque, rectified EMGs of tibialis anterior, medial head of gastrocnemius, rectus femoris and biceps femoris muscles. Dashed vertical lines are 1 s time marks.

The muscle force which is produced by electrical stimulation can be regulated by a change in recruitment (numbers of activated motor units) or by change in temporal summation (firing frequency of active units). At low frequencies the muscle twitches are not fused and the lower limit for restoring posture is approximately 16 Hz. On the other hand high frequencies are known to cause rapid fatigue of the stimulated muscle. Therefore pure frequency modulation is not suitable for regulation of muscle force. Recruitment modulation can be achieved by varying either the pulse amplitude or the pulse width. For both parameters a wide range with an approximately linear relationship between stimulation and muscle force can be found. For the standing-up and sitting-down experiments described below pulse width modulation at a constant frequency of 20 Hz was selected.

One of the most important problems of FNS is the rapid fatigue in electrically stimulated muscles.

One factor influencing fatigue involves reverse recruitment of the motor units to the physiological situation during FNS, because large motoneurones have the lowest threshold to electrical stimulation. A second factor involves the fact that all stimulated motor units are activated at the same time. Thus a relatively high stimulation frequency (12 to 20 Hz) is necessary to produce a smooth contraction. A third factor is that at a given level of stimulation the same motor units are always activated. Stimulation techniques for alternating activation of different groups of motoneurones in one nerve are still at an experimental stage. Today the most significant approach of increasing the fatigue resistance of stimulated muscles is electrical training of the muscles which induces a change of muscle fibre composition in favour of slow twitch oxidative fibres.

For the experiments in the present paper stimulation was provided through surface elec-

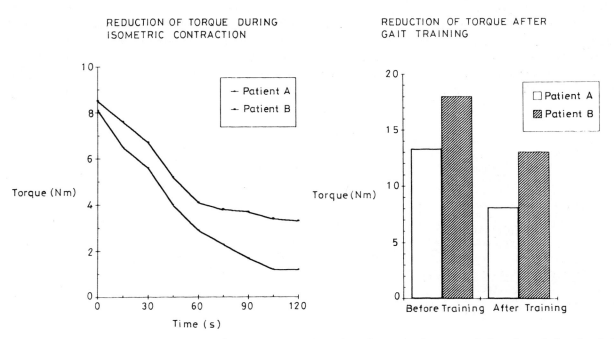

Fig. 3. Influence of fatigue on the torque produced by the quadriceps femoris muscle of two paraplegic patients during electrical stimulation. Patient AT6 complete; Patient B, T4 incomplete spinal cord injury. Knee angle was 90°, stimulation frequency 20 Hz, pulse width 300 μm, amplitude 80 mA. Left: continuous isometric contraction for 2 min. Right: torque before and after 30 min of gait training.

trodes. Two female paraplegic patients participated in the experiments. Patient A had a T6 complete spinal cord injury after a motor car accident 6 years ago. Patient B had an almost complete T4 lesion after ischaemia of the anterior spinal artery 5 years ago.

In Fig. 3 the influence of fatigue on the force output of the quadriceps muscle can be seen for two different conditions in both patients. On the left side of the figure, the time course of torque during two minutes of isometric contraction is displayed. After 2 min of continuous stimulation the torque was reduced to less than 20% of the initial value. The right side of the figure shows the torque measured before and after 30 min of gait training. Despite the much longer overall stimulation time with the same stimulation parameters there is considerably less fatigue when the muscle can rest for a while between contractions.

The maximum torque which could be produced by the quadriceps of the patients at 20 Hz was about 40 Nm for one leg. Since the peak torque values observed in normal subjects during standing-up and sitting-down were in the range of 35 to 70 Nm per leg, some patients may have to use their arms to assist the knee extensor muscles during the push-off period of standing-up and the last

second of sitting-down. Bajd et al. (1982) came to the same conclusion although they used a different model to calculate the desired torque and therefore obtained slightly higher values.

Standing-up and sitting-down in paraplegic patients with open-loop and closed-loop stimulation

In this series of experiments the quadriceps and the gluteal muscles on both sides were stimulated in the paraplegic patients to provide the torque for standing-up and slowly sitting-down. Because the lower leg muscles were not stimulated the patients had to use crutches or walking aids in order to maintain balance. The patients were instructed to use their arms mainly for balancing and only to push the body upwards if the stimulation did not provide sufficient torque. Goniometers at the ankle, the knee and hip joint were used to record movements. The data were digitized and sampled by a Victor Sirius I computer system, the sampling frequency was 20 Hz.

The same computer was used to generate pulses and to drive the battery-powered four-channel stimulator via optoisolators. For each sampling interval the pulses were delivered successively to the channels of the stimulator; the same pulse width was used for the left and right side. The stimula-

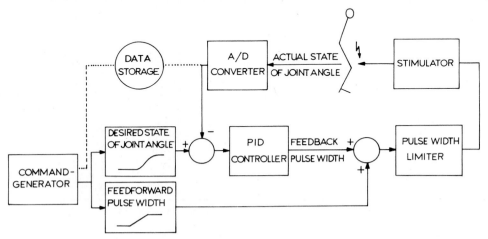

Fig. 4. Schematic diagram of the experiments with closed-loop stimulation of knee extensor muscles. The feedforward pulse width modulation and the desired joint angle are simultaneously generated. The total stimulation pulse width modulation is composed of an open-loop part (feedforward pulse width) and a closed-loop part (output of the pid-controller). For the open-loop experiments the same programme was used with the controller gain set to zero.

tion amplitude could be separately adjusted for each muscle at the stimulator. Fig. 4 is a block diagram of the feedback stimulation system. In the block labelled "command generator" the time course of the desired state of knee joint angle and the open-loop pulse widths for standing-up and sitting-down were stored. The desired state of knee joint angle was that recorded from a healthy subject. The open-loop pulse width is the feedforward part of the stimulation applied to the muscles and was either a simple ramp up or down or a more complex stimulation pattern calculated from the requested joint torque and the recruitment characteristics of the patient's muscle. The gluteal muscles were only stimulated open-loop using simple ramps during standing-up and sitting-down. With a button the posture could be toggled from a sitting to a standing position. When this button was pressed the command generator successively delivered the sequence of values for the respective movement. When the desired posture was achieved

the values were kept constant until the button was pressed again.

For the sensory feedback the error between the actual state and the desired state of joint angle and the first derivative was calculated, thus providing position and velocity feedback. A standard lead-lag feedback controller (labelled PID in Fig. 4) was selected because this controller has a wide range of adjustment and thus permits empirically acceptable performance even if the characteristics of the whole system are not completely known (Jaeger, 1986). Another reason underlying the selection of this controller design was its ability to simulate many elements of the human somatosensory feedback system. The output of the controller (feedback pulse width) was added to the feedforward pulse width. For safety reasons the total pulse width was limited to 511 μs. For the open-loop stimulation the same arrangement was used but the controller gain was set to zero so that only the feedforward pulse width was delivered to the

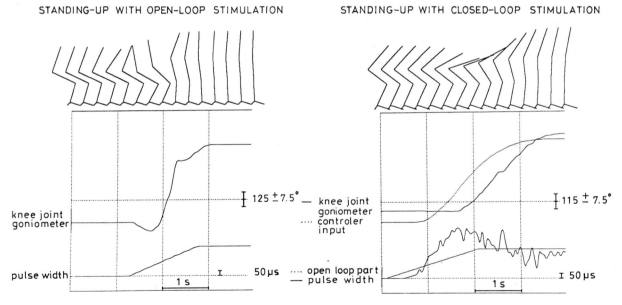

Fig. 5. Standing-up of a paraplegic subject with open-loop (left) and closed-loop (right) stimulation of the quadriceps muscle. Stick figure representations are calculated from joint angles. Left: angle of knee joint (upper trace) and stimulation pulse width. Right: the upper two curves represent the angle of knee joint (dashed, desired value; solid, actual stage). The lower two curves represent the stimulation pulse width (simple ramp, feedforward part of pulse width; complex waveform, total pulse width). Dashed vertical lines are 1 s time marks.

stimulator.

In Figs. 5 – 7 typical results from the stimulation experiments in a paraplegic subject (patient A, T6 complete) are displayed. All curves are single movements (not averaged). Only the pulse width modulation for the quadriceps muscles is shown. The stick figure representations were calculated from the joint angles. Fig. 5 (left) shows standing-up without sensory feedback (open-loop). The simple ramp which was used in this example did not provide enough torque to extend the knee during the push-off period therefore the patient made a ballistic trunk movement flinging the hip forward and thus extending the knee. The final posture was achieved by pushing the trunk forward. Fig. 5 (right) shows the same stimulation pattern modified by sensory feedback (closed-loop). A delay of about one second between the slow onset of the feedforward stimulation (open-loop part) and the trajectory of the desired knee joint angle (controller input) was selected. Because the requested torque for the push-off is very high, a considerable error built up before the stimulation provided sufficient torque to extend the knee. The following

knee extension was much smoother than with the open-loop stimulation although there were minor oscillations due to the high controller gain.

For standing-up, good performance could be achieved without sensory feedback if the time course of the stimulation pulse width was selected properly with a steep rising phase and a gradual falling phase. The most significant problem then was the timing between the patient's actions and the stimulation. If for example the patient did not put enough weight on his feet at the onset of the stimulation, then the feet were shifted forward thus preventing the patient from standing up. Another problem was that with only open-loop stimulation the speed of the movement could not be controlled. The advantages of sensory feedback are, however, much more striking in lengthening contractile movements such as sitting down.

The problem of controlling the torque provided by the muscles during sitting-down using open-loop stimulation is illustrated in Fig. 6. On the left side a simple ramp down was used. For the posture selected by the patient no knee extensor muscle torque was necessary to stand, therefore the patient

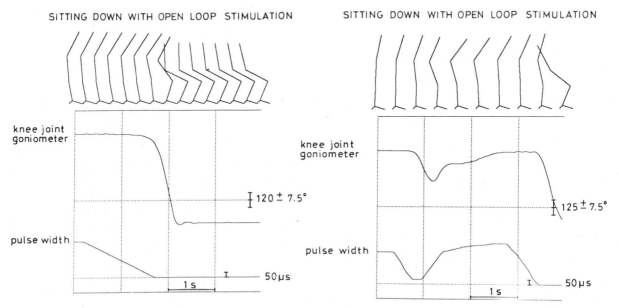

Fig. 6. Sitting-down of a paraplegic subject with open-loop stimulation of the quadriceps muscle with two different stimulation programmes. Left: simple ramp down. Right: with stimulation pause for breaking off.

remained standing until the stimulation was turned off. Without stimulation the knees buckled and the patient fell backward onto the chair. On the right side of Fig. 6 a more complex stimulation pattern was used consisting of a steep ramp down and a reduced stimulation for about one second in order to cause buckling of the knees. The second part of the stimulation pattern with a ramp up should anticipate increasing knee joint torque during the movement. This concept sometimes worked very well but most times it failed. It can be seen in the figure that the knees were first bent but the ascending ramp of stimulation was too steep and the knees were extended again. When the stimulation was finally turned off the patient dropped backwards.

In Fig. 7 a similar feedforward stimulation pattern (open-loop part) as used on the right side of Fig. 6 but with sensory feedback was employed. Because the feedback could prevent the fast bending of the knees a longer delay between the descending and the ascending ramp could be selected. The actual movement has to begin before

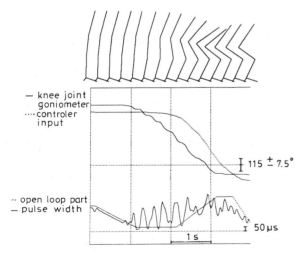

SITTING-DOWN WITH CLOSED-LOOP STIMULATION

Fig. 7. Sitting-down of a paraplegic subject with closed-loop stimulation of the quadriceps muscle. For the displayed parameters see Fig. 5, right part.

the "desired movement" in order to build up an error necessary to increase the pulse width and compensate for the increasing torque. In Fig. 7 it can be seen that sensory feedback is able to compensate for the increasing torque during sitting-down. Despite some oscillations due to high controller gain the movement is much smoother and better controlled than with open-loop stimulation only.

In all experiments best performance was achieved with proportional (position) and low derivative (velocity) feedback and with a relatively high proportional controller gain and high derivative controller gain. The system was oscillating if the overall gain was too high or if the balance between proportional and derivative control was not selected properly. However, sensory feedback could only improve the performance if the gain was high enough. For that reason some oscillations had to be taken into account. Integral control mostly impaired the stability of the system and was therefore switched off.

It was only possible to control the movements with some feedforward stimulation. Pure feedback control was unstable because an excessively high feedback gain was needed to get enough stimulation.

There is no doubt that a simple lead-lag controller with stimulation of only the agonist muscles does not represent the ultimate solution. Many improvements of the present system are possible. For example, better controller algorithms, stimulation of antagonistic muscles for increased stiffness, independent control of the left and right leg, and combination of recruitment and frequency modulation for faster response times (Petrofsky, 1978) and an increased force range. It was however not the aim of this paper to develop a perfect FNS system but to discuss basic principles of natural and artificial motor control systems.

Discussion

The important role of afferent feedback for the compensation of external disturbances is commonly accepted. There is, however, some controversy about the role of feedforward and feedback during undisturbed movements. Rothwell et al. (1982) showed that a man deafferented by a severe peripheral sensory neuropathy is not able to perform simple tasks in daily life like grasping a pen or holding a cup although normal muscle activation patterns during simple and complex motor tasks were preserved. Sanes et al. (1985) found that in deafferented patients postural control without vision was heavily disturbed even in unloaded movements. There are however other studies which support the view that spring-like behaviour of antagonistic muscles provides enough stability for undisturbed movements. Polit and Bizzi (1979) found in arm movement experiments in monkeys that deafferented animals were able to point to a target without visual control. They concluded that the correct equilibrium point between agonist and antagonist muscles which is necessary for reaching the desired posture can be found without afferent feedback. In these experiments afferent feedback seemed only to play a role when the initial postural setting was disturbed.

There is no doubt than an increased stiffness by coactivation of agonist and antagonist muscles plays an important role whenever a certain posture has to be maintained against a load. In our experiments in the neurologically intact subjects a coactivation of quadriceps and biceps femoris muscles occurred during standing-up and sitting-down. However, it is not possible to stabilize a globally unstable biomechanical system only by increasing the stiffness. Because of the torque characteristics, both movements (standing-up and sitting-down) can be regarded as a globally unstable system. A similar biomechanical configuration exists for many movements like the support phase during running or stair-climbing, but also quiet standing represents an unstable system which can be compared to an inverted pendulum (Jaeger, 1986).

It is evident that a globally unstable biomechanical system could be regulated by feedforward control only if no external disturbance occurs and if the torque provided by the muscles remains absolutely constant at the requested value. The slightest deviation from the equilibrium point would cause the system to drift to one direction. Thus, in our stimulation experiments of undisturbed movements, reproducible results could not be achieved with open-loop control. It could however be shown that the changing muscle characteristics mainly due to fatigue and the irregularities of knee joint torque due to movements of the upper body can be compensated by simple position and velocity feedback, even if this leads to local instabilities (oscillations) in the movement trajectories.

One can argue that problems concerning the coordination of different body segments do not occur in neurologically intact subjects because the movement is generated as a whole, and that therefore the time course of the joint torques and the required muscle forces can be predicted. On the other hand the problem of changing muscle characteristics is common for both electrically stimulated and physiologically activated muscles. During voluntary contractions the primary reason for a loss of contractile strength is a change in the contractile properties of the muscles (Bigland-Ritchie, 1981). It is very unlikely that the central nervous system can exactly predict the amount of fatigue in the different muscles, therefore muscle force during voluntary contractions and movements can only be regulated at a specific value with afferent feedback. This view is supported by the finding that patients with severe peripheral sensory neuropathy are unable to maintain consistent levels of muscle activity (Rothwell et al., 1982; Sanes et al., 1985). We conclude that, for the exact execution of a given trajectory during slow voluntary movements like standing up and sitting down, sensory feedback is necessary and that the spring model of motor control (Polit and Bizzi, 1979) is not an adequate description of these movements.

The next question which arises concerns the type of feedback required for the control of movements in the stimulated and the physiological situation. In the stimulation experiments the trajectory was controlled using position (proportional) and velocity (derivative) feedback, and for the controller itself, proportional and derivative gain was again used. Thus the closed-loop system provided position, velocity, and acceleration feedback. For this controller design, many analogies to physiological feedback loops exist. The proportional and derivative parts of the feedback to the controller correspond to static and dynamic sensitivity of natural proprioceptors, especially the muscle spindle afferents (Lennerstrand and Thoden, 1968; Hulliger and Noth, 1979; Houk et al., 1981; Matthews, 1981). The controller loop itself can be compared with spinal and transcortical reflex loops. Unlike a simple tendon jerk, medium latency reflexes are adapted to the specific motor task (Berger et al., 1984) and are not only dependent on the initial velocity but also on the duration of a perturbation (Gottlieb and Agarwal, 1980; Dietz et al., 1987). Dufresne et al. (1979) postulated from studies with torque-induced reflexes in human arm muscles, different loops for velocity and acceleration feedback. In these experiments position feedback did not seem to play an essential role. This could be explained by the fact that holding a specific position was not requested in the experiment. These authors suggested that the acceleration feedback was not due to an acceleration sensitivity of the muscle spindles but to a functional differentiation within the central nervous system. The properties of the reflexes postulated by Dufresne et al. (1979) are similar to the artificial feedback loops described in this paper.

It should be discussed whether it is necessary to control position, velocity and acceleration in movements like standing-up and sitting-down and if other variables like muscle force or stiffness may play a role in the performance of the system (see Stein, 1982). It is evident that joint position should be controlled if a specific trajectory of joint angle is desired. Because there is a close relationship between muscle length and joint angle and because of the large number of muscle spindles present in muscles, it is very likely that the muscle spindle afferents play a major role in the control of these movements. Furthermore it is the dynamic sensitivity of muscle spindles which provide velocity control. The main reasons for controlling not only position but also its derivative(s) are faster responses to disturbances and increased stability of the whole system. From feedback system theory it is known that an oscillation tendency can often be damped out if the feedback information is advanced in phase compared to the actual output of the system (velocity feedback is advanced in phase compared to output position). In our closed-loop stimulation experiments an acceptable performance and stability could only be achieved when the derivative gain was high with respect to the proportional gain. Additional acceleration feedback may have further improved the performance of the system. This agrees with the results of Mulder et al. (1987) showing that theoretically the knee joint angle cannot be regulated using only proportional (position) control.

If as in our experiments the controlled variable of a movement is the trajectory, then the input to the controller must be related to the movement. In the closed-loop stimulation experiments presented in this chapter a copy of the desired movement was used for comparison with the actual movement. This "efference copy", however, existed at a different level: not in the muscle activation level (like the pulse width) but in the trajectory level (desired stage of joint angle). Reflex studies during gait of healthy subjects showed that this principle of trajectory control can also be applied to natural movements. Dietz et al. (1984) showed that the reflex responses following disturbances of the normal ankle joint trajectory during different phases of the gait cycle depend not on the absolute muscle stretch but on the deviation from the normal trajectory. In muscles, the interpretation of sensory information dependent on the efferent input can already occur in the sensor itself. Coactivation of α and γ motoneurones functionally replaces the principle of efference copy for sensory information from the muscle spindles.

Another important topic of feedback is the overall gain of the system. If the gain is too low then deviations from the desired state cannot be fully compensated by the feedback loop. On the other hand, high gain can cause instability and oscillations. In our stimulation experiments the overall gain had to be set within a narrow range in order to get a satisfactory performance. Because of oscillations it was not possible to set the gain high enough to give up the feedforward part of stimulation. The gain problem can also be related to physiological feedback loops. Spinal circuits are high gain systems and oscillations like clonus occur when inhibition is lacking. Therefore inhibitory pathways are necessary to achieve postural stability (Hemami and Stokes, 1983). It has to be postulated that the nervous system changes the amount of inhibition used for afferent feedback dependent on the motor task (Morin et al., 1982; Dietz et al., 1985; Quintern et al., 1987) and that adaptation of the reflex gain occurs (Quintern et al., 1985) when a subject is learning a new motor task. The overall gain includes the input – output relationship of the muscle, therefore adaptation of the feedback gain would also be desired if changes in muscle characteristics due to fatigue are to be regulated. Because this problem plays an important role in FNS, adaptive controller designs with variable gain have been proposed (Bernotas et al., 1987).

Not only temporal changes but also other nonlinearities of the muscle characteristics are a problem for the control of movements in both open-loop and closed-loop conditions. For this reason it seems favourable to control respectively not only position and muscle length, but also muscle force in order to linearize the input – output relationship of the muscle. It can be speculated that in natural motor control the Golgi tendon organs and the inhibitory Ib afferent pathway may play an essential role for the linearization of muscle force. It has been shown that each tendon organ is most sensitive to the force produced by a single motor unit and that the threshold of tendon organs is low enough for the regulation of muscle force (Houk and Henneman, 1967; Matthews, 1981; Crago et al., 1982).

As already mentioned above, in movements with compliant loads such as standing-up and sitting-down, the main controlled variable should not be force or stiffness but rather position and velocity. This is not true for movements with isometric loads where the controlled variable should be force (Crago et al., 1980). Because both conditions are very common, future FNS systems should provide both force and position feedback.

Regarding the importance of sensory feedback the question arises as to what extent feedforward control of the muscles is necessary during FNS. In movements like standing-up and sitting-down the extensor muscle torque must be regulated within a wide range. Without feedforward activation of the muscles an extremely high feedback gain would be necessary and therefore the system would be unstable. Also, a considerable error between the desired and the actual trajectory would be necessary to produce the required muscle force, therefore the movement would be delayed and the trajectory distorted. For these reasons, in our stimulation experiments a combination of feedforward and feedback was always necessary. These considerations are also related to the natural motor control and the servo hypothesis of Merton (1953). For reasons mentioned above it is very unlikely that the command signal uses only the γ motoneurone route to control movements.

In natural motor control, afferent feedback is not only used for regulating a variable at a specific value or for maintaining a desired trajectory. Afferent feedback also plays an important role in updating the motor programme itself. Afferent feedback is used to adjust the feedforward activation and also the closed-loop gain to the requirements of the respective phase of a movement and the external conditions. For example, during sitting-down the feedforward activation and the reflex gain should decrease when cutaneous afferents signal that contact with the chair is made.

Natural motor control includes not only a variety of somatosensory information but also vestibular and visual inputs (Allum et al., 1988). Currently, many of these sensory signals cannot be incorporated within FNS systems, but may become available through further technical developements. It seems however that there are also limitations for the control strategies used by FNS systems: in healthy subjects voluntary movements are anticipated by postural responses prior to the movement itself (Lipshits et al., 1981). In the paraplegic patients using FNS two separate systems control the upper and the lower part of body: the central nervous system and the stimulator. The synchronization of the natural and the artificial motor control system will remain one essential problem of FNS.

Acknowledgement

We thank the Bodenseewerk-Gerätetechnik in Überlingen, West Germany for supporting this study.

References

Allum, J.H.J., Keshner, E.A., Honegger, F. and Pfaltz, C.R. (1988) Organization of leg-trunk-head equilibrium movements in normals and patients with peripheral vestibular deficits. In O. Pompeiano and J.H.J. Allum (Eds.), *Progress in Brain Research, Vol. 76*, Elsevier, Amsterdam, pp. 277 – 290.

Bajd, T., Kralj, A. and Turk, R. (1982) Standing-up of a healthy subject and a paraplegic patients. *J. Biomech.*, 15: 1 – 10.

Berger, W., Dietz, V. and Quintern, J. (1984) Corrective reactions to stumbling in man: neuronal co-ordination of bilateral leg muscle activity during gait. *J. Physiol. (London)*, 357: 109 – 125.

Bernotas, L.A., Crago, P.E. and Chizeck, H.J. (1987) Adative control of electrically stimulated muscle. *IEEE Trans. Biomed. Eng.*, 34: 140 – 147.

Bigland-Ritchie, B. (1981) EMG and fatigue of human voluntary and stimulated contractions. In *Human Muscle Fatigue: Physiological Mechanisms*, Pitman Medical, London, pp. 130 – 156.

Crago, P.E., Mortimer, J.T. and Peckham, P.H. (1980) Closed-loop control of force during electrical stimulation of muscle. *IEEE Trans. Biomed. Eng.*, 27: 306 – 312.

Crago, P.E., Houk, J.C. and Rymer, W.Z. (1982) Sampling of total muscle force by tendon organs. *J. Neurophysiol.*, 47: 1069 – 1082.

Dempster, W. (1955) Space requirements of the seated operator. *WAOC Tech. Rep., Wright Patterson Air Force Base, Ohio*, pp. 55 – 159.

Dietz, V., Quintern, J. and Berger, W. (1984) Corrective reactions to stumbling in man: functional significance of spinal and transcortical reflexes. *Neurosci. Lett.*, 44: 131 – 135.

Dietz, V., Quintern, J. and Berger, W. (1985) Afferent control of human stance and gait: evidence for blocking of group I afferents during gait. *Exp. Brain Res.*, 61: 153 – 163.

Dietz, V., Quintern, J. and Sillem, M. (1987) Stumbling reactions in man: significance of proprioceptive and pre-programmed mechanisms. *J. Physiol. (London)*, 386: 149 – 163.

Dufresne, J.R., Soechting, J.F. and Terzuolo, C.A. (1979) Reflex motor output to torque pulses in man: identification of short- and long-latency loops with individual feedback parameters. *Neuroscience*, 4: 1493 – 1500.

Gottlieb, G.L. and Agarwal, G.C. (1980) Response to sudden torques about ankle in man. II. Postmyotatic reactions. *J. Neurophysiol.*, 43: 86 – 101.

Hemami, H. and Stokes, B.T. (1983) A qualitative discussion of mechanisms of feedback and feedforward in the control of locomotion. *IEEE Trans. Biomed. Eng.*, 30: 681 – 689.

Houk, J. and Henneman, E. (1967) Responses of Golgi tendon organs to active contractions of the soleus muscle of the cat. *J. Neurophysiol.*, 30: 466 – 489.

Houk, J.C., Rymer, W.Z. and Crago, P.E. (1981) Dependence of dynamic response of spindle receptors to muscle length and velocity. *J. Neurophysiol.*, 46: 143 – 166.

Hulliger, M. and Noth, J. (1979) Static and dynamic fusimotor interaction and the possibility of multiple pacemakers operating in the cat muscle spindle. *Brain Res.*, 173: 21 – 28.

Jaeger, R.J. (1986) Design and simulation of closed-loop electrical stimulation orthoses for restoration of quiet standing in paraplegia. *J. Biomech.*, 19: 825 – 835.

Jaeger, R.J., Smith, R. and Scanu, M. (1986) An application of a technique for superimposition of computer graphics and video images in real time. *Med. Instrumentation*, 20: 233 – 236.

Kantrowitz, A. (1960) *Electronic Physiologic Aids. Report of the Maimonides Hospital*, Brooklyn, NY, pp. 4 – 5.

Lennerstrand, G. and Thoden, U. (1968) Position and velocity sensitivity of muscle spindles in the cat. II. Dynamic fusimotor single-fibre activation of primary endings. *Acta Physiol. Scand.*, 74: 16 – 29.

Lipshits, M.J., Mauritz, K.H. and Popov, K.E. (1981) Quantitative analysis of anticipatory postural components of a gross voluntary movement. *Fisiol. tcheloveka (Human Physiology)*, 7: 411 – 419 (in Russian).

Matthews, P.B.C. (1981) Muscle spindles: their messages and their fusimotor supply. In V.B. Brooks (Eds.) *Handbook of Physiology, The Nervous System, Vol. 2/II*, Amer. Physiol. Soc. Bethesda, pp. 189 – 228.

Mauritz, K.H. (1986) Restoration of posture and gait by functional neuromuscular stimulation (FNS). In W. Bles and T. Brandt (Eds.), *Disorders of Posture and Gait*, Elsevier, Amsterdam, pp. 367 – 385.

Merton, P.A. (1953) Speculations on the servo-control of movement. In G.E.W. Wolstenholme (Ed.), *The Spinal Cord*, Churchill, London, pp. 247 – 255.

Morin, C., Katz, R., Mazieres, L. and Pierrot-Deseilligny, E. (1982) Comparison of soleus H-reflex facilitation at the onset of soleus contractions produced voluntarily and during the stance phase of human gait. *Neurosci. Lett.*, 33: 47.

Mulder, A.J., Verheyen, J.M.E. and Nijmeijer, H. (1987) Closed loop control of stimulation during standing. In D. Popovic (Ed.), *Advances in External Control of Human Extremities, IX*, Belgrade, pp. 275 – 282.

Petrofsky, J.S. (1978) Control of the recruitment and firing frequencies of motor units in electrically stimulated muscles in the cat. *Med. Biol. Eng. Comput.*, 16: 302 – 308.

Polit, A. and Bizzi, E. (1979) Characteristics of motor programs underlying arm movements in monkeys. *J. Neurophysiol.*, 42: 183 – 194.

Quintern, J., Berger, W. and Dietz, V. (1985) Compensatory reactions to gait perturbations: short and long term effects of neuronal adaptation. *Neurosci. Lett.*, 62: 371 – 376.

Quintern, J., Berger, W. and Dietz, V. (1987) Afferent control of posture and gait. In G.N. Gantchev, B. Dimitrov, and P. Gatev (Eds.), *Motor Control*, Plenum, New York, pp. 135 – 140.

Quintern, J. and Jaeger, R.J. (1987) Analysis of modes of quiet standing in neurologically intact human subjects. In D. Popovic (Ed.), *Advances in External Control of Human Extremities, IX*, Belgrade, pp. 167 – 180.

Rothwell, J.C., Traub, M.M., Day, B.L., Obeso, J.A., Thomas, P.K. and Marsden, C.D. (1982) Manual motor performance in a deafferented man. *Brain*, 105: 515 – 542.

Sanes, J.N., Mauritz, K.H., Dalakas, M.C. and Evarts, E.V. (1985) Motor control in humans with large-fiber sensory neuropathy. *Human Neurobiol.*, 4: 101 – 114.

Stein, R.B. (1982) What muscle variable(s) does the nervous system control in limb movements? *Behav. Brain Sci.*, 5: 535 – 577.

Subject Index